The Art and Science of Cardiac Physical Examination

CONTEMPORARY CARDIOLOGY

CHRISTOPHER P. CANNON, MD
SERIES EDITOR
ANNEMARIE M. ARMANI, MD
EXECUTIVE EDITOR

Management of Acute Pulmonary Embolism, edited by *Stavros Konstantinides*, MD, 2007

Stem Cells and Myocardial Regeneration, edited by *Marc S. Penn*, MD, PhD, 2007

Handbook of Complex Percutaneous Carotid Intervention, edited by *Jacqueline Saw*, MD, *Jose Exaire*, MD, *David S. Lee*, MD, *Sanjay Yadav*, MD, 2007

Preventive Cardiology: Insights Into the Prevention and Treatment of Cardiovascular Disease, Second Edition, edited by *JoAnne Micale Foody*, MD, 2006

The Art and Science of Cardiac Physical Examination: With Heart Sounds and Pulse Wave Forms on CD, by *Narasimhan Ranganathan*, MD, *Vahe Sivaciyan*, MD, and *Franklin B. Saksena*, MD, 2006

Cardiovascular Biomarkers: Pathophysiology and Disease Management, edited by *David A. Morrow*, MD, 2006

Cardiovascular Disease in the Elderly, edited by *Gary Gerstenblith*, MD, 2005

Platelet Function: Assessment, Diagnosis, and Treatment, edited by *Martin Quinn*, MB BCh BAO, PhD, and *Desmond Fitzgerald*, MD, FRCPI, FESC, APP, 2005

Diabetes and Cardiovascular Disease, Second Edition, edited by *Michael T. Johnstone*, MD, CM, FRCP(C), and *Aristidis Veves*, MD, DSc, 2005

Angiogenesis and Direct Myocardial Revascularization, edited by *Roger J. Laham*, MD, and *Donald S. Baim*, MD, 2005

Interventional Cardiology: Percutaneous Noncoronary Intervention, edited by *Howard C. Herrmann*, MD, 2005

Principles of Molecular Cardiology, edited by *Marschall S. Runge*, MD, and *Cam Patterson*, MD, 2005

Heart Disease Diagnosis and Therapy: A Practical Approach, Second Edition, by *M. Gabriel Khan*, MD, FRCP(LONDON), FRCP(C), FACP, FACC, 2005

Cardiovascular Genomics: Gene Mining for Pharmacogenomics and Gene Therapy, edited by *Mohan K. Raizada*, PhD, *Julian F. R. Paton*, PhD, *Michael J. Katovich*, PhD, and *Sergey Kasparov*, MD, PhD, 2005

Surgical Management of Congestive Heart Failure, edited by *James C. Fang*, MD and *Gregory S. Couper*, MD, 2005

Cardiopulmonary Resuscitation, edited by *Joseph P. Ornato*, MD, FACP, FACC, FACEP and *Mary Ann Peberdy*, MD, FACC, 2005

CT of the Heart: Principles and Applications, edited by *U. Joseph Schoepf*, MD, 2005

Coronary Disease in Women: Evidence-Based Diagnosis and Treatment, edited by *Leslee J. Shaw*, PhD and *Rita F. Redberg*, MD, FACC, 2004

Cardiac Transplantation: The Columbia University Medical Center/New York-Presbyterian Hospital Manual, edited by *Niloo M. Edwards*, MD, *Jonathan M. Chen*, MD, and *Pamela A. Mazzeo*, 2004

Heart Disease and Erectile Dysfunction, edited by *Robert A. Kloner*, MD, PhD, 2004

Complementary and Alternative Cardiovascular Medicine, edited by *Richard A. Stein*, MD and *Mehmet C. Oz*, MD, 2004

Nuclear Cardiology, The Basics: How to Set Up and Maintain a Laboratory, by *Frans J. Th. Wackers*, MD, PhD, *Wendy Bruni*, BS, CNMT, and *Barry L. Zaret*, MD, 2004

Minimally Invasive Cardiac Surgery, Second Edition, edited by *Daniel J. Goldstein*, MD, and *Mehmet C. Oz*, MD 2004

Cardiovascular Health Care Economics, edited by *William S. Weintraub*, MD, 2003

Platelet Glycoprotein IIb/IIIa Inhibitors in Cardiovascular Disease, Second Edition, edited by *A. Michael Lincoff*, MD, 2003

Heart Failure: A Clinician's Guide to Ambulatory Diagnosis and Treatment, edited by *Mariell L. Jessup*, MD and *Evan Loh*, MD, 2003

The Art and Science of Cardiac Physical Examination

With Heart Sounds and Pulse Wave Forms on CD

By

Narasimhan Ranganathan
MBBS, FRCP(C), FACP, FACC, FAHA

Vahe Sivaciyan
MD, FRCP(C)
University of Toronto and St. Joseph's Health Centre,
Toronto, Ontario, Canada

Franklin B. Saksena
MD, FACC, FAHA, FRCP(C), FACP
Northwestern University School of Medicine, Chicago, IL

Humana Press
Totowa, New Jersey

© 2006 Humana Press Inc.
999 Riverview Drive, Suite 208
Totowa, New Jersey 07512

www.humanapress.com

All rights reserved. No part of this book may be reproduced, stored in a retrieval system, or transmitted in any form or by any means, electronic, mechanical, photocopying, microfilming, recording, or otherwise without written permission from the Publisher.

The content and opinions expressed in this book are the sole work of the authors and editors, who have warranted due diligence in the creation and issuance of their work. The publisher, editors, and authors are not responsible for errors or omissions or for any consequences arising from the information or opinions presented in this book and make no warranty, express or implied, with respect to its contents.

Due diligence has been taken by the publishers, editors, and authors of this book to assure the accuracy of the information published and to describe generally accepted practices. The contributors herein have carefully checked to ensure that the drug selections and dosages set forth in this text are accurate and in accord with the standards accepted at the time of publication. Notwithstanding, as new research, changes in government regulations, and knowledge from clinical experience relating to drug therapy and drug reactions constantly occurs, the reader is advised to check the product information provided by the manufacturer of each drug for any change in dosages or for additional warnings and contraindications. This is of utmost importance when the recommended drug herein is a new or infrequently used drug. It is the responsibility of the treating physician to determine dosages and treatment strategies for individual patients. Further it is the responsibility of the health care provider to ascertain the Food and Drug Administration status of each drug or device used in their clinical practice. The publisher, editors, and authors are not responsible for errors or omissions or for any consequences from the application of the information presented in this book and make no warranty, express or implied, with respect to the contents in this publication.

Cover design by Patricia F. Cleary

For additional copies, pricing for bulk purchases, and/or information about other Humana titles, contact Humana at the above address or at any of the following numbers: Tel.: 973-256-1699; Fax: 973-256-8341, E-mail: orders@humanapr.com; or visit our Website: www.humanapress.com

This publication is printed on acid-free paper. ∞

ANSI Z39.48-1984 (American National Standards Institute) Permanence of Paper for Printed Library Materials.

Photocopy Authorization Policy:
Authorization to photocopy items for internal or personal use, or the internal or personal use of specific clients, is granted by Humana Press Inc., provided that the base fee of US $30.00 is paid directly to the Copyright Clearance Center at 222 Rosewood Drive, Danvers, MA 01923. For those organizations that have been granted a photocopy license from the CCC, a separate system of payment has been arranged and is acceptable to Humana Press Inc. The fee code for users of the Transactional Reporting Service is: [1-58829-776-4/06 $30.00].

Printed in the United States of America. 10 9 8 7 6 5 4 3 2 1

eISBN 1-59745-023-5

Library of Congress Cataloging-in-Publication Data
Ranganathan, Narasimhan.
 The art and science of cardiac physical examination : with heart sounds and pulse wave forms on CD / by Narasimhan Ranganathan, Vahe Sivaciyan, Franklin B. Saksena.
   p. ; cm. -- (Contemporary cardiology)
 Includes bibliographical references and index.
 ISBN 1-58829-776-4 (alk. paper)
 1. Heart--Examination. 2. Heart--Diseases--Diagnosis. 3. Heart--Sounds. I. Sivaciyan, Vahe. II. Saksena, Franklin B. III. Title. IV. Series: Contemporary cardiology (Totowa, N.J. : Unnumbered)
 [DNLM: 1. Heart Diseases--diagnosis. 2. Heart Function Tests--methods. 3. Heart Sounds--physiology. 4. Physical Examination--methods. WG 141 R196 2006]
 RC683.R25 2006
 616.1'2075--dc22
                                                        2006009499

To
Saroja Ranganathan,
Ayda Sivaciyan,
and
Kathleen Saksena

Without their support,
this book would not have been possible.

Preface

It has been our experience that instruction in physical examination of the heart in medical schools has been deteriorating since the advent of such modern diagnostic tools as two-dimensional echocardiography and nuclear imaging. At best, the teaching has been sketchy and too superficial for the student to appreciate the pathophysiological correlates. Both invasive and the noninvasive modern technologies have contributed substantially to our knowledge and understanding of cardiac physical signs and their pathophysiological correlates. However, both students and teachers alike appear to be mesmerized by technological advances to the neglect of the age-old art, as well as the substantial body of science, of cardiac physical examination. It is also sad to see reputed journals give low priority to articles related to the clinical examination.

Our experience is substantiated by a nationwide survey of internal medicine and cardiology training programs, which concluded that the teaching and practice of cardiac auscultation received low emphasis, and perhaps other bedside diagnostic skills as well *(1)*. The state of the problem is well reflected in the concerns expressed in previous publications *(2–4)*, including the 2001 editorial in the *American Journal of Medicine* (Vol. 110, pp. 233–235), entitled "Cardiac auscultation and teaching rounds: how can cardiac auscultation be resuscitated?", as well as in the rebuttal, "Selections from current literature. Horton hears a Who but no murmurs—does it matter?" *(5)*. The latter goes to the extent of suggesting that auscultation be performed only when cardiac symptoms are encountered in patients. This appears to be based on an exaggerated concern for the waste of time and resources. Implicit in this statement, if one chooses to agree with it, will be the acknowledgment of one's failure as a physician—at least, a physician caring for patients.

On the contrary, we not only share the opinion of others that cardiac auscultation is a cost-effective diagnostic skill *(6)*, we go one step further and suggest that all aspects of cardiac physical examination are very cost effective and rewarding in many ways. A properly obtained, detailed, and complete history of the patient's problems and a thorough physical examination are never counterproductive to the interests of the patient.

Modern technological advances are here to stay. They should be an adjunct to the clinical examination of the patient, but they should not be allowed to replace the physical examination. Let's not forget that many of these tools add to the rising costs of health care all over the world. A well-carried-out physical examination of the heart often provides the critical information necessary to choose the right investigative tool and to avoid the unnecessary ones. Even if one ignores the cost factor, a physician caring for a patient where advanced technologies may not be accessible (at nights and on weekends in some institutions, in rural or otherwise remote locations, during power failure and timesof natural or other disasters) should be able to assess and diagnose cardiac function and probable underlying pathology using the five senses, a stethoscope, and a sphygmomanometer.

Mackenzie integrated the jugular venous pulse as part of the cardiovascular physical examination *(7)*. Wood further went on to show that the precise analysis of the jugular venous pulse wave forms and the measurement of the venous pressure with reference to the sternal angle is possible at the bedside *(8)*. Interpretation of the jugular venous pulse contour and the assessment of the pressure remains yet an occult art practiced only by experienced clinicians. Poor, ill-defined, and vague terms such as jugular venous distension are commonly used and written about even in reputed journals when cardiac physical findings are mentioned.

One of the satisfying features of medicine, aside from contributing to the clinical improvement of an ailing patient, is the intellectual excitement and satisfaction of arriving at the right conclusion through proper reasoning based on clues derived from the clinical examination of the patient. In addition, not surprisingly, some of the physical signs have also been shown, in this day and age of "evidence-based medicine," to be of prognostic importance. For instance, elevated jugular venous pressure and the third heart sound in patients with symptomatic heart failure have been shown to have independent prognostic information *(9)*. To understand the pathophysiological correlates of various cardiac signs and symptoms requires the same skills of logical thinking exhibited by any good clinician at work, and their development is one benefit of such a discipline. It is all the more important when the detection of an abnormal sound or sign can be related to other cardiac measurements *(10)*. Improper understanding of the pathophysiological correlates would only result in testing the wrong hypotheses and possibly obtaining a misleading conclusion.

The purpose of *The Art and Science of Cardiac Physical Examination* is to arm the student of cardiology with the proper techniques and understanding of the art and science of the cardiac physical examination, to dispel myths and confusion, and to help develop skills required of any astute clinician.

This work is a culmination of long-standing experience in teaching and training physicians and physicians-to-be, as well as other students of cardiology. In fact, we have offered annually and continually refine a course of the same title at our institution in Toronto for more than 25 years. The course has always been well received and appreciated for both teaching methods and content. We utilize audiorecordings of heart sounds and murmurs, as well as videorecordings of jugular and precordial pulsations with simultaneously recorded sounds and flow signals for timing, all from actual patients collected over many years of clinical practice. Video display of the actual sounds and murmurs provides a real-time playback effect, and multiple listening devices with infrared transmission of sounds enhances the group teaching and learning experience. Refinements in the course have been stimulated by enthusiastic and inquisitive students and trainees and aided by our own research and studies, particularly with reference to the jugular venous flows and pulsations, as well as to precordial pulsations.

The organization of the material presented in this volume, *The Art and Science of Cardiac Physical Examination,* warrants some elaboration. We believe that the presentation helps integrate the science with concepts useful for logical application in clinical situations. The teaching method adopted is somewhat unique and, we believe, totally original in some sections. This is most evident in chapters on jugular venous pulse or precordial pulsations, as well as in the chapter on arterial pulse. Our approach to the interpretation of jugular venous pulsations highlights the proper method for integrating art with science at the bedside. We believe that it is different in many ways from other books describing cardiac examination. Every important topic has a summary of salient and practical points directed toward clinical assessment. These serve as a quick review as well as pointing to concepts that need reinforcement.

Many illustrations of sounds and murmurs used in the text are derived from digital display of actual audiorecordings from patients. The pathophysiology of some of the important clinical cardiac conditions is shown in flow diagrams as well as in tabular format, permitting logical review and reinforcement. References at the end of each chapter were carefully chosen for their now classic approaches as well as for their diverse perspectives.

A special chapter covering local and systemic manifestations of cardiovascular disease, written by our colleague and friend Dr. Franklin B. Saksena, has been carefully illustrated and exhaustively documented from the literature.

The audio and the videorecordings of sounds and murmurs provided on the companion CD capture the jugular and the precordial pulsations from patients with the range of cardiac problems most likely to be encountered clinically. The CD is playable on any up-to-date computer, both Mac and PC. We intend that these videorecordings enhance learning both for an individual or a group of students and trainees in cardiology. They provide a real-time playback effect of heart sounds and murmurs displayed on an oscilloscope. Another unique feature in the videofiles is the presentation of simultaneous recordings of two-dimensional echocardiographic images with the audiorecordings of heart murmurs from a few patients with specific cardiac lesions.

Thus, we present *The Art and Science of Cardiac Physical Examination* with a firm conviction that it will be an invaluable asset in learning and teaching clinical cardiology.

Narasimhan Ranganathan,
MBBS, FRCP(C), FACP, FACC, FAHA
Vahe Sivaciyan, MD, FRCP(C)

References

1. Mangione S, Nieman LZ, Gracely E, Kaye D. The teaching and practice of cardiac auscultation during internal medicine and cardiology training. A nationwide survey. Ann Intern Med 1993;119:47–54.
2. Schneiderman H. Cardiac auscultation and teaching rounds: how can cardiac auscultation be resuscitated? Am J Med 2001;110:233–235.
3. Lok CE, Morgan CD, Ranganathan N. The accuracy and interobserver agreement in detecting the 'gallop sounds' by cardiac auscultation. Chest 1998;114:1283–1288.
4. Tavel ME. Cardiac auscultation. A glorious past—but does it have a future? Circulation 1996;93:1250–1253.
5. Kopes-Kerr CP. Selections from current literature. Horton hears a Who but no murmurs—does it matter? Fam Pract 2002; 19:422–425.
6. Shaver, JA. Cardiac auscultation: a cost-effective diagnostic skill. Curr Probl Cardiol 1995; 7:441–530.
7. Mackenzie J. The study of the pulse. London, Pentland, 1902.
8. Wood P. Diseases of the Heart and Circulation. Philadelphia, J.B. Lippincott, 1956.
9. Drazner MH, Rame JE, Stevenson LW, Dries DL. Prognostic importance of elevated jugular venous pressure and a third heart sound in patients with heart failure. N Engl J Med 2001; 345:574–581.
10.. Marcus GM, Gerber IL, McKeown BH, et al. Association between phonocardiographic third and fourth heart sounds and objective measures of left ventricular function. JAMA 2005; 293:2238–2244.

Acknowledgment

I wish to express, on behalf of all the authors, our sincere thanks and gratitude to many individuals who have helped either directly or indirectly our efforts in the teaching of bedside clinical cardiology over the years and thereby made the publication of this work possible. First, our thanks go to all the patients who kindly volunteered their time for the purpose of medical education and teaching. I wish to express also my sincere thanks to all my colleagues in the cardiology division of St. Michael's Hospital, University of Toronto, with whom I worked from 1970 to 1988, my colleagues at St. Joseph's Health Centre since 1989, as well as the administration of the St. Joseph's Health Centre for their support of our educational programs and endeavors. A special thanks is also due to Mr. John Cooper and his family, whose kind donation toward the cardiology service at St. Joseph's Health Centre allowed the acquisition of a computer with a fast processor and modern video editing capabilities that eventually helped in the conversion of old technology to modern technology. We express our thanks also to Professor Emeritus Rashmi Desai of the Department of Physics at the University of Toronto and his colleague Dr. Katrin Rohlf of the Department of Chemistry, University of Toronto, for their input and comments.

We offer our profound gratitude and sincerest thanks most especially to Mr. Roger Harris, who is the head of the audiovisual department at St. Joseph's Health Centre, without whose ingenuity and dedicated and continuing assistance, the publication of this book and its companion CD would not have been possible. Most of the audiorecordings were originally made on a four-channel Cambridge magnetic disc recorder of the 1960s. In fact, we used to play these discs—even during our annual continuing medical education courses—using a storage oscilloscope and a television camera connected to large monitors for instant display of the waveforms. In 1989, after I joined St. Joseph's Health Centre, I had the good fortune to begin my association with Roger Harris. With his assistance and advice, the audiorecordings were initially converted to videorecordings. When reliable video editing programs with good and acceptable synchrony between the audio and the video tracks became available, Roger helped to digitize and archive these videorecordings. In addition, it is through his efforts we have made the successful transition to current technology, which enables display in the Windows media player on any up-to-date computer. Furthermore, his assistance has been invaluable for the production of all of the illustrations in the text as well as the production of the companion CD. Therefore, his enthusiasm for this project and many contributions are gratefully acknowledged and very much appreciated.

Finally, we express our sincere appreciation and thanks also to Mr. Balu Srinivasan for the professional assistance in the preparation of the CD.

Narasimhan Ranganathan,
MBBS, FRCP(C), FACP, FACC, FAHA

Contents

Preface vii
Acknowledgment x
Companion CD xv
Color Plates xvii

Chapter 1
Approach to the Physical Examination of the Cardiac Patient 1

Reasons for Which Cardiac Assessment Is Sought 2
Cardiac Symptoms and Their Appraisal 2
Generation of Working List of Possible Diagnoses 4
Focused Physical Examination: *Clinical Exercise* 6
Focused Physical Examination: *Practical Points* 14

Chapter 2
Arterial Pulse 15

Physiology of the Arterial Pulse 15
Assessment of the Arterial Pulse 34
Practical Points in the Clinical Assessment of the Arterial Pulse 44
References 46

Chapter 3
Blood Pressure and Its Measurement 49

Physiology of Blood Flow and Blood Pressure 49
Physiology of Blood Pressure Measurement 50
Points to Remember When Measuring Blood Pressure 52
Factors That Affect Blood Pressure Readings 53
Interpretation of Blood Pressure Measurements 54
Use of Blood Pressure Measurement in Special Clinical Situations 56
References 64

Chapter 4
Jugular Venous Pulse 67

Normal Right Atrial Pressure Pulse Contours 68
Jugular Venous Inflow Velocity Patterns and the Relationship
  to the Right Atrial Pressure Pulse 70
Jugular Venous Flow Events and Their Relationship to Jugular Venous Pulse Contours 74
Normal Jugular Venous Pulse Contour and Its Recognition at the Bedside 81
Individual Components of the Right Atrial Pressure Pulse, Their Determinants,
  and Their Recognition in the Jugulars 82
Abnormal Jugular Venous Pulse Contours as Related
  to Abnormal Jugular Venous Flow Velocity Patterns 92
Abnormal Jugular Contours 96
Assessment of Jugular Venous Pressure 105
Clinical Assessment of the Jugular Venous Pulse 107
References 110

Chapter 5
Precordial Pulsations 113
Mechanics and Physiology of the Normal Apical Impulse 113
Physical Principles Governing the Formation of the Apical Impulse 115
Normal Apical Impulse and Its Determinants 118
Assessment of the Apical Impulse 120
Left Parasternal and Sternal Movements 133
Right Parasternal Movement 134
Pulsations Over the Clavicular Heads 134
Pulsations Over the Second and/or Third Left Intercostal Spaces 135
Subxiphoid Impulse 135
Practical Points in the Clinical Assessment of Precordial Pulsations 136
References 138

Chapter 6
Heart Sounds 141
Principles of Sound Formation in the Heart 141
First Heart Sound (S1) 142
Clinical Assessment of S1 and Components 156
Second Heart Sound (S2) 158
Normal S2 159
Abnormal S2 162
Clinical Assessment of S2 174
Opening Snap (OS) 179
Third Heart Sound (S3) 185
Clinical Assessment of S3 198
Fourth Heart Sound (S4) 200
Clinical Assessment of S4 204
References 206

Chapter 7
Heart Murmurs: *Part I* 211
Principles Governing Murmur Formation 211
Hemodynamic Factors and Cardiac Murmurs 214
Frequencies of Murmurs 214
Grading of Murmurs 216
Systolic Murmurs 216
Ejection Murmurs 217
Regurgitant Systolic Murmurs 232
Mitral Regurgitation 233
Tricuspid Regurgitation 253
Ventricular Septal Defect (VSD) 258
Clinical Assessment of Systolic Murmurs 265
References 269

Chapter 8
Heart Murmurs: *Part II* 275
Diastolic Murmurs 275
Diastolic Murmurs of Mitral Origin 275
Diastolic Murmurs of Tricuspid Origin 282
Semilunar Valve Regurgitation 283
Aortic Regurgitation 283
Pulmonary Regurgitation 290

Contents   xiii

    Clinical Assessment of Diastolic Murmurs 292
    Continuous Murmurs 294
    Persistent Ductus Arteriosus 296
    Aorto-Pulmonary Window 298
    Sinus of Valsalva Aneurysm 298
    Coronary Arteriovenous Fistulae 299
    Venous Hum 300
    Mammary Souffle 300
    Clinical Assessment of Continuous Murmurs 300
    Pericardial Friction Rub 302
    Innocent Murmurs 303
    References 304

Chapter 9

Elements of Auscultation 309

    The Stethoscope 309
    Auscultation Method 310
    References 318

Chapter 10

Pathophysiological Basis of Symptoms and Signs in Cardiac Disease 321

    Pathophysiology of Mitral Regurgitation 321
    Pathophysiology of Aortic Regurgitation 325
    Pathophysiology of Mitral Stenosis 329
    Pathophysiology of Aortic Stenosis 331
    Pathophysiology of Myocardial Ischemia/Infarction 334
    Pathophysiology of Hypertensive Heart Disease 336
    Pathophysiology of Dilated Cardiomyopathy 338
    Pathophysiology of Hypertrophic Obstructive Cardiomyopathy 340
    Pathophysiology of Atrial Septal Defect 342
    Pathophysiology of Diastolic Dysfunction 345
    Pathophysiology of Constrictive Pericarditis 347
    Pathophysiology of Cardiac Tamponade 348
    Appendix 351
    References 356

Chapter 11

Local and Systemic Manifestations of Cardiovascular Disease 361

    General Observations 361
    Congenital Syndromes/Diseases 364
    Vascular Diseases 369
    Valvular Heart Disease 372
    Endocrine and Metabolic Diseases 373
    Inflammatory Diseases 377
    Diseases of Connective Tissue and Joints 377
    Pharmacological Agents 381
    Musculoskeletal Diseases 384
    Tumors 386
    Synopsis 386
    Acknowledgment 390
    References 390

Index 397

About the Authors 413

COMPANION CD

Contents

Jugular Venous Pulse
Precordial Pulsations
Heart Sounds
Heart Murmurs (Part 1)
Heart Murmurs (Part 2)

The Companion CD is playable on any up-to-date Mac or Windows computer or laptop. On a PC, just insert in the CD drive and the program "ASCPE.exe" will launch itself. If auto-launch is disabled on your computer, start the application by double clicking the ASCPE.exe icon. On a Mac, insert in the CD drive, open the icon appearing on the desktop, and start the application by double clicking the ASCPE.exe icon. *See* Help on the CD for additional tips and guidance.

Headphones are recommended for listening to the heart sounds. Adjust the audio volume to hear some of the heart sounds properly.

System and Software Recommendations

For Microsoft Windows®:
Intel Pentium® II with 64 MB of available RAM, running Windows 98
or
Intel Pentium® III with 128 MB of available RAM running Windows 2000 or XP
Soundcard and speakers or headphones
Monitor resolution of 800 x 600 or higher

For Macintosh® OS X:
Power Mac G3 with 128 MB RAM running Mac OS X 10.1.5, 10.2.6, or 10.3, or later
Soundcard and speakers or headphones
Monitor resolution 1024 x 768 or higher

Color Plates

Color Plates follow p. 270.

Color Plate 1 Fig. 1A,B, Chapter 7: Two-dimensional echocardiographic images with Doppler color flow mapping from a normal subject in the apical four-chamber view taken in diastole (**A**) and systole (**B**). *See* complete caption and discussion on p. 212.

Color Plate 2 Fig. 2, Chapter 7: Two-dimensional echocardiographic images and Doppler color flow mapping from a patient with mitral regurgitation taken in the parasternal long axis. *See* complete caption and discussion on p. 213.

Color Plate 3 Fig. 7B, Chapter 7: Doppler color flow image showing turbulent flow across the left ventricular outflow, in apical four-chamber view. *See* complete caption on p. 223 and discussion on p. 222.

Color Plate 4 Fig. 12A,D, Chapter 7: Two-dimensional echocardiographic images in the parasternal view from a patient with hypertrophic obstructive cardiomyopathy with severe subaortic obstruction. The diastolic frame (**A**) shows the open mitral valve allowing the inflow from the left atrium (LA) into the left ventricle (LV). In (**D**), turbulent outflow as well as some mitral regurgitation. *See* complete caption and discussion on p. 226.

Color Plate 5 Fig. 3, Chapter 11: Osler–Weber–Rendu syndrome. *See* complete caption on p. 367 and discussion on p. 365.

Color Plate 6 Fig. 6, Chapter 11: Eruptive xanthoma. Skin lesions over back and chest resemble acne. *See* complete caption on p. 370 and discussion on p. 369.

Color Plate 7 Fig. 7, Chapter 11: Mitral facies and malar flush in 35-yr-old woman with mitral stenosis and mitral regurgitation. *See* complete caption and discussion on p. 373.

Color Plate 8 Fig. 12A, Chapter 11: Janeway lesions in infective endocarditis in a 50-yr-old drug addict. *See* complete caption on p. 378 and discussion on p. 377.

Color Plate 9 Fig. 13A, Chapter 11: Mixed connective tissue diseases: patient with mask facies with puckering of skin around lips and malar depigmentation. *See* complete caption and discussion on p. 379.

Color Plate 10 Fig. 17, Chapter 11: Amiodarone skin toxicity. *See* complete caption and discussion on p. 383.

1 Approach to the Physical Examination of the Cardiac Patient

CONTENTS

REASONS FOR WHICH CARDIAC ASSESSMENT IS SOUGHT
CARDIAC SYMPTOMS AND THEIR APPRAISAL
GENERATION OF WORKING LIST OF POSSIBLE DIAGNOSES
FOCUSED PHYSICAL EXAMINATION:
  CLINICAL EXERCISE
FOCUSED CARDIAC PHYSICAL EXAMINATION:
  PRACTICAL POINTS

Performance of a proper cardiac physical examination and the interpretation of the findings require a good understanding of both the physiology of the cardiovascular system and the pathophysiology involved in the abnormal states caused by various cardiac lesions and disorders. The development of good bedside skills requires not only dedication on the part of the student of cardiology, but also that the instruction methods be sound and based on both science and logic. The clinician instructor and the student clinician then come to appreciate that the whole process involves the integration of the science with the art of the physical examination.

While each aspect of the cardiac physical examination is dealt with in a detailed manner in this volume, this chapter is devoted to the general approach to the physical examination of the cardiac patient. In this chapter the following points are discussed:

1. The various reasons for which a cardiac assessment might be sought.
2. The appraisal of the various cardiac symptoms and their proper interpretation in order that an intelligent list of the various possible etiological causes of the problem can be generated.
3. The generation of the possible etiological causes of the symptoms of the patient.
4. The physical examination that is focused to derive pertinent information helpful in the differential diagnosis and thereby enables one to plan the subsequent investigation and management.
5. The material is illustrated by two different patient histories. In the first case the discussion of the physical findings is somewhat general, and in the second case it is more specific. We believe that both clinical cases can be treated as material for self-testing by the interested student or the trainee, both before and after studying the remainder of the book.

REASONS FOR WHICH CARDIAC ASSESSMENT IS SOUGHT

The patient for cardiovascular assessment generally presents for one of the following reasons:

1. For confirmation and assessment of a suspected cardiac lesion or disease
2. Because of the presence of abnormal cardiac findings on physical examination (such as a heart murmur) and/or one of the laboratory tests (such as an abnormal electrocardiogram [ECG] chest x-ray or echocardiogram)
3. Because of the presence of cardiac symptoms (such as dyspnea, chest pain, syncope)

In the patient with a suspected cardiac lesion or disease, one needs to have a clear mental picture of associated symptoms and signs and risk factors, if any. The examiner then should analyze the patient's history, symptoms, and signs from this perspective. For instance, if the patient is sent with a diagnosis of atrial septal defect, the mental picture of this lesion should be one of a precordial pulsation dominated by the right ventricle, inconspicuous left ventricle, and fixed splitting of the second heart sound. If that patient were to have a large-area hyperdynamic left ventricular apical impulse, then either the diagnosis is incorrect or the lesion is complicated by an additional condition such as mitral regurgitation, which may be significant.

If the patient was referred because of an abnormal finding on physical examination, such as a heart murmur, the examiner, in addition to confirming the finding, also needs to establish the cause and the severity of the lesion. In patients with abnormal laboratory test results, the abnormality must be identified and confirmed. One needs to have clear knowledge of the associated lesions and causes for proper evaluation of such instances. For instance, patient referred for cardiomegaly on the chest x-ray should have the x-ray reviewed to rule out apparent cardiomegaly from causes such as scoliosis or poor technique. Physical examination and, in some cases, a two-dimensional echocardiogram may be essential to determine the actual chamber dimensions and wall thickness. Sometimes a markedly hypertrophied ventricle with reduced internal dimensions can cause an increased cardiothoracic ratio on the chest radiograph.

In patients with abnormal electrocardiograms, the identification of the abnormality often can give directions to diagnosis. For instance, the presence of left ventricular hypertrophy and strain pattern should indicate the presence of left ventricular outflow obstruction, hypertrophic cardiomyopathy, or hypertensive heart disease. If the ECG were to show an infarct, one needs to consider also conditions other than ischemic heart disease that can cause infarct patterns on the ECG, such as hypertrophic cardiomyopathy or pre-excitation, as seen in Wolff–Parkinson–White syndrome.

Most patients seen for cardiac assessments are referred primarily on account of their predominant cardiac symptoms. A clear evaluation of the symptoms and their severity could lend itself to an analytical approach to diagnosis.

CARDIAC SYMPTOMS AND THEIR APPRAISAL

Symptoms can be grouped to identify underlying pathology as follows:

1. Definite orthopnea and/or nocturnal dyspnea should point to the presence of high left atrial pressure and therefore help in generating a list of possible causes to look for in the examination.
2. Triad of dyspnea, chest pain, and exertional presyncope or syncope should indicate fixed cardiac output lesions (where cardiac output fails to increase adequately during exercise) such as due to outflow tract obstruction (e.g., aortic stenosis).

Chapter 1 / Approach to Physical Examination 3

3. Low-output symptoms of fatigue, lassitude, and light-headedness could be caused by severe inflow obstructive lesions, severe cardiomyopathy of ischemic or nonischemic etiology, constrictive pericarditis, cardiac tamponade, or severe pulmonary hypertension.
4. Syncope and presyncope in addition to outflow obstructive lesions may also be caused by significant bradyarrhythmia or tachyarrhythmias, hypotension of sudden onset brought on by postural change, vagal reaction, or be of neurogenic origin.

Symptoms and signs of peripheral edema and ascites may be caused by congestive heart failure, but may also result from other causes such as severe tricuspid regurgitation and constrictive pericarditis. They may also result from other noncardiac causes related to low serum albumin of hepatic, gastrointestinal, or renal causes as well as venous obstruction. Only when the pitting edema is of cardiac origin would significant elevation in the jugular venous pressure be expected.

In the assessment of patients with symptoms described as dizziness, one needs to distinguish as far as possible between presyncopal feeling (weakness or a drained feeling as though one is about to faint) and vertiginous sensation, which often is not cardiac in origin and is related to the peripheral or central vestibular system. Vertiginous feeling should be considered if a sensation of spinning or imbalance is experienced with or without nausea.

Chest pain, which is often a common reason for cardiac referral, needs to be properly assessed with regard to character, location, duration, frequency, provoking and relieving factors, as well as the associated presence or absence of coronary risk factors (history of smoking, gender, age, diabetes, hyperlipidemia, hypertension, obesity, family history). Careful analysis should allow the chest pain to be defined as one of the three following categories:

1. Typical angina: central chest discomfort often described as tightness, heaviness, squeezing or burning sensation, or sensation of oppression or weight on the chest with or without typical radiation to the arms, shoulders, back, neck, and/or jaw with or without accompanying dyspnea related often to activity and relieved usually within a few minutes of rest or after nitroglycerin
2. Atypical angina: the chest discomfort has some features characteristic of angina and yet other features not so typical; e.g., left anterior or central chest tightness related to physical exertion but requiring a long period of rest for relief such as having to lie down for extended period of time
3. Noncardiac chest pain such as that related to musculoskeletal, pleuritic, and esophageal, etc.

Exertional angina, although commonly associated with ischemic (coronary) heart disease, could also be caused by conditions that increase the myocardial oxygen demands such as aortic stenosis, aortic regurgitation, and severe uncontrolled hypertension. Systemic factors, which could aggravate the problem, would also need to be considered, such as anemia and hyperthyroidism. Classical anginal discomfort occurring unprovoked at rest but nevertheless responding to nitroglycerin should elicit consideration of coronary vasospasm (Prinzmetal's or variant angina) as well as possible unstable coronary syndrome. Prolonged (>20 min in duration) and/or severe central chest discomfort or tightness with or without radiation should raise suspicion of acute coronary syndromes and their mimickers. Among the latter conditions, acute pericarditis and dissection of the aorta deserve special mention. The discomfort of acute pericarditis is aggravated in the supine position, and relief of the intensity of discomfort is often experienced with the patient sitting upright and leaning forward. The discomfort caused by dissection of the aorta may be described as a sudden tearing sensation or crushing feeling, often with wide radiation, particularly to the back, sometimes to the neck and arms, and occasionally to the abdomen. It may also be intermittent. Sometimes patients with acute myocardial infarction, particularly that of the inferior wall, might have discomfort primarily in the epigastrium accompanied by symptoms of nausea or vomiting. Acute infarct could of course occur without any discomfort and sometimes with minimal symptoms, such as some numbness in the arm or hand. It often requires a high index of suspicion given appropriate clinical markers to identify all of them accurately.

Angina occasionally may present as exertional belching. Occasionally exertional dyspnea and even nocturnal dyspnea, in addition to being symptoms indicative of elevated left atrial pressure, may represent anginal equivalent symptoms with discomfort being totally absent. If the angina is atypical, one should not only consider coronary artery disease, but also other conditions such as mitral valve prolapse syndrome, hypertrophic cardiomyopathy, unrecognized uncontrolled systemic hypertension, pulmonary hypertension, and hyperthyroidism.

Assessment also requires one to define the degree of severity of the cardiac symptomatic disability. This requires one to classify the severity of the cardiac symptoms such as dyspnea or angina using one of the accepted classification systems like that of the New York Heart Association classification of dyspnea or heart failure symptoms into Classes I, II, III, and IV.

Class I is defined as symptoms on severe exertion, while Class IV implies symptoms at rest. Class III implies symptoms on light or less than ordinary exertion, and Class II implies symptoms on a moderate level of exertion or ordinary exertion. The ordinary exertion that the patient could normally do without symptoms would depend on the age of the patient as well as his or her mental attitude or wishes. For instance, in two patients of similar age, one might be satisfied with walking comfortably while the other might insist on playing tennis, considering this to be a normal activity. The Canadian Cardiovascular Society classification has a Class 0, which simply means asymptomatic. It is often used for defining the severity of anginal symptoms.

GENERATION OF WORKING LIST OF POSSIBLE DIAGNOSES

In the evaluation of the cardiac patient, an analytical approach to a full and complete cardiac history should point to a working list of possible diagnoses. One can enumerate possibilities, which could produce all or most of the predominant symptoms of the patient. The enumeration should draw from broad categories of both congenital and acquired cardiac disorders. The categories can be similar to those shown in Tables 1 and 2.

In addition, one should consider possible precipitating factors, which could be causative in the presence of pre-existing cardiac disorders, which are otherwise asymptomatic. Such precipitating factors may include extracardiac factors such as:

- Infection, such as pneumonia
- Anemia
- Hyperthyroidism
- Pulmonary thromboembolism
- Hypoxemia secondary to pulmonary and ventilatory disorders such as sleep apnea

Table 1
Categories of Congenital Heart Defects

Acyanotic forms without a shunt

Outflow obstruction	– Pulmonary stenosis, aortic stenosis, coarctation of aorta	
Inflow obstruction	– Mitral stenosis	
Regurgitant lesions	– Mitral	– Congenitally corrected transposition, anomalous origin of the left coronary artery from the pulmonary artery
	– Tricuspid	– Ebstein's anomaly
	– Aortic	– Bicuspid aortic valve

Acyanotic forms with left-to-right shunts

Atrial level	– Atrial septal defect primum/secundum
Ventricular level	– Ventricular septal defect
Aortic level	– Persistent ductus arteriosus, aorto-pulmonary window
Other communications	– Coronary A-V fistulae, ruptured sinus of Valsalva aneurysm

Cyanotic forms

Eisenmenger syndrome	– Reversed shunt with pulmonary hypertension due to pulmonary vascular disease
Tetralogy/tetralogy-type lesions	– Decreased pulmonary flow
Common-mixing chamber defects	– Common atrium, single ventricle, truncus arteriosus – Total anomalous pulmonary venous drainage

Others

Conduction system disorders	– Congenital A-V block, accessory pathways

Table 2
Categories of Acquired Cardiac Disorders

1. Valvular disease
   - Stenotic lesions
   - Regurgitant lesions
2. Infective endocarditis
3. Ischemic heart disease
4. Hypertensive heart disease
5. Myocardial diseases
   - Cardiomyopthies
   - Hypertrophic, restrictive and dilated
   - Myocarditis
6. Pericardial diseases
   - Acute pericarditis
   - Pericardial effusion with or without cardiac compression (tamponade)
   - Chronic constrictive pericarditis
7. Cardiac tumors (atrial myxoma)
8. Conduction system disorders
   - Tachyarrhythmia
   - Bradyarrhythmia
9. Pulmonary hypertension

- Salt and fluid overload secondary to renal insufficiency
- Iatrogenic causes (e.g., use of nonsteroidal anti-inflammatory drugs or Cox-2 inhibitors).

The next step involves a careful examination and definition of the arterial pulses, the jugular pulsations, the precordial pulsations, as well as the peripheral and systemic signs. All of these need to be evaluated in relation to the possibilities listed from the history. When this is done properly, a clear and definitive diagnosis can often be established or arrived at even before auscultation is performed. Auscultation, which is often the last step in the physical examination of the cardiac patient, may sometimes become the confirmatory step in this process. Only mild lesions are diagnosed on the basis of auscultation alone (e.g., mitral valve prolapse, hypertrophic obstructive cardiomyopathy).

FOCUSED PHYSICAL EXAMINATION: *CLINICAL EXERCISE*

This approach can be illustrated by discussing two different patients, each presenting with specific cardiac symptoms. One could use the following sections as both pre- and posttests, namely before and after studying the remaining chapters in the book.

Patient A: A 70-Year-Old Woman, Previously Healthy, Presenting with Sudden-Onset Dyspnea, Orthopnea With Radiological Signs of Pulmonary Edema.

The symptom complex with radiological evidence of pulmonary congestion obviously indicates a pathological process associated with high left atrial pressure if high altitude and acute pulmonary injury are not involved. The latter two can be easily solved by the relevant history surrounding the onset. One can then develop a list of all possible lesions, both congenital and acquired, that can cause this problem. Then evidence in the history both in favor and against each listed condition should be considered.

CONGENITAL

The only congenital lesion that could possibly be considered is bicuspid aortic valve with stenosis and/or regurgitation. But the age of the patient is somewhat against this.

ACQUIRED

Valvular Lesions

MITRAL STENOSIS OR OBSTRUCTION. A patient with mitral stenosis may present with acute pulmonary edema due to the sudden onset of atrial fibrillation. Rapid ventricular rate, such as that accompanying uncontrolled atrial fibrillation, might be the precipitating cause of acute pulmonary edema in a patient with significant mitral stenosis which the patient otherwise is able to tolerate. The rapid heart rate, by shortening the diastolic filling time, impedes emptying of the left atrium in mitral stenosis, thereby raising the left atrial pressure acutely. But this type of presentation in rheumatic mitral disease is more likely to be seen in the fourth and the fifth decades. Mitral obstruction due to atrial myxoma, however, could occur in this patient's age group and therefore cannot be excluded. Occasionally a patient with a prosthetic mitral valve with a previous history of mitral valve replacement could present with pulmonary edema because of an acute thrombus on the prosthetic valve obstructing inflow and preventing proper prosthetic valve function.

CHRONIC MITRAL REGURGITATION. Chronic mitral regurgitation does not usually present with pulmonary edema unless its severity is suddenly markedly increased. This can happen with rupture of chordae tendineae (spontaneous or due to infective endocarditis) or may be due to other problems, which also affect the mitral valve function (such as ischemic papillary muscle dysfunction with or without avulsion of chordae or severe uncontrolled hypertension).

ACUTE SEVERE MITRAL REGURGITATION. This often is likely to present with acute pulmonary edema and may be caused by spontaneous rupture of chordae tendineae, for instance in a patient with previously unrecognized myxomatous degeneration of the mitral leaflets, sometimes resulting from avulsion of chordae secondary to papillary muscle infarction in a patient with acute coronary syndrome and rarely due to papillary muscle rupture with acute myocardial infarction. None of these could be excluded or considered low on the list based primarily on the history.

AORTIC STENOSIS. While this lesion on an acquired basis (calcific or degenerative) is more common in men, it can nevertheless present with acute left ventricular failure and usually some preceding history of the presence of a heart murmur and the classical triad of symptoms, namely dyspnea, angina, and exertional presyncope or syncope. Absence of any of these does not, however, exclude this condition from consideration.

CHRONIC AORTIC REGURGITATION. This can arise from valvular lesions (bicuspid valve, rheumatic involvement, trauma, endocarditis, etc.) or aortic root dilatation (Marfan's syndrome, syphylitic aortitis, spondylitis, etc.). The compensated state may last for a long time, and when the left ventricular failure sets in, it can be quite dramatic and associated with pulmonary edema. Therefore this needs to be seriously considered.

ACUTE SEVERE AORTIC REGURGITATION. Acute severe aortic regurgitation (often caused by endocarditis on a native valve or a prosthetic aortic valve with virulent pathogens such as staphylococci) obviously can present with acute pulmonary edema. Sometimes the symptom complex and some of the physical signs may be mimicked by ruptured sinus of Valsalva aneurysm, which also needs to be considered.

Ischemic Heart Disease

Acute myocardial infarction is by far the most common cause of sudden *de novo* acute pulmonary edema and therefore needs to be on the top of the list of all the causes of acute pulmonary edema. While the presence of chest discomfort or pain at onset and/or the presence of coexisting coronary risk factors raise the suspicion to high levels, neither the absence of chest discomfort nor the absence of significant coronary risk factors excludes it from consideration. The diagnosis would require either electrocardiographic and/or enzymatic determination of cardiac markers such as an elevated troponin level or creatine kinase MB fraction.

Hypertensive Heart Disease

Acute uncontrolled or poorly controlled hypertension can present with acute pulmonary edema. It can be seen, for instance, in younger females with complicating glomerulonephritis or pregnancy. However, these conditions need not be present. The systolic left ventricular function could be normal and yet, because of significant diastolic dysfunction, the left ventricular diastolic filling pressures could be severely elevated, causing the symptoms. This is not uncommon in the elderly female. Occasionally chronic renal failure might coexist in these patients, aggravating the fluid and volume overload. The renal failure could itself be caused by hypertensive nephrosclerosis and/or diabetic nephropathy. Thus, this is an important entity to consider.

Cardiomyopthies

Acute dyspnea and pulmonary edema could occur in patients with hypertrophic obstructive cardiomyopathy with significant resting aortic outflow tract gradient. Similar symptomatology could occasionally occur in patients with dilated cardiomyopathy (of various etiologies including idiopathic, viral, alcoholic, and others). They are therefore not excluded on the basis of the history alone. Restrictive cardiomyopathy with etiologies like those caused by infiltrative processes such as amyloid or myxedema is not likely to present with such dramatic onset.

Conduction System Disorders

These by themselves will not be implicated for this presentation, but conduction system involvement by electrocardiographic findings as part of the underlying cardiac disease may be detected; for instance, the presence of left bundle branch block on the ECG may be noted in a patient with idiopathic dilated or restrictive cardiomyopathy or in calcific aortic stenosis (Lev's disease).

Pericardial Diseases

Pericardial diseases of acute or chronic origin are not expected to cause acute symptoms of high left atrial pressure. While acute dyspnea may be caused by pericardial effusion that is causing significant cardiac compression, it is unlikely to produce radiological signs of pulmonary edema. Unilateral left-sided constriction from chronic constrictive pericarditis is extremely rare and unlikely to present acutely.

Cardiac Tumors

Primary cardiac tumors such as a myxoma, because of its location and mobility resulting from its attachment by a stalk to the underlying endocardial wall, could cause obstructive symptoms. If the myxoma is left atrial in location, it can cause acute symptoms of high left atrial pressure caused by mitral obstruction.

Pulmonary Hypertension

All lesions listed above that cause significant elevations in the left atrial pressure and symptoms thereof will more than likely raise the pulmonary arterial pressures and cause pulmonary hypertension. However, in this instance the symptoms primarily stem from the high left atrial pressure. In chronic pulmonary hypertension, the right ventricle gets the brunt of the problem and will raise the systemic venous pressures with or without secondary tricuspid regurgitation and will eventually lead to diminished right ventricular output. The former will cause systemic venous congestion and peripheral edema; the latter would only diminish the left ventricular output and cause low cardiac output symptoms but not pulmonary congestion. Therefore, this pathophysiological process is not under consideration here.

In view of the acute onset of symptoms, presumably unprovoked, some of the likely precipitating and/or aggravating factors also need to be considered in the evaluation process because these may be operative when there is pre-existing left ventricular dysfunction, which is otherwise tolerated and asymptomatic.

Precipitating or Aggravating Factors

Rapid Ventricular Rate

Rapid heart rate resulting from uncontrolled atrial fibrillation or similar supraventricular tachyarrhythmia, such as uncontrolled atrial flutter, atrial tachycardia, and occasionally even ventricular tachycardia, could precipitate onset of acute pulmonary edema in patients with pre-existing left ventricular dysfunction of varied etiologies (ischemic heart disease with prior myocardial infarction, uncontrolled hypertensive heart disease, hypertrophic or dilated cardiomyopathies), all of which might have been otherwise asymptomatic.

Acute Infection Such as Pneumonia

This needs to be considered in the elderly since both systolic and/or diastolic left ventricular dysfunction of varied and/or multiple etiologies (ischemic, hypertensive, and non-ischemic cardiomyopathies) are common in the elderly, particularly in the very old (in the eighties and above). In these individuals, systemic infection and particularly pulmonary infection might throw them into left ventricular failure because of additional hypoxemia, which can further depress cardiac function unable to meet increased demands in cardiac output.

Acute Pulmonary Embolism

This should not be expected to cause left ventricular dysfunction directly and therefore will not present as acute left ventricular failure when the left ventricular function is normal. However, when the underlying left ventricular function is already previously compromised by other pre-existing cardiac disease, it can aggravate the same leading to pulmonary edema. The mechanisms involve hypoxia, tachycardia, or atrial tachyarrhythmia, which it may produce, and increased reflex vasoconstriction (mediated by catecholamines, serotonin, etc.), which can raise the afterload.

It is of utmost importance that the patient in acute pulmonary edema be treated for the same with appropriate measures, which should include oxygenation, intravenous diuretics, morphine, as well as ventilatory support when considered essential. It is even appropriate to look at the electrocardiogram quickly for signs of an acute myocardial infarction given the fact that it is often the leading cause of acute pulmonary edema. The discussion here is not meant to be about management of the patient, but rather how one goes about considering the various possible etiologies, because it is important for the complete management of the patient.

We have listed the various possible lesions/disorders that can present with acute pulmonary edema and also indicated the precipitating factors. The physical examination of the cardiovascular system carried out in a systematic manner would bring in either positive or negative findings in relation to each of the diagnosis listed. One makes a mental note of each, as one proceeds with the examination.

First, the arterial pulse is assessed with regard to rate and rhythm. The assessment of heart rate and rhythm would help in identifying the presence of atrial fibrillation. Sometimes the irregularity in the rhythm might be picked up better by auscultation, and one may quickly use this method early on if the rhythm is thought to be irregular but not totally certain by palpation alone. Then the rate of rise of the arterial pulse, particularly the carotid pulse, will help to indicate or rule out significant outflow tract obstruction. Sometimes in the elderly, the rate of rise may be modified by reflected waves secondary to the stiff arterial system. The amplitude of the arterial pulse and its rate of rise together will help distinguish significant mitral regurgitation from aortic regurgitation. The arterial pulse of severe mitral regurgitation will have either normal or fast upstroke with normal or lower than normal amplitude or volume. Severe aortic regurgitation, however, will have a fast rate of rise with increased amplitude. Of course, when the aortic regurgitation, is severe exaggerated peripheral signs will become obvious which can all be looked for including measurement of blood pressure differences between the arms and the leg (Hill's sign). One must remember that severe aortic regurgitation might be simulated by conditions that have exaggerated early run-off as in ruptured sinus of Valsalva aneurysm. This also will give rise to similar peripheral arterial findings. If the arterial pulse is brisk in its upstroke with decreased volume, then hypertrophic cardiomyopathy with obstruction needs to be considered. Sometimes one might feel a bisferiens pulse, which might bring into consideration mixed aortic regurgitation and aortic stenosis as well as hypertrophic cardiomyopathy with obstruction. Besides the character of the arterial pulse, blood pressure measurement would give important information regarding the stroke volume as reflected in the pulse pressure whether increased, decreased, or normal as well as help with regard to the presence or absence of hypertension.

The jugular venous pressure and the venous pulse contour might not directly influence the diagnosis, but it can throw light on the presence or otherwise of secondary pulmonary hypertension and indicate the status of the right ventricular function.

The assessment of precordial pulsations is of crucial importance. When the apical impulse is palpable and considered as left ventricular, as revealed by the presence of medial retraction, then its location, its area, and its character (single, double, or triple, whether it is normal, sustained, or hyperdynamic) will all give important clues to the assessment of the problem and the function of the left ventricle. In addition, assessment for the presence of a right ventricular impulse by subxiphoid palpation, as well as assessment for systolic sternal movement (retraction or outward movement), are also important.

A displaced large-area hyperdynamic left ventricular apical impulse will suggest severe mitral and/or aortic regurgitation. Although severe mitral regurgitation may have a somewhat wider than normal area of medial retraction, the detection of a marked systolic sternal retraction would clearly point to the presence of severe isolated aortic regurgitation. Sustained left ventricular impulse with an atrial kick and a brisk rising arterial pulse would point to hypertrophic obstructive cardiomyopathy, as the presence of a delayed carotid upstroke would indicate significant aortic stenosis, whereas the same in the presence of a normally rising pulse would make one consider moderate left ventricular dysfunction (with possible underlying hypertensive heart disease, ischemic heart disease, or cardiomyopathy of nonischemic etiology). Sustained left ventricular impulse without an atrial kick, on the other hand, would make one strongly suspect the presence of severe left ventricular dysfunction and decreased ejection fraction due to either ischemic or nonischemic cardiomyopthy. If the apical impulse is normal but the first heart sound is loud and palpable, one might consider mitral obstruction (e.g., from mitral stenosis or a left atrial tumor), and this suspicion may be increased if signs of pulmonary hypertension were detected by both jugular venous pressure and jugular pulse contour abnormalities together with a sustained right ventricular impulse detected on subxiphoid palpation. None of these can be ruled out if the apical impulse is not palpable or characterizable.

After this, a careful and complete auscultation is also carried out, first paying attention to the heart sounds (both the normal and the abnormal) and later to the detection and characterization of murmurs if any. By the time one is ready to auscultate, however, if proper thinking were to accompany the physical examination and this type of analytical approach is applied to each of the things being assessed, then the examiner might have actually coned down on the possibilities (for instance, whether one is dealing with acute severe mitral regurgitation, severe aortic regurgitation, or its mimickers, hypertrophic cardiomyopathy, dilated cardiomyopthy, etc.). Then the auscultation may even be tuned and focused to further confirm or rule out suspected lesions.

Patient B: *A-35-Year-Old Man, Chronic Smoker, Previously Well, Presents With History of Two Recent Episodes of Lightheadedness (Presyncopal Feeling) While Climbing Two Flights of Stairs*

EXERCISE

1. Develop a list of possible conditions that might cause these symptoms in this patient.
2. Discuss the physical findings noted on the cardiac examination and synthesize further to narrow down the possibilities to arrive at the proper diagnosis.

Presyncopal symptoms on exertion would point to transient abrupt fall in cardiac output. The first comment that one can make regarding this particular patient is that the exertion that caused the presyncopal symptom in this relatively young man who has been "previously well" appears to be quite minimal. Therefore, the symptoms may or may not be related to the exertion. Therefore, while generating possible conditions that could have caused the symptoms, one cannot totally limit these to lesions associated with exertional syncope (namely, fixed-output lesions such as result from severe outflow obstruction) alone. Abrupt onset of any tachyarrhythmia supraventricular or ventricular if it were rapid (rate >160) and sufficiently long in duration (at least >30 s) could cause a fall in cardiac output and therefore cause symptoms. Similarly, any significant bradycardia (pauses >4.0 s or rates <35) can be associated with a fall in cardiac output, which may be symptomatic.

The ability to generate such a list requires some background knowledge of various disorders and their typical presenting features. But one can certainly think of them in general categories and add individual disorders appropriate to the level of the experience and knowledge of the physician. This likely would vary whether the individual is a beginner or student or is a cardiac fellow.

CONGENITAL ETIOLOGIES

- Obstructive outflow lesions: significant aortic/pulmonary stenosis
- Inflow obstruction: unlikely
- Severe pulmonary hypertension secondary to Eisenmenger's syndrome: with reversed intracardiac shunt from pulmonary vascular disease
- Disorders associated with significant tendency for tachyarrhythmias: Ebstein's anomaly of the tricuspid valve; arrhythmogenic right ventricle; conduction system disorders with tendency for tachyarrhythmias
- With tendency for bradyarrhythmias: congenital atrioventricular (A-V) block

Acquired Etiologies

- Left ventricular outflow obstruction: valvular aortic stenosis (unlikely at this age unless congenital in origin); hypertrophic obstructive cardiomyopathy
- Inflow obstruction such as due to atrial myxoma (mitral stenosis unlikely)
- Regurgitant valvular lesions: by themselves these are not expected to cause such symptoms. Occasionally, however ventricular tachyarrhythmias may be seen in patients with advanced mitral regurgitation. Rarely severe ventricular tachyarrhthmias might also occur in patients with mitral valve prolapse syndrome with redundant myxomatous degeneration of the valves.
- Ischemic heart disease: ischemia with ventricular arrhythmia (patient relatively young but cannot be excluded); coronary vasospasm with ventricular tachyarrhythmia or bradycardia or A-V block, depending on the coronary artery involved
- Cardiomyopathies: ventricular tchyarrhythmias, in the presence of underlying nonobstructive or obstructive hypertrophic cardiomyopathy, dilated cardiomyopathy, or bradyarrhythmias in the presence of restrictive cardiomyopathy
- Pericardial diseases: unlikely to be associated with the symptoms of presyncope unless there is severe pericardial effusion, then invariably other symptoms such as lassitude, fatigue, and dyspnea would be present.
- Conduction system disorders: with tendency for tachyarrhythmia; pre-excitation syndromes (Wolff–Parkinson–White syndrome, Lown–Ganong–Levine syndrome); long QT syndrome; re-entrant tachycardia in the absence of pre-excitation; paroxysmal atrial tachycardia
- Severe pulmonary hypertension: secondary to severe pulmonary disease, ventilatory disorders such as sleep apnea and others
- Primary pulmonary hypertension: more common in females
- Acute pulmonary embolism: can cause drop in cardiac output suddenly and may also induce arrhythmias; not very typical but cannot be excluded

Others

- Vasovagal reaction: usually occurs secondary to anxiety, acute pain somatic or visceral, and distension of viscus organ and rarely secondary to ischemia.
- Usually associated with sweating, nausea, and/or vomiting.

Cardiac Examination Findings in Patient B

- Patient slightly tachypneic, 5' 7", weighing 185 lb; BP 125/80, heart rate 95/min, respirations 25/min
- Arterial pulse: normal volume or amplitude pulse with normal upstroke in the carotids. All pulses palpable and symmetrical
- Jugular venous pulse: jugular venous pressure 8 cm above the sternal angle at 45°. The contour showed $x' = y$; the venous pressure tended to rise on inspiration.
- Precordial pulsations: apical impulse normal with medial retraction; right ventricular impulse palpable on deep inspiration by subxiphoid palpation.
- Auscultation: S2 palpable at the II LICS. S2 splitting appeared to be somewhat wide but appeared to vary normally on inspiration. S3 and S4 were both heard at the lower left sternal area and over the xiphoid area and appeared to increase slightly on inspiration. No significant murmurs. Chest was clear.

INTERPRETATIONS OF THE PHYSICAL FINDINGS OF PATIENT B

1. Mild dyspnea and increased respiratory rate should raise suspicion about possible hypoxemia.
2. The arterial pulse upstroke being normal rules out significant left-sided obstruction. It also is not suggestive of hypertrophic cardiomyopathy, where the arterial pulse upstroke is often brisk. The normal pulse volume or amplitude and the normal pressure indicate adequate stroke volume and tend to rule out any significant cardiac compression.
3. The elevated jugular venous pressure indicates rise in the diastolic pressures in the right ventricle. The abnormal contour of x' *descent* = y *descent* can occur both with and without significant pulmonary hypertension. The preservation of x' indicates preserved right ventricular systolic function. The prominent y *descent* would indicate increased v wave pressure head in the right atrium, which is usually caused by raised right ventricular diastolic pressures (the pre-a wave pressure). This contour in the absence of pulmonary hypertension can occur in pericardial effusion with some cardiac compression. The preserved y *descent*, however, excludes cardiac tamponade because early diastolic emptying of the right atrium must be free and unrestricted. The same $x' = y$ contour in the presence of pulmonary hypertension, however, would indicate significant pulmonary hypertension severe enough to alter the diastolic function of the right ventricle.
4. The palpable S2 in the second left interspace and right ventricular impulse subxiphoid together would indicate the presence of pulmonary hypertension. This will be the evidence to conclude that the jugular venous pulse contour abnormalities arise from significant degree of pulmonary hypertension.
5. The apical impulse with medial retraction suggests a left ventricular impulse. It has been described as normal, indicating presumably normal and perhaps no more than mild left ventricular dysfunction. Therefore, the left ventricular dysfunction is not the cause of the pulmonary hypertension.
6. The widely split S2 moving physiologically may indicate some right ventricular dysfunction resulting from pulmonary hypertension because pulmonary hypertension *per se*, by increasing the pulmonary impedance, would cause P2 to occur earlier and a narrower split S2. Another possibility is an electrical delay, such as a co-existing right bundle branch block.
7. The presence of S3 and S4 heard over the lower left sternal border and xiphoid area, both of which are described as slightly increasing on inspiration, suggest right-sided events compatible with right ventricular diastolic dysfunction and acute decompensation of the right ventricle.

SYNTHESIS

1. So far the predominant right-sided signs all point to the presence of significant pulmonary hypertension with right ventricular diastolic dysfunction. Because the patient is described as previously well and the history is rather of sudden and recent onset, acute cause of pulmonary hypertension, such as acute pulmonary embolism, must be considered to be present unless proven otherwise.
2. Such a conclusion is also suggested by the presence of mild tachycardia and mild tachypnea.
3. Such an analysis should lead to immediate application of appropriate measures of management, including treatment and diagnostic investigations.

FOCUSED CARDIAC PHYSICAL EXAMINATION: *PRACTICAL POINTS*

1. Proper evaluation of the cardiac symptoms and their severity would ultimately require defining the appropriate causal cardiac disorder. Therefore, it helps to group symptoms to identify underlying pathology.

2. Definite orthopnea and/or nocturnal dyspnea should point to the presence of high left atrial pressure. Triad of dyspnea, chest pain, and exertional presyncope or syncope should indicate fixed cardiac output lesions. Fatigue, lassitude, and lightheadedness may be due to low output. Significant brady or tachyarrhythmias or hypotension of sudden onset may also cause syncope and presyncope in addition to outflow obstructive lesions. Peripheral edema and ascites represent congestive symptoms resulting from high right atrial pressure.

3. Proper evaluation of cardiac symptoms includes generation of a working list of possible etiologies drawn from a broad range of cardiac disorders and lesions.

4. While a complete and thorough cardiac examination is performed, each finding, both normal and abnormal, should be analyzed with regard to its significance in relation to the etiological causes under consideration for the particular patient problem. This automatically becomes a sound tool or method for arriving at proper conclusions with regard to both diagnosis and management.

2 Arterial Pulse

CONTENTS

PHYSIOLOGY OF THE ARTERIAL PULSE
ASSESSMENT OF THE ARTERIAL PULSE
PRACTICAL POINTS IN THE CLINICAL ASSESSMENT
    OF THE ARTERIAL PULSE
REFERENCES

PHYSIOLOGY OF THE ARTERIAL PULSE

Although the arterial pulse, which is considered a fundamental clinical sign of life, has been the subject of study by many physiologists as well as clinicians in the past *(1–28)*, it received less attention by clinicians for many years after the discovery of the sphygmomanometer *(29)*. There has been a renewed interest in this field in recent years since new techniques such as applanation tonometry are now being applied for its study *(30–33)*. The physiology of the arterial pulse is, however, quite complicated, and the subject is often given only cursory description even in the most popular textbooks in cardiology. Also, the retained terminology and nomenclature do not help to clarify the issues *(21,34)*. The most detailed review of the complicated physiology of both the normal and the abnormal arterial pulse can be found in some of the excellent papers of O'Rourke and his co-workers *(21,35–38)*. The subject has, however, remained somewhat elusive even to the most interested clinicians. Therefore, in this chapter an attempt will be made to simplify some of the concepts for the sake of better understanding.

The purpose of the arterial system is to deliver oxygenated blood to the tissues but, more importantly, to convert intermittent cardiac output into a continuous capillary flow. This is primarily achieved by its structural organization *(6)*. The central vessels, namely the aorta up to the iliac bifurcation and its main branches — the carotid and the innominate arteries — are very elastic and act in part as a reservoir in addition to being conduits. The vessels at the level of the radial and femoral arteries are more muscular, whereas the iliac, subclavian, and axillary vessels are intermediate or transitional in structure. When an artery is put into stretch, the readily extensible fibers of the vessel wall govern its behavior. The more elastic the vessel, the greater is the volume accommodated for a small rise in pressure.

It is well known that the recording obtained with a pulse transducer placed externally over the carotid artery has a contour and shape very similar to a pressure curve obtained through a catheter placed internally in the carotid artery and recorded with a strain gauge manometer system (Fig. 1). While the former records displacement of the vessel transmitted to the skin through overlying soft tissues, the latter is a true recording of the internal pressure changes. The displacement in the externally recorded tracing is due to

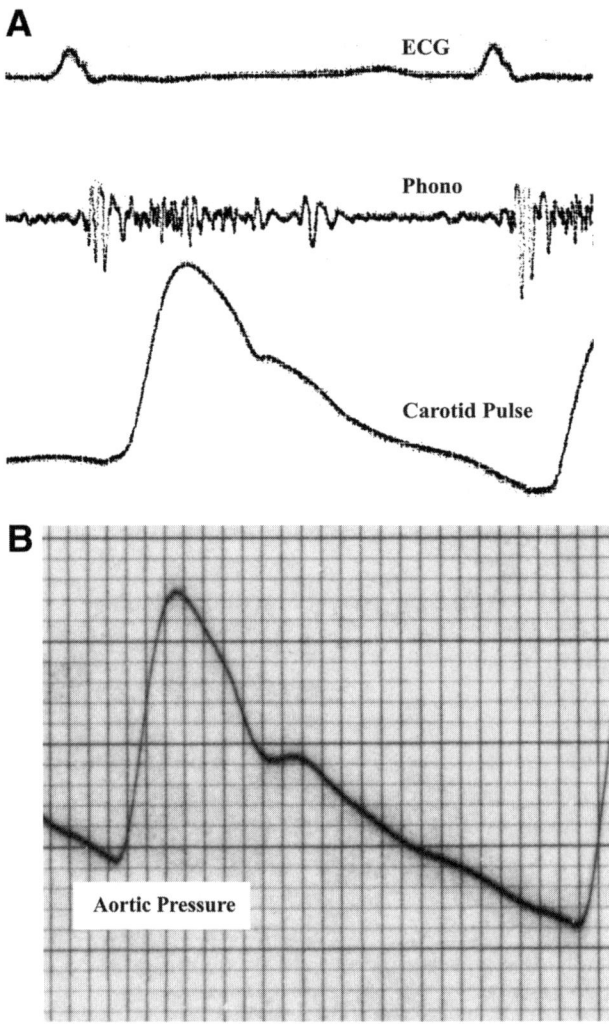

Fig. 1. (**A**) Simultaneous recordings of electrocardiogram (ECG), phonocardiogram, and the carotid pulse. (**B**) Intra-aortic pressure recording in the same patient. Note the similarity of the carotid pulse tracing and the aortic pressure recording.

changes in the wall tension of the vessel similar to the recording of an apical impulse reflecting the change in left ventricular wall tension. The wall tension is governed by the principles of Laplace relationship. The tension is directly proportional to the pressure and the radius and inversely related to the thickness of the vessel wall. Since ejection of the major portion of the stroke volume takes place in the early and mid-systole, the cause of major change in tension in early and mid-systole is a result of changes in both volume and pressure. During the later part of systole and during diastole, however, the predominant effect must be primarily due to changes in pressure, although volume may also play a part. The dominance of the pressure pulse effect on the tension of the vessel wall for the greater part of the cardiac cycle is the main reason for the similarity of the externally recorded carotid pulse tracing and the internally recorded pressure curve.

The contraction of the left ventricle imparts its contractile energy on the blood mass it contains, developing and raising the pressure to overcome the diastolic pressure in the aorta in order to open the aortic valve and eject the blood into the aorta. As the ventricle ejects the blood mass into the aorta with each systole, it creates a pulsatile pressure as well as a pulsatile flow. By appropriate recording techniques applied in and/or over an artery, one can show the pulsatile nature of the pressure wave, the pulsatile nature of the flow wave, as well as the dimensional changes in the artery as the pressure wave travels *(36)*.

What is actually felt when an artery is palpated by the finger is not only the force exerted by the amplitude of the pressure wave, but also the change in the diameter. For instance, the pressure pulse of both arteriosclerosis and hypertension in the elderly and that caused by significant aortic regurgitation will look similar when recorded. It will show a rapid rise in systole and a steep fall in diastole with an increased pulse pressure (the difference between the systolic and the diastolic pressure). However, the arterial pulse in these two different situations will feel different to the palpating fingers. The difference is essentially in the diameter change. The pulse of aortic regurgitation is associated with a significant change in diameter, whereas this is usually not the case in arteriosclerosis. The diameter change due to the high volume of the pulse in aortic regurgitation can be further exaggerated by elevating the arm, which helps to reduce the diastolic pressure in the brachial and the radial artery.

Since pressure and radius are two important factors that affect wall tension, as shown by Laplace relationship, it is probably reasonable to consider both of them together. What is actually felt when the arterial pulse is palpated can therefore be restated as the effect caused by a change in the wall tension of the artery.

Laplace's law is expressed as follows:

$$\text{Tension} = P \text{ (pressure)} \times r \text{ (radius)}$$

for a thin-walled cylindrical shell. If the wall has a thickness, then the circumferential wall stress is given by Lamé's equation, as follows:

$$\text{Tension} \propto P \text{ (pressure)} \times r \text{ (radius)} / 2h \text{ (wall thickness)}$$

Amplitude of the pulse will depend not only on the amplitude of the pressure wave, but also on the change in dimensions between diastole and systole (or simply the amount of change in wall tension).

The Volume Effect

According to Laplace's law, the volume has a direct effect on the wall tension in that it relates to the radius. The actual volume of blood received by each segment of the artery and its effect on the change in wall tension of that segment depends also on the vessel involved. The proximal elastic vessels (aorta and its main branches) receive almost all of the stroke volume of the left ventricle. The elastic nature of these vessels allows greater displacement and change in their radius. However, as one goes more peripherally, total cross-sectional area increases. Therefore, each vessel receives only a fraction of the stroke volume. In addition, the vessels are more muscular and less distensible. For similar rise in pressure, the change in vessel diameter is less. The corollary of this is that to achieve similar diameter change in the peripheral vessels, the pressure developed must be higher.

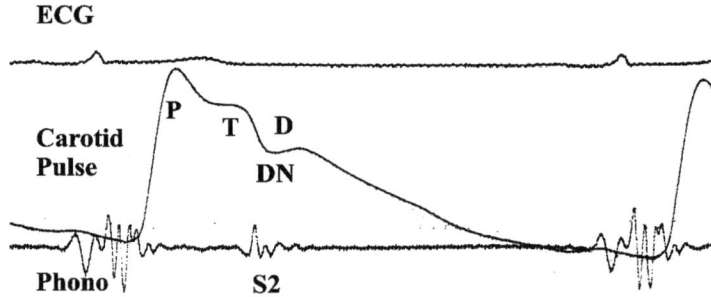

Fig. 2. Simultaneous recordings of ECG, carotid pulse tracing, and phonocardiogram. The carotid pulse shows the percussion wave (P), the tidal wave (T), and the dicrotic wave (D), which follows the dicrotic notch (DN).

Pressure in the Vessel

The pressure pulse generated by the contraction of the left ventricle is transmitted to the most peripheral artery almost immediately, and yet the blood that leaves the left ventricle takes several cardiac cycles to reach the same distance. Thus, it must be emphasized that pressure pulse wave transmission is different and not to be confused with actual blood flow transmission in the artery. The analogy that can be given is the transmission of the jolt produced by an engine of the train to a series of coaches while shunting the coaches on the track as opposed to the actual movement of the respective coaches produced by the push given by the engine. This is the classic analogy given by Bramwell *(6)*.

The mechanics of flow dictate that it is the pressure gradient, not the pressure, that causes the flow in the arteries. There is very little drop in the mean pressure in the large arteries. Almost all of the resistance to flow is found in the precapillary arterioles. This is where most of the drop in mean pressure also occurs in the arterial system *(11,12,35)*. The shape of the pressure pulse changes as it propagates through to the periphery. Although the mean pressure decreases slightly, the pulse pressure (systolic pressure minus the diastolic pressure) increases distally so that the peak pressure actually increases as the wave propagates *(11,37)*. The higher peak systolic pressure achieved in the less distensible and more muscular peripheral vessels helps to accommodate the volume received by the distal vessels.

Reflection

Experimental studies have clearly shown that pressure pulse wave generated artificially by a pump connected to a system of fluid-filled closed tubes or branching tubes with changing calibre gets reflected. The reflective sites appear to be branching points *(11,12)*. This implies that the incident pressure pulse (not flow) produced by the contracting left ventricle gets reflected back. It is reflection of the pressure pulse that gives the pulse wave its characteristic contour (Fig. 2). The pressure and the velocity waveforms vary markedly at different sites in the arteries. The peak velocity generally occurs before the peak in pressure at all sites *(17)*. As one moves to the periphery, the pulsatile pressure fluctuations increase while the oscillations of flow diminish as a result of damping. The peripheral pressure fluctuations often become amplified to the extent of exceeding the central aortic systolic pressure. This is further evidence that the pressure waves get reflected peripherally *(17,37)*.

Table 1
Determinants of Arterial Pressure Pulse and Contour

Components	Determining factors
1. Incident pressure wave	<ul><li>Compliance of aorta</li><li>Stroke volume</li><li>Velocity of ejection</li><li>Left ventricular pump<ul><li>Preload</li><li>Afterload</li><li>Contractility</li><li>Pattern of ejection</li><li>Impedance to ejection</li></ul></li></ul>
2. Pulse wave velocity	<ul><li>Mean arterial pressure</li><li>Arterial stiffness/compliance</li><li>Vasomotor tone</li></ul>
3. Intensity of reflection<ul><li>Increased</li><li>Decreased</li></ul>	<ul><li>Peripheral resistance (arteriolar tone)</li><li>Vasoconstriction</li><li>Vasodilatation</li></ul>
4. Effects of wave reflection	<ul><li>Distance from reflecting sites</li><li>Pulse wave velocity</li><li>Timing of arrival in cardiac cycle</li><li>Duration of ejection</li></ul>
• Diastolic wave	<ul><li>Compliant arteries</li><li>Slow transmission</li><li>Shortened duration of ejection</li></ul>
• Late systolic wave	<ul><li>Stiff arteries</li><li>Rapid transmission</li><li>Long duration of ejection</li></ul>

Since the pressure pulse normally travels very fast (m/s), the recorded arterial pressure wave at any site in the arterial system is usually the result of the combination of the incident pressure wave produced by the contracting left ventricle and the reflected wave from the periphery *(37,38)*.

Pulse Wave Contour

When one records the arterial pulse wave with a transducer, one may be able to identify three distinct components in its contour:
- The *percussion wave*, which is the initial systolic portion of the pressure pulse
- The *tidal wave*, which is the later systolic portion of the pressure pulse
- The *dicrotic wave*, which is the wave following the dicrotic notch (roughly corresponding to the timing of the second heart sound) and therefore diastolic.

Factors That Affect the Magnitude of the Initial Systolic Wave

Although this portion of the arterial pulse may also be influenced and modified by reflected waves from the periphery, the rate of rise and the amplitude of the incident pressure wave of the arterial pulse is still dependent on the ejection of blood into the aorta by the contracting left ventricle. Thus, the characteristics of the proximal arterial system and the effect of the left ventricular pump become pertinent (Table 1; Fig. 3).

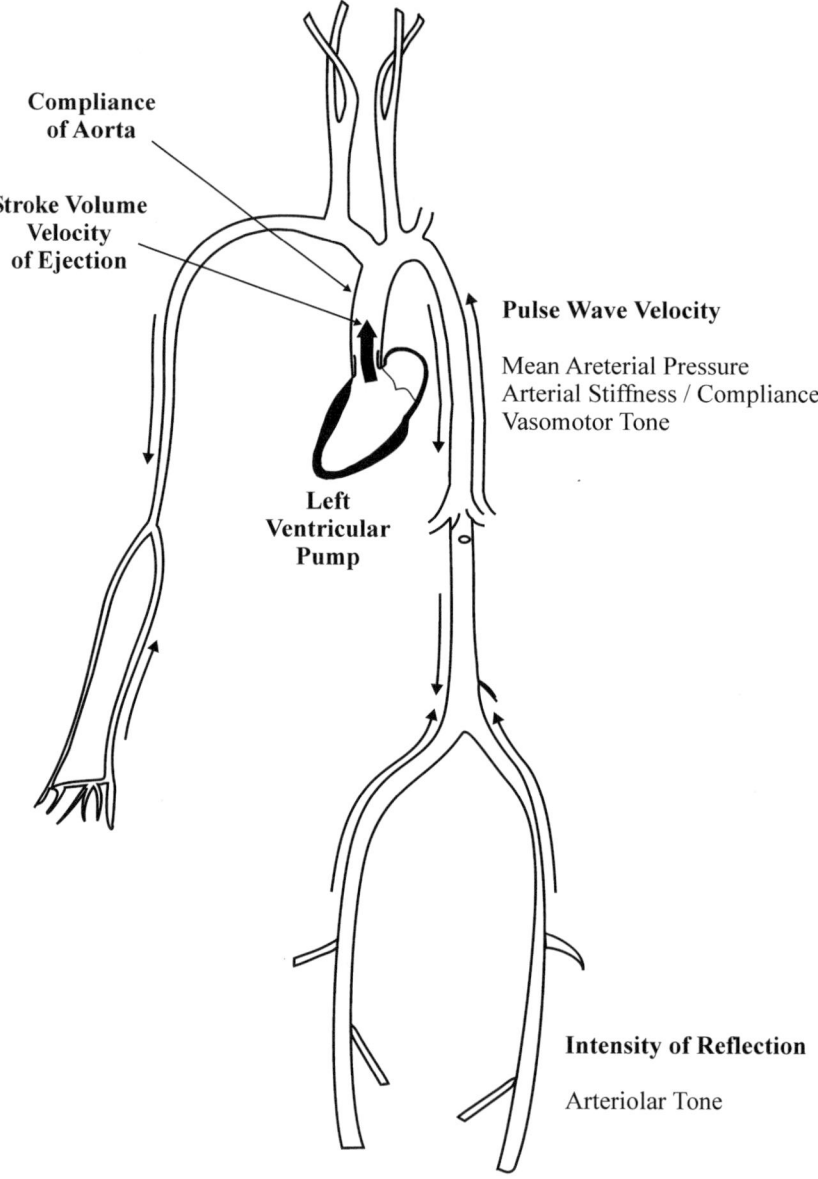

Fig. 3. Diagrammatic representation of factors involved in the arterial pressure pulse wave contour, including the incident pressure wave, pulse wave velocity, transmission, and reflection (*see* text).

CHARACTERISTICS OF THE PROXIMAL ARTERIAL SYSTEM

Ejection of blood into the aorta by the contracting left ventricle during systole leads to a rise in aortic pressure from the diastolic level at the time of the aortic valve opening to the peak in systole. The rise in aortic pressure from its diastolic to the systolic peak is determined by the compliance of the aorta as well as the stroke volume. The aorta is very compliant because of its greater content of elastin compared to the smooth muscle and the collagen in its walls. Because the walls of the aorta are compliant, it expands to accommodate the blood volume. The increase in pressure for any given stroke volume will be determined by the compliance of the aorta. Increasing age leads to changes in the structural components of the walls of the aorta and reduced compliance *(39)*. When the aorta is rigid and stiff, the pressure will rise steeply to an increased peak systolic pressure, giving rise to an increased pulse pressure.

In some elderly patients the decreased compliance of the proximal vessels could be severe enough to hide the slowly rising percussion wave of the aortic stenosis due to marked increase in pressure despite small increase in volume *(36)*. In addition, the pressure rise will be steeper and faster if the stroke volume is delivered to the aorta with a faster rate of ejection, as would be expected with increased contractility.

THE LEFT VENTRICULAR PUMP

The left ventricular output is dependent on the filling pressures (preload), the intrinsic myocardial function, and the afterload against which it pumps (determined by the vascular properties of the arterial system, which affect its compliance, the peripheral resistance, and the peak systolic pressure). When the ventricle begins to contract at the end of diastole, the intraventricular pressure rises as more and more myocardial fibers begin to shorten. When the left ventricular pressure exceeds the left atrial pressure, closing the mitral valve, the isovolumic phase of contraction begins. During this phase the rate of pressure development is rapid. The rate of change of pressure (dP/dt) during this phase usually is reflective of the contractile state of the left ventricle. It is increased when the left ventricle is hypercontractile and is usually depressed when the ventricular function is diminished. When the left ventricular pressure exceeds the aortic diastolic pressure, the aortic valve opens and the ejection phase of systole begins. Recordings of pressures in the left ventricle and the aorta obtained by special microtip sensors show that the left ventricular pressure exceeds that of the aorta in the early part of systole *(40–42)*. This pressure gradient is termed the *impulse gradient* because it is generated by the ventricular contraction. The aortic flow velocity reaches a peak very soon after the onset of systole. During the latter half of systole, the rate of myocardial fiber shortening slows and the left ventricular pressure begins to fall. When the left ventricular pressure falls below that in the aorta, the gradient reverses, and this is associated with the deceleration of aortic outflow. The initial rapid rise in the aortic outflow velocity to its peak is caused by early and abrupt acceleration of blood flow out of the left ventricle. This acceleration is achieved as a result of the force generated by the ventricular contraction. The peak aortic flow velocity achieved is dependent on the magnitude of the force (F) multiplied by the time (t) during which it acts. The physical term "*Impulse*" describes $F \times t$.

The kinetic energy imparted by the ventricular contraction to the blood mass it ejects can be viewed as the total momentum gained by the blood mass. The force of contraction and the peak rate of pressure development (dP/dt), by determining the rate of acceleration of flow, should influence the rate of rise of the incident pressure. Both the mass (m) of blood ejected, namely the stroke volume, and the velocity (v) of ejection would be expected to affect the amplitude of the incident pressure wave. The stroke volume and the velocity of ejection together represent the *momentum of ejection* (mv). The effect of the maximum momentum achieved during ejection as well as the rate of change in momentum on the rate of rise and the amplitude of the pressure pulse can be explained by an analogy. This is best understood by observing a strength-testing game in carnivals where a person hits a platform on the ground with a large wooden hammer, displacing

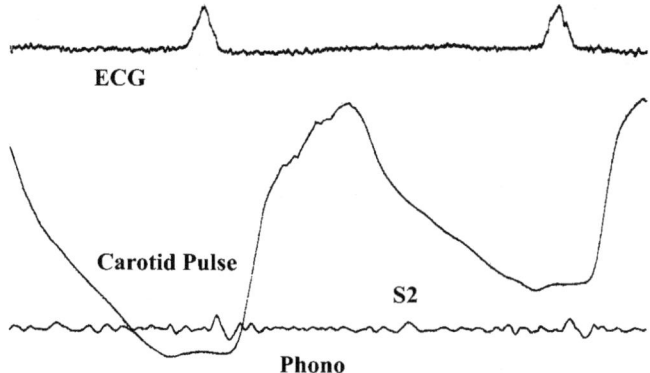

Fig. 4. Carotid pulse recording in a patient with aortic regurgitation. Note the wide pulse excursion.

a metal weight vertically. The aim is usually to raise the weight high enough to ring a bell at the top of the column to show strength and win a prize. The force with which the platform is struck results in the launching momentum. The harder the platform is struck, the faster and higher the weight will rise.

Momentum of Ejection

MASS (STROKE VOLUME)

In conditions with large stroke output, momentum of ejection will be augmented, causing increased amplitude of the pressure wave. The stroke volume will be increased in hyperdynamic and hypervolemic states such as anemia, hyperthyroidism, Paget's disease, and pregnancy. Large stroke volumes can also occur in the absence of the above in certain cardiovascular conditions such as aortic regurgitation and persistent ductus arteriosus (Fig. 4). In addition, bradycardia as seen with chronic complete atrioventricular (A-V) block by virtue of increased diastolic filling of the ventricle can also produce increased stroke volume.

Diminished stroke volume will therefore be expected to cause decreased momentum of ejection and decreased amplitude of the pressure pulse. This will occur in conditions with significant obstruction to either left ventricular outflow or inflow. Severe aortic stenosis, often with some left ventricular dysfunction, and severe mitral stenosis are examples of such states. Cardiac failure with poor pump function will also result in severe reduction in stroke volume. Severe reduction in filling of the left ventricle as seen in patients with cardiac tamponade will have a similar effect on the stroke volume and therefore on the momentum of ejection.

VELOCITY OF EJECTION

The velocity of ejection will be determined by the strength with which the left ventricle contracts as well as the by the impedance to ventricular ejection.

Contractility

Increased velocity of ejection, in the absence of outflow obstruction, will likely lead to larger amplitude of the pressure pulse in the aorta since more volume will be delivered over a shorter duration. The rapid velocity also implies a stronger contractile force and increased *dP/dt* and therefore will be expected to cause a faster rate of rise of the pressure pulse or rapid upstroke of the pulse.

In the absence of obstruction to the left ventricular outflow, the velocity of ejection is mainly determined by the pump function of the left ventricle as well as the preload and the afterload. In conditions with large stroke volume due to Starling effect, the ejection velocity would also be increased unless significant left ventricular dysfunction coexists.

In mitral regurgitation there is increased contractility as a result of the Starling effect of the increased filling of the left ventricle (from both the normal pulmonary venous return and the volume of blood that went backwards into the left atrium due to the regurgitation), resulting in faster ejection. However, there is no increased stroke volume received by the aorta, because the left ventricle has two outlets during systole, namely the aorta and the left atrium. The amplitude of the pressure pulse is expected to be normal, but the rate of rise may be rapid *(43)*.

In hypertrophic cardiomyopathy, the ventricle is hypercontractile and ejects the blood very fast. This leads to a very rapid rise of the arterial pulse. In addition, in this condition the pattern of ejection is such that the flow into the aorta often may be biphasic with a smaller secondary peak in late systole, which may partly contribute to a secondary late systolic pressure rise in the aorta *(44)*. This is more pronounced in patients who have a dynamic obstruction to the outflow when during the middle of systole the anterior leaflet of the mitral valve is pulled from its closed position and moves anteriorly towards the interventricular septum (systolic anterior motion [SAM]). While there is still controversy as to the cause of the SAM *(45)*, it has been attributed to a Venturi effect caused by the rapid outflow velocity. This septal mitral contact obstructs ejection, and the aortic flow ceases. In late systole when the intraventricular pressure begins to fall, the anterior mitral leaflet moves away from the septum, the obstruction subsides, and the ejection resumes. This will then give rise to a second peak in the pulse in late systole, which will be smaller than the first peak.

In aortic stenosis, although the ejection velocity is significantly increased due to the obstruction, the accompanying volume increment is low. Therefore the increase in radius and the tension in the aortic wall will be expected to be slow. In addition, the increased velocity of the aortic jet through the stenotic valve, by a Venturi effect, will cause a decrease in the lateral pressure *(26,46)*, thereby contributing to a slower rate of pressure rise in the aorta, giving rise to a delayed upstroke and a shoulder in the ascending limb of the pressure wave called the anacrotic shoulder (Fig. 5).

Impedance to Ejection

In addition to the factors affecting the afterload, impedance to ejection includes the vascular properties of the arterial system and the peripheral resistance. The load that the ventricle needs to handle during contraction is usually called the afterload, sometimes considered to be synonymous with intraventricular systolic pressure. In fact, afterload is more closely related to left ventricular wall tension or stress. According to Lamé's modification of the Laplace relationship, the tension is directly proportional to the pressure and the radius and is inversely related to the thickness. Thus, when the left ventricle faces a chronic pressure load (e.g., hypertension or aortic stenosis) or volume load (e.g., mitral or aortic regurgitation), eventually its walls will undergo hypertrophy. This will then tend to normalize or reduce the wall stress or tension. Since wall tension is an important determinant of myocardial oxygen consumption, increased afterload would be disadvantageous to ventricular myocardial fiber shortening.

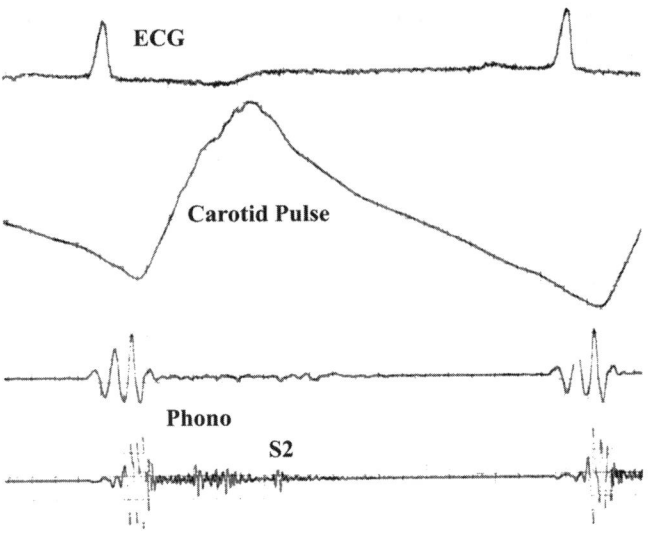

Fig. 5. Carotid pulse tracing in a patient with aortic stenosis. The delayed or slow upstroke with peak of the pulse at the end of systole, almost at the timing of the second heart sound (S2).

The vascular properties of the arterial system, especially the aorta, are also important because they determine the yield or the compliance. The peripheral resistance is a result of the combined resistance to flow of all the vessels in the arterial system. This is predominantly determined by the precapillary arteriolar tone (commonly referred to as the resistance vessels). The level of sympathetic activation generally determines this vasomotor tone. In addition, the arteries in general will offer variable resistance to flow depending on the bulk of the smooth muscle, the relative content of collagen and elastin in their walls, as well as the tone of the smooth muscle in the media *(39)*. The tone of the smooth muscle is in turn locally mediated by the endothelial function. It is well known that the normal endothelium produces nitric oxide, which causes smooth muscle relaxation *(47)*. The basal diastolic tension in the arteries is related to the tone of the vessels and the peripheral run-off. The change in wall tension caused by the pressure wave amplitude as felt by palpation is to a certain extent dependent on the basal diastolic tension in the vessel before ejection.

Low Peripheral Resistance

Low peripheral resistance may result from:

1. Peripheral vasodilatation resulting from withdrawal of the sympathetic tone as seen in patients with aortic regurgitation (large stroke volume turning off the renin–angiotensin system leading to precapillary vasodilatation), secondary to certain drugs and septic or anaphylactic shocks.
2. Development of arteriovenous communications, congenital (arteriovenous malformations), iatrogenic (arteriovenous fistulae), or resulting from pathological processes in various systemic organs (cirrhosis of the liver, chronic renal disease, chronic pulmonary disease, Paget's disease, and beriberi).

Conditions with low peripheral resistance and vasodilatation will lead to increased amplitude of the pulse because the diastolic pressure and the diastolic tension in the vessels in these states is low and therefore the effect of change in tension is better appreciated. Conditions that are associated with increased stroke output (mass augmenting momentum of ejection) with low peripheral resistance (e.g., persistent ductus or arteriovenous communications, aortic regurgitation) cause increased velocity of ejection. Both of these factors lead to a large amount of change in tension leading to greater amplitude of the pulses (bounding pulses).

High Peripheral Resistance

High peripheral resistance is usually caused by high sympathetic tone causing constriction of the precapillary arterioles. The effect of the vasoconstriction is also present on the other vessels. This will lead to decreased compliance of the proximal vessels, making them less distensible as well as causing increased basal diastolic tension in the arteries. Therefore, the change in tension during systole is less. The increased resistance to ejection will decrease ejection velocity and, to some degree, the volume.

In severe hypertension, the basal tension being high in diastole, the change in tension during systole may be poorly felt since much of the change in tension is due to pressure rise alone. It is not uncommon to find constricted and poorly felt peripheral arterial pulses in the context of significantly elevated intra-arterial pressures in some patients receiving inotropic and vasoactive agents. However, in some very elderly patients with stiffened arteries resulting from arteriosclerosis (medial degeneration and sclerosis of the media), the arterial pressure rise might be quite steep and large with large-amplitude pulses due to very marked increase in the pulse pressure *(15,35,37,38)*. The diastolic pressure and tension in these elderly patients' vessels are not usually increased.

Transmission or Velocity of Propagation of the Pulse Wave

As mentioned earlier, the velocity of pulse transmission is generally very rapid. The velocity of pulse transmission is not to be confused with the velocity of ejection or blood flow. The latter can be easily measured by Doppler and is only about 0.3 m/s at the radial, whereas at the level of the femoral, the pulse wave transmission velocity is almost close to 10 m/s. It gets faster as one moves more peripherally, because the peripheral vessels are more muscular and therefore stiffer. The pulse wave velocity is normally faster in the elderly due to the stiffness of the vessels *(4)*. Vasoconstriction and the increased tone of the vessel walls also make the arterial system stiffer and allow faster propagation. The elasticity of the arterial segments is also influenced by the distending pressure *(39)*. As distending pressure increases, the vessel becomes more tense. This is due to greater recruitment of the inelastic collagen fibers and consequently a reduction in elasticity and conversely an increase in stiffness *(27,48)*. The mean arterial pressure determines the background level of distending pressure in the arterial system. Thus, when the mean arterial pressure rises, the arteries become more tense and allow the pulse wave to travel faster *(39)*. The pressure pulse wave travels slowly when the mean arterial pressure is lower *(36,37,39)*.

The concept can also be demonstrated by plucking the middle of a string that is held steady and firm at either end. The oscillations produced by the transmission of the wave and its reflection will be grossly visible when the string is held loose. When it is held tight, the transmission is fast and the oscillations become a blur, and when the frequencies reach audible range, one can hear a tone as well. The tightness with which the string is held is analogous to the stiffness of the vessels in the arterial system.

In severe left ventricular failure with very low cardiac output and stroke volume, associated with decreased rate of pressure development, the momentum of ejection and the rate of change in momentum may be poor and lead to a low amplitude arterial pulse, and if the mean arterial pressure is low, this will tend to slow pulse wave velocity. In aortic stenosis, the velocity of ejection is increased, but the rate of change in momentum is very slow because of less mass or volume being ejected per unit time. In addition, the increased velocity of ejection caused by the pressure gradient across the aortic valve gives rise to a Venturi effect, causing a decrease in lateral pressure in the aorta *(26,46)*. This results in a slowly rising low-volume pulse with lower mean arterial pressure, which may also be transmitted slowly to the periphery. In severe aortic stenosis, one may actually feel an appreciable delay between the upstroke of the brachial arterial pulse and that of the radial arterial pulse (*brachioradial delay*) in the same arm. This is a rare sign *(49)*, which has also been observed by us in some patients with severe degree of aortic stenosis with low output. It is conceivable that the delay may also result from other factors, including more compliant arteries, which will also make the wave travel slower *(50,51)*.

Reflection

Wave of propagation would eventually die out in a completely open system. The arterial system is far from being a completely open system. Although the total collective cross-sectional area increases peripherally, because of change in caliber and branching, reflection of the incident pressure wave occurs from these sites. Complete occlusion of a vessel or a branch will result in complete and fast reflection. Under normal conditions close to 80% of the incident wave is reflected from the periphery. The main reflection site for the proximal segment of the arterial system may be the aortoiliac bifurcation *(22)*. For the more peripheral muscular portion of the arterial system, reflecting sites are at the level of the arterioles. Increase in peripheral resistance or vasoconstriction will increase the intensity of wave reflection (*reflection coefficient*) *(37,38)*. On the other hand, the effect of lowering the peripheral resistance and vasodilatation will cause a decrease in wave reflection. This can be demonstrated pharmacologically by the intra-arterial injection of nitroglycerin or acetylcholine *(25,52)* as observed by the changes in the arterial pressure pulse waveform.

The arterial pulse waveform has been studied by breaking it down into its component harmonics much like a musical wave. The majority of the energy of the pulse is contained in its first five harmonics. Vascular impedance studies relating corresponding harmonic component of pressure and flow waves have allowed quantitative analysis and have given better insights into arterial pressure and flow mechanics *(11,14,15)*.

The peripheral circulation has been considered to provide two discrete components of the reflecting sites: one representing the resultant of all reflecting sites from the upper body and the other representing the resultant of all reflecting sites from the trunk and the lower extremities. This has been described as an asymmetrical T tube in shape model. *(36,38,53)*.

The Effects of Wave Reflection on Pressure and Flow Waveforms

The effect of wave reflection is related to the time of arrival of the reflected wave during the cardiac cycle. The latter will depend not only on the pulse wave velocity, but also on the distance from the individual reflecting sites. Reflected waves from the upper limbs arrive earlier at the ascending aorta compared to those that arrive from the lower body. Reflected waves from the most peripheral reflecting sites will arrive earlier at the larger peripheral arteries before they will arrive at the central aorta.

When the reflected wave is in the same direction, as the incident wave it will facilitate flow, whereas when it has an opposite direction to the incident wave it will diminish flow. Therefore the upper and lower body reflections will have different effects on the ascending and the descending aortic flow. Reflected waves from the lower body arriving in the upper arm vessels show the effect of facilitation of forward flow, altering its contour from that seen in the ascending aorta.

Reflected pressure wave always adds to the pressure waveform.

The recorded arterial pressure waveform will depend on the incident wave, the intensity of wave reflection from the peripheral sites, and the timing of reflection during the cardiac cycle where the two meet and merge *(36,37)*. Reflection added to the incident central aortic pressure wave contributes to the shape of the central aortic pressure. In general it tends to augment the central aortic pressure. In the peripheral more muscular arteries, such as at the level of the femoral or the radial artery, the reflection from the distal sites arrive in such a way as to fuse with the peak of the incident pressure wave, giving rise to an elevated systolic pressure and a larger pulse pressure compared to the central aortic pressure wave. Such amplification of the pressure pulse peripherally is more marked in the lower extremities than in the upper extremities. The peripheral amplification in the arterial pressure appears to be somewhat related to the frequency component. In fact, transfer of pressure wave to the periphery has been studied by relating the degree of amplification of the peripheral pressure compared to the aortic pressure to the individual harmonic frequency component of the pressure pulse. The amplification appears to be least in the lower frequencies, peaking at relatively higher frequencies *(36,37)*. This must be considered in relation to the fact that most of the energy of the arterial pressure pulse is actually in the first five harmonics.

When the arteries are relatively compliant and the pulse wave velocity is relatively slow (as in young adults), reflected waves return to the central aorta in diastole augmenting diastolic pressure and therefore coronary blood flow, which occurs predominantly during diastole. In these normal young individuals, reflected wave from the periphery causes a secondary wave or hump in diastole (dicrotic wave) to the central aortic pressure (Fig. 6A). When arteries are stiffer and the pulse wave velocity is higher, as with increasing age, reflected waves arrive earlier and augment the central aortic systolic pressure, causing a second late systolic peak to the waveform (tidal wave) that is higher than the first peak *(22)* (Fig. 6B). It also adds to the duration of the pressure pulse. This would in effect increase the left ventricular workload and compromise the coronary perfusion *(54,55)*.

The duration of ejection (ejection time) also plays an important role in how the central aortic pressure contour is modified by the reflected wave from the periphery *(17,19, 35)*. When the ejection duration is increased, the reflected wave from the periphery will arrive at the central aorta during late systole and thus cause a secondary wave in late systole (Fig. 6B). When the ejection time is shortened, the reflected wave will arrive after the incisura on the aortic pressure curve (dicrotic notch on the carotid pulse), which corresponds to the aortic valve closure. This will obviously give rise to a diastolic wave (dicrotic wave) (Fig. 7A). The importance of the effect of ejection time or duration of ejection has been demonstrated in humans during the Valsalva maneuver. During this

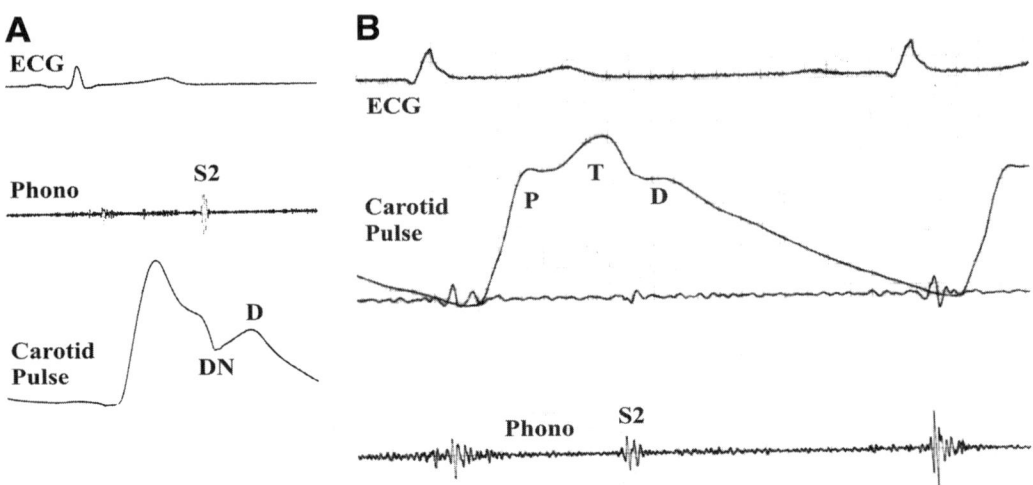

Fig. 6. **(A)** Simultaneous recordings of ECG, phonocardiogram, and carotid pulse recording. Note the prominent distolic (dicrotic D) wave, which comes after the dicrotic notch, which occurs at the time of S2 and aortic valve closure marking the end of systole. **(B)** Simultaneous recordings of ECG, phonocardiogram, and carotid pulse recording. Note the percussion (P) and the tidal (T) wave in the carotid pulse tracing. The late systolic (tidal wave) peak is higher than the initial systolic wave.

maneuver, one tries to exhale forcefully against a closed glottis. During the strain phase, there is increased intrathoracic and intra-abdominal pressure. This will lead to a decrease in venous return, accompanied by decreased stroke volume and falling blood pressure, which causes reflex tachycardia secondary to sympathetic stimulation. All of these lead to a shortened duration of ejection. When the straining phase ends, there is a sudden surge of all the damped venous return from the splanchnic and the peripheral veins. This will in turn increase the stroke output, which will be ejected into an arterial system that is constricted by the marked sympathetic stimulation that occurred during the strain phase. Ejection of a larger stroke volume into constricted arterial system leads to a sudden rise in the arterial pressure (blood pressure overshoot). This in turn will cause reflex bradycardia resulting from baroreceptor stimulation. The ejection time will therefore be increased during the poststrain phase. The pattern with late systolic peak has been observed in the beats with longer duration of ejection and the pattern with the diastolic (dicrotic) wave when the duration of ejection is short and the arterial pressure is low *(8,17,23,36, 37)* (Table 1).

Intensity of Reflection

Intensity of reflection is related to the degree of arteriolar tone. Vasoconstriction will intensify reflection, and vasodilatation will abolish the same. Vasodilatation associated with exercise will be expected to cause less amplification of pressure in the active limb, whereas in the inactive limb the amplification may in fact be greater. The amplification of brachial pressures caused by leg exercise can be abolished by reactive hyperemia of the arm *(56)*. Intra-arterial injection of nitroglycerin or acetylcholine in a single vascular bed can be shown to abolish secondary diastolic waves (usually caused by reflection) in the arterial pressure wave *(25,37)*.

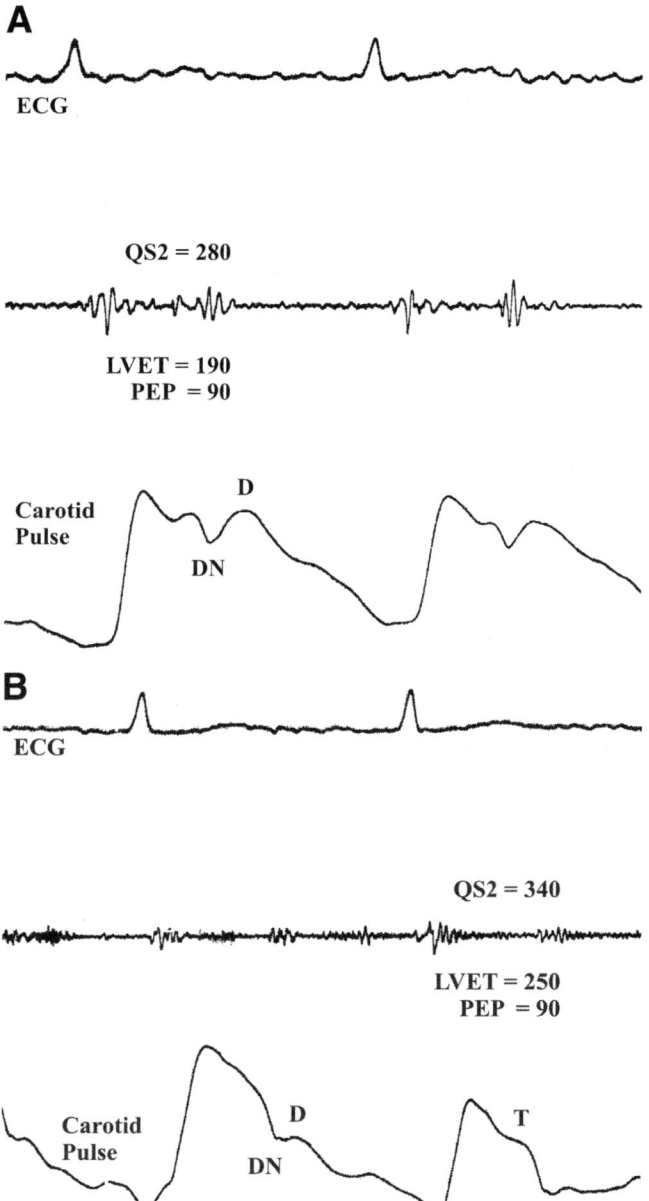

Fig. 7. **(A)** Carotid pulse in a patient with cardiac tamponade. Note the prominent dicrotic wave (D). If palpable, it could give rise to a bifid pulse. DN, dicrotic notch. Systolic time intervals QS2 (total duration of electromechanical systole), LVET (left ventricular ejection time), and PEP (pre-ejection period) are given in milliseconds. **(B)** Same patient as in Fig. 7A after pericardiocentesis. Note the change in the D. It is much smaller. The improvement in the stroke output following the relief of tamponade is evidenced by the increase in LVET.

In summary, multiple factors determine pressure pulse wave reflection and its effects, including vasomotor tone, vascular properties, mean arterial pressure, left ventricular ejection time, and the pattern of left ventricular ejection (37) (Table 1, Fig. 3).

Clinical Implications of Pressure Pulse Wave Reflection

The multiple factors that determine wave reflection and its effects are of clinical relevance in the assessment of the arterial pulse.

Wave reflection is the primary reason for the alteration of the incident pressure wave centrally in the aorta contributing to the change in its contour and duration, as stated earlier. If the reflected waves arrive in diastole and cause diastolic pressure rise, it helps in the coronary perfusion, whereas if it arrives in systole and augments the late systolic pressure, then it will add to the increased left ventricular workload, thereby increasing the systolic left ventricular wall tension, which is one of the major determinants of myocardial oxygen consumption *(37,38)*.

If the left ventricular function is relatively good, then the contracting left ventricular pump, despite the increased demand of myocardial oxygen, may sustain the increased pressure load in late systole. However, in situations where the left ventricular systolic function is severely compromised, as in late stages of myocardial dysfunction of any etiology, the left ventricle will be unable to sustain the late systolic augmentation of the pressure. In fact, the reflected pressure wave will impede forward flow from the left ventricle, causing it to diminish its output. This will in turn abbreviate the left ventricular ejection time or duration. Such patients are usually in cardiac failure with poor left ventricular function and decreased stroke output. This will not be an issue in patients with cardiac failure purely on the basis of diastolic dysfunction where the congestive symptoms are related to decreased compliance and stiffness of the ventricular myocardium resulting in elevated ventricular diastolic filling pressures. They will have normal left ventricular ejection time *(37)*.

When the initial (percussion) and the late systolic (tidal) portion of the arterial pressure pulse are well separated, one may feel a bifid or *bisferiens pulse* (e.g., bisferiens pulse of combined aortic stenosis and aortic regurgitation) *(21,35,36)*. In this situation, aortic stenosis causes slower rate of change in momentum of ejection leading to slower rate of pressure rise, as discussed previously. However, when the bisferiens pulse is felt, usually the co-existing aortic regurgitation is usually significant. The high stoke volume accompanying the aortic regurgitation will cause a large-amplitude pressure pulse wave. The increased velocity of turbulent flow at peak systole due to the obstruction will cause a decrease in lateral pressure in the aorta due to the Venturi effect similar to that seen in isolated aortic stenosis (Fig. 8) leading to a drop in pressure rise during the middle of systole, thereby separating the initial from the late systolic peak *(38,46)*. In this instance, however, the late systolic peak will be greater than the initial one. In aortic valve disease, the ejection duration is prolonged, and this may have some effect on the harmonic components of the arterial pressure pulse wave since the left ventricular pump ejects its stroke volume over a longer period of systole. The pressure pulse has been noted to have predominance of lower frequencies *(19)*.

When the dicrotic (diastolic) wave becomes large and palpable, it may mimic the bisferiens pulse. This is usually produced under circumstances of low momentum of ejection (usually due to low stroke volume), e.g., severe left ventricular failure, cardiac tamponade, and cardiomyopathy (Fig. 7A and B). In these states there may be increased sympathetic stimulation and activation of the renin–angiotensin system. Sympathetic stimulation will cause vasoconstriction. This will be accompanied by increased intensity of reflection. The pulse wave velocity could be normal or low. The activation of the renin–angiotensin system, by making the vessels stiffer, will favor increased pulse wave velocity.

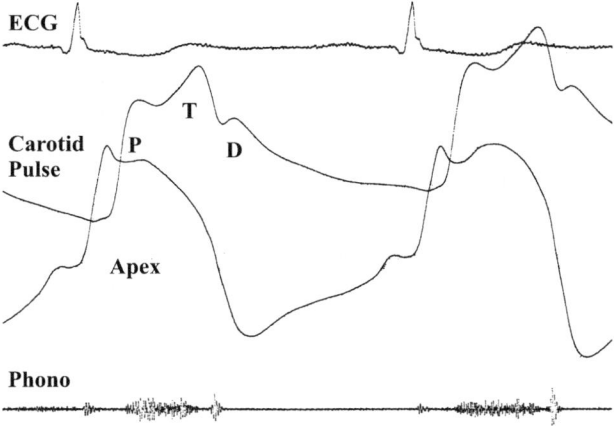

Fig. 8. Simultaneous ECG, carotid pulse, phonocardiogram, and apexcardiogram from a patient with aortic stenosis and aortic regurgitation. Carotid pulse shows a well-separated initial systolic (percussion, P) and late systolic (tidal, T) waves, which were palpable as a bisferiens pulse.

However, the poor left ventricular function and output will cause a poor momentum of ejection, resulting in a decreased rise in the mean arterial pressure. The low mean arterial pressure will make the pulse wave travel slower. The ejection time may be shortened due to the low stroke volume. Intense vasoconstriction will be associated with good intensity of reflection. Thus the reflected wave will arrive in the central aorta after the aortic valve closure, i.e., after the incisura in diastole.

The three conditions that govern reflection in severe cardiac failure are also present in low-output states such as shock and cardiac tamponade (21,37). They are:

1. The low arterial pressure, which favors slow wave travel
2. Intense vasoconstriction, which intensifies wave reflection
3. Shortened left ventricular ejection time, which makes the reflection arrive in diastole (dicrotic wave) after aortic valve closure

The importance of low stroke volume and shortened ejection duration has also been demonstrated by the fact that the dicrotic wave is exaggerated, in beats following shorter diastoles, during the strain phase of the Valsalva maneuver (8,20,37) (breathing against the closed glottis) and during amyl nitrite inhalation. Amyl nitrite is a rapidly acting arterial dilator. It is fairly quickly inactivated in the lungs, and the effect is primarily on the arterial system, which causes rapid onset of arterial dilatation with fall in blood pressure. The brisk sympathetic stimulation secondary to the hypotension produces reflex sinus tachycardia and decreased stroke output initially and decreased ejection time. The reflex sympathetic stimulation leads to vasoconstriction, which favors reflection. All three conditions are thus met to cause prominent dicrotic waves. The sympathetic stimulation also leads to venoconstrictrion, causing increased venous return. The increased venous return results in increased cardiac output (stroke volume × the heart rate /min) (Fig. 9).

Compliant arterial system (as in the younger patients, post-aortic valve replacement in patients with aortic regurgitation) with associated slow pulse wave velocity can cause the reflected wave to travel slowly enough to augment the diastolic portion of the arterial pressure wave, thereby causing a prominent dicrotic wave.

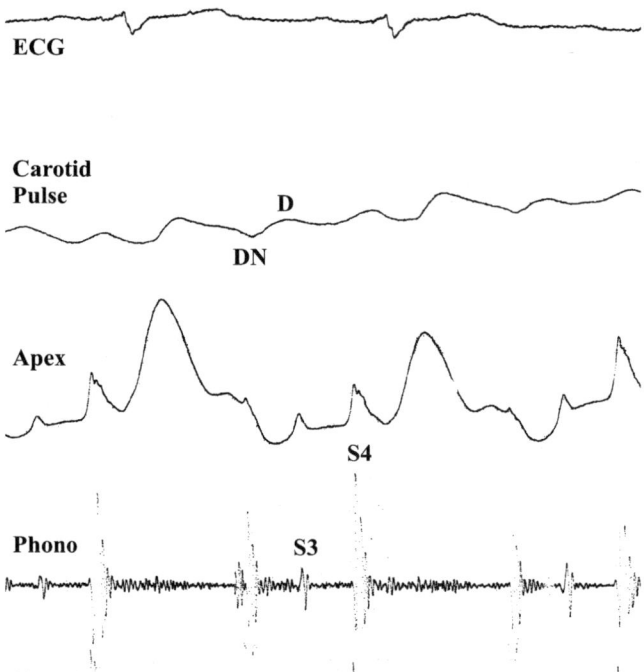

Fig. 9. Prominent dicrotic wave (D) following amylnitrite inhalation in a patient with hypertrophic cardiomyopathy. Amyl nitrite causes rapid onset of arterial dilatation with fall in blood pressure. The brisk secondary sympathetic stimulation produces increased vasoconstriction and tachycardia with shortening of ejection time. Venoconstriction with increased venous return will eventually increase the cardiac output. While the cardiac output is increased, the stroke volume may actually fall due to the tachycardia.. The exaggerated diastolic inflow in the presence of the hypertrophic cardiomyopathy brings out the third (S3) and the fourth (S4) heart sounds. Apexcardiogram (Apex) reflects these events with exaggerated rapid filling wave and atrial kick, respectively.

ARTERIAL PULSE CONTOUR IN HYPERTROPHIC CARDIOMYOPATHY

In hypertrophic cardiomyopathy, obstructive or nonobstructive, the left ventricular contractility is markedly increased. The pattern of ejection is such that the aortic outflow tends to be biphasic in systole unlike the normal monophasic outflow *(44)*. This is particularly marked in patients with obstruction to the outflow caused by the sudden *SAM* of the anterior mitral leaflet towards the interventricular septum during the middle of systole presumably caused by the Venturi effect of the rapid outflow velocity. The latter mechanism has been questioned by some, and the *SAM* has been attributed to pushing or pulling of the mitral valve by the anatomical distortion aggravated by vigorous contraction in these patients with marked hypertrophy of the left ventricular walls associated with small cavity *(45)*. In any event the flow ceases in midsystole and resumes in late systole. The biphasic outflow therefore generates a bifid contour of the pressure wave in the aorta. The late systolic pressure may also be augmented by reflected wave from the periphery. The initial part of ejection being rapid and strong is associated with a faster and greater momentum of ejection resulting in a sharply rising and peaked initial systolic (percussion) wave, which has a larger amplitude than the late systolic (tidal) wave. (Figs. 10 and 11).

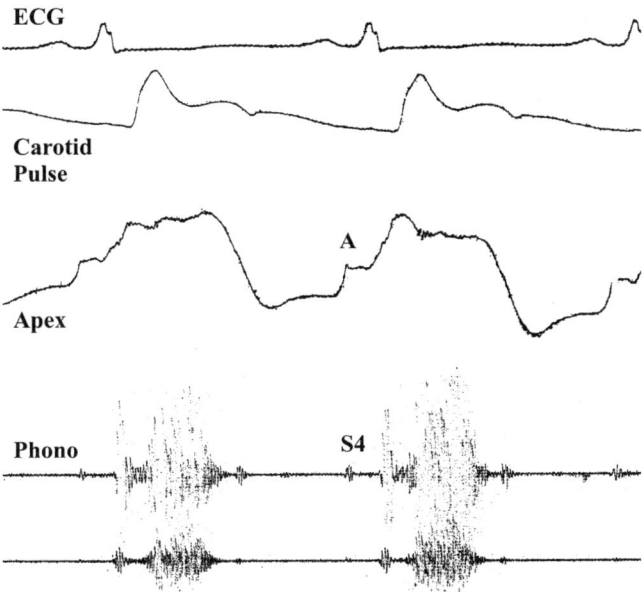

Fig. 10. Simultaneous recordings of the ECG, the carotid pulse, the phonocardiogram, and the apexcardiogram from a patient with hypertrophic obstructive cardiomyopathy. Carotid pulse shows a rapid rate of rise of the percussion wave.

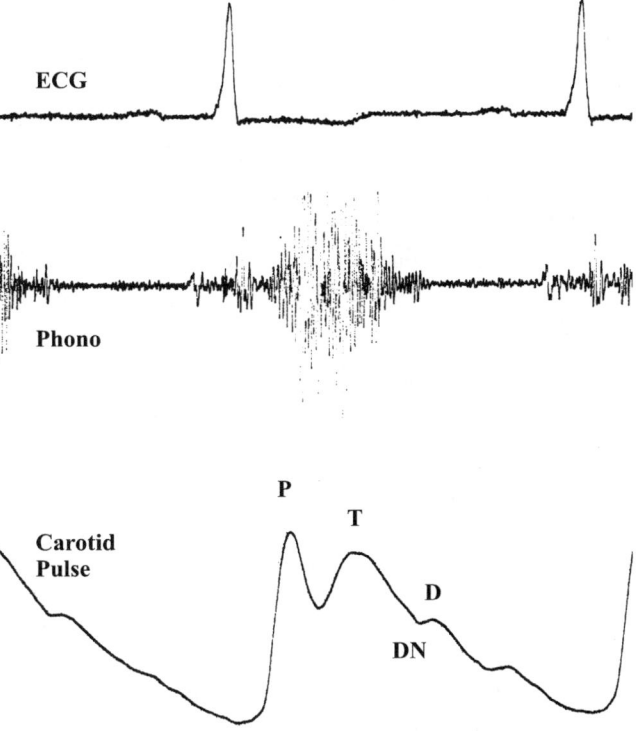

Fig. 11. Bisferiens carotid pulse in a patient with hypertrophic obstructive cardiomyopathy. The initial systolic or percussion (P) and the late systolic tidal (T) waves can be felt separately. The initial systolic wave is more prominent than the late systolic tidal wave.

ASSESSMENT OF THE ARTERIAL PULSE

The essential elements of examination of the arterial pulse should be geared towards the assessment of the volume, the upstroke, and the pulse contour abnormalities. In addition to these essential points, the observer would also be able to assess heart rate, rhythm, and arterial wall characteristics. The assessment of the arterial pulse will be discussed for the following points:

1. Rates, rhythm, and pulse deficit
2. Symmetry and radiofemoral delay
3. Vessel wall characteristics
4. Amplitude
5. Upstroke
6. Contour abnormalities
7. Bruits
8. Pulsus alternans
9. Peripheral signs of aortic regurgitation

Rate, Rhythm, and Pulse Deficit

The heart rate per minute can be quickly ascertained in most instances by counting the peripheral arterial pulse from any site for at least 15 s. When the pulse rhythm is irregular, the presence of an arrhythmia is suggested. In such instances the pulse rate may not reflect correctly the heart rate. Simultaneous cardiac auscultation and palpation of the peripheral arterial pulse will reveal a faster rate at the apex of the heart than suggested by the peripheral pulse. This difference is termed the *pulse deficit*. Simultaneous auscultation may also assist in determining the possible cause of the irregularity. A pause in the peripheral pulse due to an extrasystole or premature beat can be correctly distinguished from that caused by a dropped beat, such as seen in second-degree sinoatrial or A-V block. An exaggerated pulse deficit is most often present in atrial fibrillation, especially when the ventricular rate is not well controlled. The R-R intervals in atrial fibrillation are usually variable. This leads to varying lengths of diastole. The ventricular filling following short diastole is poor, leading to low stroke volume and ejection velocity, resulting in poor ejection momentum and poor pulse, which cannot be felt. Similar effects can also be caused by premature beats.

Symmetry and Radio-Femoral Delay

All peripheral pulses should be palpated, including the temporal arteries in the head, the carotids in the neck, the brachial, the radial, and the ulnar in the upper extremities, the abdominal aorta, the femoral, the popliteal, the posterior tibial, and the dorsalis pedis in the lower extremities. The presence of the pulse at all these sites must be ascertained. Comparison of the similar pulse at opposite sides of the body should be made. An absence of the pulse at any site and the presence of significant discrepancy between the two sides usually indicates a proximal blockage in the vessel with the absent or weaker pulse.

The temporal artery is usually felt for the presence of tenderness commonly seen in temporal arteritis. The carotid pulse, being most central and closer to the aorta, should be preferentially used for the assessment of the pulse volume, upstroke, as well as detection of contour abnormalities. It may be occasionally anatomically difficult to palpate in some patients with short and thick necks. It is usually located somewhat medially to the sternomastoid muscles.

The brachial pulse is located medially in the antecubital fossa. The brachial arterial pulse is commonly used for measurement of blood pressure in the arms. It should also be felt for the proper placement of the stethoscope for blood pressure measurement. The radial and the ulnar pulses are felt laterally and medially, respectively, on the anterior aspect of the wrist. One of these could be congenitally absent. Both of these arteries are usually connected in the hand through the anastomotic arches. In some patients these connections may be inadequate. Radial artery often is used for intra-arterial blood pressure monitoring in critically ill patients, and such instrumentation may lead to occlusion of the vessel. This is usually tolerated by most because of the anastomotic connections in the hand, which continue to be perfused through the ulnar artery. In patients with poor anastomotic connections such iatrogenic blockage may lead to gangrene of the hand. The adequacy of the anastomosis in the hand must be determined prior to any such instrumentation. This is usually determined by the radial compression test (*Allen's test*). Both the radial and the ulnar arteries should be blocked by direct compression of the vessels against the underlying wrist bones. The patient is asked to make a tight fist, thus emptying the hand of the venous blood. This should leave the hand pale until the radial artery is released from the compression. This should result in immediate hyperemia of the hand, resulting in the disappearance of the pallor and return of the normal pink appearance. The test should be repeated a second time with release of the ulnar artery. Similar result should be obtained to indicate intact anastomosis.

The abdominal aorta may or may not be palpable in the adult depending on the degree of obesity. In obese individuals mere palpability may be an indication of the presence of an aneurysm. Palpability of a wide area of pulsation over the region of the abdominal aorta, particularly when the pulsation is expansile, would indicate the presence of an abdominal aortic aneurysm. *Expansile pulsation* can be easily checked by palpating with two index fingers of each hand placed on either side of the pulsating aorta approximately 1–2 in apart. If the fingers are further separated by each pulsation, as opposed to being lifted up without separation, the pulsation can be considered expansile.

The femoral arteries should be palpated in each groin below the inguinal ligament. Diminished or absent femoral pulses indicating proximal blockage is often seen in peripheral vascular disease. Normally the femoral and the radial pulses occur simultaneously. When the femoral pulse lags behind the radial (*radio-femoral delay*), occlusion of the aorta either due to coarctation or atherosclerosis is indicated.

The differential effects of the anatomical variations in coarctation of aorta may be diagnosable at the bedside by the careful comparison of the brachial pulses between the two arms. If both the brachial pulses and the carotids are strong with delayed or diminished femoral pulses, it will indicate the coarctation to be distal to the left subclavian artery. However, when the left brachial arterial pulse is weak or diminished compared to the right, it will indicate the coarctation to be proximal to the left subclavian artery. If the right subclavian has an anomalous origin from the aorta distal to the coarctation, then the right brachial pulse will be diminished or poor.

Popliteal pulses are felt by applying pressure over the popliteal fossa with both hands encircling the knee with the thumbs on the patella and the fingertips held over the popliteal fossa with the knees very slightly bent to relax the muscles. The normal popliteal pulse is often difficult to feel, especially in heavy patients. Popliteal pulses may be more easily felt in patients with significant aortic regurgitation and in other causes of wide pulse pressure.

The dorsalis pedis and the posterior tibial can have marked anatomical variations, resulting in the absence occasionally of one or the other without proximal occlusive disease. Other signs of occlusive disease causing absence of these pulses in the feet should be looked for (temperature of the foot, color, skin perfusion assessment by blanching, presence or absence of hair on the dorsum of the toes).

Vessel Wall Characteristics

The readily accessible arteries such as the brachials and the radials can be rolled between the finger and the bone to get a feel for the thickness and the stiffness of the walls. A calcified vessel will feel hard and not easily compressible. Vessels affected by medial sclerosis would feel thicker and stiffer and less pliable.

Amplitude

The amplitude of the pulse is assessed by determining the displacement felt by the palpating fingers. The displacement is dependent on the change in tension between diastole and systole developed in the arterial wall palpated. The tension is increased according to Laplace's law as the radius and the pressure increase. The radius is increased with large stroke volumes. Patients with low output and low stroke volume will have a "thready" or weak pulse as a result of poor displacement and reduced level of tension developed. Such a low-amplitude pulse (low-volume pulse) is known as *pulsus parvus*. The peak systolic arterial pressure also contributes to the tension developed on the vessel wall. Thus the presence of a marked increase in pulse pressure could also result in increased amplitude of the pulse.

The amplitude of the arterial pulse should be assessed in general using the carotid pulse. Carotid pulse amplitude may be low in the presence of significant obstructive lesions such as severe aortic and mitral stenoses. Large stroke volumes, as seen in aortic regurgitation, would result in exaggerated pulse displacement of the carotids, which may be visible from a distance (*Corrigan's pulse*). The large-amplitude pulsation may be felt in more peripheral vessels as well and reflects the increased change in wall tension secondary to increased stroke volumes. The low basal tension due to the low diastolic pressure, low peripheral resistance, and vasodilatation is also associated with an increase in the pulse pressure (Figs. 4 and 8).

In the presence of a large stroke volume associated with low diastolic pressure as in aortic regurgitation or its mimickers (aortic sinus rupture or communication with another low-pressure cardiac chamber such as the right atrium, aorto-pulmonary window, persistent ductus arteriosus), the arterial pulse feels strong and bounding with large volume of expansion. Therefore the amplitude is often casually referred to as the volume of the pulse. In patients with significant hypertension, in the presence of severe vasoconstriction, the peripheral pulses may even be difficult to palpate due to the decreased change in radius and wall tension.

In patients with combined aortic stenosis and regurgitation where both are significant, the amplitude of the carotid pulsation often would reflect the aortic stenosis, whereas the aortic regurgitation will show its effects on the amplitude more peripherally, such as in the popliteal arteries. The amplified systolic pressures due to reflection in these more muscular and peripheral vessels together with the low diastolic pressure secondary to vasodilatation and retrograde flow into the left ventricle would cause a wide change in tension between diastole and systole, causing more prominent pulsation.

Upstroke

The arterial pulse upstroke is best judged at the carotid. This is a palpatory assessment of the rate of rise of the pulse from its onset to the peak. The normal rate of rise of the carotid arterial pulse is usually sharp and rapid and indicates unobstructed ejection by a healthy ventricle. This in essence rules out a significant fixed type of aortic stenosis. The normally rising carotid pulse transmits a sharp tapping sensation to the palpating finger. When the upstroke is delayed due to significant aortic stenosis, the rise is slow and gives a more sustained, gentle type of pushing sensation reflecting the gradual rise. In fact the sensation in some patients may be jagged and simulates a "thrill" or "shudder." In normals, most of the stroke volume is ejected during the first third of systole, causing a rapid rise in the aortic pressure giving rise to a rapid upstroke. In aortic stenosis, this rapid ejection cannot occur. In fact, it takes all of systole to eject the same volume. The decreased mass or volume ejected per unit time leads to a considerable decrease in ejection momentum despite increased velocity of ejection. In addition, the increased velocity of flow caused by the significant pressure gradient between the left ventricle and the aorta caused by the stenosis produces a Venturi effect on the lateral walls of the aorta. This has the effect of significantly reducing the net pressure rise in the aorta. Thus the rate of rise of the arterial pressure pulse is slow in aortic stenosis. The net effects on the arterial pulse in valvular aortic stenosis are diminished amplitude (small), slow ascending limb (*parvus*), and a late and poorly defined peak (*tardus*). When the stenosis is very severe and accompanied by failing ventricle, the upstroke and the pulse may be poorly felt, if felt at all (*pulsus tardus et parvus*, meaning late, slow, and small). When the carotid pulse amplitude is judged to be very low, one will have extreme difficulty in assessing the rate of rise accurately.

The decreased momentum of ejection, particularly in severe cases with decreased stroke volume, will result in a low mean arterial pressure. This may be accompanied by slow pulse wave velocity, which in rare instances may actually be felt as an appreciable delay between the brachial and the radial artery pulses (*brachio-radial delay*). In the normals, simultaneous palpation of the brachial and the radial arterial pulse of the same side will not show any delay at the onset of the pulses over the two vessels. In fact an appreciable delay between the two pulses would indicate a slow transmission of the pulse wave. This is a rare sign, which may be present in severe aortic stenosis *(49)*.

In aortic stenosis, the peripheral amplification of pressures is diminished but may be still present. This must be taken into account in assessing the gradient of pressure between the left ventricle and a peripheral artery, especially in children.

In elderly patients with stiffened arteries, even significant aortic stenosis may fail to be detected by the assessment of the upstroke. When compliance of the aorta is decreased, as seen in the elderly, even the small volume that is ejected in the early systole will cause a significant rise in pressure, thus increasing the tension in the carotids quickly enough to hide the expected effect of the stenosis on the pulse.

In some elderly patients with stiff vessels with rapid pulse wave velocity and reflection, there may be a hump or shoulder felt in the upstroke (*anacrotic shoulder*). This may mimic a delayed upstroke. These patients may be falsely diagnosed as having aortic stenosis, especially when the findings are associated with aortic sclerosis and ejection murmurs. Therefore, in the elderly, interpretation of carotid pulse upstroke should take these factors into account because of rapid transmission of the incident and the reflected pulse waves.

Very rapid or "brisk" upstroke of the carotid pulse when felt in association with a large-amplitude pulse suggests a hyperdynamic state such as due to aortic regurgitation or aortic regurgitation mimickers (aortic sinus rupture or communication with another low-pressure cardiac chamber such as the right atrium, aorto-pulmonary window, persistent ductus arteriosus). When the upstroke is brisk and the pulse amplitude is normal or low, hypertrophic cardiomyopathy with or without subvalvular muscular dynamic mid systolic obstruction must be considered (Fig. 10). In severe mitral regurgitation, the upstroke may tend to be brisk due to a Starling effect on the left ventricle secondary to the volume overload. However, the amplitude will tend to be normal *(43)*.

In supravalvular aortic stenosis, the right brachial pulse and the carotid may be stronger than the left brachial. This will be reflected in a greater pulse pressure in the right arm than in the left. It has been attributed to a *Coanda effect* (the tendency of a jet of fluid, when properly directed, to attach to a convex surface instead of moving in a straight line) *(43)*. The obstruction in the supravalvular aortic stenosis is such that the high-velocity jet is directed towards the right innominate artery and gets carried by this *Coanda effect*. It probably means that the direct impact pressure at the center of the jet is received by the right innominate artery. There may be actually a Venturi effect of lowered lateral pressure in the aorta distal to the stenosis transmitted to the left subclavian and the left brachial artery.

Contour Abnormalities

The normal arterial pulse has a single impulse with each cardiac systole. Occasionally in certain abnormal states, the pulse may be felt as a double impulse. This abnormality of the contour of the impulse is termed "*pulsus bisferiens*" or simply bifid pulse. Bifid pulse contours may be felt and recorded in arterial pulse tracings.

The conditions that may exhibit bifid pulse contours are (1) hypertrophic cardiomyopathy with obstruction (Fig. 11) and (2) severe aortic regurgitation with some aortic stenosis (Fig. 8). The mechanisms are different in these two conditions and have been dealt with previously. The arterial pulse will tend to have an increased volume and amplitude in combined aortic stenosis and regurgitation compared to hypertrophic cardiomyopathy. The effect of aortic regurgitation on the amplitude will be particularly evident in the periphery, whereas the aortic stenosis effect may be more appreciable in the carotid. The bisferiens of aortic stenosis and regurgitation also is altered in peripheral arteries, where they may not be recognizable as such. It is always best detected in the carotids, and the bisferiens is usually such that the late peak is always higher than the initial peak. This is different in hypertrophic cardiomyopathy, where the initial peak is often brisk and higher that the late peak.

Dicrotic wave, when exaggerated, may become palpable and cause a bisferiens effect on the pulse. The difference lies in the appreciation of the fact that the second impulse is diastolic and will occur after the second heart sound, as judged by simultaneous auscultation and palpation. The exaggerated dicrotic wave is usually associated with low momentum of ejection due to low stroke volume as in severe heart failure, cardiomyopathy, and cardiac tamponade. In these instances, the pulse amplitude will be expected to be low. The mechanisms and factors favoring the development of prominent dicrotic waves have been discussed previously.

Bruits

Bruits are audible noises, often systolic, caused by turbulence in flow usually resulting from partial obstruction of the lumen of the arteries and, very occasionally, from high flow. These are often heard over large arteries and detected by auscultation with a stethoscope. Routine assessment of the arterial pulse must therefore include auscultation over all large peripheral arteries such as the carotid, subclavians, vertebrals, abdominal aorta, the renals, the iliacs, and the femorals. Often a systolic murmur originating from the aortic valve and occasionally from the mitral valve may radiate to the carotids. This can be differentiated by noting the location of maximal loudness of the bruit murmur. The carotid bruit is maximally loud, as expected, over the carotids as opposed to a radiating murmur, which should be maximally loud over the precordium. In high-flow states, continuous bruit lasting throughout systole and diastole may be heard over the intercostal vessels. This could occur in situations that lead to development of collateral flow such as seen in patients with aortic coarctation. Peripheral arteriovenous shunts (congenital or acquired A-V fistulae) may also produce continuous bruits over the vessels involved.

Pulsus Alternans

When the pulse amplitude changes beat by beat, alternating between higher and lower pulse amplitude as a result of alternating stroke volume, the resulting pulse is termed *pulsus alternans*. The alternating weaker and stronger pulses can be both felt and recorded. In such patients when the intra-arterial pressures are monitored, similar changes in both systolic and pulse pressures are noted. It can be detected by palpation and can be confirmed by blood pressure recording. *Korotkoff sounds* will be heard to double in rate once the cuff pressure is lowered and the lower systolic peaks of the weaker beats are detected. Pulsus alternans, if detected clinically, usually indicates a severe degree of myocardial dysfunction and left ventricular failure.

Pulsus alternans is, however, a normal phenomenon in as much as it can be induced after a premature beat. The effect of alternans in normal subjects can only be demonstrated by measurements of the systolic time intervals (Fig. 12). Systolic time intervals consist of the following:

1. The duration of the total electromechanical systole is measured by the interval QS2 between the onset of the QRS in the ECG and the end of systole as depicted by the onset of the second heart sound (S2) on the simultaneously recorded phonocardiogram.
2. The left ventricular ejection time (LVET) is measured from the onset of the upstroke of the simultaneously recorded carotid artery pulse tracing to the dicrotic notch.
3. The third interval, which is derived from these two measurements, is the pre-ejection period (PEP). This is obtained by subtracting the LVET from the QS2.

The stronger beat has better stroke output and therefore has longer left ventricular ejection time. The increased contractility of the stronger beat is reflected in a shorter pre-ejection period. The weaker beat has the opposite, namely a longer pre-ejection period. The effect of the alternans after an extrasystole in normal subjects lasts for two beats. As left ventricular function deteriorates, the alternans effect is more pronounced and tends to persist for a longer period. When the left ventricular function is severely depressed, the alternans becomes more pronounced and may become clinically noticeable and palpable in the arterial pulse (Fig. 13). This may sometimes last for long periods of time, such as several hours or days. Pulsus alternans is often initiated by an extrasystole. Although the mechanism is not fully elucidated, it is perhaps related in some ways to the phenomenon of postextrasystolic potentiation *(57,58)*.

It is well known that the beat following an extrasystole is associated with increased contractility and stroke volume. This *postextrasystolic potentiation* is partially related

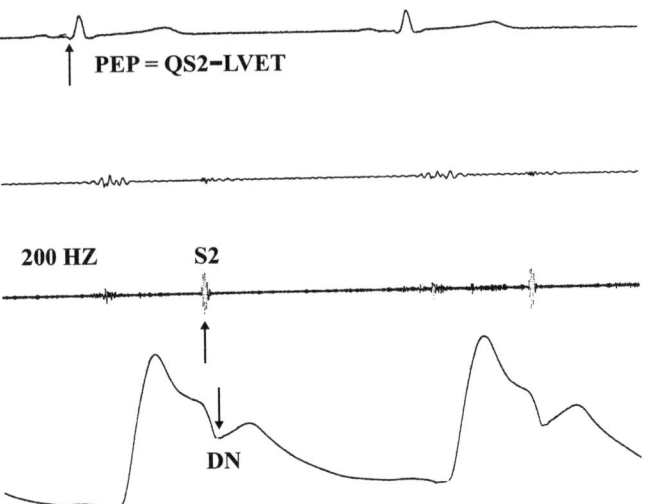

Fig. 12. Simultaneous recordings of ECG, phonocardiogram, and carotid pulse tracings showing measurement of systolic time intervals. QS2, Total electromechanical systole; LVET, left ventricular ejection time; PEP, pre-ejection period. All intervals are in milliseconds.

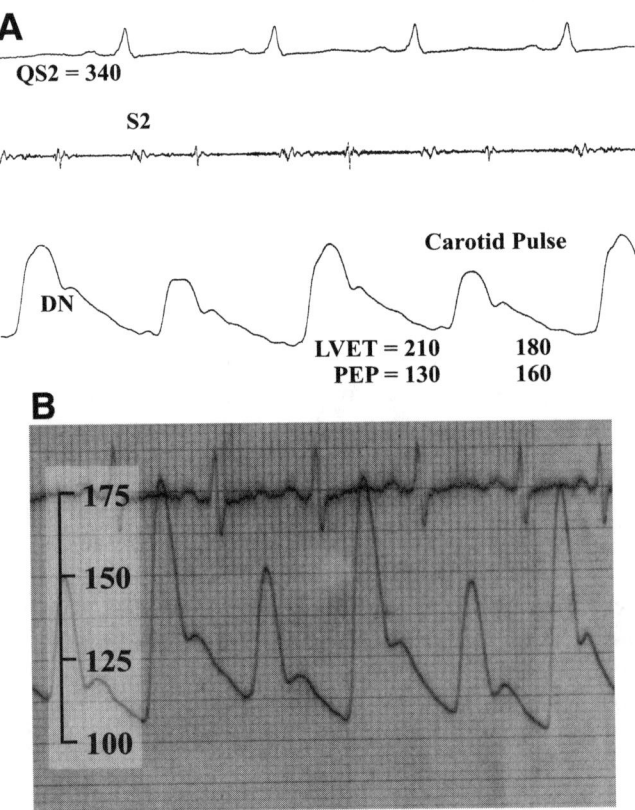

Fig. 13. (A) Carotid pulse recording from a patient with cardiomyopathy showing pulsus alternans. (B) In the same patient, intra-aortic pressures showing alternating levels of increased and decreased systolic pressures and pulse pressures.

to the compensatory pause, which follows the extrasystole, providing increased time for diastolic filling, which in turn through the Starling effect would help increase the contractility and stroke volume. The long pause will also allow more time for peripheral runoff and drop in diastolic pressure. This will in turn help the postpremature beat by decreasing the afterload. However, the postextrasystolic potentiation can be demonstrated even when there is no compensatory pause, thereby keeping both the filling and the afterload constant by pacing studies. In this instance, the increased contractility is probably due to increased levels of intracellular calcium availability for the actin-myosin interaction. The premature depolarization caused by an extrasystole is thought to release more intracellular calcium from the sarcoplasmic reticulum (SR) before all the calcium released during the previous beat could be taken back up by SR. The increased calcium is therefore available for the postpremature beat, thereby increasing its contractile force by more actin–myosin interaction. The calcium uptake and release may actually fluctuate alternatingly from beat to beat reaching the steady state in the normals after a couple of beats. However, in the severely diseased myocytes of patients with severe cardiomyopathy or end-stage heart failure, the steady state may not be reached for prolonged periods of time *(59)*. This becomes manifest as alternating strong and weak contractions of *pulsus alternans*.

Peripheral Signs of Aortic Regurgitation

The peripheral signs of aortic regurgitation are:

- Quincke's sign
- Corrigan's pulse
- Water-Hammer pulse
- Pistol-shot sounds
- Duroziez's sign
- de Musset's sign
- Hill's sign

Most of these peripheral signs of aortic regurgitation *(60)* are related to the large stroke volume, increased ejection velocity, and momentum together with decreased peripheral resistance, and widened pulse pressure with low diastolic pressure secondary to retrograde flow into the left ventricle and peripheral vasodilatation. Some of these signs may therefore be present in aortic regurgitation mimickers (aortic sinus rupture or communication with another low-pressure cardiac chamber such as the right atrium, aorto-pulmonary window, persistent ductus arteriosus) as well as other conditions fulfilling the same pathophysiological requirements (Paget's disease, arterio-venous communications, severe anemia).

QUINCKE'S SIGN

This sign refers to the capillary pulsation as detected in the nailbed. This sign is elicited by applying enough pressure at the tip of the fingernail to cause blanching of the distal nail bed while shining the penlight through the pulp of the fingertip. The observer should look for movement of the proximal edge of the blanched area. This sign is not diagnostic of aortic regurgitation and can occur in many other states with increased pulse pressure and may even be detected in normal young individuals.

CORRIGAN'S PULSE

This term refers to the visible large-amplitude carotid pulsation.

WATER-HAMMER PULSE

This term refers to a toy, which consists of a sealed tube of vacuum partially filled with water so that when it is turned upside down the water falls with a palpable slap. The peripheral arterial pulse, such as the radial, in patients with aortic regurgitation and other similar states as mentioned above, is usually peaked and with rapid rise, which is poorly sustained followed by a rapid fall. When the radial artery is palpated with the palm of the hand while the arm is held raised, which helps to lower the diastolic pressure further in the arm palpated, the sharp slapping quality may be exaggerated.

PISTOL-SHOT SOUNDS

The phenomenon responsible for water-hammer effect upon auscultation over large vessels such as the femorals produces loud slapping sounds, which mimic *pistol shots*. These are short loud sounds. The mechanism has not been clearly established, but it is thought to be due to shock waves generated when the flow velocities exceed pressure velocities locally *(35)*. It is also conceivable that they may be associated with actual reflection at these sites.

DUROZIEZ'S SIGN

This is also termed *the intermittent femoral double murmur of Duroziez (60)*. It is elicited by compressing the femoral artery by applying gradual pressure over the stethoscope, which is placed over the femoral artery. At a certain moment of pressure a double murmur will be heard. The second method is to listen over the femoral artery while applying pressure with the finger in succession first 2 cm upstream (meaning proximal to) and then 2 cm downstream (meaning distal to) of the stethoscope. The upstream pressure will produce a systolic murmur, and the downstream pressure will produce a diastolic murmur. The mechanism involved is the turbulent flow caused by the partial obstruction. The turbulence gives rise to bruit, and its presence in relation to the site of obstruction should suggest the direction of flow. The systolic bruit is easy to understand because flow is toward the periphery during systole; one would expect the bruit to be distal to site of obstruction. Because diastolic bruit is heard proximal to the obstruction, the turbulent flow must also be proximal to the obstruction, indicating retrograde flow. Retrograde flow in some major arteries, including the coronaries during diastole, has been documented by angiography in aortic regurgitation.

Duroziez's sign may be falsely positive in other high-output states such as thyrotoxicosis, severe anemia, fever, persistent ductus and arteriovenous fistula. In high-output states, the diastolic component of the bruit may be due to forward flow. The specificity of the sign can be increased by eliciting the sign slightly differently by applying the partial compression of the femoral artery with the proximal or the distal edge of the stethoscope while listening for the loudest diastolic component. In retrograde flow states (such as aortic regurgitation and persistent ductus arteriosus), as opposed to high-output states, the diastolic components are louder when the distal edge of the stethoscope is pressed.

deMUSSET'S SIGN

This sign is best elicited by watching the patient's upper body and head while seated at the edge of the examining table. The upper body and head will be seen to move back and forth rhythmically with each systole. This is the result of the exaggerated ballisto-

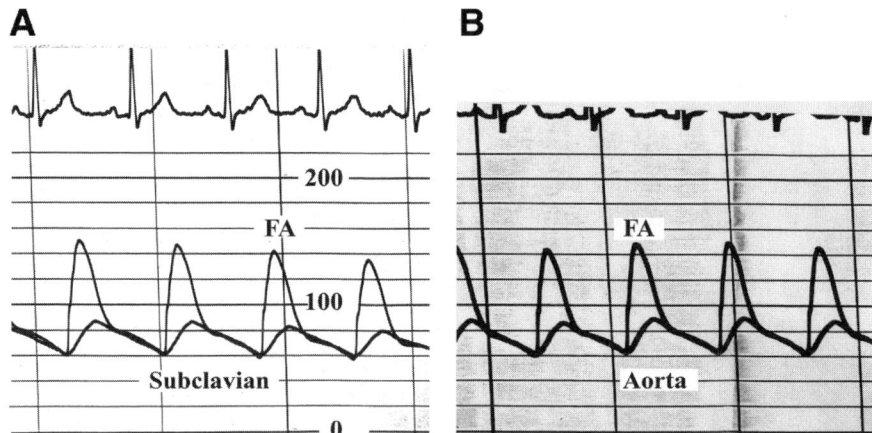

Fig. 14. (**A**) Shows simultaneous intra-arterial pressure recordings through catheters placed in the femoral artery (FA) and the subclavian artery in a patient with aortic regurgitation. Note the significant difference in the systolic pressures. (**B**) In the same patient, the catheter is withdrawn from the subclavian artery to the central aorta and simultaneous recordings of aortic and femoral arterial pressures are shown. Note that there is no significant difference of systolic pressures between the central aorta and the subclavian artery. There is, however, about a 60-mm difference in pressures between the FA and the central aorta.

graphic effect of the large stroke volume and wide pulse pressure together with low peripheral resistance. *Ballistocardiography*, an old physiological method *(61)*, involves recording of the reaction of the whole body to the action of ejection of blood into the aorta (Newton's third law of motion). The recoil of the aorta itself may play a part in contributing to the movement. Special instruments and bed are required to detect these in normal subjects with normal stroke volume. However, it is so exaggerated in aortic regurgitation that it becomes visible and detectable clinically.

HILL'S SIGN

This sign is elicited by measurement of the systolic blood pressure in the arm and the leg simultaneously or in very quick succession *(3,62)*. It must be emphasized that the *Hill's sign* refers to systolic blood pressure differential as obtained by indirect blood pressure measurements using the traditional cuff. The pressure is obtained in the usual way at the arm over the brachial artery. The pressure in the leg can be elicited over the popliteal artery or at the ankle by palpation of the posterior tibial artery. Intra-arterial pressure recordings at the femoral level are not the way to look for this difference accurately. The reason for this is that the femoral artery is probably not peripheral enough to show this exaggerated effect.

Normally the peripheral pressures are usually amplified due to the muscular nature of these vessels, allowing rapid transmission of the pulse wave in both directions resulting in summation of the reflected with the peak of the incident wave. This peripheral amplification is usually more pronounced in the leg than in the arm. In normal subjects this difference in peak pressure between the arm and the leg is in the order of 15–20 mmHg. This difference may be markedly exaggerated in patients with significant aortic regurgitation (Fig. 14).

A difference of 20–40 mmHg in peak pressure can easily be seen in other conditions with wide pulse pressures (e.g., thyrotoxicosis, anemia, fever, or Paget's disease). A difference of between 40 and 60 mm Hg is associated with a moderate degree of aortic regurgitation, whereas an excess of 60 mmHg is usually indicative of moderately severe aortic regurgitation. *Hill's sign* is therefore somewhat related to the degree of aortic regurgitation and useful in following the patients with aortic regurgitation assuming, of course, there is no significant peripheral arterial disease.

The blood pressure differential between the arm and the leg is probably multifactorial in origin even in normal subjects:

1. The reflecting sites in the lower extremities are probably more than in the arm.
2. The vessels of the lower extremities are probably more muscular.
3. It is known that the age-related change in the compliance of the arteries is less in the upper limb vessels than in the lower limb vessels *(36,37)*.
4. The upper arm vessels tend to arise anatomically at approximately 90° angle from the aortic arch. The diameter of these vessels being smaller than the aorta, the relative rapid flow in the aortic arch may cause a Venturi effect of relative suction on these cephalo-brachial vessels. This may tend to reduce the net effect of peripheral amplification of pressures caused by reflection. This effect of suction can be demonstrated in the side arm of a tap by running water through it when the side arm is of a smaller diameter and at right angles to the direction of water flow.

    This concept derives support from the fact that when direct impact pressure gets transmitted preferentially to the orifice of the innominate artery, as it happens in supravalvular aortic stenosis, the pressure is actually higher in the right arm supplied by that vessel *(43)*. Presumably here, the Venturi effect of reduction in lateral pressure does not apply since the direct impact pressure of the jet gets directed preferentially towards the orifice due to the anatomical nature of the stenosis.
5. In aortic regurgitation, the increased momentum of ejection will produce larger-amplitude incident pressure wave. The increased momentum of ejection as well as the increased duration of ejection may in fact alter the harmonic components of the wave. It has been shown that peripheral amplification is less with lower frequencies than with higher frequencies of the pressure pulse wave. It has been suggested, therefore, that peripheral amplification is generally less in aortic regurgitation *(36,38)*. While these may be valid, it is known that in echo Doppler measurements of pure aortic regurgitation, the aortic outflow velocity is quite variable. Sometimes it can be quite high without the presence of any stenosis. In patients with aortic regurgitation and high velocities of flow in the aortic arch, one can expect exaggerated result from the Venturi effect. This may explain variations seen in the sensitivitiy of the Hill sign in patients with aortic regurgitation. In patients who have a positive Hill's sign, it becomes useful in their long-term follow-up.

PRACTICAL POINTS IN CLINICAL ASSESSMENT OF THE ARTERIAL PULSE

In the clinical assessment of the arterial pulse, it is worth remembering the following points:

1. The three features of the arterial pulse that should be diligently sought for are the amplitude, the upstroke, and the pulse contour abnormalities.
2. Other features include the determination of rate, rhythm, pulse deficit, symmetry, radio-femoral delay, bruits, and specifically looking for the peripheral signs of aortic regurgitation when indicated.

3. Palpation of the carotid arterial pulsation is necessary to determine the pulse upstroke and for the detection of abnormal contours. The amplitude may be judged by palpation of the carotid as well as the more peripheral vessels.
4. The amplitude of the pulse is assessed by determining the displacement felt by the palpating fingers. The displacement is dependent on the change in tension in the artery between diastole and systole. The amplitude of the pulse must be judged as to whether it is normal, low, or increased.
5. The low-amplitude (the low-volume) pulse usually indicates low momentum of ejection due to decreased stroke volume and low pulse pressure as seen in significant obstructive lesions of the outflow or the inflow tracts (severe aortic or mitral stenoses), poor ventricular pump function as in severe cardiomyopathy or heart failure, and severe reductions in left ventricular filling as in cardiac tamponade or significant loss in the blood volume or the extracellular fluid volume.
6. In severe systemic hypertension with excessive vasoconstriction, the peripheral pulse amplitude may be poor due to decreased change in radius and wall tension.
7. If the pulse amplitude is considered increased or exaggerated ("bounding pulses"), then conditions associated with large stroke volume and low peripheral resistance must be considered. These include aortic regurgitation and aortic regurgitation mimickers (aortic sinus with a communication to a low-pressure chamber such as the right atrium, aorto-pulmonary window, and persistent ductus arteriosus).
8. The pulse amplitude will also be exaggerated in conditions associated with vasodilatation and low peripheral resistance, since in these states (e.g., septic states, drugs causing vasodilatation, arterio-venous communications congenital or iatrogenic or due to pathological processes in systemic organs as in cirrhosis of the liver, chronic renal disease, chronic pulmonary disease, Paget's disease, and beriberi) the diastolic pressure in the vessel is low and therefore the change in tension is better appreciated.
9. In patients with combined aortic stenosis and regurgitation where both are significant, the amplitude of the carotid pulsation often would reflect the aortic stenosis, whereas the aortic regurgitation will show its effects on the amplitude more peripherally such as in the popliteal arteries.
10. In the elderly with decreased compliance of the large arteries, ejection of normal stroke volume may cause significant systolic hypertension. The pulse amplitude will be high due to rapid pulse wave velocity caused by the increased stiffness and reduced compliance of the arteries, resulting in increased augmentation of central systolic and pulse pressures due to reflection. In fact, even the presence of aortic stenosis may be masked in such patients.
11. The upstroke of the pulse is best assessed over the carotid artery. The normal rate of rise is felt as a sharp tap by the palpating finger. The delayed upstroke is felt as a gentle sustained push. In some, the sensation may be jagged, simulating a "thrill" or "shudder." A normally rising carotid pulse rules out significant fixed aortic stenosis. The delayed carotid upstroke, on the other hand, is indicative of fixed left ventricular outflow obstructive lesions. Rare exceptions are, of course, elderly patients. Delayed upstroke may be masked in the elderly with stiff aorta where the pressure rise may be steep due to the decreased compliance of aorta. The elderly may also have a hump on the upstroke due to an exaggerated anacrotic shoulder mimicking a delayed upstroke without the presence of any significant aortic stenosis.

When the amplitude of the pulse is low as in low stroke output, then the rate of the rise of the pulse is often difficult to judge.

12. When the upstroke of the pulse is thought to be brisk or rapid and if the pulse amplitude is normal or low, then conditions associated with rapid left ventricular ejection such as hypertrophic cardiomyopathy with or without subvalvular dynamic muscular obstruction must be considered. If the upstroke is brisk and the pulse amplitude is normal, then rapid ejection with normal stroke volume as in significant mitral regurgitation must be considered.

13. Bifid pulse contours or pulsus bisferiens must lead one to consider hypertrophic cardiomyopathy with possible obstruction as well as combined aortic regurgitation and stenosis where the aortic regurgitation is more dominant and hemodynamically significant than the aortic stenosis. In hypertrophic cardiomyopathy with obstruction, amplitude of the pulse is low while the upstroke will be brisk and the initial peak will be brisk and taller than the late peak. In combined aortic stenosis and regurgitation with bisferiens, the amplitude will be large and the upstroke will be relatively normal. The second peak will be larger than the first peak.

14. Exaggerated dicrotic wave may occasionally be the cause of a bifid pulse contour. The second impulse in this instance will occur in diastole as timed by auscultation. The exaggerated dicrotic wave is usually associated with low momentum of ejection, usually the result of low stroke volume as in severe heart failure, cardiomyopathy, and cardiac tamponade. In these instances, the pulse amplitude will be expected to be low.

REFERENCES

1. Mahomed F. The physiology and clinical use of the sphygmograph. Med Times Gazette (London) 1872;1:62–65.
2. Mackenzie J. The Study of the Pulse, Arterial, Venous, and Hepatic, and of the Movements of the Heart. Edinburgh: Pentland, 1902.
3. Hill L, Rowlands RA. Systolic blood pressure. (1) in change of posture, (2) in cases of aortic regurgitation. Heart 1911;3:219–232.
4. Bramwell JC, Hill AV. Velocity of transmission of the pulse wave and elasticity of arteries. Lancet 1922;1:891–892.
5. Wiggers CJ. The Pressure Pulses in the Cardiovascular System. New York: Longmans Green and Company, 1928.
6. Bramwell JC. The arterial pulse in health and disease. Lancet 1937;2:239–247.
7. Kroeker EJ, Wood EH. Comparison of simultaneously recorded central and peripheral arterial pressure pulses during rest, exercise and titlted position in man. Circ Res 1955;3:623–632.
8. Kroeker EJ, Wood EH. Beat to beat alterations in relationship of simultaneously recorded central and peripheral arterial pressure pulses during Valsalva maneuver and prolonged expiration in man. J Appl Physiol 1956;8:483–494.
9. Remington JW, Wood EH. Formation of peripheral pulse contour in man. J Appl Physiol 1956;9:433–442.
10. Wood P. Diseases of the Heart and Circulation. Philadelphia: J.B. Lippincott, 1956:26–32.
11. McDonald DA. Blood Flow in Arteries. London: Edward Arnold Publishers Ltd, 1960.
12. Attinger EO, ed. Pulsatile Blood Flow. Proceedings of the First International Symposium on Pulsatile Blood Flow. New York: McGraw-Hill, 1963.
13. Ikram H, Nixon PGF, Fox JA. The hemodynamic implications of bisferiens pulse. Br Heart J 1964;26:452–459.
14. O'Rourke MF, Taylor MG. Input impedance of the systemic circulation. Circ Res 1967;20:365–380.

15. O'Rourke MF, Blazek JV, Morreels CL, Jr., Krovetz LJ. Pressure wave transmission along the human aorta: changes with age and in arterial degenerative disease. Circ Res 1968;23:567–579.
16. Barner HB, Willman VL, Kaiser GC. Dicrotic pulse after open heart operation. Circulation 1970; 42:993–997.
17. Mills CJ, Gabe IT, Gault JH, et al. Pressure-flow relationships and vascular impedance in man. Cardiovasc Res 1970;4:405–417.
18. Mills CJ, Gabe IT, Gault JH, et al. Blood velocity and pressure waveforms in the major arteries in man. Clin Sci 1970;38:10P.
19. O'Rourke MF. Influence of ventricular ejection on the relationship between central aortic and brachial pressure pulse in man. Cardiovasc Res 1970;4:291–300.
20. Meadows WR, Draur RA, Osadjan CE. Dicrotism in heart disease. Correlations with cardiomyopathy, pericardial tamponade, youth, tachycardia, and normotension. Am Heart J 1971;82:596–608.
21. O'Rourke MF. The arterial pulse in health and disease. Am Heart J 1971;82:687–702.
22. Murgo JP, Westerhof N, Giolma JP, Altobelli SA. Aortic input impedance in normal man: relationship to pressure wave forms. Circulation 1980;62:105–116.
23. Murgo JP, Westerhof N, Giolma JP, Altobelli SA. Manipulation of ascending aortic pressure and flow wave reflections with the Valsalva maneuver: relationship to input impedance. Circulation 1981;63: 122–132.
24. Murgo JP, Westerhof N, Giolma JP, Altobelli SA. Effects of exercise on aortic input impedance and pressure wave forms in normal humans. Circ Res 1981;48:334–343.
25. Hamilton WF. The patterns of the arterial pressure pulse. Am J Physiol 1944;141:235–241.
26. Dow P. The development of anacrotic tardus pulse of aortic stenosis. Am J Physiol 1941;131:432–436.
27. Roach MR, Burton AC. The reason for the shape of the distensibility curves of arteries. Can J Biochem Physiol 1957;35:681–690.
28. O'Rourke MF. Pressure and flow waves in systemic arteries and the anatomical design of the arterial system. J Appl Physiol 1967;23:139–149.
29. Ruskin A. Classics in Arterial Hypertension. Springfield, IL: Charles C Thomas, 1956.
30. Drzewiecki GM, Melbin J, Noordergraaf A. Arterial tonometry: review and analysis. J Biomech 1983; 16:141–152.
31. Kelly RP, Hayward C, Ganis J, Daley J, Avolio A, O'Rourke MF. Non-invasive registration of arterial pressure waveform using high-fidelity applanation tonometry. J Vasc Med Biol 1989;1:142–149.
32. Karamanoglu M, O'Rourke MF, Avolio AP, Kelly RP. An analysis of the relationship between central aortic and peripheral upper limb pressure waves in man. Eur Heart J 1993;14:160–167.
33. Chen CH, Nevo E, Fetics B, et al. Estimation of central aortic pressure waveform by mathematical transformation of radial tonometry pressure. Validation of generalized transfer function. Circulation 1997;95:1827–1836.
34. Glossary of cardiologic terms related to physical diagnosis. IV. Arterial pulses. Am J Cardiol 1971;27: 708–709.
35. O'Rourke MF. Arterial Function in Health and Disease. Edinburgh: Churchill Livingstone, 1982.
36. O'Rourke MF, Kelly R, Avolio A. The Arterial Pulse. Philadelphia: Lea & Febiger, 1992.
37. Nichols WW, O'Rourke MF. McDonald's Blood Flow in Arteries. London: Edward Arnold, 1998.
38. Vlachopoulos C, O'Rourke M. Genesis of the normal and abnormal arterial pulse. Curr Probl Cardiol 2000;25:303–367.
39. Oliver JJ, Webb DJ. Noninvasive assessment of arterial stiffness and risk of atherosclerotic events. Arterioscler Thromb Vasc Biol 2003;23:554–566.
40. Rushmer RF. Origins of pulsatile flow; the ventricular impulse generaotors. In: Attinger, EO, ed. Pulsatile Blood Flow. NewYork: McGraw-Hill Book Company, 1963:221–234.
41. Noble MI. The contribution of blood momentum to left ventricular ejection in the dog. Circ Res 1968;23:663–670.
42. Murgo JP, Altobelli SA, Dorothy JF, et al. Normal ventricular ejection dynamics in man during rest and exercise. In: Leon DF, Shaver JA, eds. Physiologic Principles of Heart Sounds and Murmurs, American Heart Association Monograph 46, 1975: 92-101.
43. Perloff JK. The physiologic mechanisms of cardiac and vascular physical signs. J Am Coll Cardiol 1983;1:184–198.
44. Murgo JP, Alter BR, Dorothy JF, Altobelli SA, McGranahan GM, Jr. Dynamics of left ventricular ejection in obstructive and nonobstructive hypertrophic cardiomyopathy. J Clin Invest 1980;66: 1369–1382.

45. Sherrid MV, Gunsburg DZ, Moldenhauer S, Pearle G. Systolic anterior motion begins at low left ventricular outflow tract velocity in obstructive hypertrophic cardiomyopathy. J Am Coll Cardiol 2000;36:1344–1354.
46. O'Rourke MF. Impact pressure, lateral pressure, and impedance in the proximal aorta and pulmonary artery. J Appl Physiol 1968;25:533–541.
47. Kinlay S, Creager MA, Fukumoto M, et al. Endothelium-derived nitric oxide regulates arterial elasticity in human arteries in vivo. Hypertension 2001;38:1049–1053.
48. Bank AJ, Wang H, Holte JE, Mullen K, Shammas R, Kubo SH. Contribution of collagen, elastin, and smooth muscle to in vivo human brachial artery wall stress and elastic modulus. Circulation 1996;94:3263–3270.
49. Leach RM, McBrien DJ. Brachioradial delay: a new clinical indicator of the severity of aortic stenosis. Lancet 1990;335:1199–1201.
50. Caro CG, Parker KH. Brachioradial delay and severity of aortic stenosis. Lancet 1990;335:1535.
51. O'Rourke MF, Avolio AP, Karamanoglu M, Gallagher D, Schyvens C. Brachioradial delay. Lancet 1990;336:1377–1378.
52. O'Rourke MF, Taylor MG. Vascular impedance of the femoral bed. Circ Res 1966;18:126–139.
53. O'Rourke MF, Avolio AP. Pressure and flow waves in systemic arteries and the anatomical design of the arterial system. J Appl Physiol 1967;23:139–149.
54. Bogren HG, Mohiaddin RH, Klipstein RK, et al. The function of the aorta in ischemic heart disease: a magnetic resonance and angiographic study of aortic compliance and blood flow patterns. Am Heart J 1989;118:234–247.
55. Ohtsuka S, Kakihana M, Watanabe H, Sugishita Y. Chronically decreased aortic distensibility causes deterioration of coronary perfusion during increased left ventricular contraction. J Am Coll Cardiol 1994;24:1406–1414.
56. Rowell LB, Brengelmann GL, Blackmon JR, Bruce RA, Murray JA. Disparities between aortic and peripheral pulse pressures induced by upright exercise and vasomotor changes in man. Circulation 1968;37:954–964.
57. Ranganathan N, Sivaciyan V, Chisholm R. Effects of postextrasystolic potentiation on systolic time intervals. Am J Cardiol 1978;41:14–22.
58. Voss A, Baier V, Schumann A, et al. Postextrasystolic regulation patterns of blood pressure and heart rate in patients with idiopathic dilated cardiomyopathy. J Physiol 2002;538:271–278.
59. Eisner DA, Diaz ME, Li Y, O'Neill SC, Trafford AW. Stability and instability of regulation of intracellular calcium. Exp Physiol 2005;90:3–12.
60. Sapira JD. Quincke, de Musset, Duroziez, and Hill: some aortic regurgitations. South Med J 1981; 74:459–467.
61. Eblen-Zajjur A. A simple ballistocardiographic system for a medical cardiovascular physiology course. Adv Physiol Educ 2003;27:224–229.
62. Frank MJ, Casanegra P, Migliori AJ, Levinson GE. The clinical evaluation of aortic regurgitation. With special reference to a neglected sign: the popliteal-brachial pressure gradient. Arch Intern Med 1965; 116:357–365.

3 Blood Pressure and Its Measurement

Contents
- Physiology of Blood Flow and Blood Pressure
- Physiology of Blood Pressure Measurement
- Points to Remember When Measuring Blood Pressure
- Factors That Affect Blood Pressure Readings
- Interpretation of Blood Pressure Measurements
- Use of Blood Pressure Measurement in Special Clinical Situations
- References

PHYSIOLOGY OF BLOOD FLOW AND BLOOD PRESSURE

The purpose of the arterial system is to provide oxygenated blood to the tissues by converting the intermittent cardiac output into a continuous capillary flow and this is achieved by the structural organization of the arterial system.

The blood flow in a vessel is basically determined by two factors:

1. The pressure difference between the two ends of the vessel, which provides the driving force for the flow
2. The impediment to flow, which is essentially the vascular resistance

This can be expressed by the following formula:

$$Q = \frac{\Delta P}{R}$$

where Q is the flow, ΔP is the pressure difference, and R is the resistance.

The pressure head in the aorta and the large arteries is provided by the pumping action of the left ventricle ejecting blood with each systole. The arterial pressure peaks in systole and tends to fall during diastole.

Briefly, the peak systolic pressure achieved is determined by (*see* Chapter 2):

1. The momentum of ejection (the stroke volume, the velocity of ejection, which in turn are related to the contractility of the ventricle and the afterload)
2. The distensibility of the proximal arterial system
3. The timing and amplitude of the reflected pressure wave

When the arterial system is stiff, as in the elderly, for the same amount of stroke output, the peak systolic pressure achieved will be higher. The poor distensibility causes a greater peak pressure. In addition, a stiff arterial system results in faster transmission and reflection of the pressure wave, thereby adding to the peak pressure. The narrow and peaked pressure seen in the more peripheral muscular arteries is the effect of such reflection. The level to which the arterial pressure will fall during diastole is primarily dependent on the state of the peripheral resistance, which controls the runoff. Conditions with low peripheral resistance and vasodilatation will cause the diastolic pressure to fall to low levels.

The mean arterial pressure is the average of all the pressures obtained over an entire duration of a cardiac cycle. Since diastole is longer than systole, the mean pressure is estimated as the sum of 60% diastolic pressure and 40% systolic pressure. More accurate measurement will be derived by integrating the area under a recorded pressure curve. The pulse pressure, which is the difference between the systolic and the diastolic pressure, reflects not only the stroke volume but also the state of the peripheral resistance. Conditions associated with a large stroke volume and low peripheral resistance will be expected to give rise to a large pulse pressure, and this will be reflected in the amplitude of the arterial pulse by palpation.

While the control of the cardiac output is usually determined by local tissue flow under physiological states, the control of the arterial pressure is independent of these and is regulated through a complex system, which involves nervous reflexes and neurohumoral mechanisms for short-term needs (such as "flight," "fright," and "fight" type reactions or in situations like those following acute loss of blood volume) and neuroendocrine, renin–angiotensin–aldosterone system, and renal mechanisms for long-term adaptation. These control systems in the normal as well as their alterations in hypertension and in heart failure are well discussed in standard texts for physiology and medicine. In this chapter our focus will be mainly on measurement of blood pressure by the sphygmomanometer and its use in special clinical situations.

PHYSIOLOGY OF BLOOD PRESSURE MEASUREMENT

The indirect measurement of blood pressure by the sphygmomanometer involves the application of a controlled lateral pressure by an inflatable cuff to occlude the artery by compression, thereby stopping the flow. The detection of the resumption of flow during slow deflation allows the determination of the pressure. The cuff is normally applied to the arm over the brachial artery. When the cuff pressure exceeds the systolic pressure, the brachial artery is fully occluded and the flow ceases. When the cuff is deflated to pressures just below the systolic peak, the flow begins to resume with each cardiac systole. The jet of blood coming through the partially occluded vessel is associated with tapping-type sounds, which can be recognized using a stethoscope placed over the brachial artery just distal to the cuff. These sounds, termed the *Korotkoff sounds*, help in identifying the systolic and the diastolic pressures in the artery. The detection of the first appearance of Korotkoff sounds (*Phase I*) as the cuff is being deflated corresponds to the systolic pressure, and the disappearance of Korotkoff sounds with further deflation of the cuff corresponds to the diastolic pressure. Korotkoff sounds generally become muffled first when the cuff is being deflated before they totally disappear. It is always advisable to take the diastolic pressure to the level at which the sounds disappear because it is less likely to introduce errors *(1)*.

The Mechanism of Origin of Korotkoff Sounds

The exact mechanism of origin of Korotkoff sounds is not completely established. They have been thought to result from turbulence of flow coming through the partially occluded artery. This is thought to be supported by the following: they become muffled (*Phase IV*) and eventually disappear (*Phase V*) generally when the flow resumes in diastole, i.e., when the cuff is deflated below the diastolic pressure, allowing the artery to be open throughout the cardiac cycle. In addition, before they become muffled and completely disappear, they may sound like a short bruit (initially as soft bruit in *Phase II* and louder bruit as in *Phase III*).

However, they do not always sound like murmurs and often present as sharp sounds. The Waterhammer theory was suggested (not to be confused with the water-hammer pulse in aortic regurgitation) to explain the presence of distinct sounds *(2)*. The sounds are thought to be produced by the deceleration of high-velocity flow coming through the vessel as it opens up from an occluded state against the stationary column of blood distal to the occlusion. The intensity of the sounds, however, may vary, being loud and persistent to low diastolic pressures or throughout diastole in certain situations such as in aortic regurgitation, in children, and in pregnancy. In aortic regurgitation, the stroke volume tends to be large with increased velocity of ejection. Children generally have hyperkinetic circulation, and pregnant women tend to have a high cardiac output with increased sympathetic tone. On the other hand, Korotkoff sounds tend to be poor in low-output states.

When an oversized cuff is used it may lead to underestimation of the systolic blood pressure. It has been shown that the state of the distal vasculature in the limb where the blood pressure is being measured affects the intensity of the Korotkoff sounds. Vasodilatation makes the sounds louder, and vasoconstriction softer *(3,4)*. When the peripheral resistance in the arm distal to the cuff was changed by interventions such as heating, cooling, and induction of reactive hyperemia, the amplitude of the Korotkoff sounds appeared to change. Thus, these effects may lead to either over- or underestimation of both systolic and diastolic pressures *(5)*. In fact, when the Korotkoff sounds are poorly heard, they are best augmented by raising the arm (decreasing venous distension) and having the patient open and close his or her fist on the side where the pressure is being measured a few times *(6,7)*. This is thought to increase the forearm flow.

Others have proposed that the pressure pulse wave itself may be the source of the Korotkoff sounds. The sounds may be attributed to "shock waves" where the flow velocity of blood in the narrowed segment may exceed the pulse wave propagation velocity and give rise to vibrations in the audible frequency range. This would be analogous to the sonic boom heard when the speed of a jet plane reaches and surpasses the speed of sound.

It is also possible that the Korotkoff sounds are related to energy (vibrations) that results from sudden termination of the pressure pulse wave at the site of the inflated cuff, which leads to partial occlusion of the vessel, causing this to become a terminating site favoring reflection. Between the systolic peak and the diastolic pressures during which time the Korotkoff sounds are present there is a considerable degree of termination and reflection together with beginning onward transmission of the pressure pulse wave. Once the cuff pressure is lowered below the diastolic pressure, there is no more termination or reflection at the site of the cuff application and the pressure pulse is further transmitted along the artery. Therefore, there is no sound to be heard. This may be supported by the fact that when an oversized cuff is used, it may lead to underestimation of the systolic blood pressure. In conditions where the Korotkoff sounds are loud and last longer to low levels of diastolic pressure such as aortic regurgitation, there is a more rapid and higher launching momentum to the pressure pulse wave because of the large stroke volume, which is ejected with a rapid velocity. Thus, there may be more energy for dissipation at the termination sites. In significant aortic regurgitation, one often feels "pistol shots" over the femoral arteries, which are also often sites of reflection because of bifurcation. On the other hand, this mechanism does not explain why the Korotkoff sounds are heard distal to the cuff and not proximal to it.

Tavel et al. had previously shown using invasive pressure measurements that the Korotkoff sounds correspond to the steepened portion of the anacrotic limb of the pressure pulse *(8)*. More recently Drzewiecki et al. have proposed an alternate origin for the production of the Korotkoff sounds. They relate it to the distortion of the pressure pulse under the cuff in the narrowed segment and a change in both pressure and flow distal to the cuff resulting in a nonlinear pattern of pressure–flow relationship. This results in a steeper pulse slope distal to the cuff with higher-frequency harmonics content of this steeper pulse slope reaching the audible frequency range. This interesting theory was proposed based on a mathematical model representing the structures involved, which was able to predict the range of features of the Korotkoff sounds previously reported *(9)*. However, it does not satisfactorily explain why in some people the Korotkoff sounds persist even when the cuff is fully deflated.

It is clear from the short description above that the origin of the Korotkoff sounds is far from established.

POINTS TO REMEMBER WHEN MEASURING BLOOD PRESSURE

The following points are worth noting when taking blood pressure measurements *(10–12)*:

1. First determine roughly the systolic pressure by palpation of the radial artery pulse as the cuff is gradually being deflated so that an *auscultatory gap* (during which Korotkoff sounds may disappear altogether and reappear again when the cuff is being deflated further), if present, will not be missed. This sometime occurs in some hypertensive patients *(13)*. The auscultatory gap may also be a result of venous congestion and decreased velocity of blood flow in the extremity where the blood pressure is being measured *(6)*. The systolic pressure estimated by the palpation of the distal radial artery (while compressing the proximal brachial artery) is usually 10 mmHg lower than the systolic pressure as assessed by the auscultatory method.

    Some studies have shown that assessment of central aortic pressure by measurement of the brachial blood pressure by cuff method underestimates the systolic pressure by 5–20 mmHg and overestimates the diastolic pressure by 12–20 mmHg. This has been related to interobserver variability. Specifically, for the diastolic pressure some may take *Phase IV* and others *Phase V* as the true pressure. This discrepancy is even more exaggerated during vasoconstriction *(14–16)*.
2. Keep the position of the antecubital fossa at the level of the heart to avoid the hydrostatic effect of gravity on the column of blood in the arm.
3. Deflate the cuff slowly. The recommended deflation rate is usually 3 mmHg/s. This rate should actually vary according to the patient's heart rate (relatively slow deflation rate during bradycardias and relatively faster deflation rate during tachycardias).
4. Avoid venous congestion, which tends to muffle Korotkoff sounds, by raising the arm and by inflating the cuff faster *(6)*.
5. When the blood pressure is first determined in a new patient, it should be measured in both arms. If a difference is noted, then the higher reading of the two must be considered as the patient's blood pressure. Slight variation between the two arms is common. The normal difference should not exceed 15 mmHg. The difference may be due to the fact that the innominate on the right side and the subclavian on the left side may arise from

the aorta at different angles. The relative suction due to a Venturi effect of the flow through the aortic arch between the two arms may be different for this reason. When the difference is abnormally high, it will be indicative of obstruction on the side with the lower reading. Conditions such as coarctation of aorta (one proximal to the origin of the left subclavian), atherosclerotic or embolic obstruction (rare in the upper extremities), and aortic dissection may have to be considered depending on the clinical situation. In coarctation of aorta proximal to the left subclavian, the right arm pressure will be naturally higher than the left. In supravalvular aortic stenosis the direction of the jet of flow tends to be directly directed into the innominate artery. This often results in the direct impact pressure of the central jet being transmitted to the right arm, thus making the right arm pressure higher than the left due to a *Coanda effect (17)*.

6. When Korotkoff sounds persist, take the point where they become muffled as the level of the diastolic pressure.
7. When Korotkoff sounds are poor, have the patient exercise his or her hand as pointed out earlier, thereby augmenting the intensity of the Korotkoff sounds *(7)*.
8. Always have a cuff of proper size for the arm, especially for very obese individuals. The width of the bladder in the cuff should be roughly 40% of the arm circumference. In most patients (normal size) a 5 in wide cuff would be the appropriate choice. Too wide a cuff may lead to erroneous recognition of the onset of the Korotkoff sounds because the site of auscultation may be too distal to the site of actual occlusion of the artery. This may make the Korotkoff sounds too soft to be heard and may result in underestimation of the pressure. A narrow cuff will allow overdistension of the bladder of the cuff before actual occlusion of the brachial artery can occur. Some of the pressures applied may be spent in distending the bladder rather than compressing the artery. This will lead to an overestimation of the systolic and even the diastolic pressures. A larger cuff (8 in wide) is needed in obese patients where the arm circumference is more than 35 cm *(18,19)*. The bladder of the cuff should cover at least 50% of the circumference of the limb where the blood pressure is being measured.
9. Support the arm so that the patient's arm muscles are relaxed. If not, isometric contraction may occur, which will raise the peripheral resistance, thereby raising the diastolic pressure. This would also adversely influence the blood pressure reading by muffling the Korotkoff sounds, thereby raising the diastolic pressure and most likely lowering the systolic pressure.
10. Avoid aneroid manometers, which can have problems in calibration. If an aneroid manometer is used, it is recommended that it be calibrated against a mercury manometer yearly, and ideally more frequently *(20)*.
11. Local changes in the limb are known to affect blood pressure readings. If the patient has washed his or her hands with cold or hot water just before the blood pressure measurement, the reading obtained may be higher or lower, respectively, and may not correctly reflect the central aortic pressure. When blood pressure is taken more than once, it should be done at least 5 min apart to avoid reactive hyperemic vasodilatation during the second measurement. This lowers the recorded blood pressure locally, leading to false estimation of central aortic pressure *(5)*.

FACTORS THAT AFFECT BLOOD PRESSURE READINGS

The following factors affect the results of blood pressure measurement:
1. Anxiety, stress, and/or pain Sometimes the mere fact of having the blood pressure taken by a physician can cause a nervous and anxious patient to experience a significant rise in the blood pressure (so-called *white coat syndrome*) *(21,22)*.

2. Exercise, such as climbing a couple of flights of stairs, and even mild activity involving bending or stooping in the elderly could raise the pressure. It should be noted that the transfer of energy of pulse pressure wave to the periphery is greater at low frequencies (<2.5 Hz) in patients at rest because of slower heart rates and longer ejection time. With exercise and the associated faster heart rates and shorter ejection time, the energy transfer occurs at higher frequencies (>2.5 Hz). Because higher frequencies are amplified more, the systolic brachial pressure will be elevated and may not necessarily reflect the true central aortic systolic pressure *(23–25)*.
3. Exposure to cold by causing sympathetic vasoconstriction will raise the pressures.
4. Postprandial state will tend to lower the pressure. In addition to increased vagal tone necessary for increased peristalsis, the lower pressure is likely related to vasodilatation in the mesenteric vessels diverting more blood to the gut for the purpose of proper digestion. This probably also relates to the increase in angina or postprandial decrease in exercise tolerance in patients with exertional angina. The increased demand of blood supply to the gut, increasing the work load of the heart coupled with the decreased diastolic pressure (coronary perfusion pressure), leads to mismatch between the oxygen demand and the coronary blood supply, resulting in angina.
5. Alcohol acutely will lower the pressure, whereas chronic alcohol consumption raises the pressures.
6. Both chronic and acute cigarette smoking tend to cause elevated pressures.
7. Use of illicit drugs such as cocaine may cause significant elevations in blood pressure.
8. Excessive use of liquorice can lead to sustained hypertension.
9. Distension of viscus organs, such as the urinary bladder, gall bladder, and bowels, can cause severe increase in pressures.
10. Significant drop in blood pressure may be noted on postural change from a supine to an erect position (*postural hypotension*) in patients with hypovolemia, following use of certain antihypertensive drugs, and in patients with diabetes with autonomic dysfunction. This is more common in type 1 diabetics.
11. During pregnancy the uterus can compress the inferior vena cava in the supine position and cause decreased venous return, thereby lowering the blood pressure. It is therefore always advisable to measure the blood pressure in a pregnant woman in the sitting position.

INTERPRETATION OF BLOOD PRESSURE MEASUREMENTS

Several important points need to be kept in mind in the interpretation of blood pressure recordings. Diagnosis of hypertension requires demonstration of sustained elevations of blood pressures under normal resting conditions. The normal upper level of blood pressure for adults regardless of age is 140/80. In fact, some newer studies suggest that mortality and cardiac events are less frequent in those with blood pressures of less than 125/75. Present recommendations suggest the blood pressure in diabetics be controlled to 130/80, and if renal disease or microalbuminuria is also present the pressure should be 120/70 or lower. It appears that lower is better as long as the patient does not suffer any symptoms or adverse effects of hypotension and remains asymptomatic. Documentation of sustained elevations of blood pressures therefore requires more than one observation. Sometimes self-recorded pressures at home and/or recordings using an ambulatory monitoring system may have to be resorted to, particularly in nervous and anxious individuals. In addition, one may also have to look for evidence of end-organ damage, such as the presence of retinal changes and electrocardiographic and/or echocardiographic evidence of left ventricular hypertrophy.

While one cannot make a diagnosis of hypertension in a patient with one isolated elevation in blood pressure, the significance of such elevations nevertheless should be interpreted in relation to the clinical problem. For instance, an elderly patient who has exertional angina or dyspnea with a resting blood pressure of 130/80 mmHg may have been noted to have a blood pressure reading of 180/90 soon after undressing himself, untying his shoe laces, and getting on the examining couch. Although one may not label this patient as hypertensive on the basis of that one recording of high pressures, it nevertheless indicates that the elevation in blood pressure in this patient was inappropriate to the level of exercise and most likely is a contributing factor to the exertional symptoms. Lowering of the pressure with the use of medications such as an angiotensin-converting enzyme inhibitor and/or a β-blocker would be an appropriate management strategy for such a patient.

In young patients because of peripheral amplification secondary to reflected waves in the more muscular stiffer vessels in the extremities, the systolic blood pressure obtained may not correctly reflect the systolic central aortic pressure and may in fact be 50% higher. In these patients, the diastolic pressure may more accurately reflect the diastolic pressure in the central aorta.

In the elderly because of arteriosclerosis and stiffened aorta and arteries in general, the pressure pulse wave travels faster. The wave reflection therefore tends to arrive early in the central vessels, augmenting the systolic pressure. In these patients no peripheral amplification is noted, and the brachial systolic pressure more accurately reflects the central aortic systolic pressure *(26–30)*.

In atherosclerosis there may be significant differences between the upper and lower limb pressures. Because atherosclerosis tends to involve the lower extremities more, one may actually find in these patients decreased pulse amplitude together with lower blood pressure in the lower limbs compared to the arms. This is in contrast to the usual findings in the young and/or normal patients, where the pressures in the legs are in fact 10–20 mmHg higher than the brachial pressures.

In patients without any evidence of hypertensive end-organ damage, significantly elevated systolic blood pressures may be obtained in doctors' offices. These high office blood pressure readings are at times associated with normal blood pressure readings throughout the day when 24 h ambulatory blood pressure monitoring is carried out. Not surprisingly, the first and the last readings (normally readings taken in the laboratory in the presence of the technician) during these recordings also show significant blood pressure elevations. This *white coat syndrome* is likely related to an anxiety reaction on the part of the patient. Generally this condition is felt to be relatively benign, although there always is a concern that patients may become hypertensive in the future.

White coat hypertension has been defined and classified *(31,32)* into three groups:

1. White coat hypertension: Abnormal office systolic blood pressure >150 mmHg and daytime average systolic blood pressure <140 mmHg. (Patients not on antihypertensives).
2. White coat syndrome—normotensive: Patients' blood pressures controlled on antihypertensives. Their daytime average systolic blood pressure <140 mmHg and office blood pressure reading of >150 mmHg.
3. White coat syndrome—hypertensive: Patients may be on or off antihypertensive medications with daytime average systolic blood pressure of >140 mmHg and office systolic blood pressure measurement of >150 mmHg, which is at least 15 mmHg higher than the average daytime systolic blood pressure.

White coat hypertension syndrome may not be as benign as once thought *(33)*. There appears to be higher incidence of increased mean albumin levels in the urine of some of these patients. Some show increased albumin/creatinine ratios of >30%.

USE OF BLOOD PRESSURE MEASUREMENT IN SPECIAL CLINICAL SITUATIONS

Determination of Pulsus Paradoxus

EFFECTS OF RESPIRATION ON BLOOD PRESSURE IN NORMAL SUBJECTS

The effects of respiration on the level of blood pressure in the normal must be understood in relation to the changes in the respiratory variations of the intrathoracic pressures as well as the venous return. On inspiration, there is generally a lower systolic pressure compared to the end of expiration. The intrathoracic pressure falls on inspiration, which helps to augment venous return to the heart. The inspiratory expansion of the lungs, by increasing its pulmonary venous capacity, accommodates for the extra volume of blood returned to the right side on inspiration and the consequent increase in right ventricular output. The increased venous return on inspiration is therefore not immediately available to the left heart. In fact, the return to the left heart may slightly decrease on inspiration, the expanded lungs holding the extra volume for at least a few cardiac cycles. By that time the expiratory phase usually occurs. The intrathoracic pressure on expiration becomes relatively more positive. The aorta being an intrathoracic structure, these changes in the intrathoracic pressures will also affect the aortic pressure. There is generally a fall in the systolic blood pressure with normal inspiration, and the magnitude of this fall is about 5–10 mm. This is a result of both the fall in intrathoracic pressure and the effect of the expanded lungs holding the extra venous return, thereby diminishing the return to the left heart and therefore its output. The opposite occurs on expiration—the intrathoracic pressure rises and the lungs contract in volume by exhaling air—and this aids in increased pulmonary venous inflow to the left side, increasing the stroke output. The net effect leads to an increased arterial pressure on expiration. In the normal, the expansion of the right ventricle on inspiration does not usually result in shift of the interventricular septum to the left since the normal pericardium does not limit physiological changes in ventricular volumes *(34)*.

In the normal, the effect of this inspiratory fall in the systolic blood pressure is not detectable by palpation of the arterial pulse. However, the magnitude of the inspiratory fall in the blood pressure can be easily assessed by blood pressure cuff at the bedside. When the cuff is being slowly deflated to detect the onset of the Korotkoff sounds, careful observation will reveal that initially the Korotkoff sounds are audible only at the end of expiration. With each inspiration they will be seen to become inaudible. The level of the blood pressure at the end of expiration when the Korotkoff sounds begin to be heard must be first noted. With further cuff deflation, however, it will be observed that the Korotkoff sounds are audible throughout both inspiration and expiration. The level of the blood pressure at which this begins to happen must be noted next. The difference between the two systolic levels, namely the number of mmHg to which the cuff needed to be deflated (i.e., when Korotkoff sounds no longer remain inaudible on inspiration), gives the magnitude of the inspiratory fall in the blood pressure.

PULSUS PARADOXUS IN CARDIAC TAMPONADE

In *cardiac tamponade*, there is an exaggeration of the normal inspiratory fall in the systolic blood pressure leading to a truly definable *pulsus paradoxus*. The fall in the stroke volume of the heart and consequently the systolic blood pressure despite the increased venous return to the heart caused by inspiration is the paradox that led to this term. In fact, in significant cardiac tamponade, the palpation of the arterial pulse may reveal that its amplitude is less or the pulse may not even be felt on inspiration. This of course is not the case in the normal. The mechanism of this exaggerated fall in the blood pressure on inspiration is attributable to the compressive effect of the fluid in the pericardial space, which is under high pressure. In cardiac tamponade, all four chambers of the heart are as if boxed in this tight pericardial space. In the absence of pre-existing cardiac disease, the pressures in the right and the left atria, the intrapericardial pressures, as well as the right and left ventricular diastolic pressures are all elevated to the same level. In extreme cases of tamponade, the thinner-walled structures like the right ventricle are compressed more completely than the thicker-walled left ventricle. When inspiration increases the venous return to the right heart as in normals, the expansion of the right ventricle within this enclosed tight pericardial space will of necessity push the interventricular septum to the left side, thereby further diminishing the left heart filling and its compliance. This will lead to decreased left ventricular output. The septal bulge on inspiration to the left side can in fact be demonstrated in echocardiograms of patients with tamponade.

Because the pericardium is attached to the diaphragm, the descent of the diaphragm with inspiration may also pull on the pericardium, thereby altering its global shape to a more spindle-like shape. This physically can lead to further rise in the intrapericardial pressure. The effects of the inspiratory fall in the intrathoracic pressures as well as the effects of the inspiratory expansion of the lungs and pulmonary venous pooling leading to diminished left heart filling, mentioned above in the normal, are also still operative in patients with cardiac tamponade. The net effect of these changes on the left heart filling as well as the intrathoracic pressures will cause a greater fall in the left ventricular stroke output and the blood pressure on inspiration. The opposite changes occur on expiration, leading to a higher arterial pressure on expiration. The effect of the inspiratory pulmonary venous pooling is even more dramatic when the left ventricular stroke output is already diminished due to the tamponade.

The blood pressure cuff is used in the same manner as mentioned above to determine the magnitude of fall in mmHg due to *pulsus paradoxus*. The pulsus paradoxus by blood pressure measurement must exceed 15 mmHg to be considered significant.

In the presence of significant elevations of the left ventricular diastolic pressures resulting from pre-existing cardiac disease, cardiac tamponade does not cause pulsus paradoxus. The raised diastolic pressures offer greater resistance to the compressive effects of the intrapericardial pressures. Cardiac tamponade also does not lead to pulsus paradoxus in two other conditions, namely aortic regurgitation and atrial septal defect. In the former, the extra source of left ventricular filling due to the aortic regurgitation keeps the left ventricular volumes from falling, thereby preventing the respiratory fluctuations in left heart filling. Similarly in atrial septal defect, the left-to-right shunt accommodates for respiratory changes in venous return, thereby preventing a fall in left heart filling during inspiration *(35–43)*.

CONDITIONS OTHER THAN CARDIAC TAMPONADE WITH PULSUS PARADOXUS
Constrictive Pericarditis

In constrictive pericarditis, pulsus paradoxus is much less common than in cardiac tamponade. It is more common in the effusive subacute type of constriction than in chronic cases. Pulsus paradoxus is absent in chronic cases because of poor transmission of the intrathoracic pressures to the cardiac chambers as a result of thickened and fibrosed and sometimes calcified pericardium. When pulsus paradoxus is seen, it is probably a result of a combination of two factors, namely the septal shift to the left and the increased pulmonary venous pooling on inspiration. The diaphragmatic pull on the pericardium on inspiration is also unlikely to be operative on a thickened and scarred pericardium *(38)*.

Bronchial Asthma and Chronic Obstructive Pulmonary Disease

The exaggerated swings in intrathoracic pressures may be directly transmitted to the aorta, affecting the systolic and the diastolic pressures with very little change in the stroke volume or the pulse pressure. In the presence of significant airways obstruction, there is marked increase in the intrathoracic pressures during expiration caused by the intercostal muscles to overcome the airways obstruction. This elevated intrathoracic pressure is directly transmitted to the aorta, raising the expiratory pressure in the aorta. Thus, there is an expiratory gain in blood pressure rather than the usual inspiratory fall in the normal. The net effect on the blood pressure is the same.

Hypovolemic Shock and Acute Pulmonary Embolism

In some patients with hypovolemic shock, pulsus paradoxus may be noted *(44)*. This is a result of an exaggerated effect of the inspiratory pulmonary venous pooling on the already diminished stroke volume. The change in the percentage of the stroke volume is higher compared to the normal individuals with normal cardiac output.

Similarly, the reduced capacity of the pulmonary arterial bed because of embolic obstruction in the presence of the normal pulmonary venous bed may also lead to an accentuated effect of the inspiratory pulmonary venous pooling on the left ventricular stroke volume *(45)*.

Blood Pressure Response to the Valsalva Maneuver

The *Valsalva maneuver* is basically a forced expiration against a closed glottis. This maneuver is used in our daily life when we try to bear down or strain One way of producing this maneuver is to ask a patient simply to hold the breath and imitate straining on the toilet. One can produce this also by asking a supine patient to actively push his or her abdominal wall against the palm of the examiner's hand placed on the patient's abdomen so as to offer some pressure without causing pain A more controlled way of doing the maneuver would be to have the patient blow into a hollow tube connected to an aneroid manometer to raise the pressure to about 40 mmHg and sustain it at that level for about 20–30 s.

ARTERIAL PRESSURE RESPONSE IN THE NORMAL DURING THE VALSALVA MANEUVER

Four phases are recognized with continuous arterial pressure recordings. Initially the effort of strain raises the intrathoracic pressures, which is directly transmitted to the aorta, causing an initial rise in the arterial pressure. During this first phase, the lungs contract to the lowest volume, emptying most of the pulmonary venous bed and helping to increase the left ventricular output. With the continued strain, the venous return drops as a result of damping of venous circulation from the abdominal viscera and the

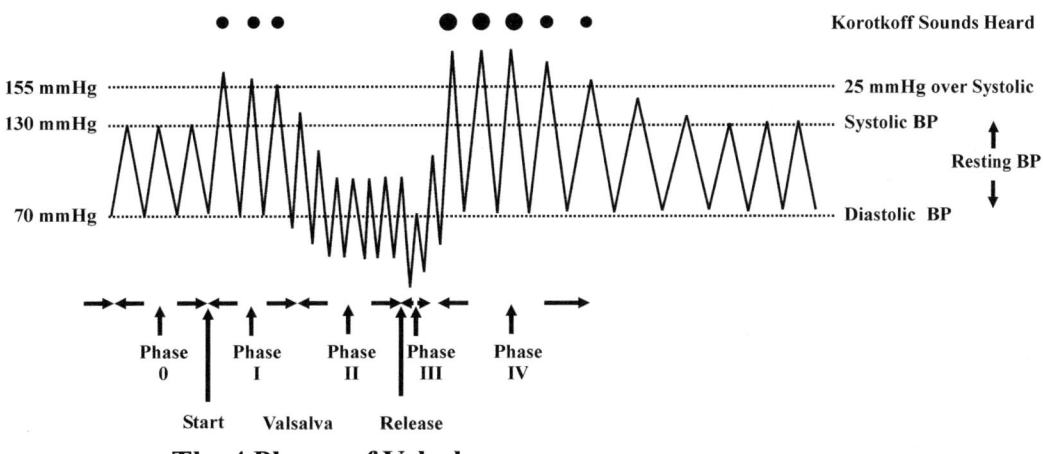

Fig. 1. The blood pressure response during the four phases of Valsalva maneuver in a patient with normal left ventricular function is shown diagrammatically. Phase 0 indicates the resting phase before the Valsalva maneuver. Phase I shows the increased blood pressure resulting from the initial increase in pulmonary venous return and the associated increased stroke volume and the increased intrathoracic pressure directly transmitted to the aorta. Phase II shows the decreased blood pressure because of decreased venous return into the thorax and therefore the heart resulting from the increased intrathoracic pressure preventing the venous return from the periphery. Note the increased heart rate secondary to the increased sympathetic tone. Phase III, immediately after the release of the Valsalva strain, shows a temporary drop in the blood pressure resulting from a sudden decrease in the intrathoracic pressure. Phase IV shows an overshoot of the blood pressure following the sudden return of peripherally pooled blood to the vaso-constricted arterial system (secondary to the increased sympathetic tone). The blood pressure then returns back to normal gradually. When the cuff is inflated to levels of 25 mmHg higher than the patient's resting systolic pressure and maintained at that pressure, the Korotkoff sounds that would be heard at the various phases of Valsalva are also depicted at the top. The size of the dots reflects the expected intensities of the sounds.

periphery. This leads to a significant drop in the stroke output, which is accompanied by a fall in the systolic and diastolic blood pressures as well as the pulse pressure (the second phase). The decreased stroke output stimulates the sympathetic system to cause a reflex increase in the heart rate at this time. Upon release of the strain, there is a sudden drop in the intrathoracic pressures, which again directly affects the aortic pressures and therefore the arterial pressure. This third phase is quite momentary and is only appreciated by continuous recordings of arterial pressure. This is almost immediately followed by a sudden surge of venous return from the splanchnic bed and the periphery augmented by the fall in the intrathoracic pressure. This leads to a significant increase in the right and the left ventricular stroke output. During this fourth phase the increased stroke volume ejected into an arterial system, which has been primed by a significant sympathetic stimulation during the earlier strain phase, causes an overshoot of the arterial pressure over and above the control level. The increased stroke volume effect is reflected in the increase in the pulse pressure as well. The rise in the arterial pressure also causes a reflex slowing of the heart rate through the baroreceptor stimulation (Fig. 1).

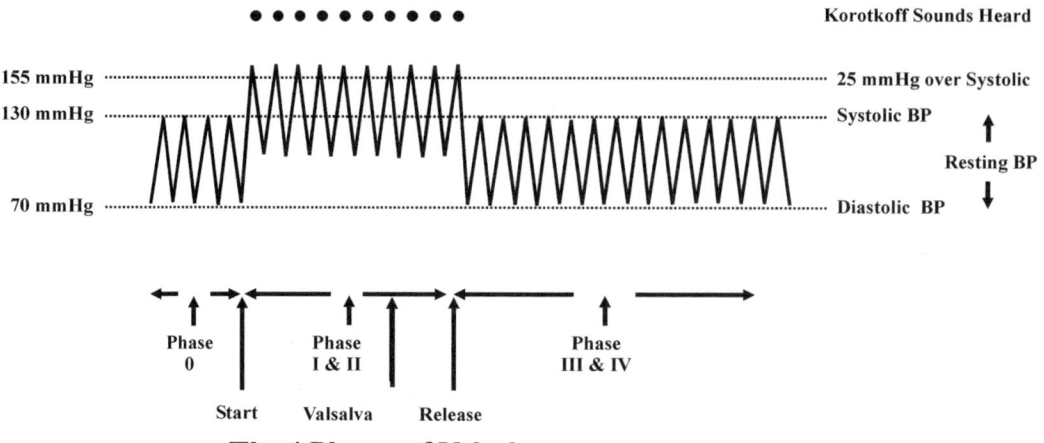

Fig. 2. Blood pressure response to the Valsalva maneuver in a patient with significant left ventricular dysfunction and heart failure is shown diagrammatically. Because of the chronically elevated venous pressures and the sympathetic tone, the blood pressure response to the Valsalva maneuver is different from that noted in the normal. During Phases I and II there is an elevation of blood pressure, and during Phase III the overshoot does not occur. The appearance of the above tracing resembles a square wave; therefore, it is called the square-wave response and indicates poor left ventricular function.

ARTERIAL PRESSURE RESPONSE TO THE VALSALVA MANEUVER IN PATIENTS WITH HEART FAILURE

The response of patients with heart failure can be described as a square-wave response as seen on a continuous recording of the arterial pressures (Fig. 2). The initial rise in the intrathoracic pressure during the strain and the immediate fall on release of strain (namely the first and the third phases mentioned above) will cause an initial rise and a later similar fall in the arterial pressure due to direct transmission effect of the intrathoracic pressures to the aorta. However, because patients with heart failure already have maximal sympathetic stimulation with vasoconstriction (both arterial and venous) and their ventricles are already operating on the flat portion of the Starling curve, whatever decrease occurs in venous return as a result of the dampening effect of strain does not drop the stroke output very much, and for the same reason following release of strain also there is no overshoot in the arterial pressure. This can also be observed in the lack of significant changes in heart rate during strain and after release of strain In other words, no significant tachycardia or bradycardia will be seen to develop during the Valsalva maneuver *(46,47)*.

BLOOD PRESSURE RESPONSE TO THE VALSALVA MANEUVER IN THE ASSESSMENT OF LEFT VENTRICULAR FUNCTION IN THE ABSENCE OF OVERT HEART FAILURE

This consists essentially of detecting the presence or the absence of the overshoot in the blood pressure following the release of a Valsalva strain The presence of the overshoot would indicate a normal left ventricular function with a normal ejection fraction (stroke volume over the end-diastolic left ventricular volume expressed as a percentage, normal being 60%). Patients with left ventricular dysfunction who are not in overt failure also often have an abnormal response. They tend to have a resting increase in sympathetic tone and fail to exhibit the overshoot in blood pressure as well as the reflex bradycardia. This can be done at the bedside with the use of a blood pressure cuff. The method involves applying a sustained additional cuff pressure of 25 mmHg over and above the detected systolic pressure in a patient who is supine and listening for the Korotkoff sounds while the patient is performing a Valsalva strain for 20–30 s. First the systolic blood pressure is determined. Then the cuff is inflated to 25 mmHg above the systolic pressure and is held there while the patient is asked to perform a Valsalva strain. During strain, if the patient has normal left ventricular function, there will be an initial rise because of transmission of the intrathoracic pressure to the aorta, and this can be detected by the appearance of the Korotkoff sounds. The fall in blood pressure, which occurs because of the decreased venous return during the strain phase, will lead to the disappearance of the Korotkoff sounds. During the postrelease phase, the Korotkoff sounds will reappear, indicating the presence of the expected overshoot in arterial pressure. In patients with left ventricular dysfunction and high sympathetic tone but not in overt failure, however, the Korotkoff sounds may initially appear during strain, but with continued strain the Korotkoff sounds will become inaudible and will never reappear because of the lack of the overshoot response. Failure to achieve an overshoot of 25 mmHg has been correlated with resting left ventricular dysfunction with decreased ejection fraction of 40 +/– 10% *(48)*.

Determination of Pulsus Alternans

Pulsus alternans has been discussed under the arterial pulse previously. The alternation of the strong and the weaker pulse can be detected while taking blood pressure. Corresponding to the alternating strength of the palpated pulse, one also can note alternating blood pressure levels. During deflation of the inflated cuff to record the systolic pressure, one will notice that initially the Korotkoff sounds begin to be heard only with every other stronger beat rather than with every beat as would occur in the normal. With continued deflation of the cuff, there will be a doubling of the rate of the Korotkoff sounds because both the strong and the weak beats will come through. In addition, one may also note an alternating intensity of the Korotkoff sounds. In general, *pulsus alternans* is associated with severe left ventricular dysfunction and low cardiac output. *Pulsus alternans* is usually precipitated by an extrasystole. The phenomenon can be shown to develop following a premature beat in almost all patients. However, in those with normal left ventricular function, it lasts only for two beats and is not noticeable clinically but may be shown by the measurement of the systolic time intervals (mentioned previously under the arterial pulse). In very severe left ventricular dysfunction, the *pulsus alternans* effect produced by a premature beat may persist for a long time (for several minutes). There may be instability of the calcium flux in the myocytes of the diseased heart, which may account for the alternating strengths of the contraction of the myocardium in the patients with myocardial disease *(49)*.

Assessment of Arterial Occlusion

ASSESSMENT OF DISSECTING AORTIC ANEURYSM

The pathology usually involves some form of degeneration of the elastic fibres of the medial layers of the aorta. The condition often starts with a sudden tear of the intima of either the ascending or the descending thoracic aorta, often precipitated by some form of excessive hemodynamic force such as a significant elevation in blood pressure. The blood under pressure in the lumen finds its way through a cleavage in the medial layers of the aorta. The process may progress at a variable rate, resulting eventually in a double lumen aorta made by the plane of dissection in the media causing a false lumen in addition to the true lumen. The difference in the blood pressures results from the impingement of the false lumen on the true lumen, causing obstruction and the consequent lowering of the blood pressure beyond the obstruction. Depending on the location and the degree of these obstructions to the true lumen, one may find significant differences in the pulses as well as the blood pressures between the two arms, between the arms and the legs, as well as between the two legs. The blood pressure differences noted may also be changing with time since dissection may further progress resulting in either more complete occlusion of the true lumen, or sometimes a distal tear of exit may reopen the previously occluded vessel. Such dynamic changes are unusual in other causes of obstruction such as chronic atherosclerotic vascular disease.

ATHEROSCLEROTIC VASCULAR DISEASE

This condition is most commonly seen in the lower extremities and much less frequently in the subclavian and the upper extremity vessels. Some of the subclavian stenoses may in fact be congenital rather than a result of acquired atherosclerotic process. The blood pressure in the arm on the side of the vascular obstruction will be lower, as expected. Normally, the lower extremity blood pressure is 10–15 mmHg higher than both the central aortic and the arm pressures. There are two reasons for this increase in pressure in the lower extremities: their thicker and muscular walls and the effect of reflection of the pressure pulses. The reasons for this increase in pressure in the lower extremities are discussed in Chapter 2.

In the lower extremity, if the blood pressure is found to be equal to or lower than in the arm, then obstructive arterial disease must be considered. The obstruction may be at the level of the aorta, the iliac, or the femoral. Blood pressure measurement in the lower extremity can be carried out by using a larger cuff (8 in wide) over the thigh and auscultating over the popliteal artery. This is best done with the patient lying prone. This method probably is more accurate but may be difficult in very obese patients. To obtain a reasonably accurate systolic blood pressure in the leg, a regular cuff can be employed above the ankle and the posterior tibial or the dorsalis pedis pulses can be palpated. When the pedal pulses are not easily felt, an ultrasound Doppler probe can be used to detect the flow and assess the peak systolic pressure. When comparisons are made, one should compare the peak pressures obtained by the same technique between the upper and the lower extremities. If one uses the Doppler technique at the ankle, then one must obtain Doppler-detected radial artery flow at the wrist with the cuff over the arm for assessment of the peak pressures in the forearm.

COARCTATION OF THE AORTA

Because *coarctation of the aorta* is a congenital condition, when blood pressure discrepancies are noted between the arm and the leg in children or young adults where atherosclerosis is not an issue, the clinician should be alerted to the possibility of the presence of this condition. If the coarctation is in the aortic arch before the take-off of the left subclavian artery, the pressure in the left arm will be significantly lower than the pressure in the right arm. Most coarctations usually occur after the take-off of the left subclavian, and the upper extremity pressures will be equal. Since coarctation also causes hypertension, in younger patients with hypertension, as detected in the arm blood pressures, lower blood pressures in the legs must suggest a diagnosis of coarctation. The amount of decrease in the blood pressures in the lower extremities will depend on the severity of the coarctation. When the coarctation is severe, the femoral pulses may not only be delayed but also poorly felt or not palpable.

Coarctation causes hypertension as a direct result of the obstruction limiting the size of capacitance of the aorta as well as directly raising the resistance. In addition, the decreased blood pressure distal to the coarctation will lead to stimulation of the juxtaglomerular cells to produce more renin The latter will increase the angiotensin II, which is a potent vasoconstrictor and will result in hypertension.

Assessment of Severity of Aortic Regurgitation and Left Ventricular Function in Aortic Regurgitation

A positive *Hill's sign* is an exaggeration of the normal blood pressure differential between the arm and the leg. This sign was discussed in Chapter 2 in relation to the peripheral signs of aortic regurgitation *(50)*. A systolic blood pressure differential of 60 mmHg or greater may be noted in the presence of moderate to severe degrees of aortic regurgitation. In those patients with aortic regurgitation when this sign is detected, serial measurements will aid in follow-up. During follow-up, if the blood pressure differential is found to be increasing, then it must be considered as a sign of worsening degree of aortic regurgitation. A gradual narrowing of the blood pressure differential, however, would not mean an improvement in the degree of the aortic regurgitation. It might indicate in fact a progressive development of left ventricular dysfunction. When significant left ventricular dysfunction and heart failure develops consequent to longstanding aortic regurgitation, the blood pressure differential between the arm and the leg will not be significant.

A Clinical Exercise: Manual Assessment of Blood Pressure

One may attempt to guess the blood pressure by manual palpation of the radial arterial pulse while applying pressure over the brachial artery with the thumb of the other hand so as to cause occlusion of the brachial artery. The pressure can be varied and applied as light, medium, or firm. When the brachial artery becomes occluded, the radial pulse will disappear. The systolic pressure must also be measured by the usual way by auscultation over the brachial artery. The amount of force that one has to exert with the thumb can be noted mentally against the recorded systolic pressures by auscultation. Generally one can learn to correlate roughly the amount of pressure required to apply with the thumb with the level of the systolic pressures recorded. On average, medium pressures will have to be applied when the systolic pressures are around 120–130. When the systolic pressures are less than 100, only light pressures will be needed. When the systolic pressures are higher than 140, it will require much firmer compression. The important part of this exercise is to make sure that one has the pressure applied directly over the palpated brachial artery; otherwise it will not be possible to occlude it. It also requires that one trains oneself to do this during routine measurements of blood pressures. The technique can be useful in situations where one has no accesss to a blood pressure cuff immediately for the purposes of a quick assessment. Caution should be exercised in patients with calcified and stiff vessels that resist compression to avoid false overestimation of the systolic blood pressure.

Blood Pressure in Assessment of Relative Intensity of the First and Second Heart Sounds

The integrity of the left ventricular function has a significant bearing on the intensity of the M1 component of the S1 (*see* Chapter 6). When S1 and S2 are not loud enough to be palpable, the assessment of their intensity must take into account the measured blood pressure of the patient. Extracardiac attenuating factors can lead to attenuations of the heart sounds. Because the degree of attenuation in any given patient will be expected to be similar on both S1 and S2, the intensity of S1 can be assessed only when compared to the intensity of the S2. The intensity or the loudness of the A2 component of the S2 is dependent to a large extent on the peripheral resistance, which is reflected in the diastolic blood pressure. A normal blood pressure would be expected to be associated with a normal intensity of A2, a high blood pressure would be expected to cause a loud A2, and finally a low blood pressure would be associated with a soft A2. The A2 intensity can be graded according to the blood pressure as probably normal, soft, or loud. Then if the intensity of the M1 is compared to that of A2, one can judge its relative intensity. It can then be graded as normal, soft, or loud depending on whether its intensity is equal to that of the A2, softer than A2, or louder than A2. While this exercise has some merit, its clinical value in the detection of left ventricular dysfunction is not established. Our preliminary observations suggest that the perception of the relative loudness of the M1 vs the A2 seems to be also influenced by the higher-frequency content of the A2.

REFERENCES

1. Levine SR. "True" diastolic blood pressure. N Engl Med J 1981;304:362–363.
2. Erlanger J. Studies in blood pressure estimation by indirect method. Part II. The mechanisms of the compression sounds of Korotkoff. Am J Physiol 1916;40:82–125.
3. Rodbard S. The significance of the intermediate Korotkoff sounds. Circulation 1953;8:600–604.
4. Cohn J. Blood pressure maesurement in shock. JAMA 1967;199:972–976.
5. Rabbany SY, Drzewiecki GM, Noordergraaf A. Peripheral vascular effects on auscultatory blood pressure measurement. J Clin Monit 1993;9:9–17.
6. Whitcher C. Blood pressure measurement. In: Weaver, CS, ed. Techniques in Clinical Physiology. New York: Macmillan, 1969:85–124.
7. Rabbany SY, Drzewiecki GM, MelbinJ, Noordergraaf A. Influence of vascular state on the Korotkoff sounds, Proceedings of the 13th Annual Northeast Bioengineering Conference, Philadelphia, 1987. IEEE Press, 166–169.
8. Tavel ME, Faris J, Nasser WK, Feigebaum H, Fisch C. Korotkoff sounds. Observations on pressure-pulse changes underlying their formation. Circulation 1969;39:465–474.
9. Drzewiecki GM, Melbin J, Noordergraaf A. The Korotkoff sound. Ann Biomed Eng 1989;17:325–359.
10. The fifth report of the Joint National Committee on Detection, Evaluation, and Treatment of High Blood Pressure (JNC V). Arch Intern Med 1993;153:154–183.
11. Perloff D, Grim C, Flack J, et al. Human blood pressure determination by sphygmomanometry. Circulation 1993;88:2460–2470.
12. Frohlich ED. Blood pressure measurement. Can J Cardiol 1995;11:35H–37H.
13. Cavallini MC, Roman MJ, Blank SG, Pini R, Pickering TG, Devereux RB. Association of the auscultatory gap with vascular disease in hypertensive patients. Ann Intern Med 1996;124:877–883.
14. London.S.B, London.R.E. Comparison of indirect blood pressure measurements (Korotkoff) with simultaneous direct brachial artery pressure distal to cuff. Adv Intern Med 1967;13:127–142.
15. Nielsen PE. The accuracy of auscultatory blood pressure measurements in the elderly. Acta Med Scand (Suppl) 1983;676:39–44.

16. Spence JD, Sibbald WJ, Cape RD. Pseudohypertension in the elderly. Clin Sci Mol Med Suppl 1978; 4:399s–402s.
17. Perloff JK. The physiologic mechanisms of cardiac and vascular physical signs. J Am Coll Cardiol 1983;1:184–198.
18. Linfors EW, Feussner JR, Blessing CL, Starmer CF, Neelon FA, McKee PA. Spurious hypertension in the obese patient. Effect of sphygmomanometer cuff size on prevalence of hypertension. Arch Intern Med 1984;144:1482–1485.
19. Manning DM, Kuchirka C, Kaminski J. Miscuffing: inappropriate blood pressure cuff application. Circulation 1983;68:763–766.
20. Chockalingam.A (guest editor). Measurement of blood pressure. Can J Cardiol 1995;11:3H–48H.
21. Mancia G, Bertinieri G, Grassi G, et al. Effects of blood-pressure measurement by the doctor on patient's blood pressure and heart rate. Lancet 1983;2:695–698.
22. Redman S, Dutch J. Cardiovascular responses during cuff inflation in subjects who have been sensitised to the measurement of their blood pressure. NZ Med J 1984;97:180–182.
23. O'Rourke MF. Influence of ventricular ejection on the relationship between central aortic and brachial pressure pulse in man. Cardiovasc Res 1970;4:291–300.
24. Karamanoglu M, O'Rourke MF, Avolio AP, Kelly RP. An analysis of the relationship between central aortic and peripheral upper limb pressure waves in man. Eur Heart J 1993;14:160–167.
25. Chen CH, Nevo E, Fetics B, et al. Estimation of central aortic pressure waveform by mathematical transformation of radial tonometry pressure. Validation of generalized transfer function. Circulation 1997;95:1827–1836.
26. O'Rourke MF. Arterial Function in Health and Disease. Edinburgh: Churchill Livingstone, 1982.
27. O'Rourke MF, Kelly RP, Avolio AP. The Arterial Pulse. Philadelphia: Lea & Febiger, 1992.
28. Nichols WW, O'Rourke MF. McDonald's Blood Flow in Arteries. London: Edward Arnold, 1998.
29. Franklin SS, Gustin W, 4th, Wong ND, Larson MG, Weber MA, Kannel WB. Hemodynamic patterns of age-related changes in blood pressure.The Framingham Heart study. Circulation 1997;96:308–315.
30. Burt VL, Whelton P, Roccella EJ, Brown C, Cutler JA, Higgins M. Prevalence of hypertension in the US adult population: results from the Third National Health and Nutrition Examination Survey 1988–1991. Hypertension 1995;25:305–313.
31. White coat systolic hypertension: definition and prevalence by 24-hour ambulatory blood pressure monitoring; Canadian Cardiovascular Congress, Halifax, Novascotia, 2001. Vol. 17(suppl C):119C.
32. Blood pressure control using 24-hour ambulatory blood pressure monitoring, Canadian Cardiovasc Congress, Halifax, Novascotia, 2001. Vol. 17(suppl C): 119C.
33. Karpanou EA, Vyssoulis GP, Mendrinos DS. Microalbuminuria in white coat hypertensives with isolated systolic hypertension, American Society of Hypertension 20th Annual Scientific Session, San Francisco, CA, May 14–18, 2005.
34. McGregor M. Pulsus paradoxus. N Engl J Med 1979;301:480–482.
35. Dornhorst A, Howard P, Leathart GL. Pulsus paradoxus. Lancet 1952; 1:746–748.
36. Wood.P. Chronic constrictive pericarditis. Am J Cardiol 1961;7:48–61.
37. Shabetai R, Fowler NO, Fenton JC, Masangkay M. Pulsus paradoxus. J Clin Invest 1965;44:1882–1898.
38. Shabetai R, Fowler NO, Guntheroth WG. The hemodynamics of cardiac tamponade and constrictive pericarditis. Am J Cardiol 1970;26:480–489.
39. D'Cruz IA, Cohen HC, Prabhu R, et al. Diagnosis of cardiac tamponade by echocardiography. Changes in mitral valve motion and ventricular dimensions with special reference to paradoxical pulse. Circulation 1975;52:460–465.
40. Schiller NB, Botvinick EH. Right ventricular compression as a sign of cardiac tamponade: an analysis of echocardiographic ventricular dimensions and their clinical implications. Circulation 1977;56:774–779.
41. Reddy PS, Curtiss EI, O'Toole JD, Shaver JA. Cardiac tamponade: hemodynamic observations in man. Circulation 1978;58:265–272.
42. Shabetai R, Mangiardi L, Bhargava V, Ross J, Jr., Higgins CB. The pericardium and cardiac function. Prog Cardiovasc Dis 1979;22:107–134.
43. Bilchick KC, Wise RA. Paradoxical physical findings described by Kussmaul: pulsus paradoxus and Kussmaul's sign. Lancet. 2002;359:1940–1942.
44. Cohn JN, Pinkerson AL, Tristani FE. Mechanism of pulsus paradoxus in clinical shock. J Clin Invest 1967;46:1744–755.

45. McDonald IG, Hirsh J, Jelinek VM, Hale GS. Acute major pulmonary embolism as a cause of exaggerated respiratory blood pressure variation and pulsus paradoxus. Br Heart J 1972; 34:1137–1141.
46. Gorlin R, Knowles JH, Storey CF. The Valsalva maneuver as a test of cardiac function. Pathologic physiology and clinical significance. Am J Med 1957;22:197.
47. Elisberg EI. Heart rate response to the Valsalva maneuver as a test of circulatory integrity. JAMA 1963;186:200–205.
48. Zema MJ, Caccavano M, Kligfield P. Detection of left ventricular dysfunction in ambulatory subjects with the bedside Valsalva maneuver. Am J Med 1983;75:241–248.
49. Eisner DA, Diaz ME, Li Y, O'Neill SC. Stability and instability of regulation of intracellular calcium. Exp Physiol. 2005;90:3–12.
50. Sapira JD. Quincke, de Musset, Duroziez, and Hill: some aortic regurgitations. South Med J 1981; 74:459–467.

4 Jugular Venous Pulse

CONTENTS

>NORMAL RIGHT ATRIAL PRESSURE PULSE CONTOURS
>JUGULAR VENOUS INFLOW VELOCITY PATTERNS AND THE
>   RELATIONSHIP TO THE RIGHT ATRIAL PRESSURE PULSE
>JUGULAR VENOUS FLOW EVENTS AND THEIR RELATIONSHIP
>   TO JUGULAR VENOUS PULSE CONTOURS
>NORMAL JUGULAR VENOUS PULSE CONTOUR AND ITS RECOGNITION
>   AT THE BEDSIDE
>INDIVIDUAL COMPONENTS OF THE RIGHT ATRIAL PRESSURE PULSE,
>   THEIR DETERMINANTS, AND THEIR RECOGNITION IN THE JUGULARS
>ABNORMAL JUGULAR VENOUS PULSE CONTOURS AS RELATED
>   TO ABNORMAL JUGULAR VENOUS FLOW VELOCITY PATTERNS
>ABNORMAL JUGULAR CONTOURS
>ASSESSMENT OF JUGULAR VENOUS PRESSURE
>CLINICAL ASSESSMENT OF THE JUGULAR VENOUS PULSE
>REFERENCES

The physiology of the normal jugular venous pulse contours and the pathophysiology of their alterations will be discussed in this chapter. Mechanisms of venous return and right heart filling have been of clinical interest from the days of Harvey and Purkinje *(1,2)*. Long before Chauveau and Marey published their recordings of the venous pulse, Lancisi had described "the systolic fluctuation of the external jugular vein" in a patient with tricuspid regurgitation *(3,4)*. Potain demonstrated the presystolic timing of the dominant wave of the normal venous pulse by simultaneous recording of the venous and the carotid artery pulses *(5)*. In the early part of the last century, the detailed studies of the venous pulse by Mackenzie helped define the waveforms, their terminology, and their origins. He called the main waves "a," "c," and "v" to denote the first letters of what he thought were their anatomical sites of origins, namely the right atrium, the carotid artery, and the right ventricle. He distinguished the "ventricular type venous pulse" of tricuspid regurgitation from the "auricular type" and associated it with atrial fibrillation, demonstrating also the progression of the former from the latter over time *(6,7)*. Since the days of Mackenzie, clinicians have studied the venous pressure and the pulse contour in different clinical conditions *(8–33)* The advent of cardiac catheterization, the recording of intracardiac pressures, and the development of techniques to study blood flow velocity all contributed substantially to our understanding of the mechanisms of venous return, right heart filling and function *(10,11,13,18,20,21,24,28,30,34–46)*.

Since right atrial pressure pulse and the venous inflow into the right heart affect the jugular contours, a good understanding of the basics of their relationship both in the normals as well as in the abnormals is very meaningful and important. The discussion will be sequential under the following headings:

1. Normal right atrial pressure pulse contours
2. Jugular venous inflow velocity patterns and the relationship to the right atrial pressure pulse
3. Jugular venous flow events and their relationship to jugular venous pulse contours
4. Normal jugular venous pulse contour and its recognition at the bedside
5. Individual components of the right atrial pressure pulse, their determinants and their recognition in the jugulars
6. Abnormal jugular venous pulse contours as related to abnormal jugular venous flow velocity patterns
7. Mechanism of abnormal jugular venous flow velocity patterns and contours in pulmonary hypertension
8. Mechanism of abnormal jugular venous flow patterns and contours in post-cardiac-surgery patients
9. Mechanism of abnormal jugular venous flow patterns and contours in restriction to ventricular filling
10. Abnormal jugular contours
11. Assessment of jugular venous pressure
12. Clinical assessment of the jugular venous pulse

NORMAL RIGHT ATRIAL PRESSURE PULSE CONTOURS

The sequential changes in right atrial (RA) pressure during the cardiac cycle can be considered starting with the beginning of diastole. In diastole when the tricuspid valve opens, the atrium begins to empty into the right ventricle (RV). The diastolic filling of the ventricle consists of three consecutive phases:

1. Early rapid filling phase when the ventricular pressure, which has fallen quite low, compared to that in the atrium (often close to 0 mmHg) begins to rise with the rapid tricuspid inflow.
2. The slow filling phase follows the early rapid filling phase when the inflow velocity begins to slow down. During this phase the ventricular pressure actually begins to equalize with that of the atrium. The pressure where this equalization occurs is determined by the compliance of the RV and the surrounding pericardium and thorax. In normal subjects the pressure during this phase is usually less than 5 mmHg. It can also be termed the *pre-a wave* pressure since this phase is immediately followed by atrial contraction. The *pre-a wave* pressure is also the baseline filling pressure over which pressure wave buildup can occur in the atrium at other periods of the cardiac cycle.
3. The last phase of ventricular filling occurs at the end of diastole during the atrial contraction, which raises the pressure in the atrium. The ventricular pressure follows the atrial pressure because the tricuspid valve is still open. The level to which the pressure might rise during atrial contraction (*a wave* pressure, named after atrial systole) would depend on the strength of the atrial contraction as well as the baseline *pre-a wave* pressure and the right ventricular distensibility (compliance).

Atrial contraction is followed not only by atrial relaxation but also by ventricular contraction. Both events follow each other in succession during normal atrioventricular (A-V) electrical conduction (during normal PR relationship). Both events lead to a fall in atrial pressure. The fall caused by atrial relaxation completes the *a wave* and is termed the *x descent*.

During ventricular contraction, which follows atrial contraction, the ventricular pressure rises, and once it exceeds the pressure in the atrium, the tricuspid valve becomes closed. As ventricular systole continues, RV pressure rises, and once it exceeds the pulmonary diastolic pressure, the pulmonary valve opens and ejection of blood into the pulmonary artery occurs. During this phase of ventricular systole, however, the atrial pressure continues to fall. This fall in atrial pressure is termed the *x' descent*. This should be distinguished from the *x descent* caused by atrial relaxation *(26)*. The *x' descent*, on the other hand, is caused by the descent of the base of the ventricle. The contracting RV actually pulls the closed tricuspid valve and the tricuspid ring, which together form the floor of the atrium *(34,37,39,46)*. This movement of the base can be easily observed when one views a cine-angiogram of the right coronary artery. The right coronary artery runs along the right A-V groove, and it can be seen to move down with each ventricular systole. Similar motion of the descent of the base can also be seen on the left side in relationship to the circumflex coronary artery, which runs along the left ventricular (LV) side of the A-V groove. The descent of the base of the ventricles can be also appreciated during ventricular systole in the four chamber views of the two-dimensional echocardiograms. The representation on the image display screen however, is usually such that the apex of the heart is at the top. Careful observation will clearly show that the A-V ring with the closed tricuspid and mitral valves moves during systole towards the ventricular side, actually causing an expansion of the atrial area and dimension. The descent of the base is particularly important for the RV for its ejection, since the interventricular septum actually moves with the left ventricle during systole, as will be readily observed in the two-dimensional echo image of the left ventricle in the long axis view as well as the short axis view (*see* Normal Subject image file in Jugular Venous Pulse, Normal on the Companion CD).

The drop in atrial pressure during ventricular systole may be facilitated by the fall in pericardial pressures that occurs when the volume of the heart decreases during systole *(27)*. The preservation of the *x' descent* in atrial standstill and atrial fibrillation further supports the concept that the *x' descent* is unrelated to atrial relaxation *(28,40,47)*. The *x' descent*, on the other hand, requires not only normal RV contraction but also an intact tricuspid valve.

Towards the later phase of systole when the ventricle has completed most of its ejection, the pull on the closed tricuspid valve and ring decreases. The venous inflow into RA from the vena cavae now is able to overcome the fall in atrial pressure caused by the descent of the base. This helps to build up the atrial pressure to a peak of the next wave, termed the *v wave*.

The *v wave* is therefore the venous filling wave in the atrium (named originally after ventricular systole). It occurs during a later phase of ventricular systole. The level to which the *v wave* pressure can be built up in the presence of an intact tricuspid valve depends not only on the right atrial distensibility or compliance, but also on the baseline filling pressure, which is the *pre- a-wave* pressure.

Occasionally one can recognize a break point on the atrial pressure curve between the *x* and the *x' descent*. This point may sometimes be termed the c point because it roughly corresponds in timing to the tricuspid valve closure. Reference to the so-called c waves is made occasionally in relation to humps seen between the *a* and the *v waves* in the

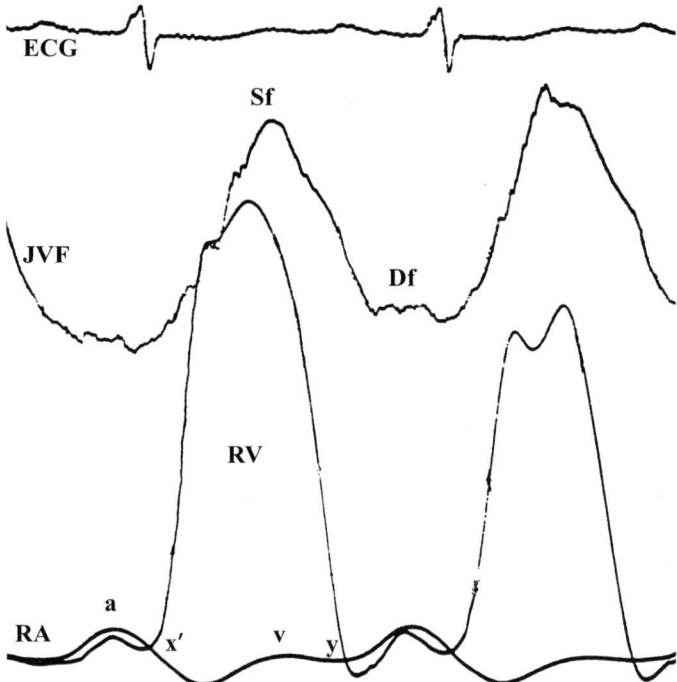

Fig. 1. Simultaneous recordings of electrocardiogram (ECG), jugular venous flow (JVF) velocity recording, right atrial (RA), and right ventricular (RV) pressures in a subject with normal right heart hemodynamics. The RA pressure curve shows the a and the v waves with x′ descent > y descent. JVF shows systolic flow velocity (Sf) > diastolic flow velocity (Df).

jugular venous pulse recordings made with transducers. These are mostly carotid pulse artifacts (c for carotid), and they are not seen in the RA pressure pulse recordings. When seen occasionally in RA pressure recordings, it may be a result of a slight tricuspid valve bulge towards the right atrium during the isovolumic phase of right ventricular contraction *(6,8,25)*.

During later phase of systole, the ventricular pressure in fact begins to fall. Once the ventricular pressure falls below the peak of the *v wave*, the tricuspid valve will open and the atrial pressure again will begin to fall. This fall in atrial pressure caused by the tricuspid valve opening and the beginning of tricuspid inflow into the ventricle is termed the *y descent*. This completes the *v wave*. The *y descent* reaches its nadir at the end of the early rapid inflow phase of the ventricular filling in diastole. This then is the sequence, which repeats itself during each normal cardiac cycle (Fig. 1).

JUGULAR VENOUS INFLOW VELOCITY PATTERNS AND THE RELATIONSHIP TO THE RIGHT ATRIAL PRESSURE PULSE

From the foregoing description of the RA pressure pulse, one can easily understand that the atrial pressure falls twice during each cardiac cycle: once during ventricular systole (*x′ descent*) and once during ventricular diastole (*y descent*). The systolic descent in the presence of normal PR intervals is usually a combination of *x* and *x′ descents*, although the *x′ descent* is more prominent and the important component. The fall during

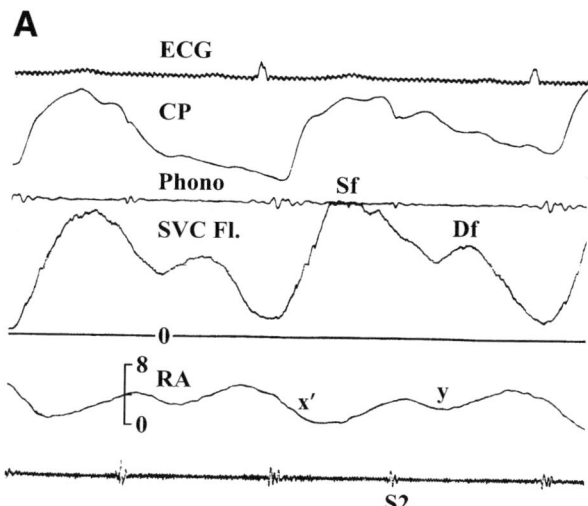

Fig. 2. **(A)** Simultaneous recordings of right atrial (RA) pressure, superior vena caval flow velocity (SVC Fl) in a normal subject. Also shown are ECG, carotid pulse (CP), and phonocardiogram (Phono) showing S2 for timing. All flow velocity recordings shown in this and all other figures are recorded in such a way that the velocities above the baseline zero (-0-) represent flows towards the right heart and all flow velocities below the baseline zero indicate flow direction away from the heart. The SVC flow is continuous and towards the heart and is biphasic with systolic flow velocity (Sf) > the diastolic flow velocity (Df). Sf corresponds to the x' descent and the Df corresponds to the y descent in the RA pressure pulse. *(Continued on next page.)*

x' descent, which is caused by active ventricular systole, is more dominant than the fall during the *y descent*, which occurs during the comparatively "passive" atrial emptying in diastole when the tricuspid valve opens (across a small pressure gradient between the atrium and the ventricle). The venous return into the atrium is actually facilitated by the fall in the atrial pressure. In fact, acceleration in venous inflow velocity can be demonstrated whenever the atrial pressure falls during cardiac cycle *(40)*.

Although the venous inflow in the jugulars is continuous, the jugular venous flow velocity, which is similar to flow velocity in the superior vena cava, in normal subjects is biphasic, with one peak in systole corresponding to the *x' descent* of the RA pressure pulse and a second peak in diastole corresponding to the *y descent* (allowing, however, for transmission delay) (Fig. 2A,B). The systolic flow (Sf) peak is normally more dominant compared to the diastolic flow (Df) peak, just as the *x' descent* is more dominant compared to the *y descent* in the normals *(40)*. Venous inflow during atrial relaxation under normal conditions can only be seen on Doppler tracings of jugular venous flow as a notch on the upstroke of the Sf velocity corresponding to the *x descent*; whereas the peak of the Sf always corresponds to the *x' descent* (Fig. 2C). Separate atrial relaxation flow as such can be demonstrated, however, during periods of A-V dissociation and when the PR interval is long *(35,36,39,40)*.

The Sf and the corresponding *x' descent* may be somewhat diminished in atrial fibrillation. This is explainable because of the lack of atrial contraction in atrial fibrillation, which may lead to a decrease in Starling effect on the ventricle, thereby diminishing the dominance of the Sf as well as the corresponding *x' descent (39,40,48)* (Fig. 3).

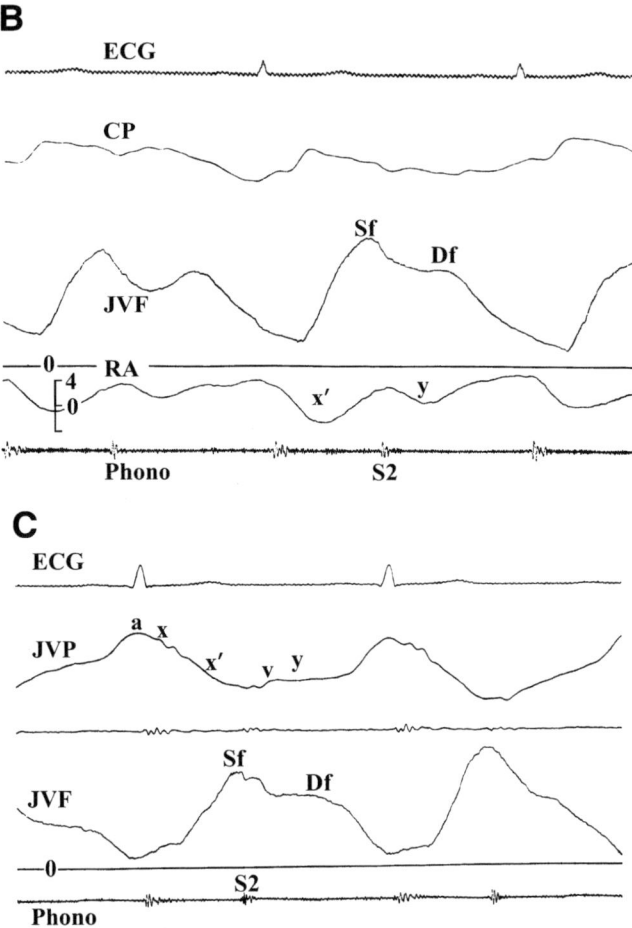

Fig. 2. *(Continued)* **(B)** In the same normal patient similar simultaneous recordings are shown except instead of the superior vena caval (SVC) flow velocity recording, transcutaneous jugular venous flow (JVF) velocity is shown. The JVF, similar to the SVC flow, also has a biphasic flow pattern with the Sf velocity > the Df velocity. The peak of Sf in the JVF occurs somewhat later than that noted in the SVC Fl, almost at the time of the second heart sound (S2). The difference is because of the delay in transmission from the heart to the jugular. **(C)** Simultaneous recordings of jugular venous flow (JVF), jugular venous pulse (JVP), ECG, and phonocardiogram (Phono) from a normal subject. Venous inflow during x descent representing the atrial relaxation is seen as a notch at the beginning of the systolic flow (Sf). Throughout the cardiac cycle the flow is always toward the heart (above the baseline zero). JVP contour in this normal patient shows a more prominent x′ descent. (Modified from ref. *40* with permission from Lippincott Williams.)

The forward flow velocity patterns in the jugulars could, however, be altered and become abnormal secondary to alterations in the right heart function. It may then lose the dominance of the Sf *(40,41,47)*. The relationship between the Sf and the Df velocity may be such that the Sf may be equal to the Df (Fig. 4). Sf may be less than the Df (Fig. 5), or it may become totally absent and may be replaced by a single Df (Fig. 6). These changes in jugular flow velocity patterns will, however, be accurately reflected by the corresponding changes in the RA pressure pulse contours of equal *x′* and *y descents*, *x′ descent* less than *y descent*, or a single *y descent (40,47)*.

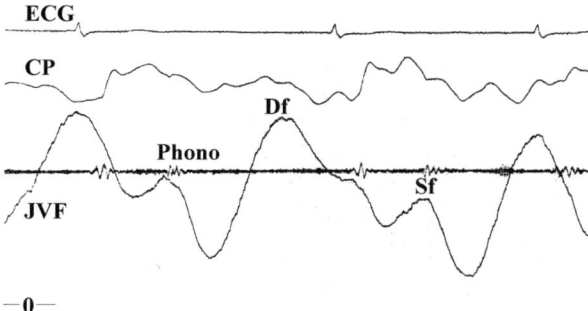

Fig. 3. Simultaneous recordings of electrocardiogram (ECG), carotid pulse (CP), phonocardiogram (Phono), and jugular venous flow (JVF) velocity in a patient with mitral regurgitation and atrial fibrillation. Because of lack of atrial contribution, the Starling effect is diminished leading to a decreased systolic flow. JVF shows a dominant diastolic flow (Df) compared to the less pronounced systolic flow (Sf).

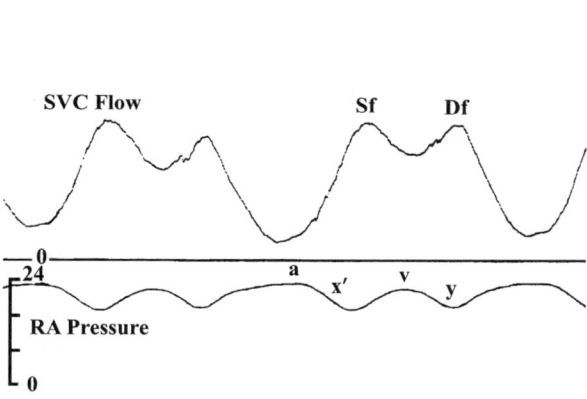

Fig. 4. Simultaneous recordings of electrocardiogram (ECG), right atrial (RA) pressure, and superior vena cava (SVC) flow velocity from a patient with constrictive pericarditis. Note the variations from the normal. The RA pressure is high. The x' and y descents in the RA pressure tracing are equal, unlike the normal, and the corresponding SVC flow velocity shows a biphasic flow where the Sf and the Df are also equal.

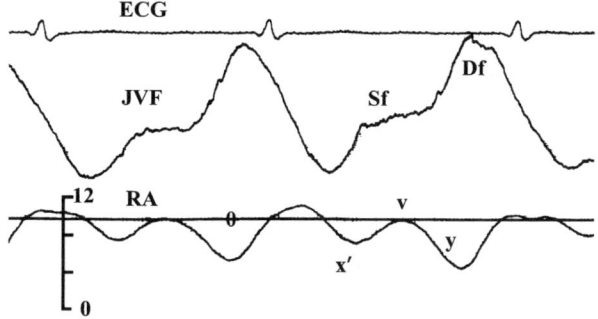

Fig. 5. Simultaneous recordings of electrocardiogram (ECG), right atrial (RA) pressure, and jugular venous flow (JVF) velocity from another patient with constrictive pericarditis. The y descent is more prominent, compared to the x' descent, on the RA pressure tracing. The corresponding JVF shows a more dominant Df compared to the Sf.

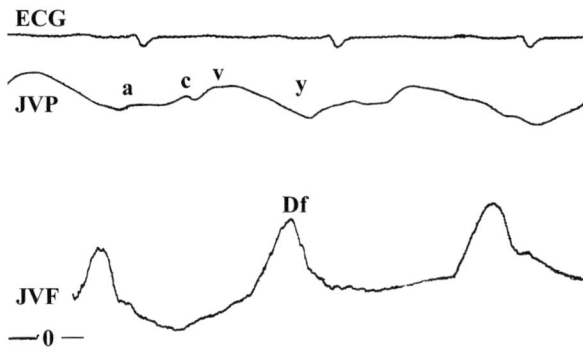

Fig. 6. Simultaneous recordings of electrocardiogram (ECG), jugular venous pulse (JVP), and jugular venous flow (JVF) velocity from a patient with cardiomyopathy. The flow pattern is conspicuous for the absence of a systolic flow, and the JVP shows no x′ descent. Instead, a single peak in diastole (Df) is seen. It corresponds to a single descent in the JVP also in diastole and therefore is the y descent. (*See* ECG for timing.) (Modified from ref. *40* with permission from Lippincott Williams and Wilkins.)

JUGULAR VENOUS FLOW EVENTS AND THEIR RELATIONSHIP TO JUGULAR VENOUS PULSE CONTOURS

Next we shall consider the jugular venous flow events as related to the jugular venous pulse contours. Although the jugular venous column is in direct continuity with the right atrium, the venous system is innervated by the sympathetic system, which can influence the tone of the smooth muscles in their walls *(19)* and as such affect the level to which the column will rise for any given volume status of the individual and the corresponding right atrial pressure. With that background we shall consider the jugular flow events as they relate to the jugular venous pulse contour.

It is important to note that the descents or fall in pressure cause acceleration of venous inflow, as stated earlier. Although more volume of blood enters the heart during diastole, the flow is slower over a longer period of time. In systole, however, the flow is much faster over a shorter period of time (first half of systole). The column of blood in the jugulars is in direct continuity with the blood in the right atrium and the right ventricle in diastole. During systole, the tricuspid valve is closed, and therefore the ventricle is excluded from this system. During the slow filling phase of diastole, the flow into the jugulars at the top of the system is matched to that entering the ventricle (Fig. 7). This represents the baseline state, at which time whatever pressure is developed is mainly determined by the ventricular distensibility (compliance) assuming that the blood volume status of the patient is normal (*pre-a wave* pressure) (Fig. 7A).

With the onset of right atrial contraction, the right atrium becomes smaller and, in fact, is emptying. Therefore, it is unable to accept any venous return. The flow in the superior vena cava and the jugulars decelerates and almost ceases. The continuous inflow from the periphery into the system will raise the volume and the pressure, thus causing the buildup of the normal a wave in the jugular (Fig. 7B). The level to which this may rise will depend on the degree of deceleration of forward flow. This, in fact, will depend on the strength of the right atrial contraction and the pressure generated by it. During atrial relaxation, the atrium expands causing its pressure to fall leading to flow acceleration in the jugulars.

Chapter 4 / Jugular Venous Pulse

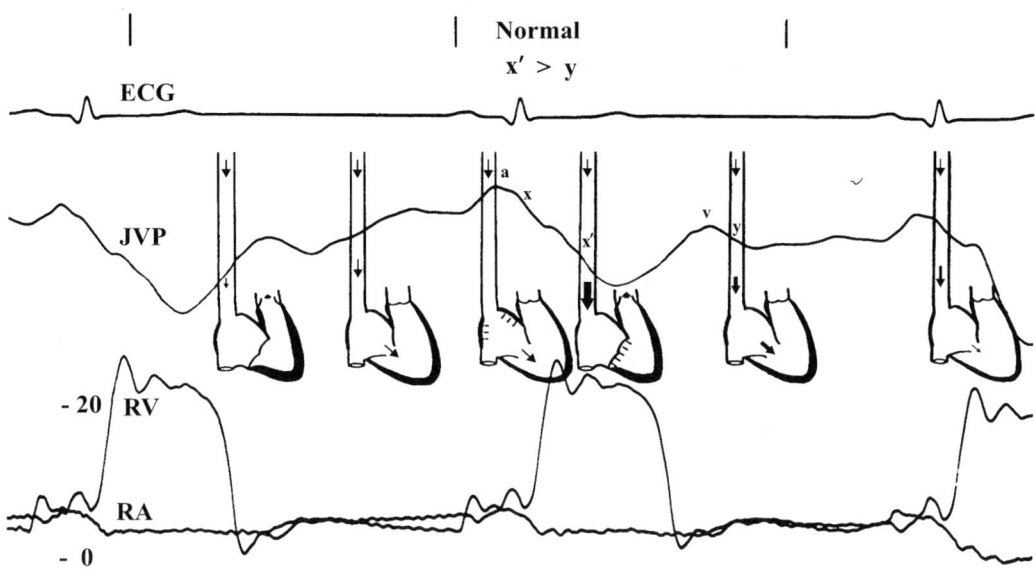

Fig. 7. Simultaneous recordings of electrocardiogram (ECG), jugular venous pulse (JVP), and right atrial (RA) and right ventricular (RV) pressure tracings from a patient with normal right heart hemodynamics. Superimposed are diagrammatic representations of right atrium and right ventricle during various phases of the cardiac cycle. The arrows represent blood flow velocities and help explain the changes in the JVP contour relating them to right heart physiology. The thickness of the arrows relate to the velocity of flow. The columns extending upward from the heart represents the superior vena cava and the jugular complex. The arrows at the top of the columns represent steady flow from the periphery into the vena cava. Each section is shown separately in Fig. 7A–F. (Modified and reprinted from ref. *42*. Copyright 2005 with permission from Excerpta Medica Inc.)

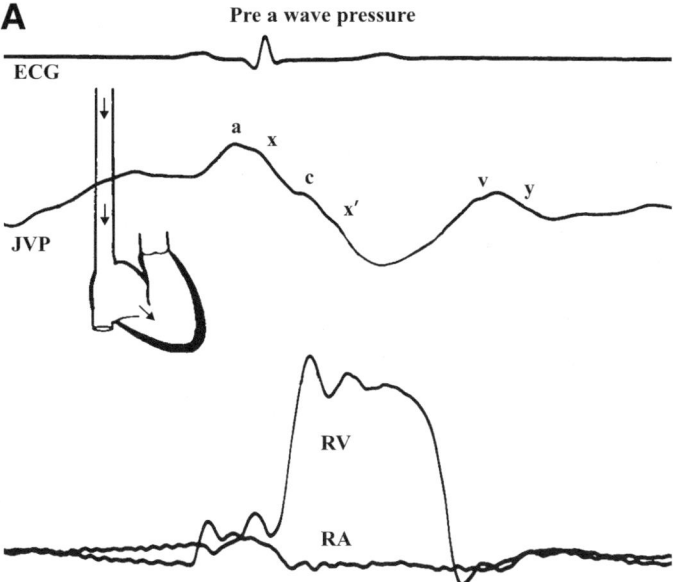

Fig. 7. (**A**) In mid diastole (slow filling phase), the tricuspid valve is open and right ventricle (RV) and right atrium (RA) with superior vena cava (SVC) form a single chamber. The ventricle is almost full, having gone through the rapid filling phase. The slow dilatation of RV causes slow flow rate in SVC, which is matched by inflow from the periphery.

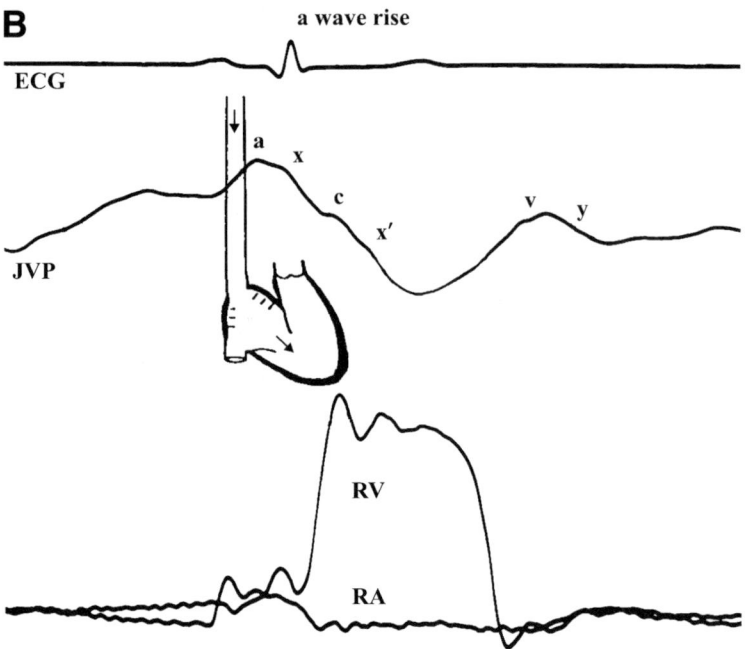

Fig. 7. (**B**) When the right atrium (RA) contracts, it is emptying and getting smaller and cannot accept any blood at that point in time. Flow into the heart in the superior vena cava (SVC) ceases. The blood coming into the system from the periphery causes a rise (a wave rise) in the jugular venous pulse.

This is a passive flow across a pressure gradient between the higher jugular pressure and lower right atrial pressure. Since the flow velocity into the atrium at this time is faster than the continuous inflow from the periphery, the jugular contour falls, causing the *x descent* (Fig. 7C).

The next event to follow is ventricular systole. As explained previously, this causes an active sudden drop in right atrial pressure, almost like a suction effect. This accelerates the flow into the right atrium markedly. This also will lead to a further fall in the jugular contour (*x' descent*) (Fig. 7D). Although this corresponds to the right atrial *x' descent*, there is a transmission delay *(40)*. The latter is accounted for by the time taken for the flow acceleration to develop in the superior vena cava and the jugulars.

During the latter half of systole, the descent of the base comes to a halt, thereby eliminating any further suction effect and/or drop in right atrial pressure. This will lead to a reduction in flow acceleration towards the heart. The venous inflow from the periphery will now exceed the flow into the right atrium, thereby filling the system. This will lead to a rise in jugular and atrial pressures, causing the *v wave* to build up (Fig. 7E). Assuming normal blood volume, the level to which this will rise in the jugulars will depend on three factors:

1. The baseline "*pre-a wave pressure*" in the system
2. The compliance or distensibility of the right atrium
3. The systemic venous tone, which is predominantly influenced by the state of the sympathetic tone

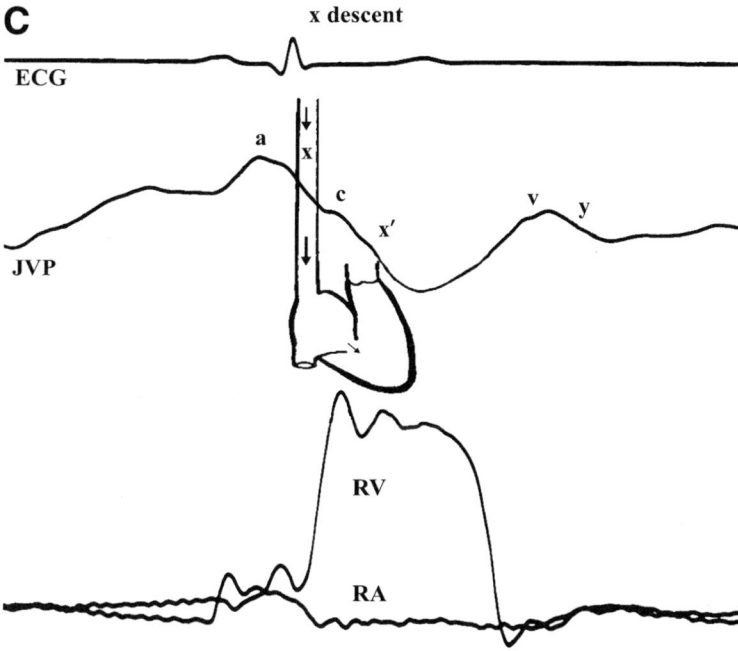

Fig. 7. (**C**) After atrial systole, the right atrium (RA) relaxes (x descent), thus increasing its capacity and allowing blood to flow in. This flow rate in the superior vena cava (SVC) is faster than the rate at which blood is flowing into the system from the periphery, therefore the jugular pulse is seen to fall.

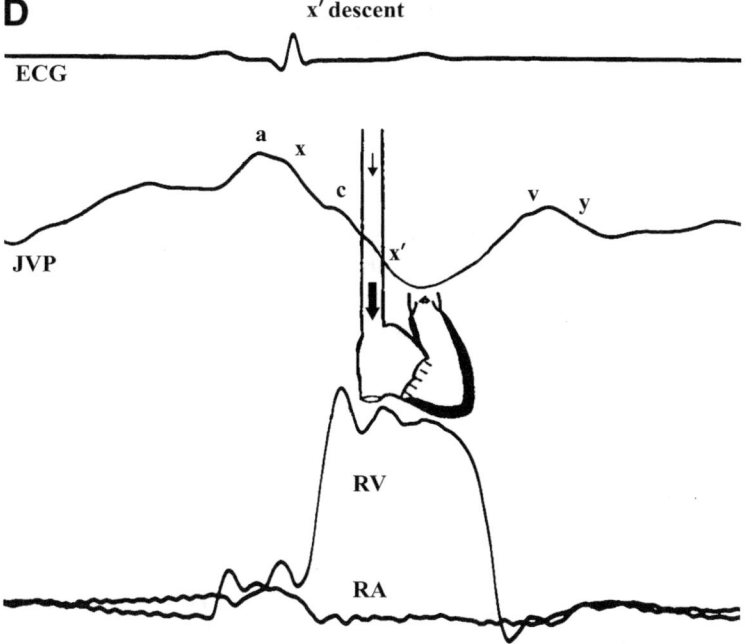

Fig. 7. (**D**) In early systole as the right ventricle (RV) contracts, it gets smaller and pulls down the base. This causes almost a suction effect (x' descent) and blood rushes into the right atrium (RA). This rate of flow is much faster than the rate of peripheral inflow. This causes a sudden fall in the jugular pulse contour.

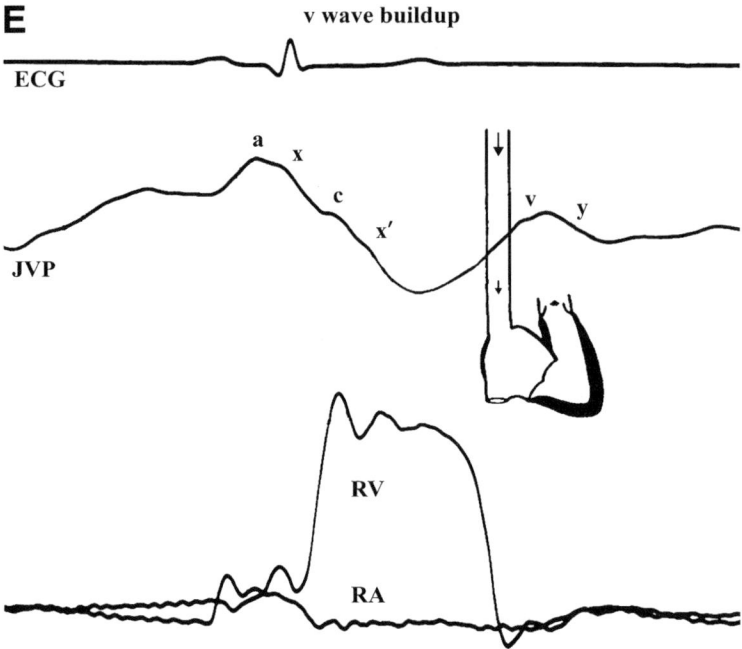

Fig. 7. (**E**) Most ejection out of the ventricle occurs during the first third of systole, and the maximum decrease in right ventricle (RV) dimension occurs during this phase. During the later part of systole, the RV size does not decrease much further. The pull on the base of the RV also is not significant at this time. By this time the RA also is full and therefore the flow in the superior vena cava (SVC) is very slow and certainly slower than blood coming from the periphery. This leads to a rise in the jugular column (v wave).

When the tricuspid valve opens with the onset of diastole, the ventricular pressure having fallen to zero allows flow through the development of a pressure gradient in the system. The acceleration of flow during this early phase of diastole is not as prominent as that which occurs during systole and therefore leads to a less prominent fall in pressure contour in the right atrium. In addition the right atrium, being a capacitance chamber, will get smaller in the process of emptying into the ventricle, and therefore the full flow velocity at the tricuspid valve is not reflected in the superior vena cava and the jugular system. This will result in the less prominent fall in the jugular contour (the *y descent*) (Fig. 7F).

The normal *a wave* caused by the atrial contraction and the normal *v wave* caused by the venous filling of the atrium during later part of ventricular systole are associated with slow and small rises of pressure. They do not exceed generally 5 mmHg and are often closer to 2–3 mmHg. Such small and slow pressure buildup in the RA does not affect the jugular venous inflow velocity significantly except to cause deceleration. They do not ever cause reversal of forward flow.

Retrograde flow into the jugulars from the superior vena cava is always abnormal. No matter the mechanisms of origin, such reversal can always be shown to be associated with abnormal pressure rises in the atrium *(40)*. This could happen during systole in the presence of normal A-V conduction because of tricuspid regurgitation if it is significant *(40,49)*.

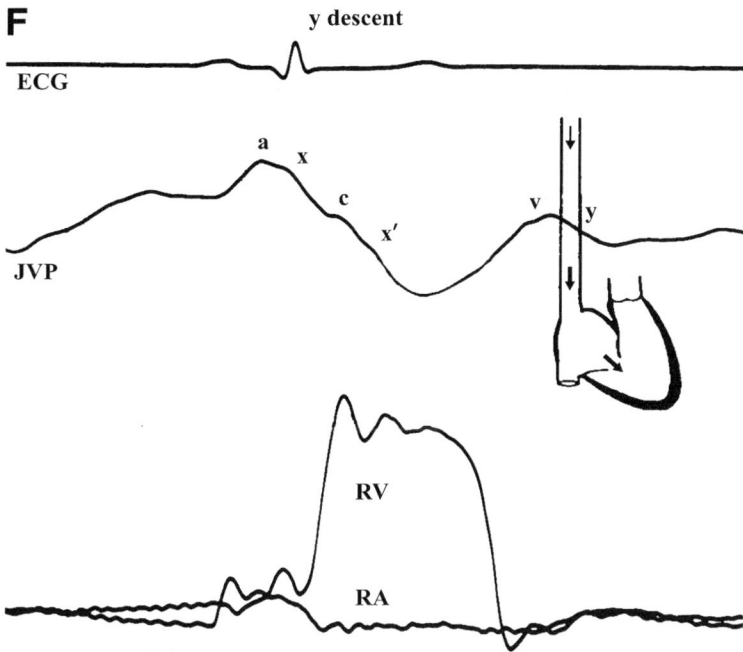

Fig. 7. (**F**) As the tricuspid valve opens in early diastole, blood flows passively across a pressure gradient into the right ventricle (RV) from the right atrium (RA). The pressure in the RA is the v wave pressure, and the pressure in the RV is close to zero because of active right ventricular relaxation. The flow at the tricuspid valve is, however, not fully reflected in the superior vena cava (SVC) because of the capacitance of the RA, which can shrink as it were in size as it empties into the RV. The flow in the SVC is only minimally faster than the flow coming from the periphery. The difference of the two being small, the y descent is not very prominent in the jugulars.

It can then eliminate the *x′ descent* and cause an early abnormal *v wave* pressure rise in the atrium (Fig. 7G).

When atrial and ventricular contraction are dissociated as in certain abnormal heart rhythms (e.g., complete A-V block with a ventricular rhythm independent and often slower than the blocked atrial complexes of sinus node origin), simultaneous atrial and ventricular contraction could occur, resulting in abnormal pressure waves termed the "*cannon*" waves. The atrial contraction occurs against a closed tricuspid valve, leading to sudden development of high atrial pressure. During the *cannon* waves, the high atrial pressure is associated with reversal of flow in the jugulars in systole *(40)*. The reversed flow into the jugulars added to the normal inflow from the periphery cause increased filling of the jugular-superior vena caval system, resulting in the abnormally prominent waves (Fig. 7H).

Flow reversal can also occur in diastole. Very powerful atrial contractions may occasionally result in high *a wave* pressure in the RA (often in the range of 15 mmHg or more), which could also be shown to be associated with reversal of forward flow during the end-diastolic phase *(40)*. This could happen in tricuspid stenosis, which is a rare condition,

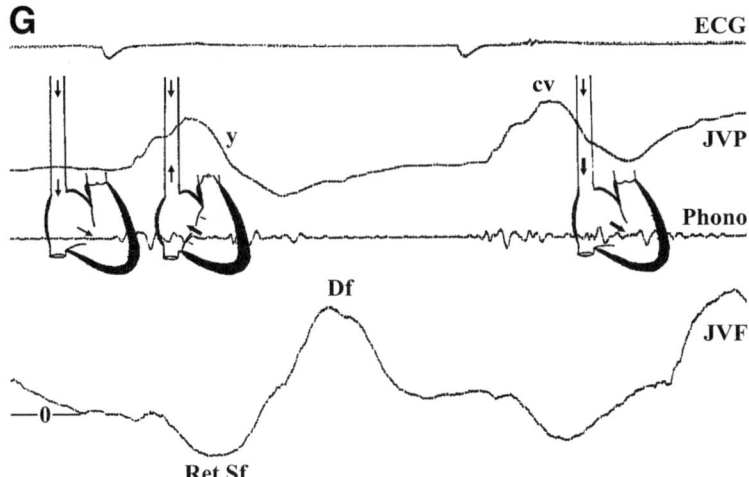

Fig. 7. (G) Simultaneous recordings of electrocardiogram (ECG), phonocardiogram (Phono), jugular venous pulse (JVP), and the jugular venous flow velocity (JVF) from a patient with tricuspid regurgitation. It shows the systolic retrograde flow (Ret Sf) from the right ventricle (RV) into the right atrium (RA). This reverses the flow in superior vena cava (SVC), giving rise to a prominent rise in jugular pulse contour ("cv" wave). The Ret Sf abolishes the effect of the descent of the base during RV contraction. In addition, the retrograde flow into the RA because of RV contraction raises the v wave pressure to higher levels. During the early filling phase of diastole when the RV pressure falls to zero, there is a higher gradient of pressures between the RA and the RV, which makes the fall steep (prominent y descent).

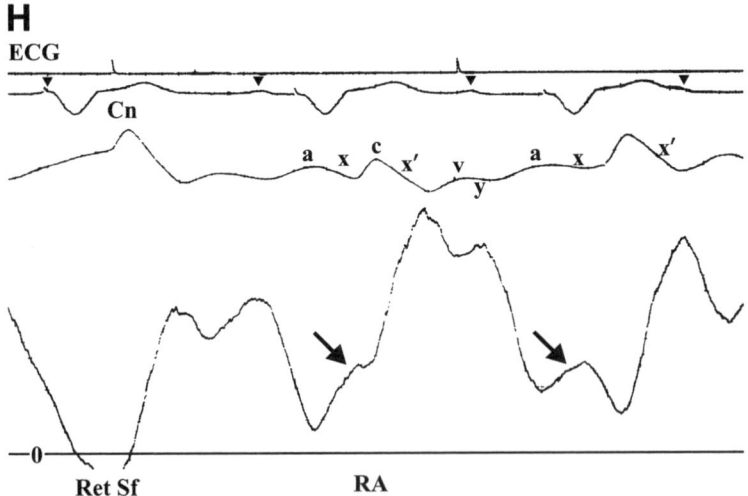

Fig. 7. (H) Simultaneous recordings of electrocardiogram (ECG), jugular venous pulse (JVP), and jugular venous flow velocities (JVF) from a patient with a permanent pacemaker. It shows a regular ventricular rhythm caused by ventricular pacing with independent P waves with atrioventricular dissociation. Arrows on ECG point to P waves. The bigger arrows on JVF indicate atrial relaxation flows corresponding to x descents. In the first beat, P and QRS are synchronous, giving rise to retrograde flow into SVC and causing a cannon wave. Note that the duration of the cannon wave is shorter than the duration of the v wave of tricuspid regurgitation shown in Fig. 7G. Because of the varying P and QRS relationship, the x, x', and y descents change from beat to beat. In the second beat the P and QRS relationship is basically normal with a normal PR interval, and the x, x', and y descents are normal. In the last beat the PR is long and the x descent is well separated from the x' descent.

Chapter 4 / Jugular Venous Pulse

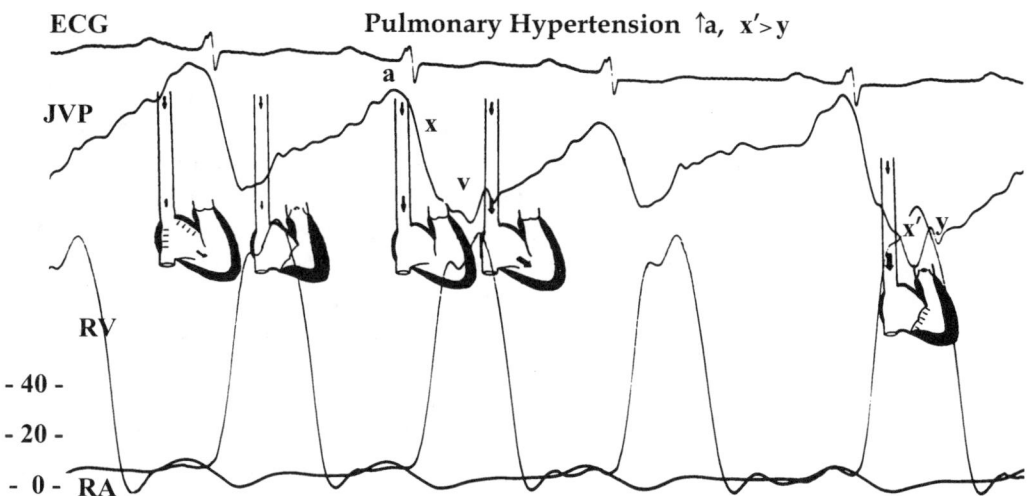

Fig.8. Jugular venous pulse (JVP) from a patient with well-compensated severe pulmonary hypertension with right ventricular (RV) hypertrophy and decreased compliance. The RV systolic pressure is between 90 and 100 mmHg. Note the prominent a wave on the JVP. The a wave rise is almost as fast as the descent. The overlying diagrams depict the events at different phases of the cardiac cycle. The first diagram shows the retrograde flow into the SVC during atrial contraction. The x – x′ descent combination is still the most prominent descent. (Modified and reprinted from ref. *41*. Copyright 2005 with permission from Excerpta Medica Inc.)

and in patients with severe decrease in RV compliance. In the latter patients, the RV is unable to dilate completely to accept blood from the contracting right atrium and the blood has no choice but to flow back into the venae cavae (Fig.8).

NORMAL JUGULAR VENOUS PULSE CONTOUR AND ITS RECOGNITION AT THE BEDSIDE

The RA pressure pulse is transmitted through the superior vena cava to the internal jugular vein. The internal jugular vein runs underneath the sternomastoid muscle. It extends in direction from the angle of the jaw to the hollowness between the two heads of the sternomastoid muscle attachments to the upper sternum and the medial portion of the clavicle. Often positioning the patient with a comfortable tilt of the neck with adequate light coming from the sides will make the jugular pulsations more easily visible. Sometimes having the patient lie in the left lateral decubitus position again with the head tilted somewhat also helps bring out the jugular pulsations. Directing the light source in such a way as to cause a shadow of a fixed nonmoving object to fall on the skin overlying the sternomastoid will reveal the pulsations of the jugulars underneath it since the edge of the shadow can be shown to move because of the jugular movement. The object could be the patient's chin, an observer's finger, or a pen held at a fixed point on the neck of the patient by the observer. Often if the light source is appropriate, one may be able to have the shadow of the laterally placed clavicular head of the sternomastoid fall on the hollow space between the two heads of that muscle.

Since normal RA pressure waves (the *a* and the *v waves*) have slow rises and are often of low amplitude, they are usually not appreciated in the jugulars. On the other hand, the descents in the RA pressure pulse are better transmitted and appreciated in the jugulars. They are generally rapid movements moving away from the eye and thus easily seen. In addition, their appreciation is made easier in that they reflect acceleration of flow velocity *(40,47)* The descents in the internal jugular vein reflect a fall in pressure in the right atrium during cardiac cycle. The reflected light intensity on the hollow area between the two heads of the sternomastoid varies when the jugular pressure rises as opposed to when the jugular pressure falls, and this is easily appreciated at the bedside as well as in video recordings of jugular pulsations. When the descents occur, there is less reflected light overlying the jugulars and the area looks darker. Slight anatomical variations from patient to patient may occur. The descents may be sometimes appreciated more anteriorly at the medial edge of the sternomastoid. Sometimes it could be somewhat lateral. In others it may be seen over a wide area in the neck.

The descents can be timed to either the radial arterial pulse or the second heart sound. The *x′ descent* corresponds to the systolic flow. Because of transmission delay this descent falls almost on to the second heart sound, and it coincides with the radial arterial pulse. The diastolic *y descent* is out of phase with the arterial pulse and occurs after the second heart sound, reflecting the diastolic flow velocity *(40)*.

In normal subjects, a single dominant descent is noted during systole (x') because of the descent of the base corresponding to the dominant systolic flow. The *y descent* is often not visible in the adult, although it may be noted in young subjects, pregnant women, and thyrotoxic and anemic patients. In these the *y descent* may become visible because of its exaggeration due to rapid circulation and increased sympathetic tone. However, in these conditions the right ventricular systolic contraction is often normal and the *x′ descent* will still be the dominant descent.

As stated previously, the normal *a* and *v wave* rises are not seen, but their presence can be inferred by the descents that follow. During normal sinus rhythm, the wave preceding *x′ descent* is the *a wave* and the one that precedes the *y descent* is the *v wave*.

Generally the external jugular vein will not always reflect the descents. This vein usually runs superficially over the mid- portion of the sternomastoid muscle. If it should exhibit the descents that could be timed to the cardiac cycle, then one could use them for assessment of waveform and pressure much as one would normally use the internal jugular pulsations. Jugular pulsation is easily distinguished from the arterial pulse in the neck because it moves in the opposite direction due to the usually dominant *x′ descent* (Figs. 2 and 9) (*see* JVP Videofiles [1st–4th patient] in Jugular Venous Pulse, Normal on the Companion CD).

INDIVIDUAL COMPONENTS OF THE RIGHT ATRIAL PRESSURE PULSE, THEIR DETERMINANTS, AND THEIR RECOGNITION IN THE JUGULARS

Pre-a wave Pressure

This is the pressure in diastole during the slow filling phase when the RV and the RA pressures become equal. During this phase the atrium and the right ventricle are one chamber on account of the open tricuspid valve. The level at which this equalization is achieved is determined by the compliance of the RV and the surrounding pericardium (Fig 7A).

The RV compliance implies the distensibility of the endocardium, myocardium, as well as epicardium. It can become abnormal and less distensible whenever pathological

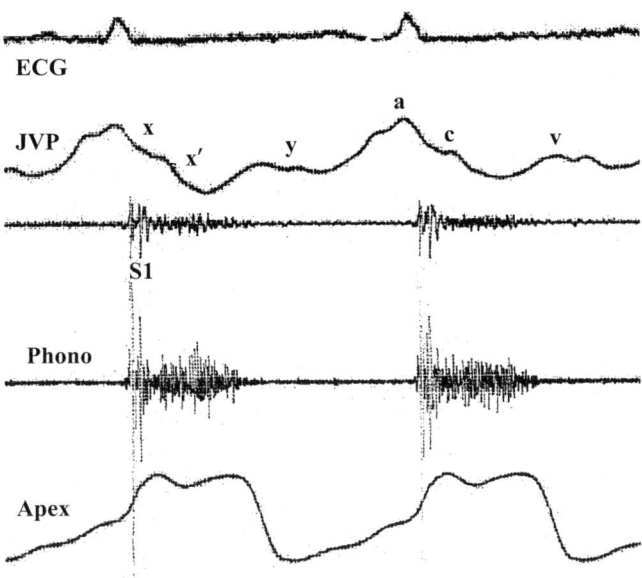

Fig.9. Normal Jugular Venous Pulse (JVP), showing a dominant fall during systole due to the x and the x′ descents. The c wave in the JVP is usually a carotid pulse artefact unlike the c wave noted on the RA pressure tracing.

processes develop in any portion of the RV wall. These processes could be in the form of hypertrophy (thickening of the myocardial fibres) such as those caused secondary to excessive pressure load (e.g., pulmonary hypertension or pulmonary stenosis). It could be in the form of inflammatory process such as myocarditis, of an infiltrative nature as in amyloidosis, ischemia, and infarction (RV infarction is usually rare but could occur when the right coronary artery becomes occluded quite proximally before the RV branch origin; this is usually associated with an infero-posterior wall LV infarction), or fibrosis, which may supervene in the course of any of the pathological processes. This diastolic dysfunction can coexist with or without a systolic dysfunction (Figs. 10 and 11).

If the RV has in fact developed systolic dysfunction and failure, this will further aggravate the diastolic dysfunction, which often precedes systolic dysfunction. If the systolic emptying is poor, the ventricular volume will be higher at the end of systole and therefore its pressure will rise quickly to high levels with diastolic inflow.

If the RV wall is surrounded by a thick and fibrotic or calcific pericardium (e.g., chronic constrictive pericarditis) or a pericardial sac filled with fluid under some pressure (e.g., acute or subacute pericarditis with pericardial effusion), easy diastolic expansion of the ventricle will not be possible, leading to a higher *pre-a wave* pressure for any degree of filling.

The *pre-a wave* pressure sets the baseline for the *a wave* and *v wave* pressures *(47)*. If it becomes elevated, as under the conditions listed above, one would expect higher *a wave* and *v wave* pressures in the atrial pressure pulse.

Elevated *pre-a wave* pressure would be reflected in the jugulars as an elevated jugular venous pressure as judged by the assessment of the level of the top of the jugular pulsations in relation to the sternal angle (*see* JVP Videofiles 2–4 in Jugular Venous Pulse on the Companion CD).

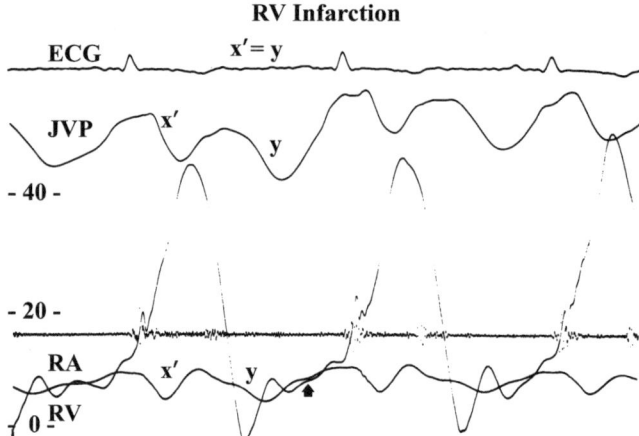

Fig.10. Simultaneous recordings of RA and RV pressures in mmHg. from a patient with Right Ventricular (RV) infarction, along with Jugular Venous Pulse (JVP). Note the double descents x' = y pattern in both the JVP and the RA pressure curve. Arrow points to the pre a wave pressure (Reproduced with kind permission from ref. *47*.)

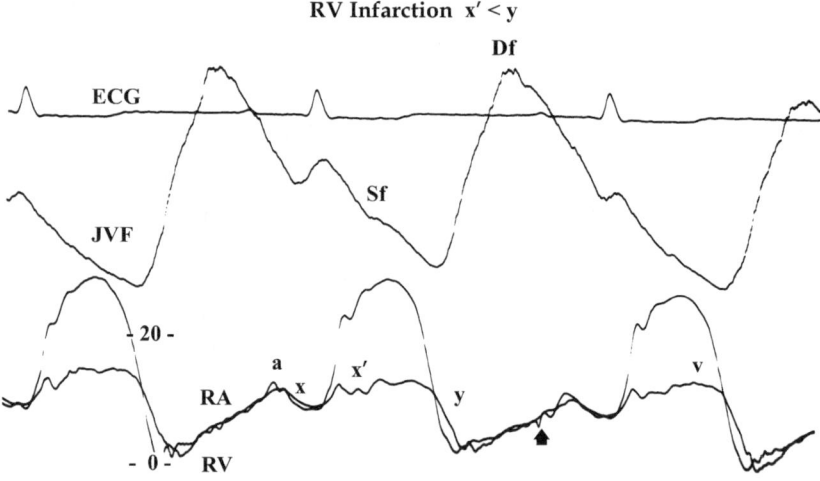

Fig. 11. Simultaneous recordings of jugular venous flow (JVF) velocity and right ventricular (RV) and right atrial (RA) pressures from a patient with RV infarction. Note the prolonged PR interval on electrocardiogram (ECG). Because of RV infarction, the RV contractility is poor and the x' descent is also poor. The x descent is well separated from the x' descent because of the long PR. Note the atrial relaxation flow on JVF corresponding to x descent. The y descent is dominant and so is the corresponding Df in JVF. Small arrow indicates pre-a wave pressure. (Reproduced with kind permission from ref. *47*.)

a Wave

Irrespective of what the *pre-a wave* pressure is, the *a wave* height in the atrial pressure is determined by the strength of the atrial contraction first and foremost because the *a wave* rise results from atrial contraction. In atrial fibrillation, both the atrial contraction and relaxation become ineffective and disorganized and feeble, leading to loss of the *a wave* peak and the *x descent (40)*.

The atrium tends to contract strongly when there is resistance to ventricular filling. The extreme form of resistance to ventricular filling would occur in tricuspid stenosis or obstruction because of a tumor (e.g., a myxoma in the right atrium). These would be expected to cause very high *a wave* pressures *(18)*. In fact they do. However, these conditions are extremely rare and therefore not to be thought of first when considering causes of prominent *a wave*.

The most common reason for resistance to ventricular filling is decreased ventricular compliance. The decreased compliance may be the result of any pathological process that affects the wall of the RV, such as hypertrophy, ischemia, infarction, inflammation, infiltration and/ or fibrosis (Fig. 8).

If the atrium itself becomes involved in the disease process, which leads to a decrease in its systolic contraction, high *a wave* pressure may not be generated despite the presence of decreased ventricular compliance.

Whereas the normal *a wave* pressure rise is slow and small and therefore not appreciated in the jugulars, a strong atrial contraction causing a quick and rapid rise in pressure may actually cause flow reversal in the jugulars and become recognizable in the jugulars as an abnormal sharp rising wave preceding the *x′ descent*, which can be timed with the radial pulse. The short duration of this wave is another distinguishing feature (*see* JVP Videofile [1st–4th patient] in Jugular Venous Pulse, Normal and JVP Videofile 8 on the Companion CD).

If atrial contraction were to occur in a haphazard relationship to ventricular systole as in atrioventricular dissociation (as in complete A-V block with a ventricular pacemaker driving the ventricles with atria beating on their own from sinus depolarizations), a fortuitous relationship could develop that could result in simultaneous atrial and ventricular contraction. Because atrial contraction would be occurring at the time of a closed tricuspid valve due to ventricular systole, it would result in a sharp and quick rise in atrial pressures, termed "*cannon waves*." These will cause flow reversal in the jugulars *(40)* and be recognizable as sharp rising waves of short duration at the time of the radial pulse. They will be irregular. Rarely regular cannon waves may occur in junctional rhythms with retrograde P waves and very short PR interval (Fig. 7H).

x Descent

The presence of atrial relaxation is the foremost prerequisite for the pressure fall termed *x descent*. A strong healthy atrial contraction can be expected to be followed by a good *x descent* (Fig. 7C).

In terms of timing, the *x descent* comes just before the more dominant systolic *x′ descent*. It usually precedes the *x′ descent* as a minor hesitation before the major fall during systole, as observed in the jugulars during periods of normal PR relationship. If the PR interval is prolonged, it could occur long before ventricular systole and, in fact, before end-diastole. When it becomes diastolic in timing, it may be difficult to distinguish this at the bedside from the usual diastolic y descent in the absence of an electrocardiogram *(40,47)* (Figs. 2C, 9, and 11).

x′ Descent

This is the major fall in atrial pressure in systole and is caused by RV contraction pulling on the closed tricuspid valve and ring *(26,40)*.

Its presence requires:

1. A good RV systolic function
2. An intact tricuspid valve

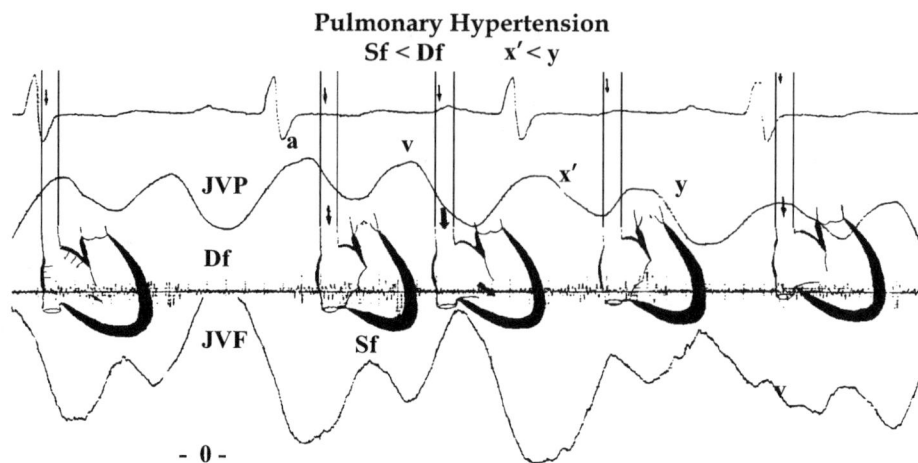

Fig. 12. Jugular venous pulse (JVP) and jugular venous flow (JVF) velocity recordings from a patient with pulmonary hypertension in a decompensated state. Note the more prominent y descent compared to the x' descent in the JVP. It corresponds to the dominant diastolic flow (Df) compared to the systolic flow (Sf). The added diagrams of the heart help explain the pathophysiology of the JVP contour abnormality. Thickness of arrows refers to flow velocities. (Modified and reprinted from ref. *41*. Copyright 2005 with permission from Excerpta Medica Inc.)

In fact, a good and dominant x' *descent* in the jugulars indicates good RV systolic function. The flow velocity peak in the jugulars during the x' *descent* is always dominant (Figs. 2C and 7D). When there is RV systolic dysfunction, the x' *descent* is diminished and eventually may become totally absent when RV function becomes poor. In pulmonary hypertension, during the late stages when decompensation sets in, the x' *descent* becomes diminished and eventually becomes lost (Figs. 12 and 13) *(41)*. In acute LV failure such as caused by acute myocardial infarction, the RV function may still be good, as indicated by the presence of a good x' *descent*. In patients with cardiomyopathy with poor ventricular function, if the x' *descent* is preserved it would indicate sparing of the RV as might be the case in ischemic cardiomyopathy *(47)*.

While mild to moderate degrees of tricuspid regurgitation with normal RV systolic pressure (usually <25 mmHg) could still be consistent with the presence of a preserved x' *descent*, more than moderate degrees of tricuspid regurgitation particularly, in the presence of elevated RV systolic pressure, is incompatible with a well-preserved x' *descent*. Significant degrees of tricuspid regurgitation would clearly lead to early buildup of RA pressure and therefore counteract or abolish the x' *descent*. The loss of x' *descent* and early buildup of the large-amplitude *v wave* (sometimes termed the "*cv*" *wave*) followed by the diastolic y descent are characteristic of significant tricuspid regurgitation (Fig. 7G). The *v wave* of tricuspid regurgitation is characteristically associated with systolic flow reversal in the jugulars. The *v wave* in the right atrium is clearly in such cases a result of the actual regurgitant flow into the atrium. Because of its large amplitude of rise together with retrograde flow into the jugulars, it can be recognized from a distance in the jugulars as the large *v wave* ascent followed by the *y descent*, which can be timed. The rise will be systolic and can be timed with the radial pulse. Unlike the *a wave*, it tends to last longer, and much longer than the duration of the arterial pulse *(40)*.

The lack of atrial contraction in atrial fibrillation leads to a decrease in Starling effect on the ventricle. This leads to a decrease in ventricular contraction and function causing

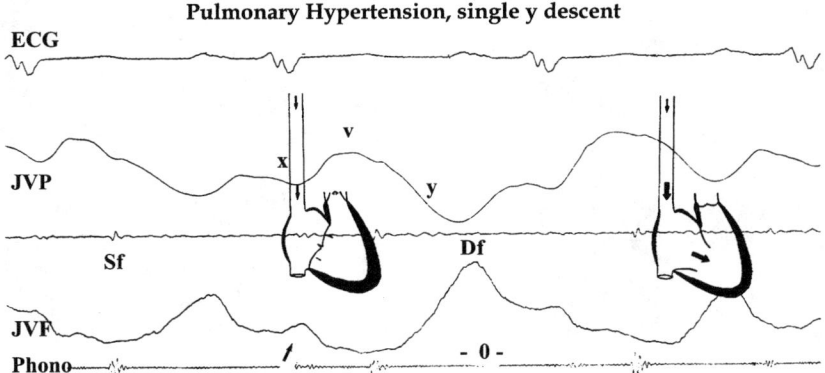

Fig. 13. Jugular venous pulse recording from a patient with right ventricular (RV) decompensation with pulmonary hypertension secondary to significant mitral regurgitation associated with ischemic heart disease. Note the x descent and the corresponding atrial relaxation flow (arrow). The x′ descent cannot be seen, and there is a prominent y descent and a corresponding Df. There may be mild tricuspid regurgitation but not enough to overcome the buffering effect of the right atrium (RA), and no systolic retrograde flow can be seen on the jugular venous flow (JVF). The JVF tracing does not fall below the zero flow line. Diagrams have been added to explain the pathophysiology of the flow pattern. (Modified and reprinted from ref. *41*. Copyright 2005 with permission from Excerpta Medica Inc.)

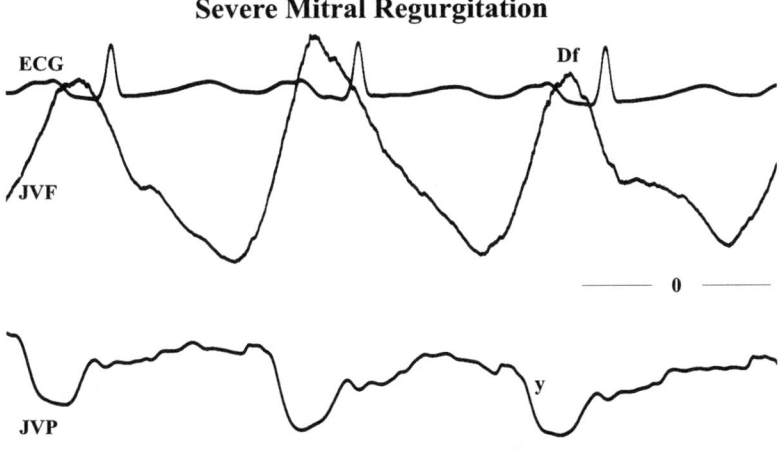

Fig. 14. Recordings from a patient with severe mitral regurgitation. Single diastolic flow (Df) in the jugular venous flow (JVF) velocity, corresponding to a single y descent on the jugular venous pulse (JVP). This is because of the Bernheim effect. (Reproduced with kind permission from ref. *47*.)

a diminished *x′ descent* (Fig. 3). In recent onset atrial fibrillation with preserved RV function, the *x′ descent* may be still recognized in the jugulars. However, in longstanding atrial fibrillation, the *x′ descent* tends to be absent because of co-existing RV dysfunction and some degree of tricuspid regurgitation.

Very rarely in patients with severe mitral regurgitation, the interatrial septum may be seen to bulge into the right atrium during systole. This would tend to diminish the full effect of the descent of the base on the right atrium. This decreases the *x′ descent* (systolic flow). This effect is termed the *Bernheim effect* on the atrial septum *(9,40,47,50)* (Figs. 14, 15A,B) (Table 1).

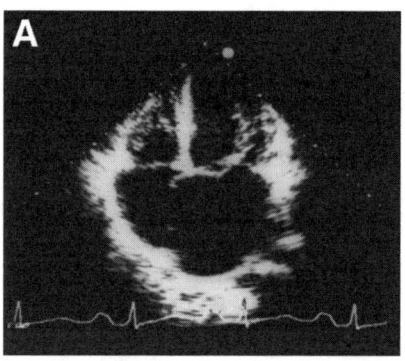 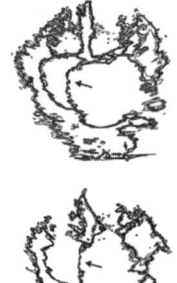 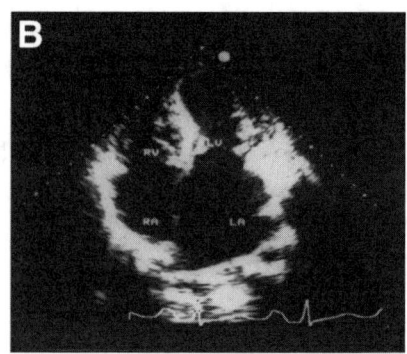

Fig. 15. Four chamber views of the two-dimensional echocardiograms from the same patient with severe mitral regurgitation with freeze frames in systole (**A**) and diastole (**B**) together with their line diagrams. In systole (**A**) indicated by the closed mitral and the tricuspid valves, the bulge of the interatrial septum into the right atrium (RA) decreasing the volume in RA is well seen. In diastole (**B**), as shown by the open mitral and tricuspid valves, the interatrial septum is more straight and the right atrial dimension is larger (*see* the text).

Table 1
Causes of Decreased *x'* Descent

1. Diminished right ventricular (RV) contraction, e.g.,
   - RV failure in pulmonary hypertension
   - Post-cardiac surgery RV damage
   - RV infarction
2. Atrial fibrillation because of loss of Starling effect
3. Bernheim effect in severe mitral regurgitation[a]

[a] Rare occurrence.

v Wave

The *v wave* rise in the RA pressure in the absence of significant tricuspid regurgitation is almost always a result of venous filling of the right atrium in the later part of systole whether the actual pressure is normal or high. The normal right atrium, being a capacitance chamber, has good distensibility. The venous inflow from the venae cavae augmented by the *x' descent* tends to build up a pressure that is often quite low, not exceeding 5 mmHg. In children the circulation is rapid because of high sympathetic tone, and the rapid venous inflow coming into an atrium, which is relatively small, could build up a relatively good *v wave* pressure. Rapid circulatory states with high sympathetic tone may also exist in conditions such as pregnancy, thyrotoxicosis, and anemia *(19)*, which also favor buildup of relatively high *v waves*. In pregnancy, in addition, the blood volume is usually expanded. Hypervolemia, however, could raise the v wave pressure. Occasionally in some patients with atrial septal defect, the extra source of venous return from the left atrium across the defect together with some changes in RA distensibility could also lead to a higher than normal *v wave* pressure *(14,17,24)*.

Because the *pre-a wave* pressure sets the baseline over which the *a wave* and *v wave* buildups naturally occur, the most common reason for pathologically high *v wave* pressure is an elevated high *pre-a wave* pressure. The reasons for this, discussed previously, include conditions such as pericardial effusion with any degree of restriction, constrictive pericarditis, pulmonary hypertension with elevated RV diastolic pressure, ischemia, and/or infarcted right ventricle and cardiomyopathy. For any given degree of elevation of *pre-a wave* pressure and right atrial distensibility, any rise in venous tone (sympathetic tone) will allow a much further rise in the jugular v wave.

In the jugulars, the *v wave* can be inferred to be present whenever a *y descent* is recognized. The *v wave* is the wave preceding the *y descent*, which can be timed to be diastolic. Normal *v wave* is not usually seen in the jugulars in the adult, as recognized by the fact that the *y descent* is absent. The rise of even an abnormal and elevated *v wave* (e.g., heart failure, constrictive pericarditis) is not usually as prominent to the observer's eyes as the fall of the *y descent* that follows it. The reason for this is an absence of any flow reversal in the jugulars under these conditions. This is in contrast to the *v wave* of tricuspid regurgitation, which always causes systolic flow reversal *(40)* (Figs. 11 and 7G) (*see* JVP Videofiles 5–7 and 9 in Abnormal Jugular Contours on the Companion CD).

The *v waves* have a larger duration and, therefore, when elevated are associated with higher mean right atrial pressure. Normally on inspiration the intrathoracic pressure falls, leading to an increase in the venous return. The right atrium, being an intrathoracic structure, is also influenced by the fall in intrathoracic pressure. In addition, the capacitance function of the right heart accommodates for the increased venous return without a rise in the RA pressure. In fact, inspiration leads to a fall in the RA pressure reflecting the fall in intrathoracic pressure. However, sometimes the RA and therefore the jugular venous pressure may actually rise with inspiration. This is termed the *Kussmaul's sign (20,21,51)*. This sign may be identified by the fact that the *v wave* is more prominent during inspiration. The latter may be recognized by the inspiratory augmentation of the *y descent*. The *Kussmaul's sign* is generally indicative of decreased compliance of the right heart and/or its surrounding structures. Thus, it may be seen in a variety of conditions including heart failure, restrictive pericardial pathology with or without effusion, and occasionally thoracic deformities such as kyphoscoliosis.

y Descent

Because the *y descent* is the fall in the RA pressure in diastole immediately following the opening of the tricuspid valve, it is necessary that the RV pressure in fact falls close to zero as it does normally with the early rapid filling phase of diastole. In other words, the ventricle should not have any restriction during this early rapid filling phase of diastole, even if it does have restriction during the later phases of diastole. This automatically excludes cardiac tamponade, which implies total diastolic restriction resulting from high fluid pressure in the pericardial sac, which allows very little or no expansion of the ventricle during diastole.

The steepness of the *y descent* will depend on the *v wave* pressure head that is present at the time of the tricuspid valve opening. The higher the *v wave* pressure head, the steeper and more prominent is the *y descent*, assuming of course that there is no tricuspid obstruction as in tricuspid stenosis (Fig. 11). The latter condition is very rare, and if significant it could be expected to slow the *y descent (18)*.

The normal *v wave* pressure being low, the *y descent* is usually not very prominent (Fig. 9). The corresponding diastolic flow velocity in the jugulars is also slow and low. Although the small *y descent* may be seen in the RA pressure pulse, it is not usually seen in the jugular venous pulse. This is because of the capacitance function of the normal

Table 2
Causes of Exaggerated *y Descent*

1. Increased *v wave* pressure head with NO restriction to ventricular filling during rapid filling phase, e.g.,
   a. High sympathetic tone as in young children, anxiety, anemia, pregnancy, thyrotoxicosis
   b. Hypervolemia
   c. Extra source of venous filling as in atrial septal defect
   d. Pericardial effusion with some restriction
   e. Constrictive pericarditis
   f. Pulmonary hypertension with elevated RV diastolic pressure
   g. Ischemic and/or infarcted RV
   h. Cardiomyopathy

Excludes cardiac tamponade:

2. Decreased right atrial capacitance function, e.g.,
   a. Post-cardiac surgery
3. Bernheim effect in severe mitral regurgitation[a]

[a] Rare occurrence.

right atrium. The reservoir function of the atrium is such that it is able to empty into the ventricle without the top of the column actually falling much. When the right atrium gets stiff and behaves like a conduit as in post-cardiac surgery patients who have had their right atrium cannulated during surgery and therefore traumatized, this capacitance function is lost. In these patients even the normal *v wave* pressure allows recognition of the *y descent* in the jugulars *(17,29,42,52)* (*see* JVP Videofiles 1–3 on the Companion CD).

Exaggerated y Descent

The *y descent* is exaggerated when there is:

1. An increased *v wave* pressure head
2. No restriction to ventricular filling during the early rapid filling phase of diastole

This mechanism necessarily excludes cardiac tamponade, in which condition ventricular filling is restricted throughout diastole including the early rapid filling phase, despite the high *v wave* pressure.

Both of these conditions, namely increased *v wave* pressure head and absence of restriction to filling during rapid filling phase, are met under the following circumstances (Table 2):

1. High sympathetic tone with rapid circulation as in children and young adults, anxiety, anemia, pregnancy, thyrotoxicosis, Paget's disease, and other similar conditions
2. Hypervolemia as in renal failure, following rapid and large fluid infusion and pregnancy
3. Extra source of venous filling as in some patients with atrial septal defect as mentioned under *v wave*
4. Pericardial effusion with some restriction but without tamponade
5. Constrictive pericarditis which restricts expansion of RV because of thickened or sometimes calcified pericardium (Figs. 16 and 17)
6. Pulmonary hypertension with elevated RV diastolic pressure (Fig. 12)
7. Ischemic or infarcted RV with elevated RV diastolic pressures (Fig. 11)
8. Cardiomyopathy with elevated RV diastolic pressures.

Chapter 4 / Jugular Venous Pulse

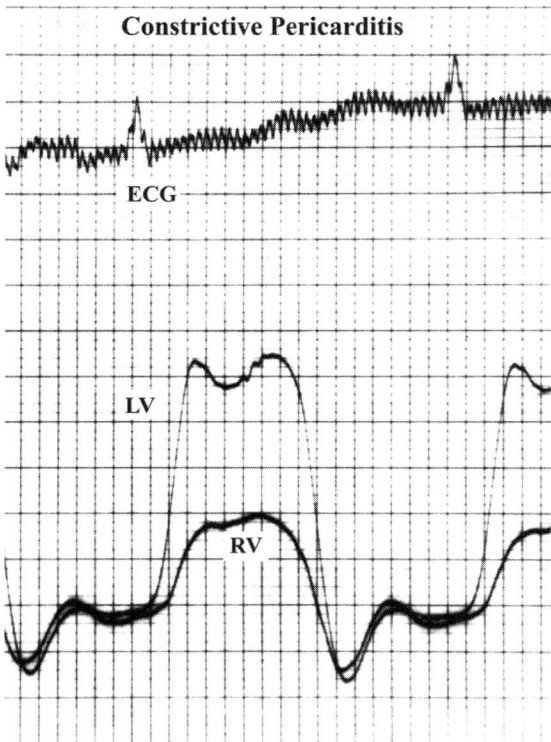

Fig. 16. Simultaneous recordings of the left ventricular (LV) and the right ventricular (RV) pressures from a patient with constrictive pericarditis showing the equalization of the diastolic pressures between the two sides with the typical dip followed by the plateau pattern.

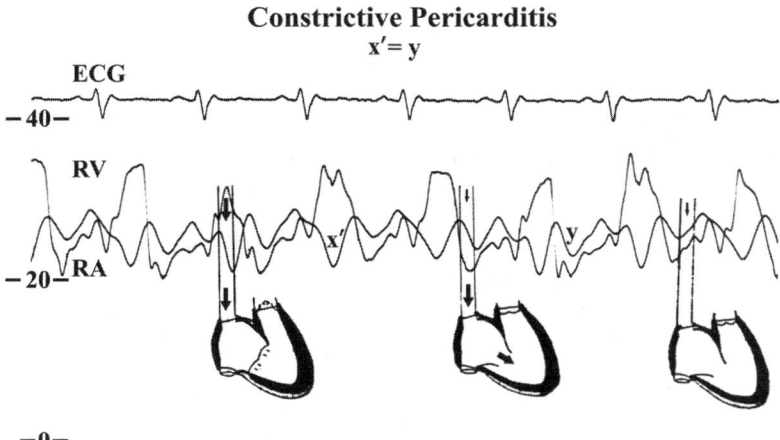

Fig. 17. Simultaneous right vericular (RV) and right atrial (RA) pressures in a patient with constrictive pericarditis. Note the high RA and RV diastolic pressures. On the RA pressure tracings both the x' and the y descents are equally prominent, and this would also be reflected in the jugular pulse contour. The added diagrams explain the pathophysiology. The first shows the x' descent, the second the y descent ,and the third the pre-a wave period. (Reproduced with kind permission from ref. *47*.)

In the rare patient with severe mitral regurgitation and atrial Bernheim effect, an exaggerated *y descent* without elevation of the *v wave* pressure may occur. This is explainable by the sudden emptying of the left atrium during early diastole, which causes a quick reversal of the systolic bulge of the inter-atrial septum *(47)*.

The *y descent* is easily identifiable in the jugulars by its timing in diastole being out of phase with the radial arterial pulse. It can be considered exaggerated when it is equal to the *x′ descent* in its prominence or when it becomes more dominant compared to the *x′ descent* and also when it is the only descent present.

ABNORMAL JUGULAR VENOUS PULSE CONTOURS AS RELATED TO ABNORMAL JUGULAR VENOUS FLOW VELOCITY PATTERNS

Studies from our laboratory using Doppler jugular venous flow (JVF) velocity recordings and their correlation to right heart hemodynamics had established that when the forward flow velocity patterns in the jugulars lose their normal systolic dominance, they can be termed abnormal *(40,47)*. The flow velocity patterns of $Sf = Df$, $Sf < Df$, and Df alone are abnormal forward flow velocity patterns. These correspond to the right atrial and the jugular venous pulse contours of $x' = y\ descent$, $x' < y\ descent$, and single *y descent*. Decrease in peak Sf would imply decreased RV contractility (decreased x'). Increase in Df velocity would imply increased *v wave* pressure head without restriction to forward flow in early diastole. This greater pressure gradient would cause faster emptying of the RA. This would be reflected in the jugulars as a greater diastolic forward flow velocity (increased *y descent*).

Mechanism of Abnormal JVF Patterns and Contours in Pulmonary Hypertension

The majority of patients with abnormal flow patterns and pulmonary hypertension had increased RA *v wave* pressure, implying that the Df velocity was increased (exaggerated *y descent*). The increased *v wave* pressure was shown to be a result of an increased RV early diastolic and *pre-a wave* pressure. The incidence of congestive heart failure was higher in patients with $Sf < Df$ and Df alone compared to the pattern of $Sf = Df$. This indicated that decreased RV systolic function (decreased *x′ descent*) also played a part. This seems to be a later phenomenon in serial observations *(41)* (Fig. 18).

Mechanism of Abnormal JVF Patterns and Jugular Pulse Contours in Post-Cardiac Surgery Patients

In most patients who have undergone cardiopulmonary bypass, the altered flow velocity patterns are not associated with alterations in right heart pressures. Postoperatively, the right atrium seems to behave as a conduit rather than a capacitance chamber. Its capacitance function may be attenuated initially because of edema and later probably due to stiffness caused by scarring. The loss of buffering function of the atrium as a capacitance chamber leads to full reflection of the diastolic flow velocity at the tricuspid valve to the superior vena cava and the jugulars, thus exaggerating the y descent (Fig. 19). When the flow velocity pattern was $Sf < Df$ ($x' < y\ descent$), RV dysfunction and decreased ejection fraction was demonstrated *(42)* (Fig. 20).

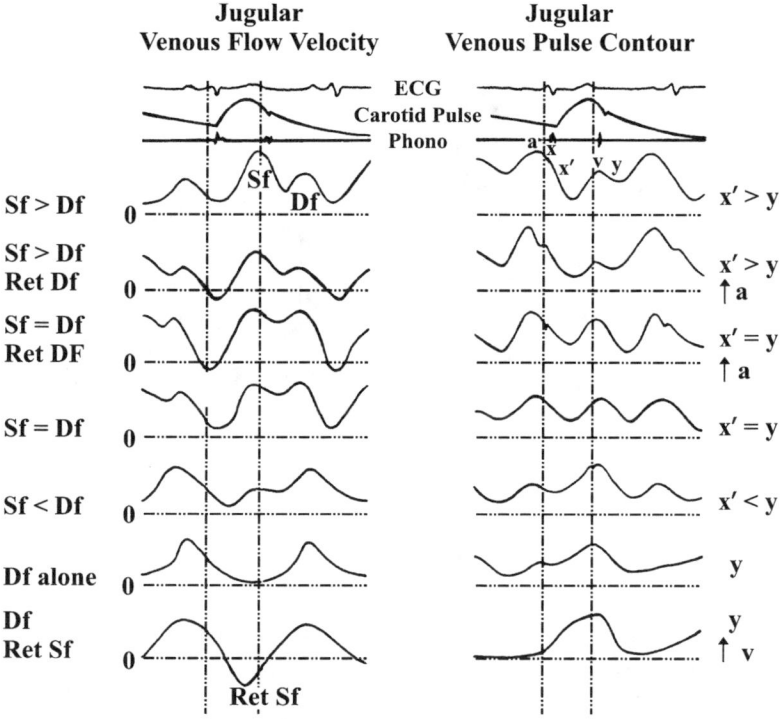

Fig. 18. Diagrammatic representation of the serial changes observed over time in the jugular venous pulse contour and the corresponding jugular venous flow patterns in pulmonary hypertension. as the right ventricle (RV) begins to decompensate. (Modified and reprinted from ref. *41*. Copyright 2005 with permission from Excerpta Medica Inc.)

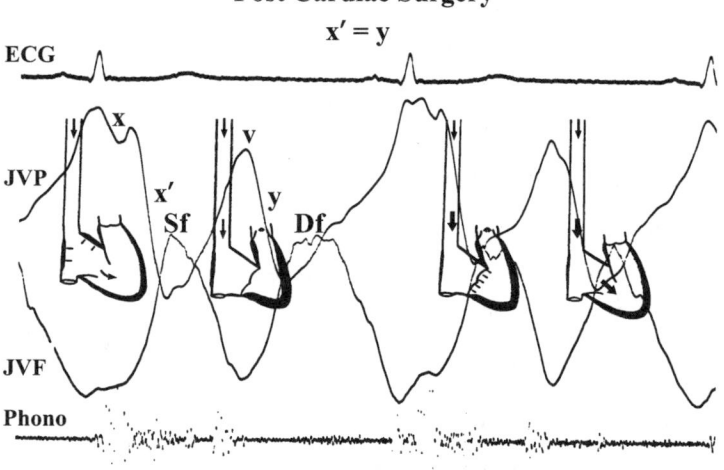

Fig. 19. Simultaneous jugular venous pulse (JVP), the jugular venous flow velocity (JVF), phonocardiogram (phono), and electrocardiogram (ECG) in a post-cardiac surgery patient showing equal x' and y descents. This is an abnormal JVP contour. Superimposed diagrams help explain the pathophysiology. The right atrium (RA), rather than acting as a capacitance chamber, acts only as a conduit. The size of the arrows depicting flow at the tricuspid valve and at the superior vena cava (SVC) during early diastole is equal to indicate this. (Modified and reprinted from ref. *42*. Copyright 2005 with permission from Excerpta Medica Inc.)

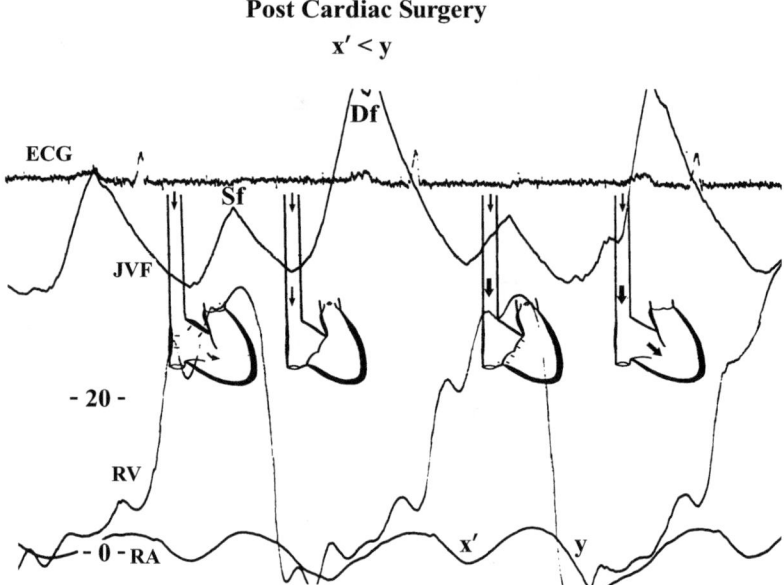

Fig. 20. Simultaneous recordings of electrocardiogram (ECG), jugular venous flow velocity (JVF) and the right atrial (RA) and right ventricular (RV) pressures in a post-cardiac-surgery patient. The y descent on the RA pressure is more prominent than the x' descent, with the corresponding dominant diastolic flow (Df) peak in JVF. (Reproduced with kind permission from ref. *47*.)

Mechanism of Abnormal JVF Patterns and Jugular Pulse Contours in Restriction to Ventricular Filling

Restriction to ventricular filling may vary in degree and may be pericardial, myocardial, or endocardial in origin. Restriction in its mild form may be apparent only at the end of diastole during the atrial contraction phase. It may involve both mid and late diastole when more severe, and when very severe it may involve almost all phases of diastole beginning with the rapid filling phase (Fig. 21).

LATE DIASTOLIC RESTRICTION

If the restriction is limited to late diastole, the only abnormality seen in right heart hemodynamics will be elevation of right atrial *a wave* pressure. This will be reflected in the jugular venous pulse as a prominent a wave (Fig. 8) (*see* JVP Videofile 8 on the Companion CD).

MID AND LATE DIASTOLIC RESTRICTION

When restriction to ventricular filling encroaches more and more into mid to early diastole, elevation of all RV diastolic pressures would result and lead to elevations of both mean RA and *v wave* pressures. The increased *v wave* pressure head during early diastole will lead to augmented Df (exaggerated *y descent*). As long as ventricular function is preserved, the increased Df will equal Sf ($x' = y$). In contrast, patients with myocardial dysfunction and diminished contractility will have flow patterns of Sf < Df and jugular contours of $x' < y$ (Figs. 4 and 5) (*see* JVP Videofile 4 on the Companion CD).

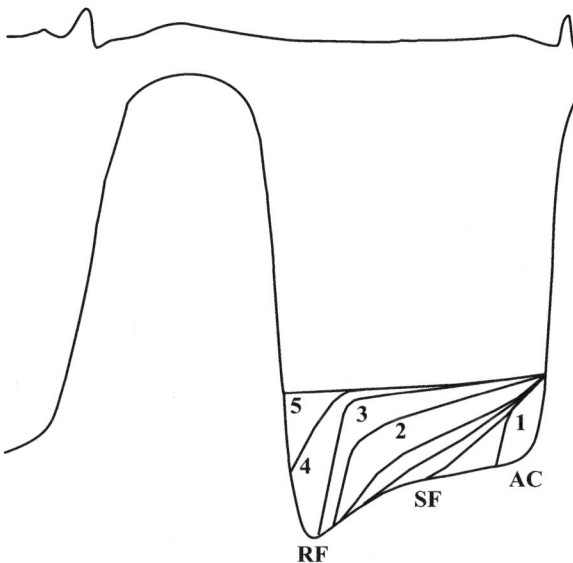

Fig. 21. The varying severity of restriction to diastolic ventricular filling is shown with lines to indicate the ventricular diastolic pressure elevations and their timing in diastole. In mild form, the pressure increase is during atrial contraction (AC) at end diastole (line #1). As restriction gets worse, the pre-a wave pressure starts to rise gradually and earlier and earlier in diastole. This progression is shown as four successive lines (lines #2). When severe, it may be total during mid and late diastole, restricting flow into the RV beginning with the slow filling phase (SF). There will be very rapid inflow only during early diastole or the rapid filling phase (RF) followed by a rapid rise in pressure with no further flow producing the classic dip and plateau or the square root pattern (line #3). This is typical for chronic constrictive pericarditis. If the restriction is severe and involves also the RF phase, the pressures rise quickly in the RV in early diastole limiting inflow altogether. This can occur in severe pericardial effusion leading to cardiac tamponade where the high intra-pericardial pressure will limit ventricular expansion altogether. Line #4 depicts pre-tamponade, and line #5 is full tamponade with no diastolic inflow possible. Such severe elevations in diastolic pressures may rarely also occur in severe cardiomyopathy, cardiac failure, and in some patients with severe right ventricular infarctions.

TOTAL DIASTOLIC RESTRICTION

When restriction is severe and occurs throughout diastole as in tamponade, no inflow can occur into the atrium during this phase. This totally abolishes diastolic flow into the atrium. In cardiac tamponade, the four chambers of the heart are boxed within a pericardial sac under high fluid pressure. During diastole no new blood can enter the heart, but blood is shifted from the atrium to the ventricle with the total volume in the boxed four chambers constant. The only time new blood can enter the heart is when blood leaves this enclosed box, namely during systole. Patients with tamponade, therefore, exhibit inflow only during ventricular systole, when the ventricular sizes are the smallest, thus allowing some expansion and filling of the atria within the pericardial sac *(47)* (Fig. 22).

Jugular flow recordings in patients with cardiac tamponade are extremely hard to obtain because of diminished flow velocity. Thus, the only recordable forward flow would occur in systole and only during inspiration with a corresponding *x′ descent* in the jugular pulse *(40,44)*. Jugulars distend in tamponade and hardly show any descent. If a descent is recognizable at all it will be an *x′* and may be seen only during inspiration.

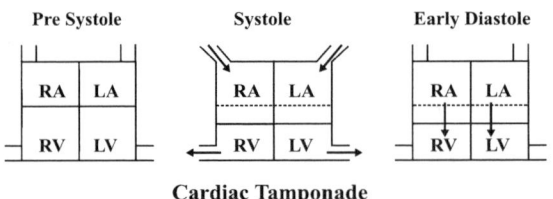

Cardiac Tamponade

Fig. 22. A diagrammatic representation of the pathophysiology of the cardiac inflow and outflow in cardiac tamponade. The extracardiac pressure is so high that the heart is as if encased in a solid box at all times. The only time flow into this "box" can occur is when blood leaves the "box." This occurs during systole as blood is ejected out of the ventricles. Flow into the heart (atria) can occur only at that time (the middle diagram). In early diastole, the blood is shifted from the atria into the ventricles, but new blood cannot enter the heart. (Reproduced with kind permission from ref. 47.)

Usually the venous pressure is so high that the pulsation at the top of the column would be higher than the angle of the jaw. Therefore, the pulsations cannot be seen, but flow may be recorded by Doppler to show single systolic flow. In fact, the occurrence of a steep *y descent* in patients with pericardial effusion excludes tamponade.

If the RV filling pressures are severely elevated even in the early rapid filling phase, as might happen in rare instances of constrictive pericarditis and severe cardiomyopathy, poor diastolic inflow (and correspondingly poor *y descent*) will result despite high RA mean and *v wave* pressures for the simple reason that there is not enough pressure difference between the RA and RV during the early rapid filling phase. If this should happen in constrictive pericarditis, it would be accompanied by good Sf (and a corresponding x' *descent*) *(16)*, whereas in cardiomyopathy such a severe elevation of filling pressures would be associated with poor RV systolic function and therefore poor x' *descent*.

ABNORMAL JUGULAR CONTOURS

Double Descents in the Jugular Venous Pulse

If two descents are visible in the jugular venous pulse for each cardiac cycle, it is usually a result of the x' and the *y descents* unless the *x descent* is far separated from the x' *descent* as with long PR intervals. The wave preceding the x' *descent* is the *a wave* during sinus rhythm, and the wave preceding the y descent is the *v wave*. In cases where double descents (x' and *y*) are noted, the relative dominance of the x' vs *y* (systolic vs diastolic descent) will easily help in identifying the flow pattern.

The relative dominance of x' and *y descents*, as with relative dominance of the flow velocities, is not volume dependent (Fig. 23A,B) *(47)*. Therefore, even when the patient had received therapy such as diuretics with consequent fall in venous pressure, the relationship was unaltered and therefore still useful in assessment of the patient. In the adult, it must be emphasized that it is uncommon to see both descents in the jugular venous pulse. Double descents where x' is still dominant would generally imply that the *y descent* is exaggerated. Double descents where $x' = y$ or $x' < y$ generally arise either because x' *descent* is decreased or the *y descent* is exaggerated or both, similar to the corresponding flow velocity peaks.

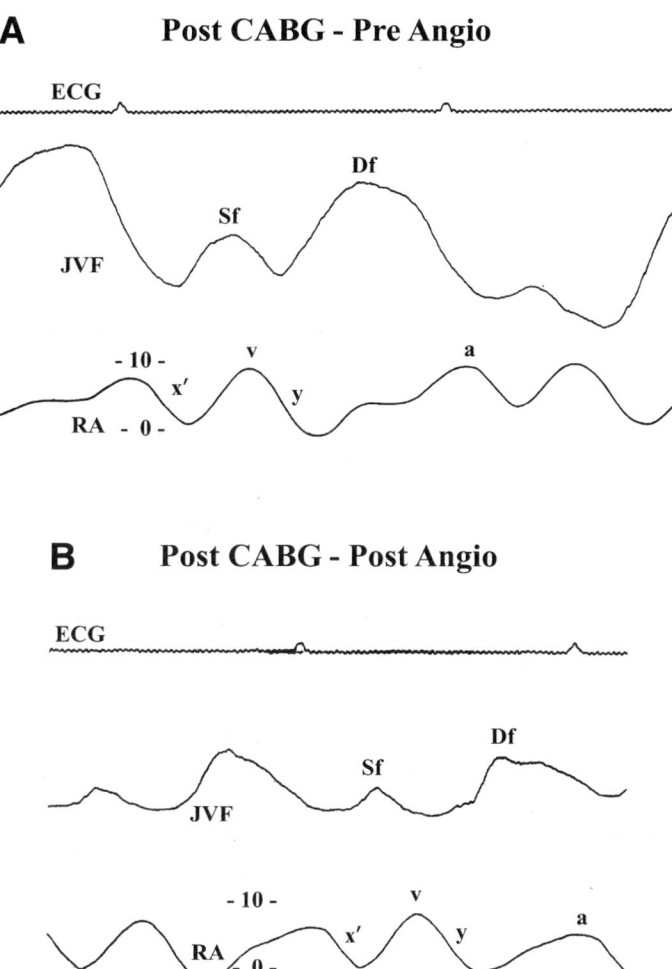

Fig. 23. (A) Simultaneous recordings of right atrial (RA) pressure and jugular venous flow velocity (JVF) in a patient who has had coronary artery bypass grafting (CABG) taken before LV angiogram. In this patient, the JVF pattern is Sf < Df and the corresponding RA pressure tracing shows x' < y. This tends to indicate some damage to the right ventricle (RV). (B) Similar recordings in the same patient postangiogram. The contrast material used for the angiogram presents an osmotic load and increases blood volume. This did not change the Sf < Df or x' < y relationship. This relationship is maintained despite the level of hydration of the patient, thus rendering a useful means of assessing RV function.

Causes of decreased *x' descent* as well as causes of exaggerated *y descents* are shown in Tables 1 and 2. Consideration of these in any given individual situation will usually help in the delineation of the problem.

Differential Diagnosis of Double Descents

A schema for the differential diagnosis and the significance of the double descents is shown in Table 3, both in the presence and the absence of pulmonary hypertension.

Table 3
Differential Diagnosis of Double Descents in Jugular Venous Pulse

In pulmonary hypertension	In the absence of pulmonary hypertension
$x' > y$: Indicates good right ventricular (RV) function	
Compensated RV function	• Normal young adult
	• Hypervolemia
	• Increased sympathetic tone
	• Early pericardial effusion
	• Extra source of venous return, e.g., ASD
$x' = y$: Increased v wave pressure with NO restriction to rapid filling	
Early RV decompensation	• Pericardial effusion
	• Constrictive pericarditis with good myocardial function
	• Early or mild RV infarction
	• Early cardiomyopathy
	• Post-cardiac surgery resulting from decreased right atrial capacitance
$x' < y$: Indicates decreased RV function	
RV failure	• Late stage of constriction
Mild tricuspid regurgitation	• RV infarction
	• Cardiomyopathy
	• Post-cardiac surgery (RV damage)

ASD, Atrial septal defect.

WITH PULMONARY HYPERTENSION

In patients with pulmonary hypertension, the jugular pulse showing only an x' or a dominant x' *descent* would imply a compensated RV function. In addition, if the wave preceding the x' *descent* is large and rising fast, this would indicate a strong atrial contraction causing reversal of flow in end-diastole implying decreased RV compliance (Figs. 8 and 24).

If the pulmonary hypertension is severe and of long duration, the jugular pulse will change to the pattern $x' = y$ *descent*. This would imply raised RV *pre-a wave* pressure and a secondary rise in RA and jugular *v wave* pressure (Fig. 24).

With progression of pulmonary hypertension, the pattern $x' < y$ will emerge (Fig. 12). At this stage, the RV contractility is significantly reduced and RV failure has begun *(41)*. Eventually RV dilatation and tricuspid regurgitation together with RV failure lead to markedly diminished or even absent x' *descent* and emergence of single dominant y *descent* (Fig. 13 and Table 3).

If the wave preceding the *y descent* is large and its rate of rise is prominent (the *"cv" wave*) it would indicate systolic flow reversal of tricuspid regurgitation. During this progression, before significant tricuspid regurgitation develops, the prominent *a wave* may in fact disappear as a result of deteriorating right atrial function.

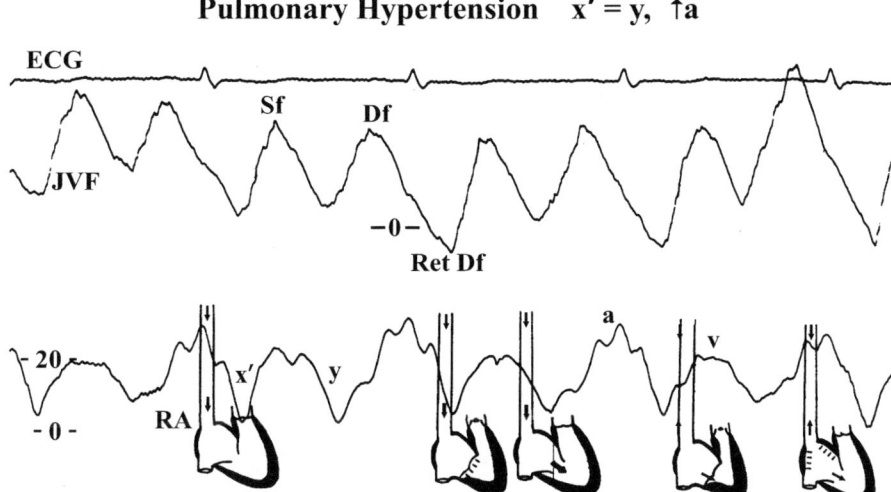

Fig. 24. Simultaneous recordings of electrocardiogram (ECG), jugular venous flow velocity (JVF), and right atrial (RA) pressure in a patient with pulmonary hypertension. Superimposed diagrams depict the altered pathophysiology at different phases of the cardiac cycle. The systolic and the diastolic flow peaks (Sf = Df) are equal with the corresponding RA pressure showing $x' = y$ descents. While the right ventricular (RV) systolic function is still preserved (good x' descent), the raised diastolic pressures in the RV secondary to RV hypertrophy and decreased diastolic compliance cause elevated RA v wave pressure, which leads to a prominent y descent. The strong contraction of the RA causes also a prominent a wave (retrograde end-diastolic flow [Ret Df] in the JVF).

WITHOUT PULMONARY HYPERTENSION

In the absence of pulmonary hypertension also, the pattern of $x' > y$ implies normal right ventricular function. This can be seen in some of the conditions that lead to an exaggeration of the *y descent* such as the first four causes in Table 2.

In the absence of pulmonary hypertension $x' = y$ can be seen in:
1. Pericardial effusion
2. Constrictive pericarditis with good myocardial function
3. Early and mild right ventricular infarction
4. Early cardiomyopathy
5. Some patients with atrial septal defect
6. This pattern is quite common in post-cardiac-surgery patients. It tends to develop quite early after the pump run and may persist for the life of the patient.

The dominant *y descent* ($x' < y$) pattern with or without pulmonary hypertension implies right ventricular dysfunction. In post-cardiac-surgery patients this pattern is less common and would imply right ventricular damage. The pattern, if noted in constrictive pericarditis, implies a late stage of constriction with myocardial dysfunction. In the presence of acute inferior infarction, this jugular pulse contour would imply right ventricular involvement *(30)*. The dominant *y descent* pattern is not usually seen in pure LV failure of acute myocardial infarction (*see* JVP Videofiles 4, 5, 9, and 10 on the Companion CD).

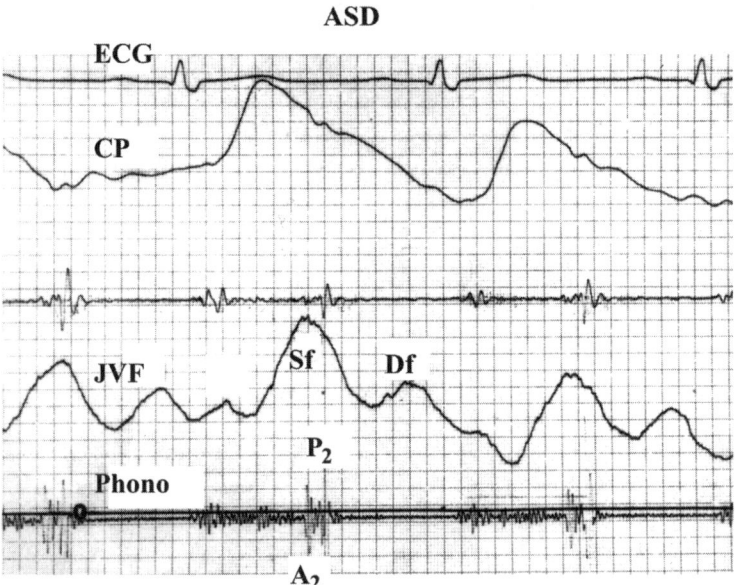

Fig. 25. Simultaneous recordings of electrocardiogram (ECG), carotid pulse (CP), phonocardiogram (Phono), and jugular venous flow velocity (JVF) in a patient with atrial septal defect (ASD). Note the splitting of S2 (A2 and P2). The important fact is that the Sf > Df flow pattern is maintained in ASD despite increased venous return to the right heart (double source of blood — normal venous return plus shunt flow). (Reproduced with kind permission from ref. 47.)

Venous Pulse Contour in Atrial Septal Defect

In adult patients with atrial septal defect, although the *y descent* may be visible, the *x′ descent* remains dominant. This is a result of the fact that the right ventricular volume overload provides a strong Starling effect augmenting its contraction (Fig. 25). In some adult patients with atrial septal defect, the pattern of *x′* = *y descent* may be observed. This is usually due to large defects with equalization of the right atrial and the left atrial pressures with elevated RV diastolic pressures.

Venous Pulse Contour in Constrictive Pericarditis

Elevated venous pressure with the sharp *y descent* and deep "*y trough*" in constrictive pericarditis has been known as the diastolic collapse of Friedreich for more than a century *(20)*. However, atypical cases, some with rapidly evolving "constrictive pericarditis," have been described, which show only a dominant *x′ descent* despite high venous pressure *(16,53)*. As expected in these patients, the RV early diastolic pressure was quite high, with very little pressure difference between the right atrium and the right ventricle at the time of tricuspid valve opening to account for the lack of a good *y descent*. This would be almost a hemodynamic imitation of tamponade to the extent that the restriction to ventricular filling also involved the early rapid filling phase.

Such a high elevation of early diastolic RV pressures in the absence of true extrinsic compression as in tamponade would imply poor systolic emptying of the right ventricle and decreased right ventricular systolic function (Figs. 4, 5, 16, and 17). Rarely such a situation could occur in severe cardiomyopathy. Such patients have poor *x′ descent*.

Ischaemic Cardiomyopathy

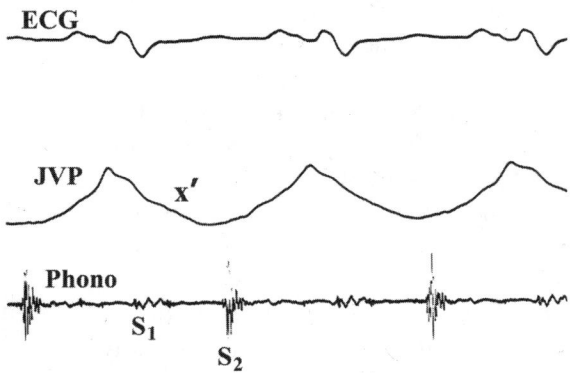

Fig. 26. Simultaneous recordings of electrocardiogram (ECG), jugular venous pulse (JVP), and phonocardiogram (Phono) in a patient with ischemic cardiomyopathy. The right ventricle (RV) is spared and the right heart function is normal, as evidenced by the good x' descent in the JVP. (Reproduced with kind permission from ref. 47.)

In fact, in patients with severe cardiomyopathy, preservation of a good *x' descent* would imply an ischemic etiology involving predominantly the left ventricle (Fig. 26).

Venous Pulse Contour in Severe Heart Failure

Patients with severe cardiac failure and poor RV systolic function will have high jugular venous pressure as a result of elevated *pre-a wave* and *v wave* pressures. The latter will be further raised in the jugulars secondary to high venous tone caused by the co-existent sympathetic stimulation *(19)*. The *x' descent* will be poor or lost. This may be aggravated by tricuspid regurgitation that may develop as a result of right ventricular dilatation. Atrial fibrillation may set in due to atrial overdistension. This will further diminish the *x' descent* as a result of the loss of the Starling effect. If early diastolic pressure in the RV falls to close to zero, as it should normally, then the y descent will be either dominant or the only descent noted (Fig. 6).

If the early diastolic RV pressures were also elevated during the rapid filling phase, as may happen in severely compromised RV with very poor compliance, then the *y descent* may be also poor even though the *v wave* pressure is elevated because of very little gradient of pressure between the atrium and the ventricle. The overall effect could be such that one would have high jugular pressure with poor descents.

Venous Pulse Contours in RV Infarction

RV infarction may complicate acute infero-posterior infarction, particularly when there is acute occlusion of a dominant right coronary artery in its proximal segment close to its origin. The RV, because of its thin walls and lower systolic pressure, has favorable systolic tension, which imposes less demands on oxygen compared to the left ventricle. If the hemodynamic failure is not severe with marked persistent hypotension and shock, the RV might recover most of its function. Nevertheless, during the acute phase, the ischemic dysfunction will alter both its diastolic compliance and systolic function. The extent of the functional derangement will depend on the acuteness and the extent of the ischemic insult. The latter may be modified by the severity and the chronicity of the underlying coronary atherosclerotic disease as well as the development of coronary collaterals. The hemodynamic compromise may be further complicated by disturbance in the sinoatrial (S-A) node and A-V nodal function caused by ischemia. The S-A nodal artery is often the first branch of the right coronary artery. The A-V nodal branch, however, arises further down where the right coronary artery takes the u-bend past the crux. The resulting arrhythmic disturbance may manifest as failure of sinus mechanism with development of junctional rhythms, first, second, or higher degrees of S-A and/or A-V block. If the right atrial branches, which arise from the proximal segment of the right coronary artery, are involved in the acute occlusion, it may cause atrial infarct, compromise the right atrial function, and may result in atrial arrhythmias such as atrial fibrillation.

In addition, the LV infero-posterior walls are often invariably the site of infarction and in severe cases often involve the posterior part of the interventricular septum. Acute RV dilatation might be accompanied by paradoxical septal motion. During diastole, the interventricular septum might encroach on the left side, restricting its filling, and during systole bulge towards the RV and move thus paradoxically. Acute and abrupt RV as well as the LV posterior wall dilatation might also cause intrapericardial pressures to rise. The pericardial constraint might further impair both RV and LV compliance and filling. Both the posterior septal infarct and pericardial constraint would be contributing to the paradoxical septal motion noted in severe cases.

When RV systolic dysfunction is significant, the *x' descent* will be diminished or absent. If the arterial supply to the right atrium is not compromised, there could be augmented and forceful contraction of the right atrium to support RV filling. Strong atrial contraction and the accompanying good atrial relaxation would cause the a wave and the *x descent* to be prominent. The latter also would help to accelerate venous inflow. The altered diastolic function and decreased compliance of the RV will lead to elevation of the *pre-a wave* pressure. This will raise the right atrial *a wave* and *v wave* pressures and consequently the mean right atrial pressure. The raised right atrial pressures will be reflected in the jugulars as well. As long as the RV diastolic dysfunction is not severe enough to raise the early diastolic pressure in the RV, the raised *v wave* will be accompanied by an exaggerated *y descent*. Therefore, the jugulars in these patients would show a diminished or absent *x' descent* with a dominant or single *y descent*. If the *x descent* is exaggerated because of forceful right atrial contraction and relaxation in the presence of normal PR interval, it would be indistinguishable from the *x' descent* at the bedside. This might actually cause the double descents with equal *x* and *y*. Sometimes the RV annular dilatation with or without right ventricular papillary muscle dysfunction could lead to tricuspid regurgitation of variable degree, raising further the right atrial *v wave* pressure.

When the diastolic dysfunction is severe, even the early diastolic pressure in the RV might become raised, blunting the *y descent* despite elevated *v wave* pressures. Such a profound elevation in the RV filling pressures is often indicative of severe RV infarction. This means that RV diastolic filling is compromised even in the early rapid filling phase. This of course is a hemodynamic imitator of cardiac pre-tamponade-like state with total diastolic restriction. This situation might be accompanied by RV dilatation as well as LV posterior wall dilatation. The pericardial constraint will lead to very high right atrial and jugular venous pressures. The blood can enter the tight space only when the blood can leave the space, namely during systole. In these patients one would see very little descent in the highly elevated venous column at the bedside. With recording of right atrial pressure, one may actually show some drop in the intra-atrial pressure during systole.

Looking for "w" and "m" patterns of waveforms described by some authors in relation to the right atrial pressure recordings, in the jugulars at the bedside will not be a fruitful exercise. In this context, because they also attribute the mechanism of the normal x' *descent* to the fall in intrapericardial pressure due to ventricular systolic emptying, a comment again on the mechanism of the normal x' *descent* needs to be made prevent confusion. The normal x' *descent* is essentially due to the descent of the base and not because of drop in intrapericardial pressure caused by ventricular systole. On the two-dimensional echocardiographic images, one can see the atrial area and consequently the volume expand with each systole as the contracting right and the left ventricles pull on the tricuspid and the mitral annulus, respectively (*see* Normal Subject image file in Jugular Venous Pulse, Normal on the Companion CD). Furthermore, the right atrial and therefore the jugular x' *descent* is selectively diminished gradually and eventually lost in chronic pulmonary hypertensive patients when RV failure sets in. In these patients, left atrial recording will confirm the presence of the normal left atrial pressure pulse contour with preserved x' *descent*. This disparity between the two sides should not be there if fall in the intra-pericardial pressure because of ventricular systole is the mechanism of the x' *descent*. Similarly, one can observe in patients with severe LV dysfunction with preserved right ventricular function, the x' *descent* will be preserved until pulmonary hypertension develops and begins to alter RV function. Intrapericardial pressure will play an important part when the pericardial space is compromised as in cardiac tamponade or situations that mimic the hemodynamics of cardiac tamponade with impediment to filling throughout diastole. This could arise in severely dilated hearts with failure and severely elevated filling pressures, rare patients with constrictive pericarditis, and some patients with severe RV infarction and shock.

Venous Pulse Contours in Ebstein's Anomaly

Ebstein's anomaly is a rare congenital defect in which the tricuspid valve is abnormally displaced downward towards the right ventricle. This implies that in this condition, the basal part of the right ventricle becomes atrialized. This results in a large right atrium, thereby increasing its capacitance. Sometimes the right atrium may be huge in size. The tricuspid valve may often be incompetent and lead to variable degrees of tricuspid regurgitation. In addition, the right ventricular systolic function will often be diminished. The effects of the diminished right ventricular function can be expected to decrease the x' *descent*. The tricuspid regurgitation, on the other hand, depending on its severity, can be expected to raise the right atrial v *wave* and cause the y *descent* to be exaggerated. Despite these changes in the right atrial pressure pulse contours, the jugulars may not reflect these adequately because of the large right atrial capacitance, which may have a buffering effect. In fact, the descents in the jugulars and the jugular pulsations may be hard to see even in the relatively young patients with this defect. It is important to consider a large sized right atrium with high capacitance effect as part of a differential diagnosis for an inconspicuous jugular contour in the young adult.

Rare Types of Double Descents

In the presence of a long PR interval, atrial relaxation and consequently the *x descent* is well separated from ventricular systole and therefore occur in diastole. This type of double descent (*x* and *x'*) may mimic the common *x'* and *y descents*. The second of a pair of descents per cardiac cycle, however, will be systolic and correspond to the radial pulse upstroke. With rapid heart rates, the diagnosis will require an ECG.

Two Descents in Diastole (Double Diastolic Descents)

Two descents in diastole imply the presence of an exaggerated *y descent* and an *x descent*, the latter because of long PR interval. This pattern is occasionally seen in heart failure with a dominant *v wave* and absent *x' descent* due to poor right ventricular function. The *a wave* is smaller and occurs early because of prolonged PR interval (Fig. 11) (*see* JVP Videofile 11 on Companion CD).

Triple Descents

Very rarely all three—*x*, *x'*, and *y—descents* may be separately visible simulating flutter waves. This again implies prolonged PR interval.

Flutter Waves

Flutter waves may be occasionally seen in patients with atrial flutter. In this rhythm, the atria contract generally 300 times per min with a varying ventricular rate, which in most untreated patients is usually about 150. Flutter waves are more likely to be seen only when the ventricular rate has been slowed spontaneously or secondary to therapy. In contrast to atrial fibrillation, the atrial contraction in patients with atrial flutter is often better organized and may generate pressure, and the atrial relaxation that follows may cause visible descents.

Single y Descent

This usually indicates poor right ventricular function. It is commonly seen in patients with chronic atrial fibrillation and congestive heart failure. When noted with a large amplitude and fast rising *v wave* before it, it would indicate tricuspid regurgitation. In tricuspid stenosis, the elevated *v wave* pressure has been described to be followed by so-called slow *y descent*. The slowing of the rate of fall of the *y descent*, even if truly present, is not usually striking enough to be detected in the jugulars (*see* JVP Videofiles 6 and 9 on the Companion CD).

Exaggerated Ascents of Waves

The normal *a* and *v wave* ascents representing low amplitude and slow rate of rise are not easily seen at the bedside. If the rise in waves is as rapid as the descents that follow and is associated with increased amplitude, it indicates retrograde flow in the jugulars, as in tricuspid regurgitation, *cannon waves* of atrioventricular dissociation, and in some cases with diminished right ventricular compliance and strong atrial contraction (giant *a wave*). A large-amplitude jugular *a wave* with rapid rise may occur in tricuspid stenosis, which is quite rare.

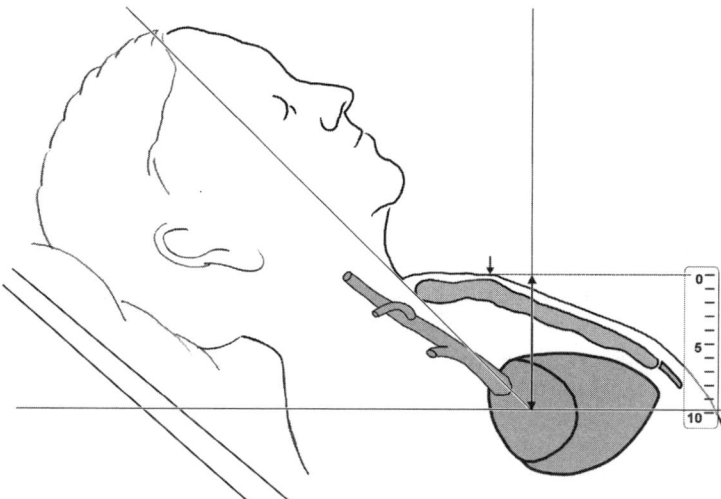

Fig. 27. Diagram showing a patient lying supine with the head tilted upward at 45° from the horizontal. The jugular venous pressure is measured by noting the level of the top of the moving jugular column in cm in vertical height from the external reference point of the sternal angle (SA). In this position the mid right atrium is about 8–10 cm in vertical height from the SA.

ASSESSMENT OF JUGULAR VENOUS PRESSURE

The normal right atrium functions as a capacitance chamber. The mean RA pressure is often quite low, often less than 5 mmHg. When assessed externally in relationship to the sternal angle with the patient's head placed at 45° upward tilt from the horizontal, the top of the moving jugular column does not exceed 4–5 cm in vertical height above the sternal angle. The recognition of the descents and their contour will make assessment of the jugular venous pressure quite easy. The top of the pulsations in the jugulars as transmitted to the skin overlying the sternomastoid muscle must be noted. Since the jugular and superior vena cava are in direct continuity with the right atrium, the estimation of the jugular venous pressure helps in the assessment of the central filling pressure in the right heart. The latter reflects the adequacy of the volume status of the patient as well as the right heart function. One must, however, always remember that the systemic venous or sympathetic tone influences the jugular column in addition to the right atrial pressure. For any given volume status or filling pressure in the right atrium, the level to which the jugular column will rise will depend on the degree of the venous tone as well.

The derivation of the right atrial mean pressure from the jugular venous pressure usually takes into account the approximate location of the mid right atrium from the sternal angle. The sternal angle is a surface anatomical mark. The right atrium can be at a variable distance from this external reference point, depending on the position of the patient. In the usual 45° upward tilt from the horizontal in which the patient is assessed, this distance in vertical height from the surface sternal angle can vary between 8 and 10 cm. The higher the tilt, the higher is this distance. When assessed at 90° tilt, the distance is almost 12 cm *(54)* (Fig. 27). This distance in cm is added to the level of jugular column in vertical height above the sternal angle in cm to derive the right atrial pressure in cmH$_2$O. The total can then be divided by 1.36 to get mmHg of pressure.

The jugular contour, unless associated with very high venous pressure, will not be visible if the patient is tilted too much upward from the horizontal. In fact, in many normal individuals the jugular descents will be observed only when they are almost lying flat. In some of the normals, the top of the jugular column may only be visible with patient lying flat or only slightly tilted, if at all. While estimation of the right atrial pressure from the jugular venous pressure by adjusting for the vertical height of the right atrium from the sternal angle may be of interest, it is not absolutely necessary. One can simply have a normal range of jugular venous pressure in vertical height in cm from the usual external reference point of the sternal angle. Based on this normal range one can decide whether in a given patient the jugular venous pressure is normal, low, or high. A simple figure for the normal range is 4–5 cm above the sternal angle at 45° of upward tilt. In fact, this level is usually obtained only in younger subjects. In the elderly, this level is generally even lower.

Hepato-Jugular Reflux

When compression is applied to the abdomen during normal respirations, the jugular venous pressure will be seen to increase transiently in normal subjects. Usually within a few cardiac cycles the pressure falls back to the precompression level. When the same maneuver is performed in a patient with heart failure, the venous pressure will increase and stay increased until the pressure is released. This is termed a positive *hepato-jugular reflux (12,32,55)*.

This test should be performed with care to avoid discomfort or pain to the patient. If pain is produced, then it may cause the test to become falsely positive. In addition, the patient should not hold the breath or perform a Valsalva maneuver during the compression. Finally, the compression should be applied for at least 30 s.

The rise in venous pressure has been attributed to a rise in the intra-abdominal pressure causing a rise in intrathoracic pressure. Subsequently, others have attributed this effect to high sympathetic tone. A positive *hepato-jugular reflux* is known to occur in conditions with high sympathetic tone even in the absence of heart failure (e.g., thyrotoxicosis, anemia, hypoxemia).

With compression of the abdomen, the intra-abdominal pressure rises. The diaphragm is therefore forced towards the thorax. In patients with normal vital capacity and normal lung reserve this does not significantly change the respiratory pattern. The rise in the intra-abdominal pressure increases the venous return from the viscera in the abdomen to the thorax. In normal subjects this increased volume is easily accommodated without any sustained rise in pressure in the venous capacitance system, including the superior vena cava and the jugulars. The initial rise is usually because of a transient rise in sympathetic tone caused by some apprehension on the part of the patient when compression is applied. In states with sustained elevation in sympathetic tone, the capacitance of the thoracic great veins is reduced due to veno-constriction. This will result in sustained rise in venous pressure. In patients with heart failure, the sympathetic tone is increased, therefore always resulting in a positive test *(55)*. If pain is caused during compression, this may raise the sympathetic tone and result in a false positive test.

In patients with chronic obstructive lung disease, a false positive test may be seen because of high intra thoracic pressure created by the change in the patient's breathing pattern, which opposes the upward movement of the diaphragm. This is also a sign of decreased lung reserve.

Obstruction of the Superior Vena Cava

When there is partial obstruction of the superior vena cava, the jugular venous pulsations may be still noted although the venous pressure may become elevated. When there is complete obstruction, the venous pressure will become markedly elevated, and the veins in the arms may also become distended. Superficial collateral flow will become easily visible with the flow directed towards the abdomen. At this stage no jugular pulsations will be observed.

CLINICAL ASSESSMENT OF THE JUGULAR VENOUS PULSE

The foregoing principles of jugular physiology and pathophysiology can be simply and very easily brought to the bedside if certain points are kept in mind and applied when assessing a patient. Jugular pulse recordings obtained with electronically amplified transducers often cause artificial exaggeration of the *a*, *c*, and *v waves*. Recognition of the jugular pulse contours and interpretation become difficult only if the usual textbook description of the *a*, *c*, and *v waves* based on such jugular recordings are searched for at the bedside.

Points to remember are:
1. Descents in the jugular venous pulse are easy to see because they are fast movements down. Objects moving away from the eyes of the observer are better seen than ones moving towards the observer. The descents reflect flow acceleration. Normal jugular wave ascents are slow rises of pressure and therefore are hard to see. If the wave rises are prominent as well and easily seen, then they are abnormal and reflect retrograde flow in the jugulars.
2. Technique of recognition of the descents: Internal jugular pulsations are often transmitted to the skin overlying the sternomastoid and sometimes over a wide area of the skin adjacent to it and above the clavicle. One should not get too close to the neck of the patient. In fact, standing at the bedside with the patient properly positioned and feeling the radial artery pulse at the same time, one should look for any fast movement down overlying the jugulars, as mentioned. Rapid downward movements that synchronize with the radial arterial pulse upstroke will immediately be identified as the jugular *x′ descent*. Simultaneous palpation of the radial arterial pulse, even when one searches for the jugular pulse, must be encouraged because this way the normal *x′ descent* is quickly identified. Movements of the soft tissues of the neck related to respiration can easily be distinguished as well. Sometimes the descents may be observed to move even a chain or necklace that the patient may be wearing. Throwing shadows over the skin overlying the jugulars and the sternomastoid muscle using natural light or an artificial light source and watching the movement of the shadow also helps in identifying the movement. Occasionally descents may also be seen in the external jugulars because of inadequacy of the venous valves.
3. Arterial pulse has a fast rise, whereas the jugulars have a fast fall. That is the best way to distinguish the arterial pulsation in the neck from the jugular movement. External pressure applied below the pulsations over the sternomastoid will help to occlude the venous pulsations and not the carotid pulsation. When the venous pressure is high with marked tricuspid regurgitation, this technique will not work.

Arterial pulsation does not last long, whereas the *v wave* of tricuspid regurgitation lasts longer.

4. Once the descent or descents are noted, one should time them with the radial arterial pulse or the second heart sound (S2). Radial arterial pulse upstroke is the easiest and the simplest for timing. This timing with the radial pulse is not by any means like timing an Olympic photo finish or microsecond timing. In other words, one should be simply able to call each time a descent is seen as "down," " down" while feeling the pulse at the same time. This can be easily demonstrated even while teaching a group of several students at the bedside. One can be made to call the descent each time it is seen while another calls the pulse each time the upstroke is felt. The descent which is simultaneous with the pulse is the x' *descent*, while the descent which is out of phase with the pulse is the *y descent*. The x' *descent* falls onto the S2, while the *y descent* comes after the S2.

5. In most normal adults what one will see is simply one large downward movement or descent, which will be synchronous with the pulse. This jugular contour of the normal adult can be simply described as showing single x' *descent*. It immediately implies a normal contour. In young subjects one may see a major descent in systole with the pulse and a much smaller descent slightly after the pulse, indicating the pattern of the x' *descent* followed by a small *y descent*. This contour can be described as a dominant x' *descent*. This description implies the presence of a small *y descent*. Occasionally there may be a slight hesitation in the systolic descent because of the presence of an *x descent* (caused by atrial relaxation) quickly followed by the x' *descent*, which is of course caused by the descent of the base. The combined movement will still be synchronous with the pulse, indicating a normal contour.

6. The presence of the x' *descent* in normal regular sinus rhythm implies the presence of the *a wave* before it, although not seen to rise prominently. The presence of even a small diastolic or *y descent* (as compared to the x' or systolic descent) implies that there is a *v wave*, although not rising prominently. Therefore, one needs to simply describe the descent pattern alone when the wave rises are not prominent.

7. Single x' *descent* or the dominant x' *descent* patterns in the jugulars imply good right ventricular systolic function and in addition indicate the absence of significant tricuspid regurgitation.

8. If two descents are seen for each cardiac cycle, these will be generally because of a combination of the x' and the *y descents*. Rarely it may be because of the combination of an *x descent* well separated from the x' *descent* because of the presence of a long PR interval. This can only be diagnosed with the help of an ECG. This is usually not the common cause of the double descents in the jugular pulse. The more usual combination is because of the presence of both the x' and the *y descents*. This is identified by the fact that the first of each pair will be systolic in timing, i.e., occurring with the radial pulse.

9. When two descents are seen to each cardiac cycle, then one must observe the relationship of the two to decide the relative dominance of the descents. If both descents are equally prominent, then the pattern is $x' = y$. If one of them is less prominent than the other, the pattern will be either $x' > y$ or $x' < y$.

10. Double descents are clearly abnormal in the adult, even when they are $x' > y$. This could be normal in young subjects or pregnant women. However, in these situations the pattern has to be $x' > y$.

11. In all cases of double descents one should consider causes of decreased x' *descent* as well as factors that may exaggerate the *y descent*.
12. The x' *descent* is decreased if there is right ventricular dysfunction in the presence of atrial fibrillation because of lack of atrial kick and in the presence of significant tricuspid regurgitation.
13. Exaggerated *y descent* requires an increased v wave pressure head with no restriction to ventricular filling in early diastole. This mechanism excludes cardiac tamponade in which filling restriction occurs throughout diastole.
14. Because double descents can occur with and without the context of pulmonary hypertension, they may be approached accordingly. These are discussed in detail in the text. Since jugular contour abnormalities are not specific for pulmonary hypertension, diagnosis of pulmonary hypertension must be made on the basis of other clinical findings, such as a loud or palpable pulmonic component of the second heart sound, sustained subxiphoid right ventricular impulse, and/or electrocardiographic evidence of right ventricular hypertrophy. Absence of these signs does not necessarily exclude the presence of pulmonary hypertension, and therefore further tests may have to be taken to exclude or confirm the presence of pulmonary hypertension. Two-dimensional echocardiogram, particularly with the Doppler assessment for tricuspid regurgitation jet, if identified, will often help in this respect. Peak tricuspid regurgitation velocity, if identified, can be related to the pressure difference between the right ventricle and the right atrium. The pressure difference is approximately four times the velocity squared (pressure gradient = $4 \times v^2$).
15. In the presence of pulmonary hypertension, the relative dominance of the x' vs the *y descent* reveals the adequacy or otherwise of the right ventricular systolic function. The $x' > y$ pattern is indicative of compensated right ventricular function. When it is $x' = y$, it probably means beginning right ventricular dysfunction. The pattern $x' < y$ definitely is a late pattern indicating right ventricular decompensation.
16. In the absence of pulmonary hypertension $x' = y$ is usually normal for a post-cardiac-surgery patient. In the patient who has not had previous cardiac surgery, other conditions such as pericardial effusion with some restriction, constrictive pericarditis, cardiomyopathy, or mild or early right ventricular infarction in the context of acute inferior myocardial infarction need to be considered. Similar pattern can also be seen in some patients with atrial septal defect. If the pattern were $x' < y$, it would in addition indicate significant right ventricular systolic dysfunction.
17. If the descent is single and is out of phase with the radial pulse, the pattern can be described as single *y descent*. It indicates significant right ventricular dysfunction. This is the common pattern seen in patients with chronic atrial fibrillation and heart failure with right ventricular dysfunction.
18. Prominent rises of either the *a wave* or the *v wave* in the jugulars imply flow reversal in the jugulars. If it is seen to precede the x' *descent*, it must be the *a wave*, and if it precedes a *y descent*, then it must be the *v wave* of tricuspid regurgitation.
19. The *a wave* as opposed to the *v wave* has a shorter duration, like a flicker. They occur regularly in the context of resistance to ventricular filling with a strong atrial contraction causing end-diastolic flow reversal. They can occur irregularly because of simultaneous right atrial and right ventricular contraction in

situations of atrioventricular dissociation. In this instance they are termed *cannon waves*.

20. The *v wave*, on the other hand, precedes the *y descent*. When a single *y descent* is noted, one must try to assess the prominence of the wave rise preceding it. If it were of large amplitude and rising actively as well, it would indicate the presence of tricuspid regurgitation. It will be seen to rise with the arterial pulse but will last longer than the arterial pulse in duration. The *v wave* of tricuspid regurgitation is often visible from a distance and may be seen well with the patient sitting up. It indicates quite clearly systolic flow reversal in the jugulars (*see* JVP Videofiles 1–11 on the Companion CD).

REFERENCES

1. Harvey W. Exercitatio Anatomica de Motu Cordis et Sanguinis in Animalibus, Frankfurt, Gugliemi Fitzeri, 1628 (English translation by Leake CD. Springfield, IL: Charles C Thomas, 1949).
2. Purkinje JL. Über die Saugkraft des Herzens Übersicht der Arbeiten und Veränderungen der schlesischen Gesellschaft für vaterländische Kultur im Jahre. 1843:147.
3. Chauveau A, Marey E. Appareilles et experiences cardiographiques par l'emploi des instruments enregistreures a indications continues. Mem Acad Med 1863; 26:268.
4. Lancisi JM. Motus Cordis et Aneurysmatibus. Rome: 1728.
5. Potain PCE. Des mouvements et des bruits qui se faissent dans les veines. Mem Soc Med Hop Paris 1867; 4:3.
6. Mackenzie J. The Study of the Pulse. London: Pentland, 1902.
7. Mackenzie J. The interpretation of the pulsations in the jugular veins. Am J Med Sci 1907; 134:12.
8. Wiggers CJ. Modern Aspects of the Circulation in Health and Disease. Philadelphia: Lea & Febiger, 1923.
9. Russek HI, Zohman BL. The syndrome of Bernheim. Am Heart J 1945;30:427.
10. Bloomfield RA, Lauson HD, Cournand A, Breed ES, Richards DW, Jr. Recording of right heart pressures in normal subjects and in patients with chronic pulmonary disease and various types of cardio-circulatory disease. J Clin Invest 1946;25:639.
11. Hansen AT, Eskildsen P, Gorzsche H. Pressure curves from the right auricle and the right ventricle in chronic constrictive pericarditis. Circulation 1951;3:881.
12. Burch GE, Ray CT. Mechanism of the hepatojugular reflux test in congestive heart failure. Am Heart J 1954;48:373.
13. Wilson RH, Hoseth W, Sadoff C, Dempsey ME. Pathologic physiology and diagnostic significance of the pressure pulse tracing in heart in patients with constrictive pericarditis and pericardial effusion. Am Heart J 1954;48:671–683.
14. Reinhold J. Venous pulse in atrial septal defect: a clinical sign. Br Med J 1955;1:695.
15. Cossio P, Buzzi A. Clinical value of the venous pulse. Am Heart J 1957;54:127.
16. Gibson R. Atypical constrictive pericarditis. Br Heart J 1959;21:583.
17. Hartman. H. The jugular venous tracing. Am Heart J 1960;59:698–717.
18. Perloff JK, Harvey PW. Clinical recognition of tricuspid stenosis. Circulation 1960;22:346–364.
19. Sharpey-Schafer EP. Venous tone. Br Med J 1961;2:1589.
20. Wood P. Chronic constrictive pericarditis. Am J Cardiol 1961;7:48.
21. Lange RL, Botticelli JT, Tsagaris TJ, Walker JA, Gani M, Bustamante RA. Diagnostic signs in compressive cardiac disorders. Constrictive pericarditis, pericardial effusion, and tamponade. Circulation 1966;33:763–777.
22. Colman AL. Clinical Examination of the Jugular Venous Pulse. Springfield, IL: Charles C Thomas, 1966.
23. Wood P. Diseases of the Heart and Circulation. Philadelphia: J.B. Lippincott, 1968.
24. Tavel ME, Bard RA, Franks LC, Feigenbaum H, Fisch C. The jugular venous pulse in atrial septal defect. Arch Intern Med 1968;121:524–529.
25. Rich LL, Tavel ME. The origin of the jugular C wave. N Engl J Med 1971;284:1309–1311.

26. Constant J. The X prime descent in jugular contour nomenclature and recognition. Am Heart J 1974;88:372.
27. Holt JP, Rhode EA, Kines H. Pericardial and ventricular pressure. Circ Res 1960;8:1171.
28. Harley A. Persistent right atrial standstill. Br Heart J 1976;38:646.
29. Matsuhisa M, Shimomura K, Beppu S, Nakajima K. Post-operative changes of jugular pulse tracing. J Cardiography 1976;6:403.
30. Jensen DP, Goolsby JP, Jr., Oliva PB. Hemodynamic pattern resembling pericardial constriction after acute inferior myocardial infarction with right ventricular infarction. Am J Cardiol 1978;42:858–861.
31. Coma-Canella I, Lopez-Sendon J. Ventricular compliance in ischemic right ventricular dysfunction. Am J Cardiol 1980;45:555–551.
32. Constant J. Bedside Cardiology, 3rd ed. Boston: Little Brown, 1985.
33. Matsuhisa M, Shimomura K, Beppu S, Nakajima K. Jugular phlebogram in congenital absence of the pericardium. Am Heart J 1986;112:1004–1010.
34. Brecher GA. Cardiac variations in venous return studied with a new bristle flowmeter. Am J Physiol 1954;176:423.
35. Brawley RK, Oldham HN, Vasko JS, Henney RP, Morrow AG. Influence of right atrial pressure pulse on instantaneous vena caval blood flow. Am J Physiol 1966;211:347–353.
36. Pinkerson AL, Luria MH, Freis ED. Effect of cardiac rhythm on vena caval blood flows. Am J Physiol 1966;210:505–508.
37. Wexler L, Bergel DH, Gabe IT, Makin GS, Mills CJ. Velocity of blood flow in normal human venae cavae. Circ Res 1968;23:349–359.
38. Froysaker T. Abnormal flow pattern in the superior vena cava induced by arrhythmias. A peroperative flowmetric study in man. Scand J Thorac Cardiovasc Surg 1972;6:140–148.
39. Kalmanson D, Veyrat C, Chiche P. Atrial versus ventricular contribution in determining systolic venous return. A new approach to an old riddle. Cardiovasc Res 1971;5:293–302.
40. Sivaciyan V, Ranganathan N. Transcutaneous doppler jugular venous flow velocity recording. Circulation 1978;57:930–939.
41. Ranganathan N, Sivaciyan V. Abnormalities in jugular venous flow velocity in pulmonary hypertension. Am J Cardiol 1989;63:719–724.
42. Ranganathan N, Sivaciyan V, Pryszlak M, Freeman MR. Changes in jugular venous flow velocity after coronary artery bypass grafting. Am J Cardiol 1989;63:725–729.
43. Shabetai R, Fowler NO, Guntheroth WG. The hemodynamics of cardiac tamponade and constrictive pericarditis. Am J Cardiol 1970;26:480–489.
44. Rittenhouse EA, Barnes RW. Hemodynamics of cardiac tamponade: early recognition from jugular venous flow velocity. J Surg Res 1975;19:35–41.
45. Nelson RM, Jenson, C.B., and Smoot, W. M.: Pericardial tamponade following open heart surgery. J Thorac Cardiovasc Surg 1969;58:510.
46. Gabe IT, Gault JH, Ross J, Jr., et al. Measurement of instantaneous blood flow velocity and pressure in conscious man with a catheter-tip velocity probe. Circulation 1969;40:603–614.
47. Ranganathan N, Sivaciyan V. Jugular venous flow velocity pattern, application to bedside recognition of jugular venous pulse contour and right heart hemodynamics. Am J Noninvas Cardiol 1993;7:75–88.
48. Kalmanson D, Veyrat C, Chicke P. Venous return disturbances induced by arrhythmias. A transcutaneous, instantaneous, flowmetric study at the site of the jugular vein. Cardiovasc Res 1970;4:279–290.
49. Froysaker T. Anomalies of the superior vena caval flow pattern in patients with tricuspid insufficiency. Scand J Thorac Cardiovasc Surg 1972;6:234–245.
50. Bernheim P. De la stenose ventriculaire droite. Rev Gen Clin Ther J Pract. 1915; 29:721.
51. Bilchick KC, Wise RA. Paradoxical physical findings described by Kussmaul: pulsus paradoxus and Kussmaul's sign. Lancet 2002;359:1940–1942.
52. Wann LS, Morris SN, Tavel ME. Effects of cardiopulmonary bypass on the jugular venous pulse. Am Heart J 1977;94:262–264.
53. Kesteloot H, Denef B. Value of reference tracings in diagnosis and assessment of constrictive epi- and pericarditis. Br Heart J 1970;32:675–682.
54. Saunders DE, Jr, Adcock DF, Head DS. Relationship of sternal angle right atrium in clinical measurement of jugular venous pressure. J Am Coll Cardiol 1988;11, No.2:89A.
55. Constant J, Lippschutz EJ. The one minute abdominal compression test or "the hepatojugular reflux," a useful bedside test. Am Heart J 1964;67:701.

5

Precordial Pulsations

CONTENTS

MECHANICS AND PHYSIOLOGY OF THE NORMAL APICAL IMPULSE
PHYSICAL PRINCIPLES GOVERNING THE FORMATION
  OF THE APICAL IMPULSE
NORMAL APICAL IMPULSE AND ITS DETERMINANTS
ASSESSMENT OF THE APICAL IMPULSE
LEFT PARASTERNAL AND STERNAL MOVEMENTS
RIGHT PARASTERNAL MOVEMENT
PULSATIONS OVER THE CLAVICULAR HEADS
PULSATIONS OVER THE SECOND AND/OR THIRD LEFT
  INTERCOSTAL SPACES
SUBXIPHOID IMPULSE
PRACTICAL POINTS IN THE CLINICAL ASSESSMENT
  OF PRECORDIAL PULSATIONS
REFERENCES

In this chapter the pulsations of the precordium will be discussed in relation to their identification, the mechanisms of their origin, and their pathophysiological and clinical significance.

Precordial pulsations include the "apical impulse," left parasternal movement, right parasternal movement, pulsations of the clavicular heads, pulsations over the second left intercostal space, and subxiphoid impulses.

MECHANICS AND PHYSIOLOGY OF THE NORMAL APICAL IMPULSE

Since during systole the heart contracts, becoming smaller and therefore moving away from the chest wall, why should one feel a systolic outward movement (the apical impulse) at all? Logically speaking there should not be an apical impulse.

Several different methods of recording the precordial motion have been used to study the apical impulse going back to the late 19th century [1,2]. Among the more modern methods, the notable ones are the recordings of the apexcardiogram [3–17], the impulse cardiogram [18], and the kinetocardiogram [19–21]. While apexcardiography records the relative displacement of the chest wall under the transducer pickup device, which is often held by the examiner's hands, the proponents of the impulse cardiography and kinetocardiography point out that these methods allow the recording of the absolute movement of the chest wall because the pickup device is anchored to a fixed point held in space away from the chest. Kinetocardiography uses a flexible metal bellows probe coupled by air transmission to the manometer. The impulse cardiogram, on the other hand, utilizes a light metal rod with a flag at one end, held by light metal springs attached to a Perspex cone. The light metal rod with the flag is coupled directly to a photoelectric cell, the instrument being held rigidly in a metal clamp fixed to a stand. Despite its limitations, apexcardiography has been extensively studied with simultaneous left ventricular pressures obtained through high-fidelity recordings with the use of catheter-tipped micromanometers *(8,14,15)*. These studies have demonstrated clearly that the upslope of the apexcardiogram corresponds closely to the rise of the pressure in the left ventricle during the isovolumic phase of systole. The summit of the systolic upstroke of the apexcardiogram (the E point) occurs about 37 ms after the opening of the aortic valve and roughly 40 ms after the development of the peak *dP/dt* of the left ventricular pressure in normal subjects *(15)*. These observations are also consistent with the findings obtained using kinetocardiography *(20)*. When the apical impulse is recorded by kinetocardiography, it is seen to begin about 80 ms after the onset of the QRS in the electrocardiogram and about 10 or 20 ms before the carotid pulse upstroke. These observations indicate, therefore, that the apical impulse begins to rise during the pre-ejection phase of the left ventricular contraction and must therefore involve part of the isovolumic phase of systole, and the peak movement must involve the early rapid ejection phase of systole.

Timed angiographic studies of Deliyannis and co-workers *(22)* show that the portion of the heart underlying the apex beat is usually the anterior wall of the left ventricle, which moves forward during early systole and moves away and backward from the chest wall during mid-late systole. They suggest that the forward movement of the left ventricle in early systole is caused by the contraction of the middle circular fibers, which are confined to the upper three-fifths of the normal heart. The falling away of the apex of the left ventricle in late systole is attributed to the contraction of the spirally oriented fibers overlying the apex of the left ventricle, since in the normal heart the middle circular fibers do not extend to the apex. They further suggest that in left ventricular hypertrophy, the middle circular fibers extend to the apex completely, thereby preventing the movement away of the apex from the chest wall in mid-late systole (according to these authors accounting for a sustained duration of the apical movement when there is underlying left ventricular hypertrophy).

A variety of explanations have been given for the presence of the normal apical impulse. The common explanation is that the heart rotates counterclockwise along its long axis during contraction, causing the left ventricle to swing forward to hit the chest wall *(23–25)*. This twisting motion has been observed in the beating heart when exposed at surgery. This rotation is along the axis of the left ventricle. Torsional deformation of the left ventricular midwall in human hearts with intramyocardial markers has in fact been demonstrated. This appears to have some regional nonuniformity. Torsional deformation appears to be maximal in the apical lateral wall, intermediate in the apical inferior wall, and minimal in the anteroapical wall. Torsional changes were less at the midventricular level compared to the apical segments with similar regional variation. The exact cause of the regional variations is not defined. The possible causes suggested by these authors include variations in the left ventricular fiber architecture as well as the asymmetrical attachment of the left ventricle to the mitral annulus posteriorly and the aortic root anteriorly *(26)*. The papillary muscles together with the underlying left ventricular myocardium contract during systole to keep the mitral leaflets together in the closed position, preventing their eversion into the left atrium with the rising intraventricular pressure. In the process, the closed mitral apparatus must exert an opposite pull on the individual papillary muscle groups. It is possible that the asymmetrical attachment of the mitral apparatus to the left ventricle may result in an asymmetrical pull on the papillary muscles with a stronger pull on the antero-lateral papillary muscle group and the underlying left ventricular myocardium compared to the pull exerted on the postero-medial papillary muscle group. This might also be a contributory factor in the accentuated torsional changes seen in the apical lateral walls. In addition, during the phase of isovolumic contraction, it has been shown that there is an increase in the external circumference of the left ventricle together with a decrease in the base-to-apex length *(27)*. However, these changes during systole alone are still insufficient to explain the apical impulse, which must result from hitting of the inside of the chest by the left ventricle.

Because during systole all fibers contract and the ventricular walls thicken all around, the overall size becomes smaller the moment ejection begins, and therefore the heart would not be expected to come closer to the chest wall. Thus, the genesis of the apical impulse is poorly explained by these mechanisms alone.

The formation of the apical impulse is perhaps better understood when simple principles of physics are also considered, since they are applicable in relation to the heart and the great vessels. Stapleton refers to these indirectly when he states that the apical impulse "probably represents recoil movement which develops as left ventricular output meets aortic resistance"*(20)*.

PHYSICAL PRINCIPLES GOVERNING THE FORMATION OF THE APICAL IMPULSE

The heart is essentially a pump connected to the aorta and the pulmonary artery, both of which are conduits of fluid (blood). Therefore, pure physical principles of hydrodynamics should be sufficient to explain the mechanism of the apical impulse formation with one important anatomical consideration, which is the fact that the aorta is essentially a coiled pipe (aortic arch) and fixed posteriorly at the descending segment.

Newton's third law of motion indicates that for every action there is equal and opposite reaction. This effect is easily demonstrated in a simple physics experiment (Figs. 1A,B and 2). Similarly, as the left ventricle contracts and the intracavitary pressure rises during the isovolumic contraction phase (after the mitral valve closure and before the aortic valve opening), this pressure is equally distributed on all the walls of the left ventricle, including the apex and the closed aortic valve. There could be some change in shape and possibly torsional deformation during the time of the peak acceleration of the left ventricular pressure development. No appreciable motion of the heart occurs, however, because forces on the opposing walls balance out. This equilibrium is disturbed once the aortic valve opens and ejection begins. As in the physics experiment, similar to the beaker's movement in the direction opposite to the flow of water, the unopposed force on the apex of the left ventricle will move the left ventricle downward (Figs. 3A,B).

Ejection of fluid under pressure into a coiled pipe will have a tendency to straighten out the pipe as is commonly observed with the coiled garden hose as the water is turned on. With the aorta representing a coiled pipe, ejection of the left ventricular stroke volume into the aorta under pressure will have a tendency to straighten the aortic arch.

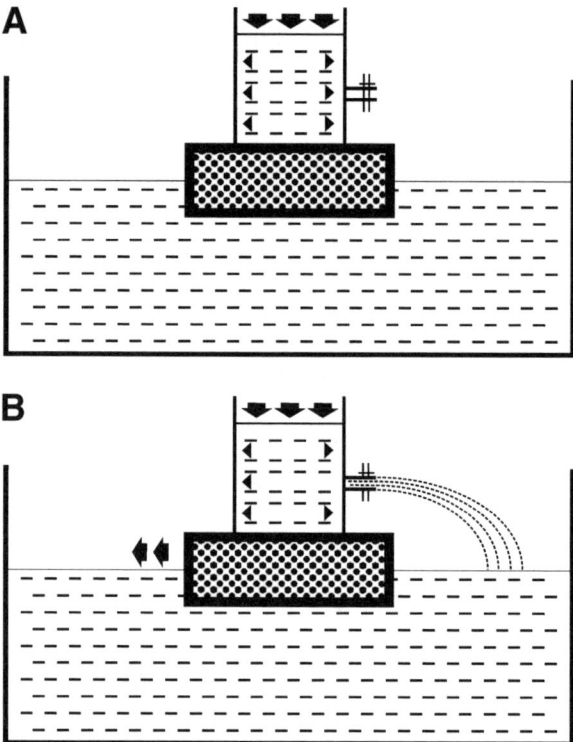

Fig. 1. (**A**) Atmospheric pressure (bold arrows) exerted on water in the beaker is evenly distributed on all sides of the beaker (short arrows in beaker), and the system is in equilibrium. (**B**) When the tap on the beaker is opened and the water runs out, the forces pushing on the left side of the beaker are no longer balanced by equal and opposite forces; therefore, the beaker and the cork it is sitting on will move to the left.

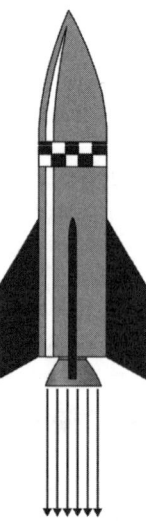

Fig. 2. Rocket propulsion is also based on the same principle of Newton's third law of motion. As the pressure escapes from the bottom of the combustion chamber of the rocket, the forces pushing up are no longer balanced by equal opposing forces and push the rocket upward.

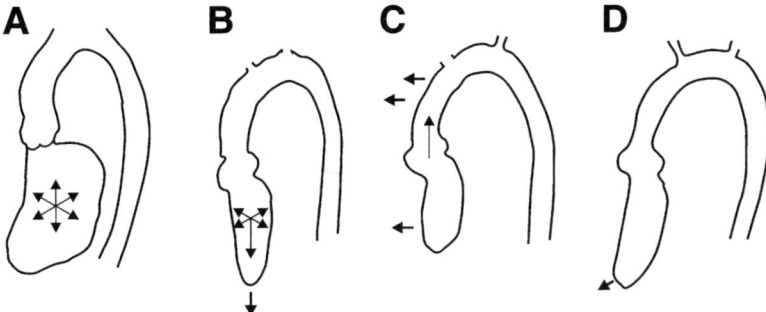

Fig. 3. (A) During isovolumic contraction, pressure in the left ventricle rises and is equally distributed on all walls of the left ventricle and no appreciable movement occurs. (B) As the aortic valve opens and blood is ejected out into the aorta, the force against the apex is no longer balanced by equal and opposite force and pushes the heart downward. (C) As the aortic valve opens and a large volume is ejected under pressure into the aorta during systole, the aortic arch being a coil will have a tendency to uncoil (recoil), thus pulling the left ventricle, which is attached to it, outward and forward with it. (D) The combined effect of the two forces on the left ventricle cause it to move downward and forward, giving rise to the apical impulse.

The aortic arch being anatomically fixed posteriorly (descending segment of the arch), only its anterior portion (the ascending segment of the arch) can recoil. This recoiling force will move the left ventricle upward and forward toward the chest wall [20] (Fig. 3C).

The resultant effect of the two forces described above will move the apex of the left ventricle toward the chest wall during systole despite the fact that the left ventricle is contracting and becoming smaller (Fig. 3D). The force and the extent of the resultant impulse that is felt on the chest wall by the examining hand as the apical impulse will be determined by both the cardiac function as well as the extracardiac attenuating factors.

The force with which the heart will move and hit the inside of the chest wall will depend on the two physical principles discussed above. The velocity of ejection, which is a reflection of the force of myocardial contractility under any given preload and afterload or impedance to ejection, is an important determinant of the momentum attained by the heart as it moves toward the chest wall according to Newton's third law of motion. The amount of blood ejected into the aorta for each beat (the stroke volume), as well as the peak systolic pressure reached, will determine the amount of recoil of the aorta, thus adding to the momentum of the heart. The force of the moving heart will compress the soft tissues between the ribs, allowing the impulse to be transmitted to the outside, where it is felt.

The transmission of the apical impulse can be affected by the characteristics of the chest wall. It is well known that the apical impulse may not be felt in patients with certain chest wall deformities, obese patients with thick chest walls, and those with stiff and fixed rib cage (e.g., ankylosing spondylitis and some elderly patients) [23,24]. Intervening lung tissue may also interfere with proper transmission of the impulse by absorbing the force as a cushion as it commonly happens in patients with chronic lung disease [24]. Similarly large pericardial and/or pleural effusion on the left side can cushion the force and prevent its transmission.

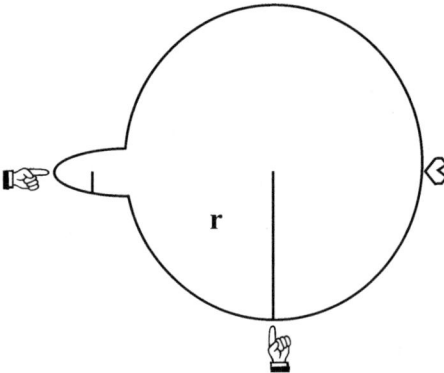

Fig. 4. A partially inflated balloon has the same pressure in the body of the balloon as well as in the nipple. However, the resistance felt by the poking finger is different in the body compared to the nipple. This is because of differences in the wall tension caused by differences in the radii (r) by Laplace's law.

NORMAL APICAL IMPULSE AND ITS DETERMINANTS

If an iron ball caused the impact on the inside of the chest wall, it would maximally compress the soft tissues of the chest wall, transmitting all the momentum to the outside of the chest wall. On the other hand, if the impact on the inside of the chest wall were caused by a cotton ball, it would become compressed by the impact, resulting in no appreciable impulse on the outside.

The same difference of transmission would be noted if the inside of the chest wall was to be impacted by the side of a balloon as opposed to the nipple at the tip of a balloon, which is not fully inflated. The nipple, being soft, cannot compress the tissues and instead will be compressed easily. Both the nipple and the inflated portion of the balloon form one single chamber having the same pressure. Applying *Laplace's law* where,

$$\text{Tension} = P \text{ (pressure)} \times r \text{ (radius)}$$

for a thin-walled cylindrical shell, and if the wall has a thickness, the circumferential wall stress is given by *Lamé's equation*, as follows:

$$\text{Tension} \propto \frac{P \text{ (pressure)} \times r \text{ (radius)}}{2h \text{ (wall thickness)}}$$

It becomes obvious that the difference in the radii of the nipple and the body of the balloon account for the difference in their wall tensions and therefore their respective compressibility (Fig. 4). The apical impulse that is felt during systole is similarly a reflection of the relative noncompressibility of the wall of the left ventricle because of the developed wall tension.

In a normal left ventricle during a normal cardiac cycle, the left ventricle has maximum volume or radius at the end of diastole. However, because the end-diastolic pressure is relatively low (around 12 mmHg), the wall tension is relatively low and also there is no appreciable motion of the heart. As the pressure rises during the isovolumic contraction phase, the left ventricular wall tension will also rise, reaching a peak just before the opening of the aortic valve (Fig. 5).

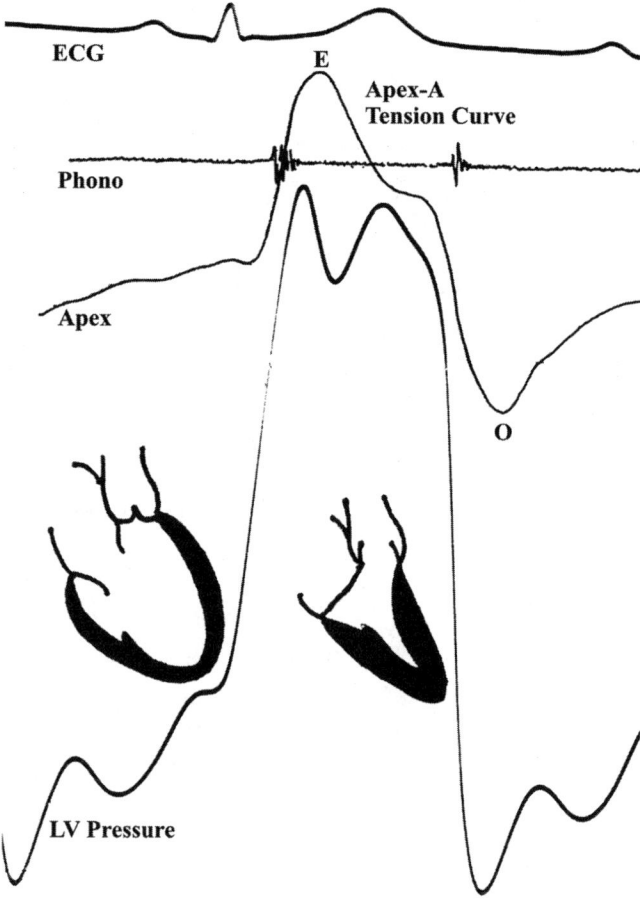

Fig. 5. Simultaneous recording of electrocardiogram (ECG), phonocardiogram (Phono), apexcardiogram (Apex), and left ventricular (LV) pressure curve. Also shown is the left ventricular outline in diastole and systole. The apexcardiogram, which is a recording of the apex beat normally felt, basically depicts a tension curve taking into account both the pressure and the radius of the LV.

Once ejection begins, the heart moves as explained previously, bringing the tense left ventricular wall against the chest wall. The left ventricular wall tension, however, will begin to fall with onset of ejection and decrease as the ventricle becomes smaller in systole. The systolic thickening of the wall during this phase also will tend to reduce the wall tension further. Because the left ventricle ejects most of its volume during the early part of systole (first third), the tension will have reached a low level by the end of this phase. The wall tension will continue to fall in late systole as a result primarily of fall in the ventricular pressure as the myocardium begins to relax.

The apical impulse in the normal heart reflects faithfully the tension curve just described *(17)*. The impulse, therefore, is felt during the first third of systole only, reaching a peak at the approximate timing of the first heart sound and moving away from the palpating hand long before the second heart sound is heard *(18)*.

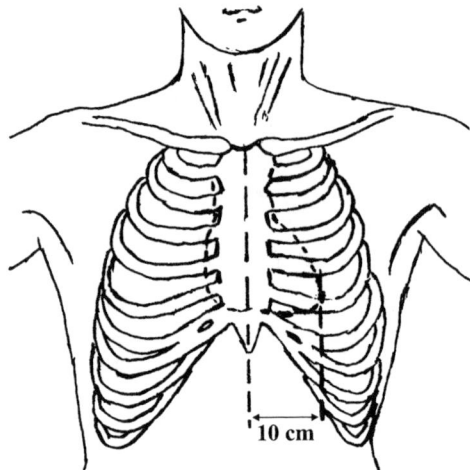

Fig. 6. The position of the normal apex beat is about 10 cm from the mid-sternum.

ASSESSMENT OF THE APICAL IMPULSE

The *apical impulse* by definition is the lateral most point of systolic outward motion that can be felt on the chest wall *(23)*. The term "point of maximal impulse" should not be confused with this and in fact should not be used to describe the apical impulse *(20)*.

The following features should be ascertained when assessing the apical impulse:

1. Location
2. Area
3. Ventricle causing the impulse
4. Character:
   - Dynamicity
   - Duration
   - Extra humps and timing
5. Palpable sounds and murmurs in the area of the apical impulse.

Location

The normal apical impulse, being formed by the left ventricle, is generally felt at the fifth intercostal space in the midclavicular line. The location should be assessed in the supine position or, better still, with the patient sitting erect. In the erect position the normal apex is usually located about 10 cm to the left from the mid-sternal line *(22–24)*. Because the mid-sternal line is easily definable and the erect position corresponds to the way in which a chest x-ray is taken to assess the cardiac silhouette, this is probably more accurate when one tries to ascertain whether or not there is cardiomegaly (Fig. 6). In the left lateral decubitus position, the heart may be slightly displaced laterally because of gravity and may give the false impression of a laterally displaced apical impulse. Therefore, this position is not useful in determining the actual location. The implication of a truly laterally displaced apical impulse is that the heart is enlarged *(23)*. In very large and dilated hearts, the apical impulse may be displaced to the posterior axillary line, and this area may be better approached from behind the patient. Medially placed apical impulse may be observed in some thin patients with vertical hearts, which is a normal variant.

Area

The normal apical impulse occupies a small area approximately the size of a quarter (2.5–3.0 cm in diameter). Its width usually fits two fingerbreadths horizontally and felt over one intercostal space vertically. This small area stems from the fact that the normal left ventricle is conical in shape and probably the apex of the cone with its small area comes into contact with the chest wall. When the left ventricle is enlarged, its shape becomes more spherical and allows greater area of contact with the chest wall, resulting in an enlarged area of the apical impulse. As opposed to the location of the apical impulse, the area or the size can be assessed in the left lateral decubitus position. This maneuver, bringing the heart closer to the chest wall, accentuates the impulse, allowing more precise determination of its characteristics. In fact, it is recommended that all features to be assessed regarding the apical impulse be carried out in the left lateral decubitus position except, of course, its location. A wide area apical impulse (>3.0 cm in diameter) is a more valuable indicator of cardiomegaly than its actual location *(28)* (e.g., left ventricular aneurysm involving the anterior wall, abnormal and enlarged right ventricle forming the apex; a thin patient with a vertical heart developing cardiomegaly may have a wide area apical impulse still placed in the "normal" location).

Which Ventricle Is Causing the Apical Impulse?

The heart during systole, becoming smaller, generally withdraws from the chest wall except for the apex for the reasons explained above. The effect of this withdrawal on the chest wall can be observed as an inward movement of the chest wall during systole called "*retraction*." Although the heart is basically comprised of two separate pumps (right and left ventricles), these two pumps operate normally at two vastly different pressures. Left ventricular systolic pressures being approximately five times higher than that of the right ventricle, its wall tension is much higher, resulting in the increased wall thickness of the left ventricular chamber. The effect of the increased muscle mass on the left side leads to dominance of the left-sided hydrodynamic forces described above. This results in the left ventricular apex as the only area of normal contact during systole. The rest of the heart essentially retracts from the chest wall. In a normal heart, this retraction of the chest wall can be observed to be located medial to the apical impulse and involving part of the left anterior chest wall *(20)*. Even the right ventricle, which is anatomically an anterior structure, is normally pulled away from the chest wall because of its own contraction (becoming smaller) and, more importantly, the septal contraction also pulling the right ventricle posteriorly. This retraction observed in normal patients is located medial to the apical impulse *(23,24)*. It can be best appreciated with patients in the left lateral decubitus position with a palpating finger only on the apical impulse with clear view of the rest of the precordium for proper observation of the inward movement of the retraction (opposite in direction to the outward movement of the apical impulse). This "*medial retraction*" identifies and indicates that the left ventricle forms the apical impulse. The extent of the area of medial retraction may be variable depending on both cardiac and extracardiac factors such as the compliance of the chest wall. It may sometimes be noted only over a small area very close to the apex beat. Nevertheless, if it is medial to the apical impulse, it still identifies the apex beat to be that caused by the left ventricle (Figs. 7A–C). (*See also* Apex Videofiles 1, 2, and 3 under Precordial Pulsations on the Companion CD.)

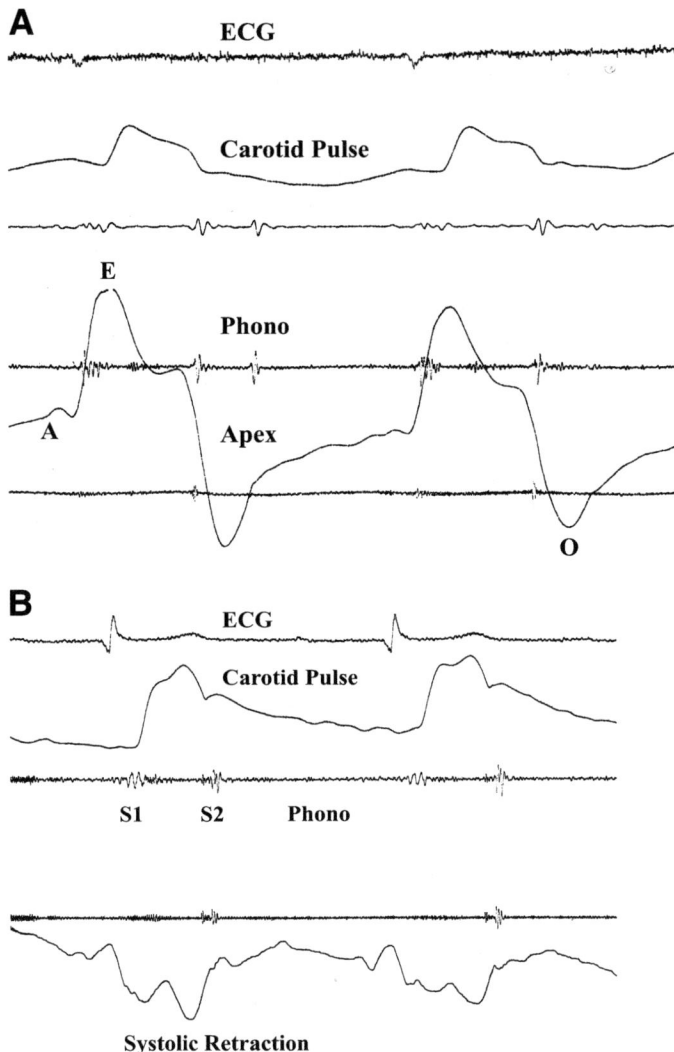

Fig. 7. **(A)** Normal apexcardiogram (Apex) showing a small A wave caused by atrial contraction (not palpable). This is followed by a rapid rise peaking at point E (onset of ejection), corresponding to the onset of the carotid pulse upstroke. The apex beat moves rapidly away from the recording transducer as well as the palpating hand during the last two-thirds of systole, ending at O point, corresponding to mitral valve opening. **(B)** Simultaneous recordings of electrocardiogram (ECG), carotid pulse tracing, phonocardiogram (Phono), and recording from an area medial to the apex beat showing systolic retraction, indicating that, in this patient, the apex beat is formed by the left ventricle. *(Continued on next page)*

When right ventricular forces are exaggerated and become dominant because of high pressures, as in pulmonary hypertension and/or excess volume in the right ventricle causing an enlarged right ventricle (as may be seen in conditions of left-to-right shunt through an atrial septal defect where the right ventricle receives extra volume of blood because of the shunt flow in addition to the normal systemic venous return), the right ventricle may form the apical impulse. Usually in these states the left ventricular forces are also dimin-

Chapter 5 / Precordial Pulsations

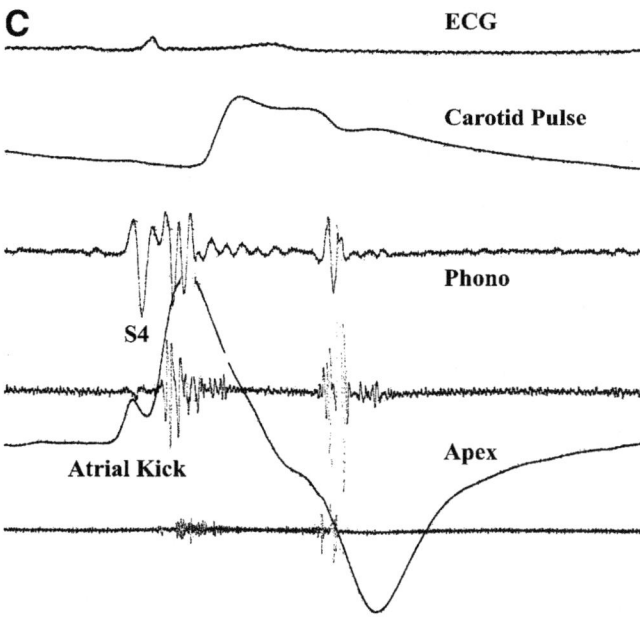

Fig. 7. *(Continued)* **(C)** Apexcardiogram of a patient with coronary artery disease with normal left ventricular systolic function. The amplitude and the duration of the systolic wave of the apex beat are normal. The downstroke of the apex starts at the upstroke of the carotid pulse (very early systole). The A wave is exaggerated (atrial kick) because of a strong atrial contraction evoked by the increased stiffness of the left ventricle (decreased diastolic compliance) producing the S4 recorded on the phonocardiogram.

ished because of underfilling of the left ventricle (e.g., atrial septal defect, pulmonary hypertension). In this situation the hydrodynamic forces, which lead to the formation of the apex beat being right ventricular, result in elimination of normal area of medial retraction. They may in fact be replaced by an outward movement of the precordium from the sternum to the apex area. In such patients, the area of the chest wall lateral to the apical impulse will have the inward movement during systole *(20,23,29)*. This *lateral retraction* is again best observed when care is taken to have a clear view of the lateral chest wall with the palpating finger on the apex beat. The presence of *lateral retraction* identifies the apical impulse to be formed by the right ventricle, which is an abnormal state.

The usefulness of identifying the retraction and thereby determining the ventricle forming the apical impulse lies in the fact that all information derived from the assessment of that apex beat pertains to that ventricle (e.g., a wide area apex beat with medial retraction implies left ventricular enlargement).

When both the right and the left ventricles are enlarged, both of them may produce palpable impulses, each having its own characteristics (the left ventricular impulse with an area of retraction that is medial to it and the right ventricular impulse overlying the lower sternal area with an area of retraction lateral to it) *(23)*. The apical impulse, being the lateral most impulse, will be left ventricular. The retraction will therefore be in between the two impulses, therefore termed the *median retraction*. (*See* Apex videofile 7 under Precordial Pulsations on the Companion CD.)

Character

The character of the apex beat is assessed in terms of its dynamicity; duration, and whether the impulse is single, double, or triple.

If the apical impulse cannot be felt or seen, it stands to reason that one cannot assess its character. This may be because of both cardiac and extracardiac factors. In fact, in patients with thick chest walls, obese patients, and patients with chronic obstructive pulmonary disease where one does not expect to be able to feel the apical impulse, mere palpability alone may indicate cardiomegaly.

DYNAMICITY

The normal apical impulse is generally felt as a short and quick outward movement, which is usually barely visible but often better felt than seen. Once the impulse is felt, it becomes easier to see the movement of the palpating finger along with the underlying chest wall in contrast to the surrounding area of the chest wall. Unless this method is followed, mistakes are often made, confusing a palpable loud heart sound in the apical area as the apical impulse. Sometimes beginners describe such palpable sounds as "diffuse apex beat." This term should never be used to describe the apical impulse in any circumstance because it does not convey any useful information.

When the movement of the apical impulse is exaggerated with large amplitude as well as being rapid, then the impulse is described as "*hyperdynamic*." Placing a stethoscope head on the area of the impulse and observing its movement can easily confirm this feature. In contrast to the normal, hyperdynamic apical impulse can be easily seen without having to palpate. In very thin-chested young adults, exaggerated amplitude may be present, but this should not be confused with hyperdynamicity.

A hyperdynamic apical impulse implies "*volume overload*" state of the ventricle involved. This usually results from a large stroke volume being ejected with increased force and velocity because of Starling mechanism. A hyperdynamic left ventricular impulse therefore suggests conditions that are associated with increased diastolic volumes *(24,25)*. The conditions that cause this may be systemic or cardiac. The systemic causes are usually associated with increased cardiac output such as seen in anemia, thyrotoxicosis, Paget's disease, pregnancy, beriberi, and arteriovenous fistulae. The cardiac causes are usually not accompanied by high cardiac outputs. These include mitral regurgitation, aortic regurgitation, ventricular septal defect, and aorto-pulmonary communications (e.g., persistent ductus arteriosus). In these conditions the left ventricle receives extra volume of blood during diastole in addition to the normal pulmonary venous return (Fig. 8). (*See also* Apex Videofiles 2 and 3 under Precordial Pulsations on the Companion CD.)

If the apical impulse is right ventricular and is hyperdynamic, then volume overload of the right ventricle must be considered as in tricuspid regurgitation, atrial septal defect, and pulmonary regurgitation.

DURATION

The duration of the apical impulse (how long the outward movement lasts during systole) can only be assessed properly by simultaneous auscultation during palpation of the apex beat. By relating the time at which the apical impulse moves away from the palpating hand to the timing of the second heart sound is heard, one can assess whether the duration of the apical impulse is normal or prolonged *(17,18,23,24)*. The apical

Chapter 5 / Precordial Pulsations   125

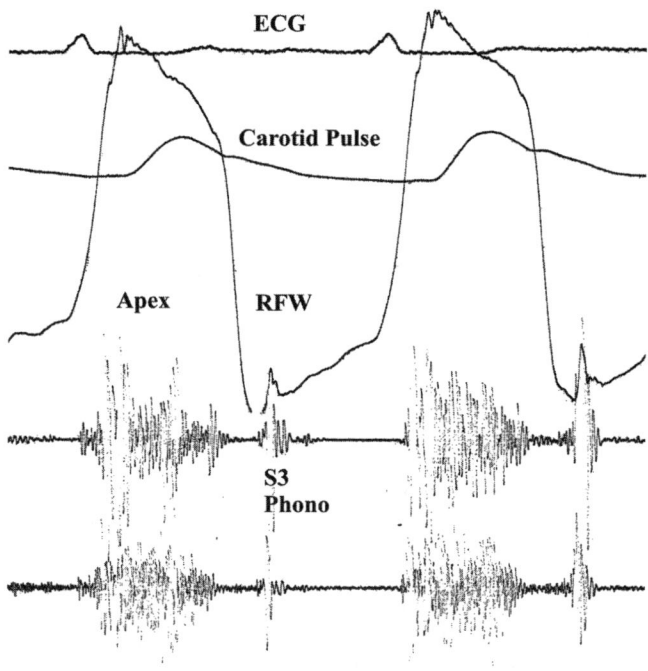

Fig. 8. Apexcardiogram (Apex) of a patient with severe mitral regurgitation with a hyperdynamic left ventricular apical impulse. Prominent rapid filling wave (RFW) in early diastole and a corresponding S3 recorded on the phonocardiogram together with the systolic murmur of mitral regurgitation.

impulse with a prolonged duration is termed "*sustained*." The term "heave" should never be used to describe the apical impulse because it conveys no clear-cut meaning and is interpreted differently by different observers.

Normal apical impulse rises rather quickly and reaches a peak at the time of the first heart sound and moves away rapidly from the palpating hand so that the second heart sound is heard long after the apex beat has disappeared. If an apical impulse is not palpable in the supine position, it is crucial to repeat the examination in the left lateral decubitus position. In our experience this does not affect the duration of the impulse *(24)*. In fact, we recommend that the duration of the apical impulse be determined in this position in all patients.

When the impulse is felt to recede from the palpating hand as the second heart sound is being heard, then the duration is prolonged and the apical impulse is sustained. Sustained left ventricular thrust during the second half of systole has been noted to be associated with an increase in left ventricular mass and volume *(7,30,31)*. In addition, sustained apical impulse has been known to be associated with significant left ventricular dysfunction *(6,7,17,31)*.

The sustained duration of the apical impulse implies that the wall tension in the ventricle forming the apex (usually the left ventricle) is maintained at a high level for the greater part of systole *(17)*. This can occur as a result of increased pressure or increased volume being maintained throughout systole. This is contrary to the general belief and

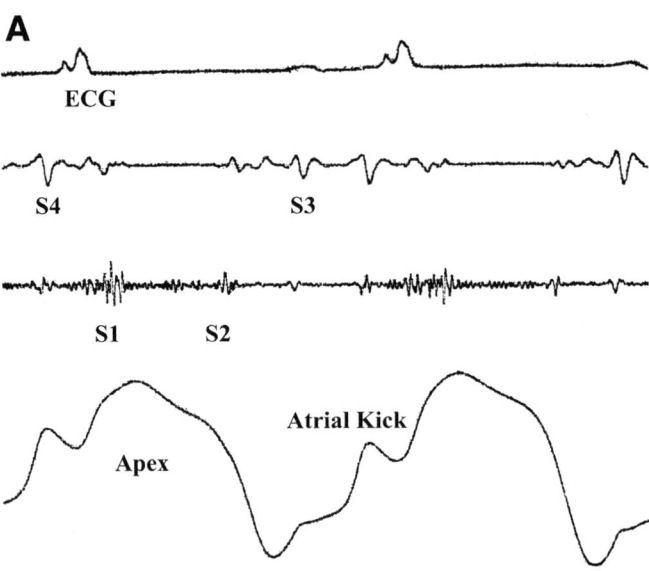

Fig. 9. **(A)** Apexcardiogram of a patient with aortic stenosis with a sustained apical impulse. The fall occurs beginning with the second heart sound (S2). A prominent atrial kick and a corresponding S4 are noted. Also, S3 was heard in this patient with some early signs of heart failure. *(Opposite page)* **(B)** Simultaneous recordings of electrocardiogram (ECG), phono- (Phono), and apexcardiograms (Apex), with its first derivative *(DD/dt)* in a patient with aortic stenosis. The recording of the left ventricular (LV) and aortic pressures show the significant systolic gradient because of the obstruction. Also shown are the LV outlines in diastole and systole depicting the hypertrophied LV with normal systolic decrease in LV size. Note the atrial kick and the sustained apical impulse with the downstroke starting at the timing of S2. **(C)** Simultaneous recordings of electrocardiogram (ECG), phonocardiogram (Phono), and apexcardiogram (Apex) and left ventricular (LV) pressure in a patient with coronary artery disease and left ventricular dysfunction. LV outlines in diastole and systole depict the lack of decrease in LV dimensions reflecting significant LV dysfunction and decreased EF. Apex recording shows sustained duration with the downstroke beginning close to S2.   *(Continued on page 128)*

teaching that sustained impulse results from a hypertrophied ventricle *(18,22,23,25)*. If one relates wall tension according to Lamé's modification of Laplace's formula, hypertrophy, if anything, should help normalize increased wall tension caused by either pressure or volume increase during systole. While the increased wall tension is a powerful stimulus for hypertrophy to occur, sometimes such hypertrophy may not fully normalize the wall tension.

The wall tension may be kept at a high level during systole by increased intraventricular systolic pressure. This is encountered in patients with significant outflow obstruction (e.g., aortic stenosis) or severe systemic hypertension. This can occur even when the ejection fraction (EF; the percentage of the diastolic ventricular volume that the ventricle ejects with each systole) is normal. The normal left ventricle ejects at least 60% of its contents with each systole. In other words, the normal EF is about 60% in these patients (Fig. 9A,B). Because there is increased impedance to ejection in such cases, the ventricle takes longer to eject its volume as opposed to normal, when most of the volume is ejected by the first third of systole.

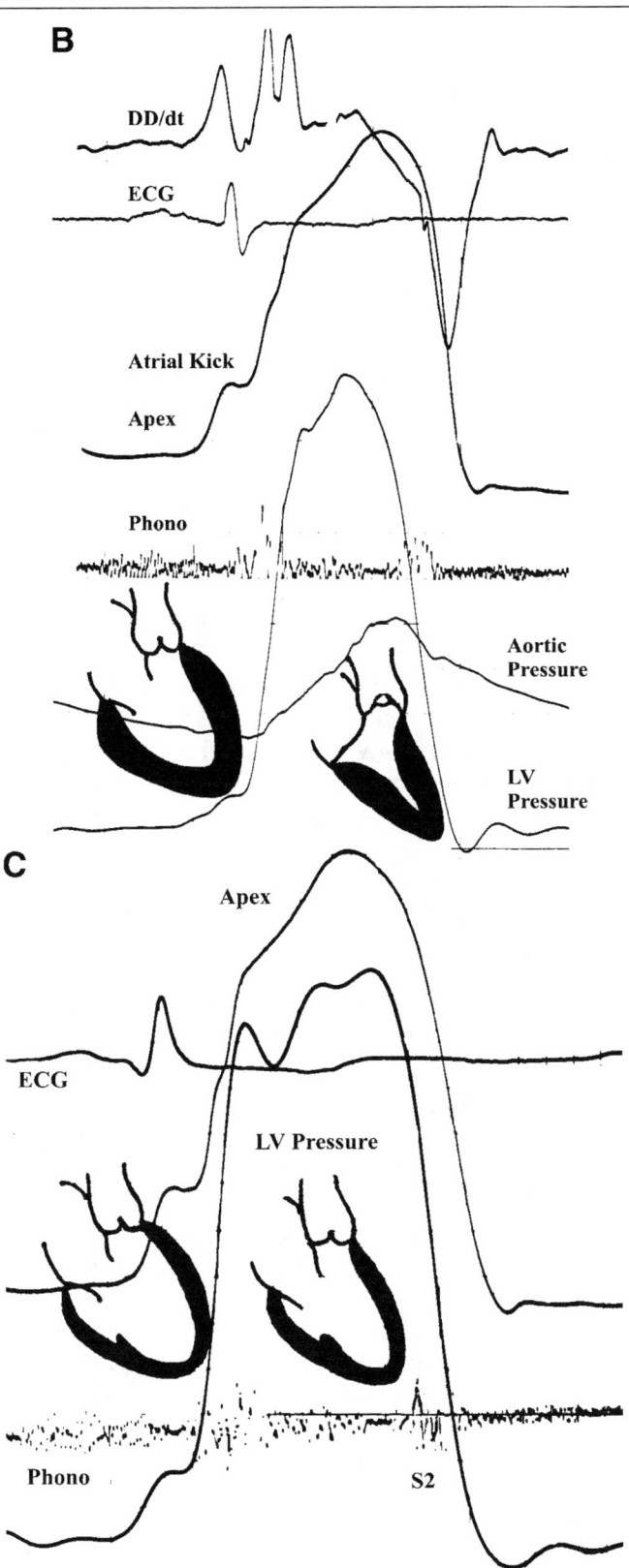

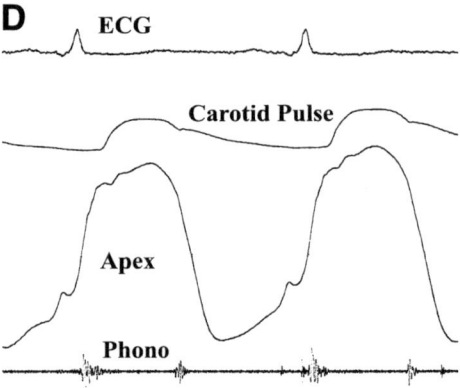

Fig. 9. *(Continued)* **(D)** Sustained apex in a patient with ischemic heart disease and significant left ventricular dysfunction.

In the absence of significant outflow obstruction and/or severe hypertension (systolic pressures >180 mmHg.), a sustained apical impulse would imply the second important cause of prolonged duration of elevated wall tension, which would result from poor systolic emptying. This is seen for instance in patients with left ventricular dysfunction (Grade III with EF of 30–49% and Grade IV with EF of <30%) (Fig. 9C,D) *(17)*. The most important corollary of this is that a nonsustained apical impulse implies normal left ventricular ejection fraction *(17)*.(*See* Apex Videofiles 3 and 4 under Precordial Pulsations on the Companion CD.)

Extra Humps and Their Timing

ATRIAL KICK

The normal apical impulse has a single outward movement, which is palpable. The rise in left ventricular wall tension during the end of diastole caused by atrial contraction, which may be recorded even in the normal subjects by sensitive instruments ("A" wave in the apexcardiogram), is not palpable (Fig. 7A). However, in patients with decreased ventricular compliance (stiff ventricles, which offer resistance to expansion in diastole), the atrium compensates for this by generating a stronger or forceful contraction, resulting in higher pressure. This produces an exaggerated A wave, which may become palpable as an extra hump, giving a double apical impulse, also called an *"atrial kick or hump"* *(9,23)*. While this corresponds to an audible fourth heart sound (S4), it is not a palpable S4. This type of double apical impulse is easily recognized at the bedside as a step or hesitation in the upswing of the apical impulse. It can also be brought out by holding a tongue depressor over the apical impulse. The length of the tongue depressor helps to amplify the movement making it visible. The presence of an atrial kick therefore implies decreased ventricular compliance. The latter can occur as a result of hypertrophy, scarring, infiltrative process, ischemia, or infarction. The forceful atrial contraction acts as an effective booster pump, enhancing the contractility and output of the ventricle *(25,32)*. It also implies a healthy atrium, sinus rhythm, and no obstruction to ventricular inflow (no mitral stenosis in case of a left ventricular apex and no tricuspid stenosis in

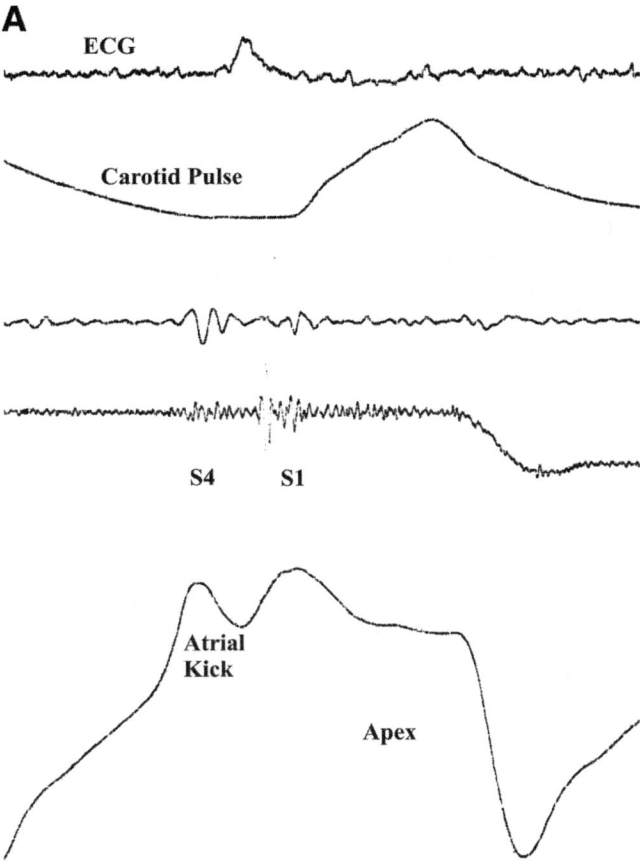

Fig. 10. **(A)** Apexcardiogram (Apex) in a patient with aortic stenosis (AS) and palpable atrial kick. Note the corresponding S4. The duration of the apex is sustained and the upstroke of the carotid pulse is delayed because of AS. *(Continued on next page)*

case of right ventricular apex). The presence of an atrial kick in patients with aortic valvular stenosis and/or hypertension would imply significant stenosis or hypertension *(33)* (Fig. 10A,B). Atrial kick may sometimes give the impression of a sustained apical impulse if assessed casually *(17,20)*. Therefore, care should be taken to assess the duration of the impulse in the presence of an atrial kick because it has a significant implication with regard to the assessment of systolic ventricular function. In ischemic heart disease, atrial kick may be the only palpable abnormality. This indicates decreased ventricular compliance and preserved systolic left ventricular function and EF (Grade I with EF ≥60% or Grade II left ventricular function with EF of 50–59%). If the atrial kick is associated with a sustained apical impulse, it indicates moderate left ventricular dysfunction (Grade III with EF 30–49%). In patients with sustained apical impulse without atrial kick who are still in sinus rhythm, the degree of left ventricular dysfunction is generally severe (Grade IV with EF <30%) *(17)*. This occurs as a result of poor atrial function secondary to overdistension or fibrosis of the left atrium. (*See* Apex Videofile 1 under Precordial Pulsations on the Companion CD.)

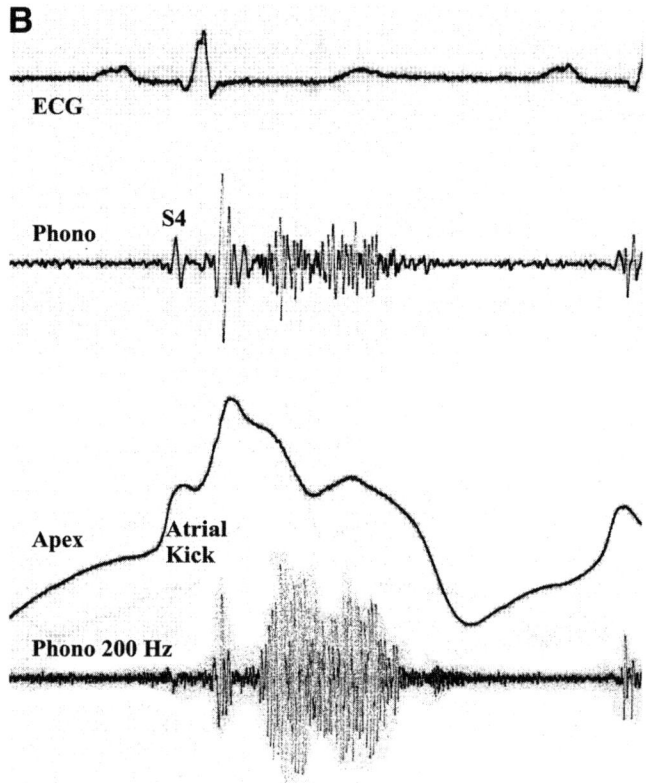

Fig. 10. *(Continued)* **(B)** Apex recording in a patient with hypertrophic obstructive cardiomyopathy with palpable atrial kick. Phonocardiogram (Phono) shows the corresponding S4 as well as the murmur caused by the left ventricular outflow obstruction.

RAPID FILLING WAVE

The second cause of a double apical impulse is the presence of an exaggerated rapid-filling wave, which becomes palpable. The ventricular filling during diastole occurs in three phases. When the atrioventricular valves open in diastole, the initial inflow from the atria into the ventricles is quite rapid, and so this phase is termed the rapid filling phase. The second phase of filling is the slow filling phase, when the inflow volume and velocity slow down and the pressure in the ventricle becomes equalized to the atrial pressure. This slow filling phase lasts until the atrial contraction occurs toward the end of diastole. When a large volume of blood enters the ventricle during the early rapid filling phase, it can cause an exaggerated rapid filling wave, thereby producing an extra hump in early diastole. This is seen in ventricular volume overload states (e.g., severe mitral or aortic regurgitation) *(25)*. This is felt as a gentle rebound after the initial rapid downstroke of the apical impulse from the palpating hand (as "a step" in the downswing of the apex beat) (Figs. 8 and 11). It may be associated with a third heart sound (S3) or short diastolic inflow rumble (not mitral stenosis). But it is not a palpable S3.

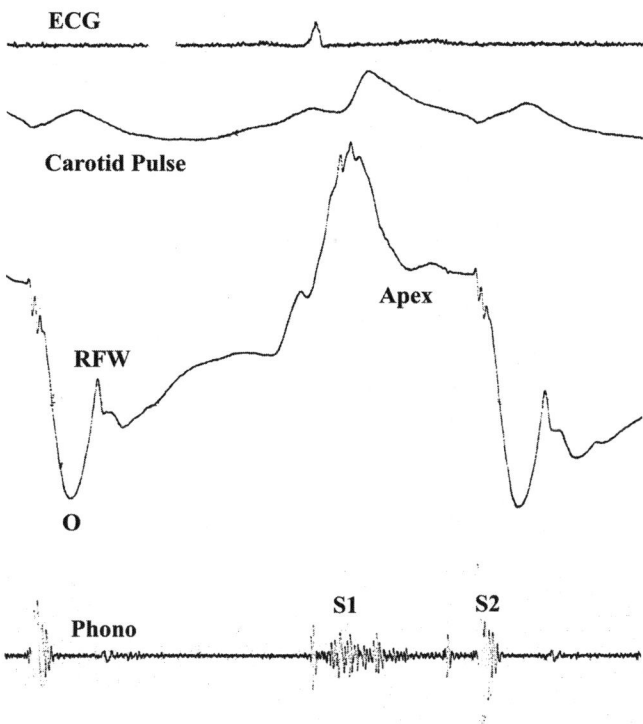

Fig. 11. Apexcardiogram (Apex) in a pregnant woman showing an exaggerated rapid filling wave (RFW) indicating an increased volume returning to left ventricle in early diastole.

MIDSYSTOLIC RETRACTION

The third cause of a double apical impulse is "*midsystolic retraction*" giving rise to two systolic humps instead of the usual single systolic impulse. This type of double impulse is noted only in some patients with hypertrophic obstructive cardiomyopathy (HOCM) with significant subaortic dynamic obstruction and rarely in some patients with severe prolapse of the mitral valve leaflets with insignificant mitral regurgitation *(20)*. This is detected by appreciating the fact that both humps occur during systole. In HOCM, the initial hump is a result of the rapid early ejection. In mid-systole, as obstruction develops because of the sudden anterior motion of the anterior mitral leaflet coming into contact with the interventricular septum, ejection momentarily stops. This causes the left ventricle to fall away from the chest wall, thus causing the mid-systolic retraction. In late systole as the ventricle starts relaxing, the obstruction disappears, leading to resumption of ejection of blood into aorta. This causes the second hump in systole.

Similar momentary and sudden decrease in ejection into the aorta may occur in mitral valve prolapse. This results from large redundant leaflets, which suddenly prolapse into the left atrium when the ventricular size becomes smaller during ejection. The blood in the ventricle preferentially goes in the direction of the left atrium because of the lower pressure in the atrium in comparison to the pressure in the aorta.

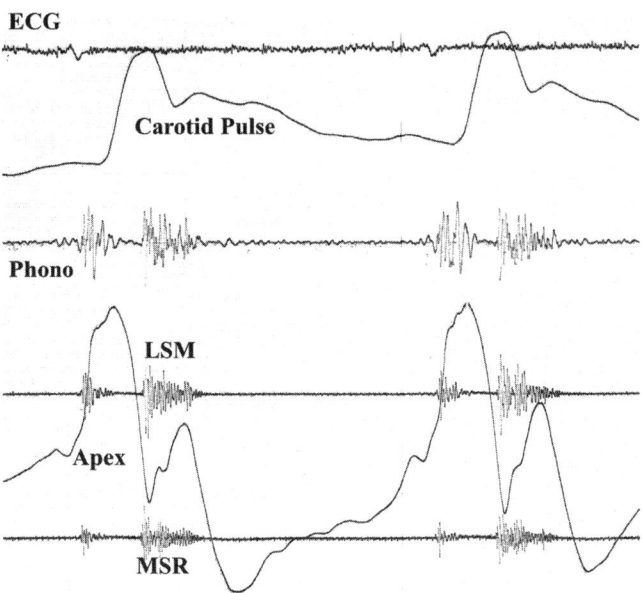

Fig. 12. Apexcardiogram (Apex) of a patient with mitral valve prolapse showing mid-systolic retraction (MSR). Note the late systolic murmur (LSM). The two peaks may be felt as a double impulse.

If the prolapse is not associated with significant mitral regurgitation, then ejection into aorta resumes once the prolapse reaches its anatomical limits, causing the second systolic hump (Fig. 12).

In very rare instances one may actually feel a *triple apical impulse (20)*. This is usually because of a combination of an atrial kick together with the presence of a mid-systolic retraction. Such combination is only possible in HOCM and therefore is diagnostic of this condition (Fig. 13). This indicates decreased compliance because of the idiopathic hypertrophy and the significant subaortic dynamic obstruction. The triple impulse is not seen in mitral valve prolapse because the ventricular compliance is not decreased in this disorder. Although one may think that a triple impulse may be possible in mitral prolapse as a result of mid-systolic retraction and a palpable rapid filling wave, this combination is not likely because palpable rapid filling wave requires significant mitral regurgitation. This, in turn, will preclude the presence of a mid-systolic retraction.

Palpable Sounds and Murmurs in the Area of the Apical Impulse

Occasionally, a loud first heart sound may be palpable in the region of the apex beat and may actually be mistaken for the apex beat itself. This may occur in patients with mitral stenosis, which has led to the description of the so-called tapping apical impulse of mitral stenosis *(18)*. In general, the apical impulse, when properly identified in uncomplicated mitral stenosis, will be expected to be a normal left ventricular impulse.

Palpation in the apex area may also help in detecting loud murmurs, which cause palpable thrills. The significance of this is in the grading of the loudness of the murmurs.

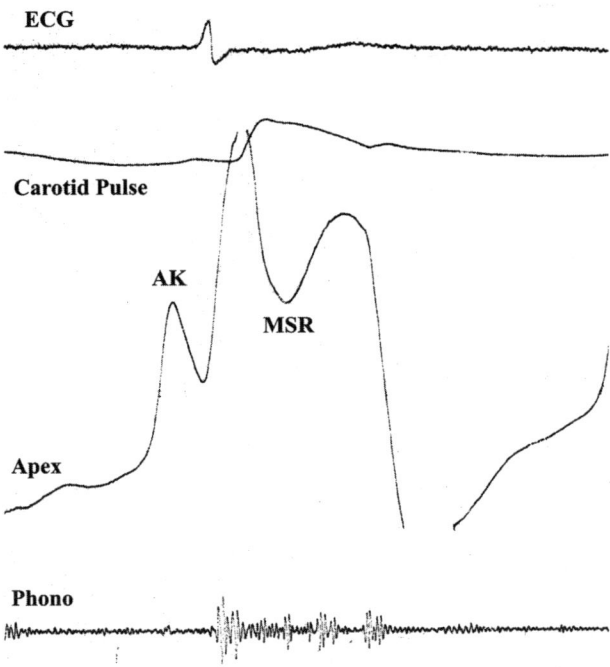

Fig. 13. Apexcardiogram (Apex) of a patient with hypertrophic obstructive cardiomyopathy showing triple apical impulse. The first impulse is the atrial kick (AK) followed by early and late systolic humps separated by a mid-systolic retraction (MSR).

LEFT PARASTERNAL AND STERNAL MOVEMENTS

Both the sternal and the left parasternal regions should be carefully assessed for either visible or palpable movements. The movements can be either an outward systolic impulse or an inward systolic retraction *(20)*. The recognition of whether it is outward or inward during systole is best assessed with timing of systole by the simultaneous palpation of the arterial pulse.

Causes of the Outward Systolic Left Parasternal/Sternal Movement

1. A right ventricle that has either high pressures (e.g., pulmonary hypertension) or high volume load (e.g., atrial septal defect)
2. A right ventricle held forward by a large left atrium (e.g., mitral stenosis).
3. A right ventricle pushed forward by systolic expansion of the left atrium in severe mitral regurgitation *(20,34)*
4. Abnormal left ventricular anterior wall expansion in systole because of an aneurysm or akinetic/ dyskinetic segments during ischemia *(20,24)*.
(*See* Apex Videofile 5 on the Companion CD.)

Causes of the Left Parasternal/Sternal Systolic Retraction

1. Normal systolic retraction in some patients
2. When the area of retraction is wide and exaggerated, then left ventricular volume overload, as with mitral regurgitation or aortic regurgitation, must be suspected. In these

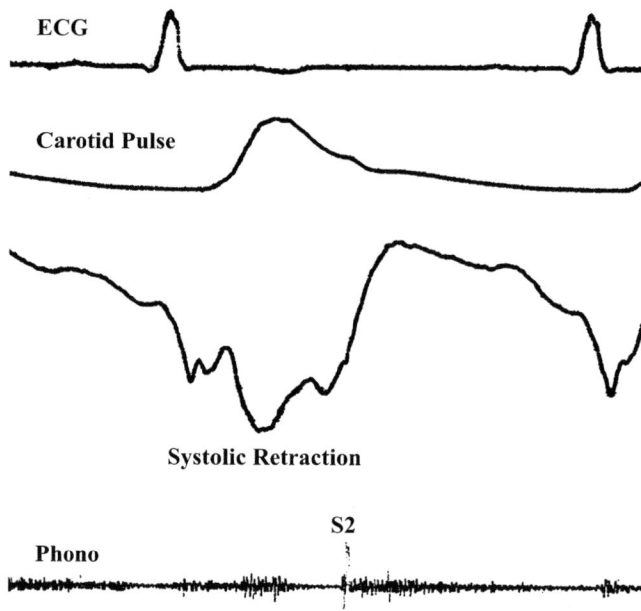

Fig. 14. Marked systolic retraction in a patient with significant aortic regurgitation. The recording was made with the transducer medial to the apical impulse over the lower left parasternal area.

conditions the left ventricle receives extra volume of blood (regurgitant volume) in diastole in addition to the normal pulmonary venous return. The retraction tends to be more exaggerated in patients with isolated aortic regurgitation as opposed to mitral regurgitation for similar degrees of volume overload. This is because of the systolic expansion of the left atrium in mitral regurgitation, which opposes the retraction caused by left ventricular systole. In fact, excessive sternal retraction rules out severe mitral regurgitation. On the other hand, it may be commonly observed in significant aortic regurgitation (Fig. 14) *(20)*.
3. When the sternum is made flail because of trauma or surgery (postmedian sternotomy), it may exaggerate the normal systolic retraction.
4. Sometimes the only visible or palpable precordial movement will be a systolic retraction without a definable apical impulse. This occurs in two conditions: *constrictive pericarditis* and *Ebstein's anomaly*. In both of these the left ventricle is relatively underfilled. In constrictive pericarditis, the systolic retraction of the chest overlying the ribs in the left axilla has been known as the *Broadbent sign (32)*. In Ebstein's anomaly, the right atrium is usually huge because of partial atrialization of the right ventricle resulting from a congenital downward displacement of the tricuspid valve attachment and the tricuspid regurgitation that accompanies it.

RIGHT PARASTERNAL MOVEMENT

Any outward systolic impulse in this region should imply aortic root dilatation as in aortic aneurysm and/or dissection.

PULSATIONS OVER THE CLAVICULAR HEADS

Pulsations of the clavicular heads indicate the presence of abnormal dilatation of the aortic arch (e.g., aneurysm).

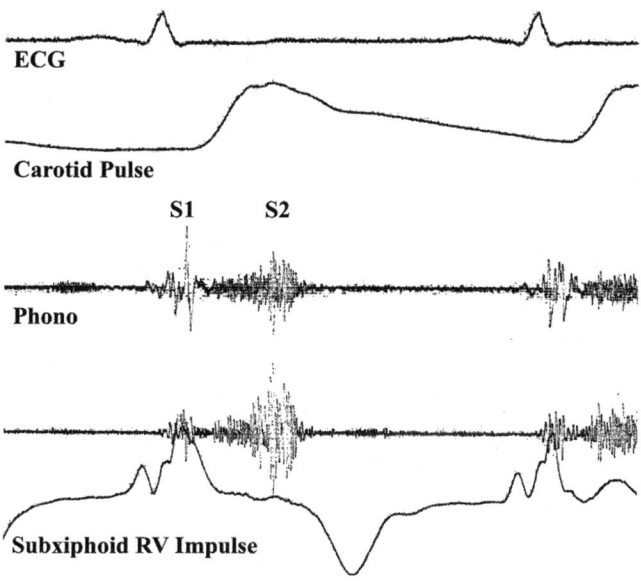

Fig. 15. Recording of a subxiphoid right ventricular impulse in a patient with combined aortic stenosis and hypertrophic obstructive cardiomyopathy and severe secondary pulmonary hypertension. It is similar to the apical impulse in its characteristics.

PULSATIONS OVER THE SECOND AND/OR THIRD LEFT INTERCOSTAL SPACES

This region anatomically overlies the pulmonary outflow tract. Pulsations in this area may be felt in patients with pulmonary artery dilatation with or without pulmonary hypertension. Pulmonary artery dilatation may occur either on an idiopathic basis or because of excess pressure (pulmonary hypertension irrespective of the cause) or excess volume flow through the pulmonary outflow (e.g., atrial septal defect with large volume flow due to left to right shunt at the atrial level).

SUBXIPHOID IMPULSE

The subxiphoid region should be palpated by placing the palm of the hand over the epigastrium with the fingertips pointing up toward the patient's head. Gentle pressure is applied downward (posteriorly) and upward towards the head. The patient should be asked to take a deep inspiration in order to move the diaphragm down. This facilitates the palpation of the right ventricle *(2,25)*. If the impulse were palpable pushing the fingertips downward (toward the feet) as opposed to lifting the palmar aspect of the hand, it would indicate a palpable right ventricular impulse. Transmitted abdominal aortic pulsations will cause the impulse to strike the palmar aspect of the hand. Unlike the sternal and parasternal movements discussed previously, subxiphoid palpation is very specific for a right ventricular impulse.

In the normal adult there is never a detectable right ventricular impulse by subxiphoid palpation. Therefore, if a right ventricular impulse is detected subxiphoid in an adult, it should indicate either a pressure and/or volume overload of the right ventricle. Its character should be determined as discussed previously in relation to the apex beat, namely, the dynamicity, duration, and whether the impulse is single or double (Fig. 15). (*See* Apex Videofile 6 under Precordial Pulsations on the Companion CD.)

PRACTICAL POINTS IN THE CLINICAL ASSESSMENT OF PRECORDIAL PULSATIONS

1. Traditional methods of inspection and palpation together with auscultation are necessary for the proper assessment of the precordial pulsations and in particular the apical impulse. In the supine position, with the patient's precordium well exposed under proper lighting conditions (preferably natural light from the sides), one should inspect carefully for movements of the chest wall over all areas of the precordium, including the sternal area, the left parasternal area, the right parasternal area, the apical area, the basal portions overlying the second and third interspaces, and the sterno-clavicular junction. Any observed movement should then be timed with simultaneous palpation of the radial pulse upstroke to determine whether the observed movement is outward during systole or inward during systole. If the movement is outward during systole, then it will be synchronous with pulse upstroke.

2. In normal patients it is uncommon to see exaggerated movements over the precordium inward or outward during systole. Rarely in very young and thin-chested subjects, one may see active movements over the apical area. The parasternal and sternal regions in most normals are very quite. The normal inward retraction of this region is usually difficult to feel. It may only be seen over a small area adjacent and medial to the apex area or the apical impulse.

3. When the area of retraction overlies a larger area of the parasternum or the sternum, then conditions that may predispose to such situations must be considered. These include left ventricular volume overload states such as aortic and mitral regurgitations. The retraction of the parasternal and the sternal region may, in fact, be excessive and easily visible in significant and isolated aortic regurgitation because in these patients the excess diastolic volumes of the left ventricle (due to both the normal pulmonary venous return coming through the mitral inflow as well as the additional regurgitant flow coming from the insufficient aortic valve) provide a strong Starling effect, increasing the force of left ventricular contraction. In addition, in isolated aortic regurgitation, the left atrium will not be enlarged and therefore will not offset the degree of the retraction as it often does in mitral regurgitation, which will cause left atrial expansion during systole. The left atrium being the posterior chamber, its expansion will tend to push the rest of the heart forward during systole. This will limit the degree of the retraction seen in mitral regurgitation. The excessive sternal retraction seen in patients with significant aortic regurgitation may be mistaken for right ventricular movement with sternal lift if one does not take care to time the movement with simultaneous palpation of the carotid or the radial arterial pulse. The timing with the arterial pulse will show the sternal movement to be inward during systole.

4. In severe mitral regurgitation, the left atrial expansion may cause a sternal lift, but this will tend to be slightly delayed in onset when compared to the onset of the left ventricular apical impulse in the same patient if both impulses are simultaneously palpated. This will be in contrast to a true right ventricular movement over the sternum, which will rise at the same time as the left ventricular apical impulse.

5. The following points are important to remember while assessing the apical impulse:
   a. The apical impulse is the lateral-most point of systolic outward movement felt over the precordium. The apical impulse, which is palpable, must be an area of

the chest wall that can be both felt and seen to move forward during systole as assessed by a palpating finger. The apical impulse may be palpable only intermittently because of respiratory variations. It may be felt well most often at end-expiration when the lungs are deflated. However, in some patients the descent of the diaphragm with respirations may have an effect on the mediastinum. This may variably affect the palpability of the apex beat. It may, however, be best felt only when it is against an intercostal space as opposed to being behind a rib. This may happen at any phase of respiration.

b. While defining the apical impulse one must be able to conclude as follows:
- It is palpable (meaning that the area can be both seen and felt to move under the palpating finger).
- It is barely palpable (meaning that one feels a sensation of outward movement but not enough to see it clearly).
- It is not palpable.

Mistaking a palpable sound over the apical area (mostly caused by a loud first heart sound) for the apical impulse can be avoided if one looks for the actual area of movement of the chest wall underneath the palpating finger. Often the loud sound may be picked up by the palm of the whole hand over the apical area and the lower left sternal region.

c. The location of the apical impulse is best assessed with the patient sitting upright. When palpable it will give some clue regarding the presence or absence of cardiomegaly. However, in a substantial number of patients, the apical impulse will be palpable only in the left lateral decubitus position.

d. All other important points to be determined regarding the apical impulse (e.g., its area or dimension, the location of the retraction, whether medial or lateral to the apex, the character, whether it is sustained in duration, its dynamicity, the determination of extra humps, and even the detection of any palpable sounds or murmurs over the apical area) are best felt and determined in the left lateral decubitus position of the patient.

e. The presence of medial retraction identifies a left ventricular impulse, whereas lateral retraction indicates a right ventricular impulse. One can sometimes stick one end of a tongue blade with a tape over the area of the apical impulse or hold it against it while observing for the area of retraction adjacent to it. The tongue blade is a valuable simple tool and can also be used to observe for the contour of the apical motion for the detection of the presence of any extra humps such as an atrial kick.

f. Retraction may sometimes be median with two areas of outward systolic impulse. One of these will be laterally placed and is obviously the apical impulse formed by the left ventricle, and the other will be the right ventricular impulse, which will be medial to the area of retraction. In such a situation both impulses will rise simultaneously. Each of the two respective impulses must be assessed further in the same manner in which the apical impulse is characterized.

g. The duration of the apical impulse is best determined with the whole palm of the hand palpating and timing at the same time by auscultation over the nearby area or the third or the fouth left interspace near the left sternal border. The normal apical impulse comes out with the first heart sound and recedes away from the palpating hand very rapidly, and it is therefore hard to latch onto it for any length of time. One cannot even know when it recedes because it does so swiftly. If one can tell when it begins to fall away from the palpating hand, then its duration is already prolonged. If it is felt to recede as one hears the second heart sound, then it is definitely sustained. A sustained left ventricular impulse in the absence of significant hypertension (systolic blood pressure >180) or aortic stenosis often picked up by delayed upstroke of the carotid pulse would be indicative of decreased left ventricular systolic function (Grade III with EF between 30 and 49% or Grade IV with EF <30%). (Left ventricular function can be graded by measurement of EF, which is obtained by dividing the stroke volume by the end-diastolic volume of the left ventricle.)

A nonsustained impulse would favor normal systolic function with normal EF (60% or more) or only mild dysfunction with EF between 50 and 59%.

h. The dynamicity of the apex beat can be best appreciated by placing the head of a stethoscope over it to see how large and rapid the movement of the chest wall is underneath it. If the movement is large and rapid, then it will be reflected by the movement of the stethoscope head.

i. While palpating for the contour and the detection of the presence of any extra humps such as the atrial kick, it is important to feel gently because excessive pressure could fail to detect them by filtering out lower-frequency vibrations. The atrial kick is detected by the presence of a hesitation or a step in the outward movement of the apical impulse. The exaggerated rapid filling wave during diastole is felt on the other hand, as a gentle rebound after the initial rapid downstroke of the apical impulse from the palpating hand (as "a step" in the downswing of the apex beat).

6. Left parasternal and sternal areas must be inspected carefully for movement with simultaneous palpation of the radial pulse. This will help in the appreciation of any exaggerated retraction over these areas, if present. Parasternal and, in particular, sternal movement must be assessed further with palpation using the palm of the hand and having the patient breathe out, holding his or her breath at end-expiration. This helps to deflate the lungs and reduce the attenuation caused by the expanded lungs.

7. Subxiphoid palpation, on the other hand, for right ventricular movement is done with the palm of the hand placed with the tips of the fingers pointing toward the head of the patient. The patient should be asked to take a deep breath so that the diaphragm can descend and with it the right ventricle. If the right ventricle is palpable, then it will produce an active motion, which will hit the fingertips. If the impulse hits the palmar aspect of the fingers, it indicates transmitted aortic pulsation and not the right ventricular impulse. In the adult, the normal right ventricle never produces a palpable subxiphoid impulse, whereas one may feel this in children and adolescents.

REFERENCES

1. Potain.C. Du rhythme cardiaque appele' bruit de galop. Bull Soc Med Hop Paris 1875;s2:12:137–166.
2. Mackenzie J. The Study of the Pulse, Arterial, Venous, and Hepatic, and of the Movements of the Heart. Edinburgh: Young J Pentland, 1902.
3. Benchimol A, Diamond E. The normal and abnormal apexcardiogram. Its physiological variation and its relation to intracardiac events. Am J Cardiol 1963;12:368.

4. Tafur E, Cohen LS, et al. The normal apexcardiogram, its temporal relationship to electrical, acoustic and mechanical cardiac events. Circulation 1964;30:381.
5. Tavel ME. CRW, Feigenbaum H, Steinmetz EF. The apexcardiogram and its relationship to hemodynamic events within the left heart. Br Heart J 1965;27:829.
6. Lane FJ, Carrroll JM, Levine HD, Gorlin R. The apexcardiogram in myocardial asynergy. Circulation 1968;37:890.
7. Sutton GC, Prewitt TA, Craige E. Relationship between quantitated precordial movement and left ventricular function. Circulation 1970;41:179–190.
8. Craige E. Clinical value of apexcardiography. Am J Cardiol 1971; 28:118–121.
9. Gibson TC, Madry R, Grossman W, McLaurin LP, Craige E. The A wave of the apexcardiogram and left ventricular diastolic stiffness. Circulation 1974;49:441–446.
10. Mc Ginn FX, Gould L, Lyonn AF. The phonocardiogram and apexcardiogram in patients with ventricular aneurysm. Am J Cardiol 1968;21:467.
11. Prewitt T, Gibson D, Brown D, Sutton G. The 'rapid filling wave' of the apexcardiogram. Its relation to echocardiographic and cineangiographic measurements of ventricular filling. Br Heart J 1975;37: 1256–1262.
12. Wayne HH. The apexcardiogram in ischemic heart disease. Calif Med 1972;116:12.
13. Venco A, Gibson DG, Brown DJ. Relation between apexcardiogram and changes in left ventricular pressure and dimension. Br Heart J 1977;39:117–125.
14. Willems JL, De Geest H, Kesteloot H. On the value of apexcardiography for timing intracardiac events. Am J Cardiol 1971;28:59-66.
15. Manolas J, Rutishauser W, Wirz P, Arbenz U. Time relation between apexcardiogram and left ventricular events using simultaneous high-fidelity tracings in man. Br Heart J 1975;37:1263–1267.
16. Manolas J, Rutishauser W. Diastolic amplitude time index: a new apexcardiographic index of left ventricular diastolic function in human beings. Am J Cardiol 1981;48:736–745.
17. Ranganathan N, Juma Z, Sivaciyan V. The apical impulse in coronary heart disease. Clin Cardiol 1985; 8:20–33.
18. Mounsey JP. Inspection and palpation of the cardiac impulse. Prog Cardiovasc Dis 1967;10:187–206.
19. Eddlemann EE. Kinetocardiographic changes in ischemic heart disease. Circulation 1965;31:650–655.
20. Stapleton JF, Groves BM. Precordial palpation. Am Heart J 1971;81:409–427.
21. Schweizer W, Bertrab RV, Reist P. Kinetocardiography in coronary artery disease. Br Heart J 1965; 27:263–268.
22. Deliyannis AA., Gillam PMS., Mounsey JPD, Steiner RE. The cardiac impulse and the motion of the heart. Br Heart J 1964;26:396.
23. Constant J. Inspection and palpation of the chest. In: Bedside Cardiology, 2nd Ed. Boston, MA: Little Brown and Co, 1976:100–133.
24. Abrams J. Precordial palpation. In: Horwitz LD, Groves BM, eds. Signs and Symptoms in Cardiology. Philadelphia, PA: J.B. Lippincott, 1985:156–177.
25. Perloff JK. The physiologic mechanisms of cardiac and vascular physical signs. J Am Coll Cardiol 1983;1:184–198.
26. Hansen DE, Daughters GT 2nd, Alderman EL, Ingels NB Jr, Miller DC. Torsional deformation of the left ventricular midwall in human hearts with intramyocardial markers.regional heterogeneity and sensitivity to the inotropic effects of abrupt rate change. Circ Res 1988;62(5):941–952.
27. Hawthorne EW. Dynamic geometry of the left ventricle. Am J Cardiol 1966;18:566–573.
28. Eilen SD, Crawford MH, O'Rourke RA. Accuracy of precordial palpation for detecting increased left ventricular volume. Ann Intern Med 1983;99:628–630.
29. Boicourt OW, Nagle RE, Mounsey JP. The clinical significance of systolic retraction of the apical impulse. Br Heart J 1965;27:379–391.
30. Conn RD, Cole JS. The cardiac apex impulse. Clinical and angiographic correlations. Ann Intern Med 1971;75:185–191.
31. Mills RM, Jr., Kastor JA. Quantitative grading of cardiac palpation. Comparison in supine and left lateral decubitus positions. Arch Intern Med 1973;132:831–834.
32. Wood PW. Diseases of the Heart and Circulation. Philadelphia, PA: J.B.Lippincott, 1956:411.
33. Epstein EJ, Coulshed N, Brown AK, Doukas NG. The 'A' wave of the apexcardiogram in aortic valve disease and cardiomyopathy. Br Heart J 1968;30:591–605.
34. Basta LL, Wolfson P, Eckberg DL, Abboud FM. The value of left parasternal impulse recordings in the assessment of mitral regurgitation. Circulation 1973;48:1055–1065.

6 Heart Sounds

CONTENTS

> PRINCIPLES OF SOUND FORMATION IN THE HEART
> FIRST HEART SOUND (S1)
> CLINICAL ASSESSMENT OF S1 AND COMPONENTS
> SECOND HEART SOUND (S2)
> NORMAL S2
> ABNORMAL S2
> CLINICAL ASSESSMENT OF S2
> OPENING SNAP (OS)
> THIRD HEART SOUND (S3)
> CLINICAL ASSESSMENT OF S3
> FOURTH HEART SOUND (S4)
> CLINICAL ASSESSMENT OF S4
> REFERENCES

PRINCIPLES OF SOUND FORMATION IN THE HEART

In the past, many theories have been advanced to explain the origins of sounds during the cardiac cycle. These included simple concepts of sound originating from the actual contact of valve cusps upon closure. When it was realized that the strength of contraction of the left ventricle had a significant effect on the intensity of the first heart sound, the myocardial theory of the origin of the sound was postulated. Some even had suggested extracardiac origin of sounds such as the third heart sound. It is now, however, well established by several investigators and accepted that the formation of all sounds in the heart can be explained by a *"unified concept" (1–10)*.

It is a common experience to hear sound produced when a pipe half-filled with water is moved back and forth, splashing the water against the two palms of the hands held against the ends of the pipe. We have all heard banging sounds sometime produced in the water pipes of the plumbing systems of our homes when air is introduced into the plumbing. In both examples, the mechanism of sound production is the same. When the moving column of water in either case comes to sudden stop or marked deceleration, the energy of the column dissipates and in the process generates vibration of the pipes as well as the column of water. These vibrations, when they are in the audible range, are heard as sounds. The intensity of the sound will very much depend on the initial energy of the moving column of water. Of the two examples, the sounds in the second case are usually very loud and may be heard throughout the whole house. This is mainly because the water pressure in the system is approximately 40 lb/in^2.

Similarly, all heart sounds are formed when a moving column of blood comes to a sudden stop or decelerates significantly. The intensity of a heart sound will depend on the level of energy that the moving column of blood has attained. The sudden deceleration causes dissipation of energy, which results in the production of vibrations affecting the contiguous cardiohemic mass *(3)*. The factors affecting the acceleration and deceleration of columns of blood involved in the formation of the various heart sounds are different and may be many. These will have to be considered for each sound separately, taking into account the physiology and the pathophysiology of the phase of the cardiac cycle involved.

FIRST HEART SOUND (S1)

The first heart sound occurs at the onset of ventricular contraction. To better understand the physiology of the first heart sound, one needs to know the cardiac events that occur around the time of the first heart sound. At the end of diastole, the atrium contracts and gives an extra stretch and filling to the ventricle. This is immediately followed by the ventricular contraction. When the ventricular pressure rises and exceeds the atrial pressure, the mitral and the tricuspid valve leaflets become apposed and close. As the ventricular pressures continue to rise and exceed that of the aorta and the pulmonary artery, the semilunar valves open and the ejection phase begins. All these events occur in rapid succession over a short period of time and contribute to the production of the first heart sound. As a result, S1 is relatively wide and is made of many components, which overlap each other. These components are "atrial," "mitral," "tricuspid," and "aortic" *(2, 5,7,10–14)*.

Atrial Component

The energy of the column of blood pushed by the atrial contraction becomes dissipated as the column decelerates against the ventricular walls. This deceleration is gradual in most normal subjects because of good compliance and distensibility of the ventricles. Therefore, the sound generated by this has a very low frequency and is not audible. This will be discussed further in relation to the fourth heart sound. However, when the PR interval on the electrocardiogram is short, this component can occur very close to the onset of the ventricular contraction and actually be part of the first heart sound and contribute to its duration. Aside from this, it has no clinical significance *(11,14)*.

Mitral Component

This is the most important component of S1. It corresponds in timing to the closure of the mitral valve leaflets *(10,12)*. However, the mere apposition of the valve leaflets does not produce the sound. As the ventricle starts contracting, the pressure rises and imparts energy into the mass of blood within its cavity. When the pressure in the ventricle just exceeds that of the atrium, the column of blood is put into motion. Since the aortic pressure is much higher than the atrial pressure and the aortic valve remains closed at this time, the blood contained in the ventricle can only rush toward the atrium. Because of the anatomical construction of the mitral valve similar to that of a parachute, the leaflets are lifted by the moving blood into a closed position. The papillary muscles contracting and pulling on the chordae tendineae prevent leaflet eversion into the atrium. The closed leaflets held back by the papillary muscles, reaching the limits of their stretch, stop the column of blood from moving into the atrium. This sudden deceleration of the column of blood causes the mitral component, or M1 (Figs. 1 and 2A,B). The energy dissipation

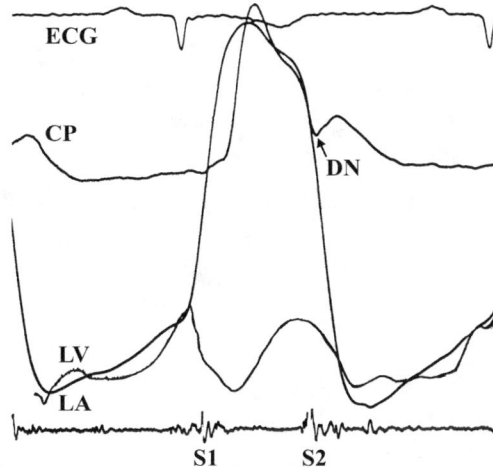

Fig. 1. Simultaneous recordings of electrocardiogram (ECG), carotid pulse (CP), left ventricular (LV), and left atrial (LA) pressures. When the rising LV pressure exceeds the LA pressure, the column of blood contained in the ventricle is put into motion because the aortic valve is still closed at this time. Because the LA pressure is relatively low, the column of blood will tend to rush toward the LA. The anatomical construction of the mitral valve is such that the leaflets close and are prevented from eversion by the contraction of the papillary muscles. The valve closure leads to sudden deceleration of the moving column of blood. The resulting dissipation of energy leads to the production of the mitral component of the S1. The rise of CP indirectly reflects aortic pressure rise. However, there is a transmission delay. DN, Dicrotic notch.

causes vibrations of the column of blood as well as the entire surrounding structures, i.e., the mitral valve structures and the ventricular wall *(15)*. The mechanism of sound formation of this M1 is very similar to the sound produced by the parachute filling with wind as it stretches and causes the deceleration of the moving mass of air or by the sail of a sailboat that snaps when filled with a gust of wind.

Tricuspid Component

This component is obviously similar in origin to the M1 for similar cardiac events occur involving the right-sided structures, namely, the tricuspid valve leaflets and the right ventricular wall. However, these events occur at much lower pressures and slightly delayed. The effects of the mechanical events of the right ventricle begin slightly later than that of the left ventricle. Therefore, the tricuspid component (T1) follows the M1 *(13)*. It must be noted that this component because of the lower pressures is usually low in frequency. The T1 in the normal adult subjects, although it may be recordable, may contribute to the duration of S1 but not be audible as a distinct component *(16,17)*.

Aortic Component

The aortic component (A1) is usually the second component of audibly split S1 in adults *(7,17)*. After mitral and tricuspid valve closures, the ventricular pressure continues to rise during the phase of isovolumic contraction. When the pressure exceeds the aortic and pulmonary diastolic pressures, the ejection phase begins as the semilunar valves open. The column of blood ejected into the aorta as it hits the aortic walls decelerates and when the deceleration is significant will result in an audible sound *(18)* (Fig. 2C).

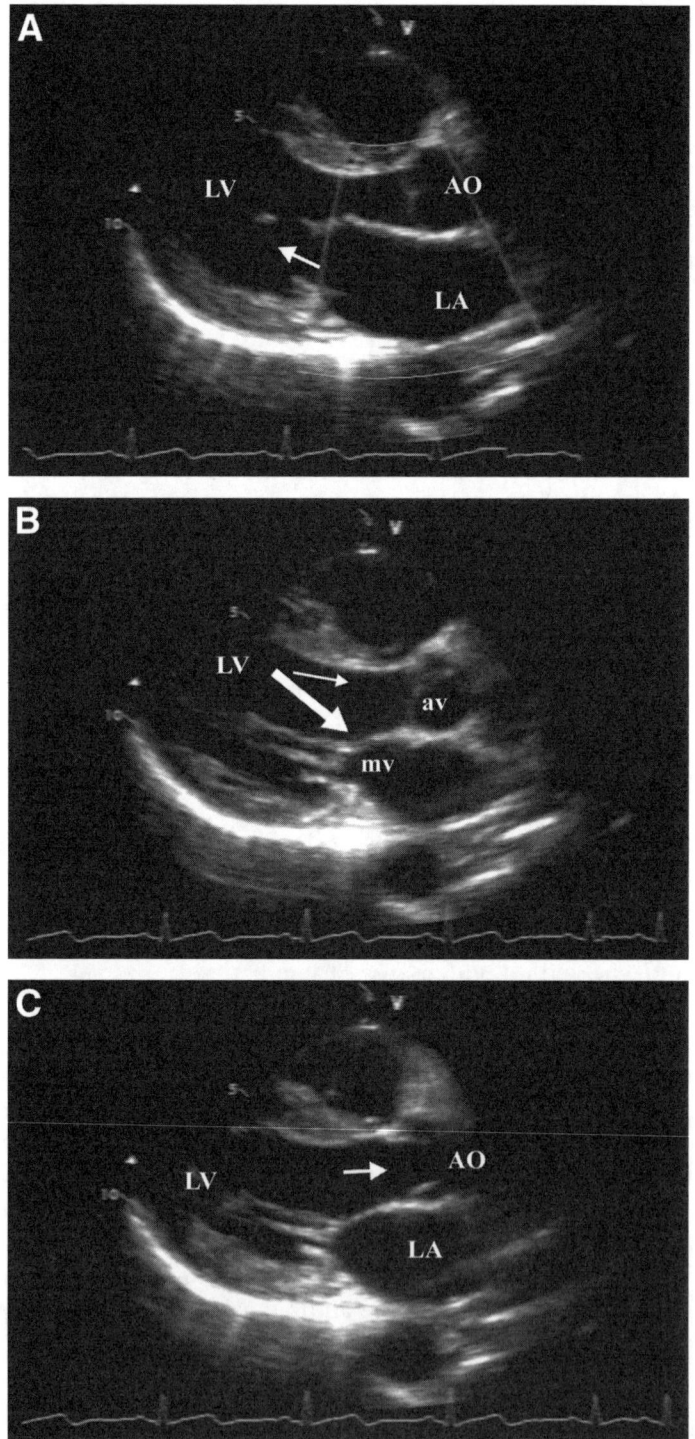

Fig. 2. Stop frames from the two-dimensional echocardiographic recordings taken in the parasternal long axis from a normal subject showing the left ventricle (LV), mitral valve (mv), left atrium (LA), aorta (AO), and aortic valve (av) at end-diastole (**A**), onset systole (**B**), and onset ejection (**C**).
(Continued on next page)

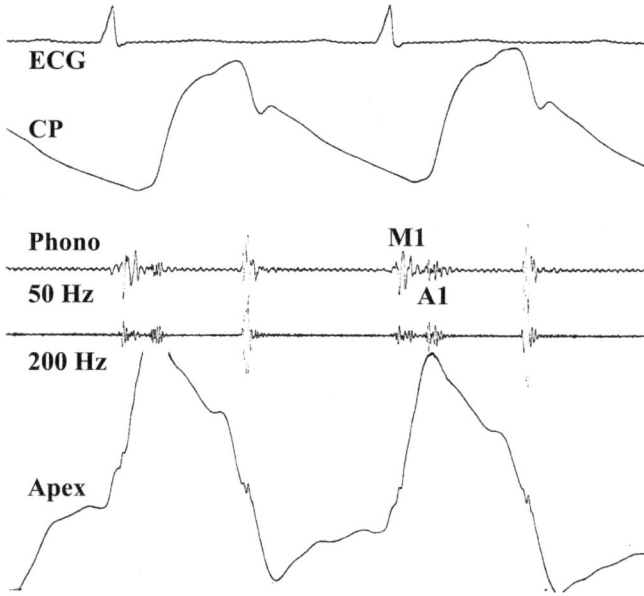

Fig. 3. Phonocardiogram (Phono) recorded at the lower left parasternal area close to the apex showing two distinct components of the normal S1, namely the mitral component M1 and the aortic component A1. The M1 precedes the onset of the carotid pulse, whereas the A1 occurs with it. Note the externally recorded carotid pulse tracing has a pulse transmission delay. Simultaneously recorded electrocardiogram (ECG), carotid pulse (CP), and apexcardiogram (Apex) are shown to indicate the timing.

Normal S1

Because the major and the most important component of S1 is M1, the S1 is usually heard loudest at the apex and the lower left sternal border around the fourth left intercostal space. The sound is usually low pitched and longer in duration compared to the sharper, shorter, and higher-frequency second heart sound (S2). It can be timed to occur at the onset of a carotid pulse or the apical impulse and is a useful way of distinguishing it from S2. It can be mimicked by the syllable "Lubbb" as opposed to the sharper S2, which sounds like "dub." It may be audibly split into two components in some patients when the separation exceeds at least 20 ms. When such a split is heard it could be because of M1-T1 in children and young adolescents and is usually due to M1-A1 in the adults (Fig. 3). The T1 component tends to be maximally heard over the sternum and the left sternal border and not usually over the apex, which is formed by the left ventricle in the

---

Fig. 2. *(Continued)* The heads of the arrows indicate the direction of movement of the column of blood in the left heart. At end-diastole, the diastolic filling of LV is nearly completed. With onset of systole, the rising LV pressure puts the column of blood into motion, with the main direction (thicker arrow) toward the low-pressure LA, where it is decelerated by the closure of the mv. This leads to production of the mitral component M1. When the rising LV pressure exceeds the aortic pressure with further contraction of the ventricle, the aortic valve opens and ejection phase begins. When the ejected column of blood hits the walls of the aorta, deceleration occurs again, leading to the production of the A1.

normal subjects. T1 also tends to get louder on inspiration because of greater volume and Starling effect during inspiratory phase of respiration on the right side. The A1, on the other hand, does not vary with respiration and is just as loud over the apex.

It must be pointed out that not all patients have a split S1 that is audible. This may be because of various factors involved in the production of the T1 and the A1. The normal T1 may not be loud enough to be audible. The A1, which occurs after the isovolumic contraction phase, may be too narrowly split to be heard as a separate distinct sound, especially when the isovolumic phase is short. The other reason may be that the orientation of the left ventricular axis in relation to the aortic axis may be such that the ejected blood easily flows out into the aorta without much deceleration at the walls. When the axial orientations form a less obtuse angle, the chances for greater deceleration and formation of audible A1 component increase. Such variations in the axial orientations can be observed in angiographic or two-dimensional echocardiographic studies in most patients.

Intensity of S1 (Loudness)

The intensity of S1 is obviously related to the intensity or loudness of the individual components, namely M1, T1, and A1. Since the major determinant of S1 intensity is M1, we shall consider this first.

M1 Intensity

Because the M1 component corresponds to the mitral valve closure and is produced by sudden deceleration and dissipation of energy of the moving column of blood in the left ventricle, its intensity will depend on the energy imparted to that column of blood by the contracting ventricle. The level of energy imparted will depend on the degree of acceleration achieved by the contracting myofibrils at the time of mitral valve closure. As the ventricle begins to contract, more and more myofibrils are recruited, which help in achieving faster rate of pressure rise (dP/dt) in the ventricle.

The mitral valve will close only when the pressure in the contracting left ventricle reaches and just surpasses the pressure in the left atrium. If the atrial pressure were high at the time of mitral valve closure, the ventricle would have achieved a high dP/dt. If the atrial pressure were low, on the other hand, at the time of mitral valve closure, the dP/dt achieved by the left ventricle would be similarly low. The energy in the moving column of blood in the left ventricle, which is dissipated upon closure of the valve, is dependent on the dP/dt achieved by the left ventricle at the time of closure. *The higher the* dP/dt *achieved by the contracting left ventricle at the time of mitral valve closure (the pressure crossover point), the louder will be the intensity of the M1 (6,12,19,20).* The corollary of this implies that the lower the dP/dt is at the time of mitral closure, the softer will be the intensity of M1.

The dP/dt achieved at the time of mitral closure will depend on the contractility of the left ventricle and the left atrial pressure. The left atrial pressure at the time of mitral valve closure may be high for one of the following reasons:

1. Mitral stenosis or mitral obstruction
2. Incomplete atrial relaxation at the time of valve closure (short PR interval)
3. Short diastoles in atrial fibrillation
4. Heart failure
5. Mitral regurgitation

However, not all of the above are associated with a loud M1.

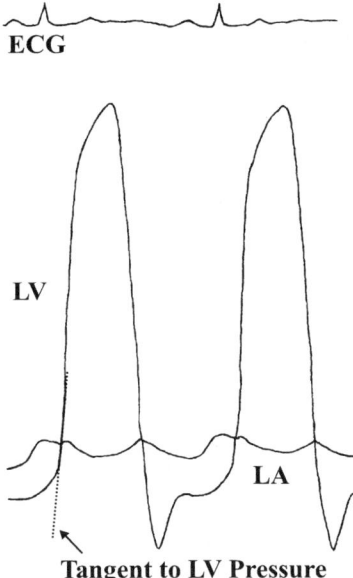

Fig. 4. Diagrammatic illustration of the left ventricular (LV) and left atrial (LA) pressure curves in a patient with mitral stenosis showing the diastolic pressure gradient between LA and the LV reflecting the mitral stenosis. When the rising LV pressure with onset of systole exceeds that of the LA, the mitral valve will close. Note that the tangent to LV pressure drawn at the point of the crossover of the two pressure curves during this phase of LV systolic pressure rise is steep, showing that the ventricle has achieved a faster rate of contraction and higher dP/dt.

M1 IN MITRAL STENOSIS OR OBSTRUCTION SECONDARY TO ATRIAL MYXOMA

It used to be thought that the loud S1 (M1) characteristic of severe mitral stenosis was caused by closure of the valve that was kept wide open by high left atrial pressure. Some even may have thought that calcification of the leaflets contributed to the intensity upon closure.

In mitral stenosis, S1 (M1) is loud because the valve closure occurs at a time when the dP/dt in the ventricle is high as a result of a higher pressure crossover point (Figs. 4 and 5). In some patients with very severe mitral stenosis, usually associated with heavily calcified valves, the M1 may not be loud. This probably stems from the fact that the left ventricles in such patients are grossly underfilled from the mitral obstruction and therefore are unable to achieve good contractility and dP/dt.

In left atrial myxoma, which causes mitral obstruction, the M1 will be loud for the same reason as in mitral stenosis.

M1 AND PR INTERVALS

After left atrial contraction, if the left ventricle begins to contract before the left atrium has a chance to fully relax, the left atrial pressure will be high at the time of pressure crossover and mitral closure. This is likely to occur when the PR interval is short. This will result also in a louder M1 component (Fig. 6A). The corollary to this means that a long PR interval will result in a soft M1 (Fig. 6B). This is because of complete relaxation

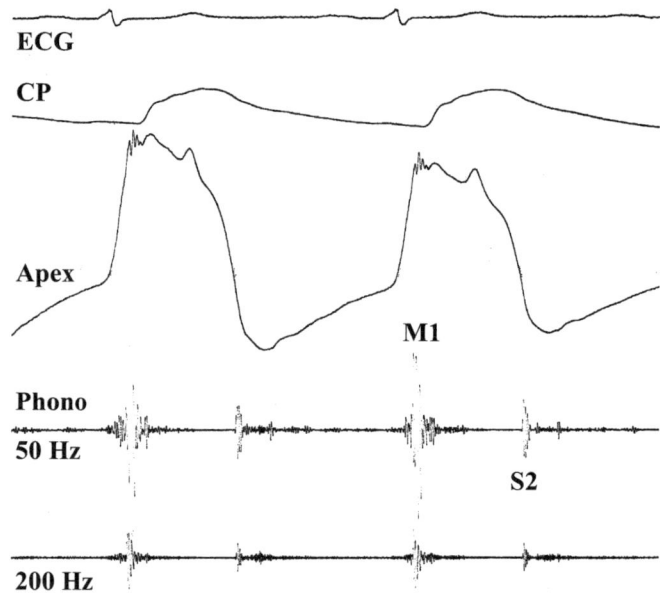

Fig. 5. Phonocardiographic (Phono) recording from a patient with mitral stenosis showing the loud intensity first heart sound caused by the loud mitral component M1.

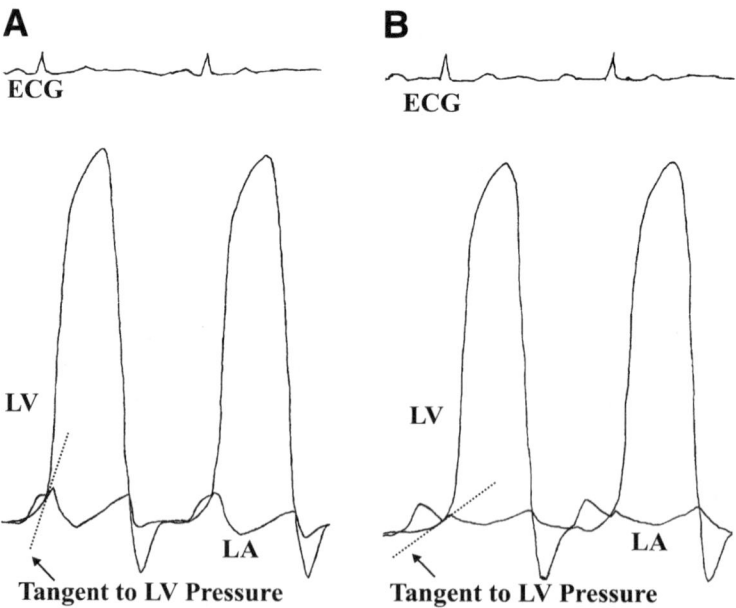

Fig. 6. Diagrammatic illustrations of the superimposed left ventricular (LV) and left atrial (LA) pressure curves to show the differences in the slope of the LV pressure rise at the point of the crossover of the two pressures with onset of systole caused by short PR interval (**A**) and long PR interval (**B**). The slope is steeper when the PR is short, whereas it is flatter when the PR is long. This will result in M1 being loud when the PR is short, but soft when the PR is long.

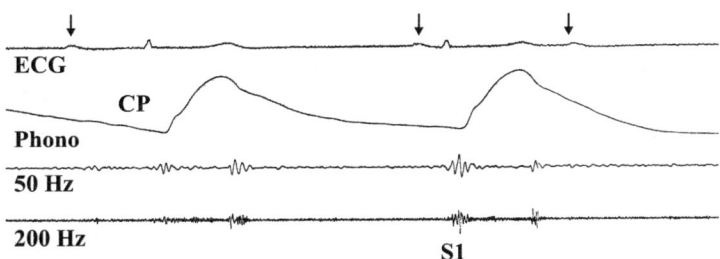

Fig. 7. Phonocardiographic (Phono) tracing from a patient with complete atrioventricular (A-V) block recorded from the apex area. Arrows show the nonconducted P waves in the electrocardiogram (ECG). The effect of the variations in the PR interval caused by the A-V block on the S1 intensity can be seen. The first beat with long PR has a poor-intensity S1, whereas the second beat with a shorter PR has much better S1 intensity.

of the left atrium before the left ventricular contraction and maximal fall in the left atrial pressure, resulting in a very low-pressure crossover point where the dP/dt achieved by the left ventricle will be low.

When the PR interval changes, as in atrioventricular (A-V) dissociation (e.g., complete A-V block) or type I second-degree A-V block (Wenckebach), the intensity of M1 will also vary according to the PR interval. It will be louder with shorter interval and softer with longer intervals (Fig. 7).

M1 AND SHORT DIASTOLES IN ATRIAL FIBRILLATION

Variable M1 intensity is also characteristic of atrial fibrillation. The mechanism, however, relates to the varying diastolic filling and its effect on contractility as well as varying levels of atrial pressure at the time of mitral closure. Following shorter diastoles, while the filling of the left ventricle may be poor leading to decreased Starling effect and contractility, the left atrial pressure does not have a chance to fall to lower levels. This results in a higher left atrial pressure. Since these two will have opposing effects on M1 intensity, usually the higher left atrial pressure effect dominates, causing louder M1 with shorter diastoles.

M1 IN HEART FAILURE

Although the left atrial pressure in heart failure is invariably elevated, this does not always result in a loud S1. The marked decrease in contractility of the left ventricle results in a poor dP/dt development at the time of mitral closure. In these patients there is often a high sympathetic tone and high levels of catecholamines. These tend to compensate and attempt to improve the contractility of the myocardium. At times this may in fact succeed in improving the initial rise in left ventricular pressure, although the effect may not be sustained throughout systole. This may be sufficient to produce a reasonable intensity of S1. In very severely damaged hearts such compensation often does not result in any significant improvement in the dP/dt, and therefore the S1 (M1) is very soft and sometimes inaudible.

M1 IN MITRAL REGURGITATION

Because the intensity of M1 is dependent on sudden deceleration of the moving column of blood in the left ventricle, the presence of significant mitral regurgitation would preclude such sudden deceleration. This in effect may lead to a softer M1. On the other hand, the mitral regurgitation may raise the mean left atrial pressure and therefore the pressure crossover point. It also presents a volume overload effect for the left ventricle, thereby increasing its contractility through the Starling mechanism. These two effects will tend to increase the intensity of the M1. Therefore, the M1 intensity in mitral regurgitation in any given patient will depend on the severity of the mitral regurgitation, the acuteness of its onset, and the underlying left ventricular function. The opposing effects of these on the M1 may result in a normal M1 intensity.

In acute mitral regurgitation, the left atrial pressure usually rises much higher because of a relatively noncompliant left atrium. This in a patient with ruptured chordae with relatively normal left ventricular function may tend to favor production of a good intensity of M1 as long as the mitral regurgitation is not too severe. In severe mitral regurgitation, however, hardly any deceleration will be possible because of the valvular insufficiency. Similarly, in a patient with ruptured papillary muscle and acute myocardial infarction, the M1 will be inaudible. This is not only because of decreased myocardial contractility, but also mainly because of the wide-open nature of the mitral regurgitation and poor or no deceleration of the column of blood.

Lesions That Interfere With the Integrity of the Isovolumic Phase of Systole

The importance of the integrity of the isovolumic systole for the preservation of the intensity of the M1 has been pointed out by Shah *(12)*. This essentially pertains to the fact that for a good-intensity M1 to occur the column of blood needs to accelerate toward the mitral valve for it to be decelerated by the closure. The cited examples of lesions that interfere with the integrity of the isovolumic phase of contraction include significant mitral regurgitation, significant aortic regurgitation, large ventricular septal defect, and large ventricular aneurysm. In these entities, the moment the left ventricular pressure rises the ejection phase begins to transfer the blood out of the contracting left ventricle. The M1 in wide-open mitral regurgitation will be soft, as pointed out earlier. M1 in aortic regurgitation is of particular interest.

M1 in Aortic Regurgitation

Aortic regurgitation, being also a volume overload situation for the left ventricle, will lead to increased contractility and therefore would be expected to have a good amplitude of S1 (M1). In severe and acute types of aortic valve regurgitation, however, the left ventricular diastolic pressures often rise to very high levels to the point that the pressure in the left ventricle may equal the aortic diastolic pressure and exceed that in the left atrium before ventricular systole begins. This will essentially result in premature mitral valve closure. In some instances, the mitral leaflets could be incompletely closed with perhaps some diastolic bulging into the left atrium under the high left ventricular diastolic pressure, allowing some diastolic mitral regurgitation. However, with the onset of ventricular systole, the leaflets may be fully closed with papillary muscle contraction even before significant pressure rise, at a time when the developed *dP/dt* in the left ventricle will be still low. Because the left ventricular and aortic diastolic pressures are often equal, there will be very little or no isovolumic phase of contraction. The moment the ventricular pressure begins to rise faster, the ejection will occur with the column of blood essentially moving toward the aorta. Because the mitral valve is already closed,

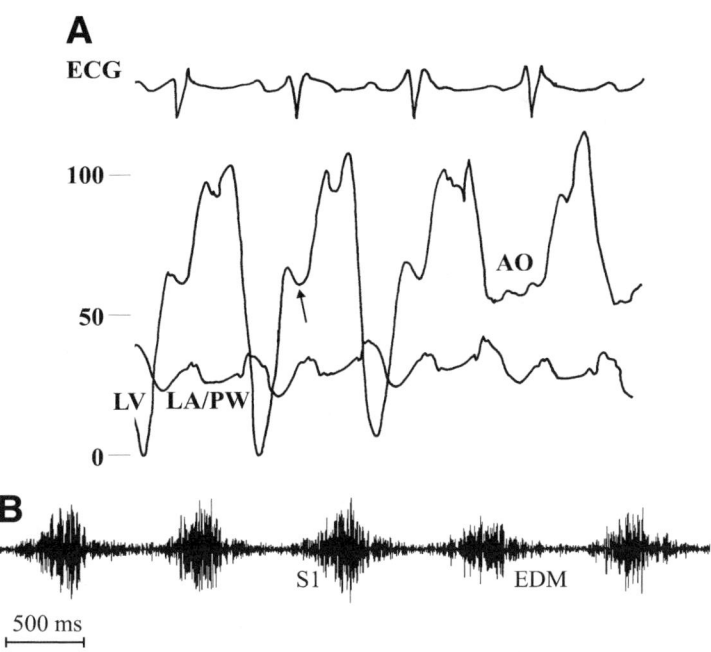

Fig. 8. **(A)** Simultaneous recordings of indirect left atrial (LA) pressure (the pulmonary capillary wedge [PW] pressure) and the left ventricular (LV) pressure from a patient with acute severe aortic regurgitation (shown in the first two beats). The recording catheter is withdrawn to the aorta to show the aortic (AO) pressure (fourth beat). The arrow points to the end-diastolic pressure in the LV, which is almost equal to the diastolic pressure in the AO. The diastolic pressure in the LV rises quite abruptly and in the middle of diastole exceeds the level of the LA pressure, thereby closing the mitral valve prematurely before the onset of systole. This will result in a poor intensity S1 (*see* Fig. 8B). **(B)** Digital display of the magnetic audio recording from a patient with severe aortic regurgitation recorded close to the apex area. Note the crescendo–decrescendo systolic ejection murmur followed by the early diastolic murmur (EDM) of the aortic regurgitation. The former is due to large stroke volume ejected from the left ventricle as a result of the volume overload. The S1 is soft and is poorly recorded.

there will be no acceleration of column of blood toward the left atrium and therefore no deceleration to cause a sound. This will lead to a very soft and inaudible M1 (S1) *(20–23)* (Figs. 8A,B).

T1 Intensity

The T1 intensity is usually soft in the normal adults and therefore not easily audible. However, its intensity may be increased under certain circumstances.

INCREASED RIGHT VENTRICULAR CONTRACTILITY

T1 intensity may be increased when there is increased right ventricular contractility, as may be seen with right ventricular volume overload causing increased Starling effect (Fig. 9). These states most commonly include left-to-right shunt through an atrial septal defect. In tricuspid regurgitation, although the volume overload is present, the regurgitation does not allow adequate deceleration of the column of blood, therefore the T1 intensity is not

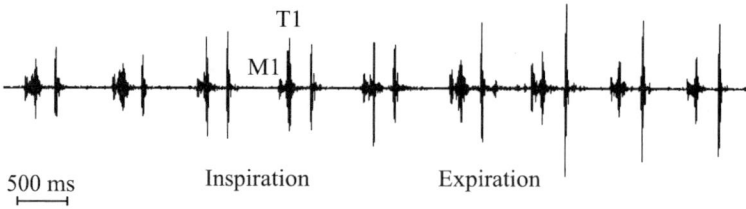

Fig. 9. Digital display of the magnetic audio recording from a 16-year-old man with a large and slightly redundant tricuspid valve taken at the lower left sternal border area. Two components (M1 and T1) of the S1 are seen, the second component of which is intensified on inspiration showing that it is the T1.

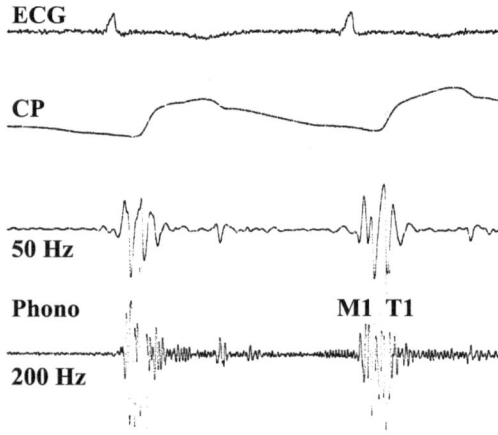

Fig. 10. Phonocardiogram (Phono) recording from a patient with Ebstein's anomaly of the tricuspid valve recorded from the lower left sternal area showing a delayed louder-intensity T1.

generally increased. In congenital pulmonary regurgitation with normal pulmonary pressures and normal right ventricular function, the T1 intensity will be increased. With iatrogenic pulmonary regurgitation, as may often occur following operative repair of tetralogy of Fallot, the T1 intensity may not be increased particularly if there is associated right ventricular damage. Similar consideration will apply also in patients with pulmonary regurgitation secondary to pulmonary hypertension.

HIGHER RIGHT ATRIAL PRESSURE AT THE TIME OF TRICUSPID VALVE CLOSURE

In tricuspid obstruction caused by either tricuspid stenosis (which is rare) or by tumors such as atrial myxoma, the right atrial pressure will be elevated and this will lead to a higher pressure crossover point on the right side. This will result in higher *dP/dt* achieved by the right ventricle at the time of tricuspid valve closure, resulting in loud T1.

When the tricuspid valve is abnormally large and redundant, as seen in some patients with *Ebstein's anomaly*, the actual deceleration of the column of blood may occur slightly later because of the redundancy. By this time the right ventricular *dP/dt* may have reached a steeper slope contributing to an increased intensity of T1 (Fig. 10). The *sail sound* described in some patients with Ebstein's anomaly represents the louder delayed T1 *(24)*.

A1 Intensity

The A1 may or may not be present depending on whether or not the ejected jet during onset of ejection decelerates sufficiently against the wall of the aortic root to cause a sound. This is perhaps purely determined by the anatomy. When present it usually is coincident with the onset of pressure rise in the central aorta. The only controlling factor determining its intensity will be the left ventricular contractility.

A1 may be increased in the presence of hyperdynamic states such as anemia, thyrotoxicosis, and Paget's disease.

Aortic Ejection Sound and Click

Certain conditions may lead to effective deceleration of the ejected jet at onset of systole, resulting in loud, sharp, and clicky sounds. These may either arise from the aortic root, as in normal A1, or from the aortic valve. Sometimes, however, the sound may not be as clicky. This may occur at the usual timing of normal A1 or slightly later. When it arises as a result of exaggeration of the normal A1, it will occur at the onset of aortic pressure rise. Strong inotropic agents (e.g., isoproterenol and norepinephrine) can be shown to increase the amplitude of the aortic root ejection sound. On the other hand, methoxamine, which lacks the inotropic effect, will decrease the amplitude *(18)*.

The most common causes of these aortic ejection sounds and/or clicks are:

1. *Bicuspid aortic valve* where the cusps are often unequal in size and the opening may be eccentric, resulting in an *eccentric jet*. The latter would therefore be expected to decelerate against the wall of the aorta. The direction of the jet may be almost perpendicular to the aortic wall, resulting in a sharper and louder sound. The timing of this is usually similar to the normal A1 or delayed only to a slight degree (Figs. 11A–C).
2. In *congenital aortic valvular stenosis*, the aortic valve is often domed. When the aortic valve is domed and stenosed and does not freely open, the deceleration may occur against the *doming valve* itself *(25)*. The sound in these instances will often be clicky. The aortic ejection clicks have been shown to correspond to the timing of the maximal doming. The click precedes the onset of the aortic stenosis murmur and occurs 20–30 ms after the onset of the aortic pressure rise. It occurs at the anacrotic shoulder of the aortic pressure pulse (Fig. 12). When the stenosis is severe and the valve is immobile and calcified, aortic ejection clicks are not heard. The presence of the ejection click in obstruction of the left ventricular outflow tract will suggest a valvular origin of the stenosis *(18,26)*.
3. In *aortic root aneurysm*, the column of ejected blood will make close to a 90º angle with the wall of the aorta because of distortion caused by the aneurysmal dilatation (Fig. 13). The aorta may also be noncompliant. This will result in more of a clicky sound, usually later than the normal A1 (Fig. 14).

Aortic ejection sounds and clicks, when present, are usually heard over the left sternal border and the apex. However, when caused by aortic root aneurysm they may be louder at the second and third right intercostal space at the sternal border.

Pulmonary Ejection Sound and Click

Because the normal pulmonary pressures are low, there is no audible or recordable normal pulmonary ejection sound. Therefore, when a pulmonary ejection sound or click is heard, it is always pathological.

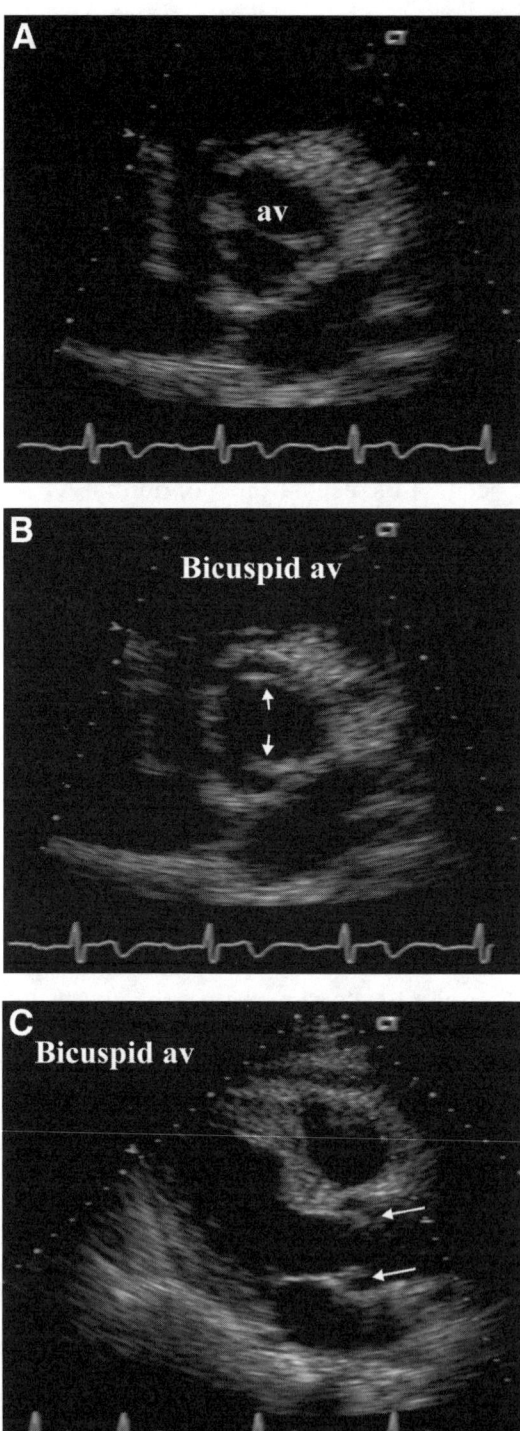

Fig.11. Stop frames from two-dimensional echocardiogram taken from a patient with a bicuspid aortic valve and aortic ejection click. The short axis shows the two cusps (**A**) in the closed position and (**B**) in the open position. The aortic valve cusps are seen to be slightly domed in systole (arrows) as observed in the parasternal long axis (**C**).

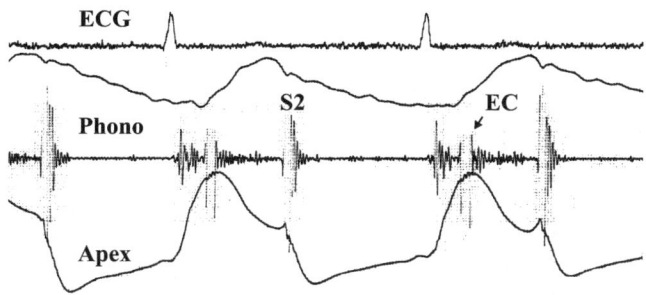

Fig. 12. Phonocardiogram (Phono) recording from a patient with congenital aortic valve stenosis with domed bicuspid aortic valve. Note that the aortic ejection click (EC) is slightly delayed and seen to correspond to the anacrotic hump on the carotid pulse (CP).

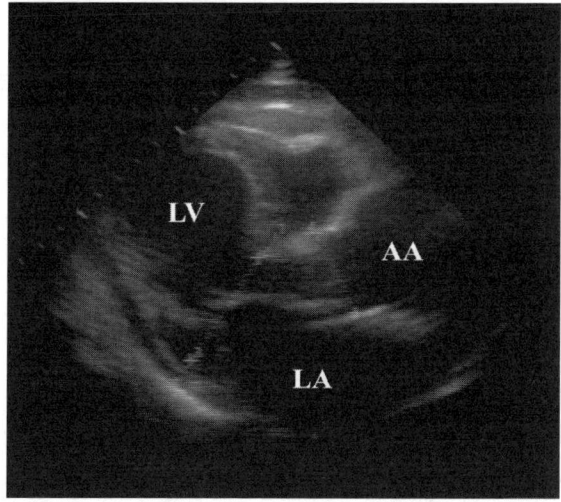

Fig. 13. Stop frame from two-dimensional echocardiogram from a patient taken in the parasternal long axis showing dilated aneurysmal ascending aorta (AA) just above the aortic valve. Note that the orientation of the AA is such that it is at a 90° angle to the longitudinal axis of the left ventricle (LV).

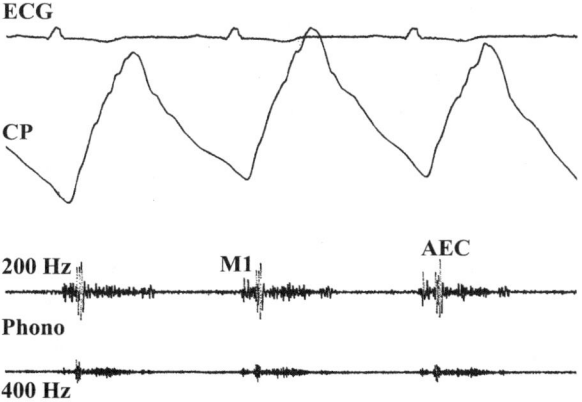

Fig. 14. Phonocardiogram (Phono) recording from a patient with hypertension and dilated aortic root taken at the lower left sternal border area showing an aortic ejection click (AEC).

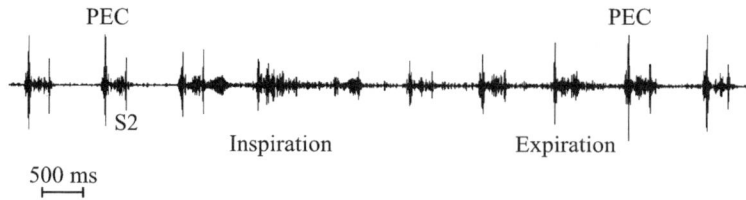

Fig. 15. Digital display of magnetic audio recording from a patient with congenital pulmonary valve stenosis taken from the lower left sternal area showing the pulmonary ejection click (PEC). Note that the sharp sound that begins the systolic murmur (PEC) is seen to become very soft and almost disappear on inspiration, becoming clicky and sharp on expiration.

There are usually two causes of pulmonary ejection clicks *(27)*:
1. Dilated pulmonary artery: The pulmonary artery may become dilated as a result of severe longstanding pulmonary hypertension or be of idiopathic origin with normal pulmonary pressures. The ejected column of blood because of distortion caused by dilatation of the root will be decelerating against the wall of the pulmonary artery causing a clicky sound. This click—as with all other right-sided events—will increase in intensity with inspiration.
2. Congenital pulmonary valvular stenosis: In congenital pulmonary valvular stenosis, the click occurs with the maximal doming of the valve. The deceleration of the column of blood is against the domed valve. The mechanism is similar to that observed in aortic valvular stenosis, except it is present invariably in all patients. The pulmonary valve is usually very pliable and never calcified. *This click, however, has a unique variation with respiration, which in fact helps to identify its origin. The click becomes softer or even inaudible on inspiration* (28) (Fig. 15). *This is the only exception to the rule that the right-sided events become exaggerated with inspiration.* In these patients the pulmonary artery pressure is usually very low. During inspiration the increased venous return into a hypertrophied and somewhat noncompliant right ventricle raises the right ventricular end-diastolic pressure during right atrial contraction. This may exceed the pulmonary artery diastolic pressure. This in effect would cause the doming of the pulmonary valve even before the ventricular contraction starts. Thus, with ventricular systole as the column of blood is set into motion, the valve being maximally domed, there is no sudden deceleration against the valve itself, and therefore no sound.

Pulmonary ejection clicks are maximally loud over the second and third left intercostal spaces at the left sternal border. However, when they are loud they can be heard over a wide area of the precordium, including the xiphoid region.

CLINICAL ASSESSMENT OF S1 AND COMPONENTS

When assessing the S1 at the bedside, one should assess the following:
1. Intensity or loudness
2. Variability of intensity (loudness)
3. Presence of more than one component (split S1)
4. Quality
5. Location of maximal loudness
6. Effect of respiration

Intensity or Loudness

Because loudness can vary due to noncardiac factors such as body shape or chest wall deformities or the presence of pulmonary disease, these should be taken into account in assessing the true loudness, which may be attenuated.

The loudness of the sound, however, can be graded using the system of grading murmurs. The system allows six categories of loudness. Grades I–III are not loud enough to be palpable, whereas grades IV–VI are loud and palpable. Grade I requires tuning in to mentally filter out room noise from the actual sound. The grade II sound is audible the moment the auscultation is begun even without having to concentrate and eliminate the room noise. This is the usual intensity heard by beginners. The grade III sound is the loudest sound audible, which, however, is not palpable. The grade IV sound, although palpable, requires full contact of the stethoscope against the chest wall for audibility. The grade V sound requires only the edge of the stethoscope to touch the chest wall to hear the sound. The grade VI sound, however, can be heard with the stethoscope slightly but completely off the chest wall.

When S1 intensity is graded using the above system, all grades IV–VI are abnormal. Even grade III may be significant in some patients. However, it is difficult to diagnose a true decrease in S1 intensity because of extracardiac factors, which attenuate the sound. Other methods to overcome part of this problem were discussed in Chapter 3 in relation to the blood pressure and the assessment of ventricular function.

When S1 is loud, it is important to locate the area of maximal loudness, which may be possible by palpation. If the apical impulse is left ventricular as defined by the presence of medial retraction and the maximal loudness of S1 is at the apex, then one can safely assume that the M1 is the loud component. But it is important to remember that the other components of S1 can at times be the loudest and may become palpable. Occasionally ejection clicks (both aortic and pulmonary) when very loud may also become palpable. These will have to be identified by other features on auscultation.

Variability of Intensity

Variations in S1 intensity from cycle to cycle are usually a result of variations in M1. There are four basic causes for variations in M1 intensity.

1. A-V dissociation, where the P-R relationship may vary haphazardly from beat to beat. The shorter PR intervals will have louder M1, whereas the longer PR will have softer M1. This phenomenon can occur in complete A-V block, patients with electronic pacemakers, and also in ventricular rhythms.
2. In Mobitz type I second-degree A-V block, the S1 intensity may become progressively softer as the PR lengthens before the dropped beat and pause.
3. Atrial fibrillation, where the diastolic filling periods keep changing constantly, causing various degrees of Starling effect and variations in left atrial pressure at the time of mitral valve closure.
4. Pulsus alternans, where because of instability of intracellular calcium shifts, the contractility alternates between weak and strong beats. This usually occurs only in severe cardiomyopathies.

Components of S1 and Quality

One should on auscultation determine whether or not more than one component of S1 is audible (split S1). Then one should try to ascertain the origin of each component and compare their relative loudness. At the same time, any clicky quality of the components should also be noted. Such clicky quality to S1 or one of its components should alert one to the presence of aortic or pulmonary ejection click. Normal M1 is not clicky, although a mechanical mitral prosthetic ball valve usually would cause a clicky M1 at the time of its closure.

When one of the components of S1 is very loud it can have a masking effect on the other component, thereby appearing on auscultation to have only a single component. When the S1 is loud one should not always assume this to be because of loud M1. It is important to identify its features thereby identifying its origin. The M1 and the A1 will be maximally loud at the apex and will not change with respiration. The same rule applies to the aortic ejection click, although it may be equally loud at the second right intercostal space. The T1, on the other hand, is loudest at the lower left sternal border and over the xiphoid area and can be noted to increase in loudness on inspiration. Occasionally when the right ventricle is very large and forms the apex of the heart (lateral retraction present), the T1 may be loudest over the apex.

It is also important to note that a loud pulmonary ejection click, being very close in timing to the normal S1, may be mistaken for one of its components. However, this can be easily solved by the fact that it will get softer on inspiration and may sometimes be audible only on expiration. The maximal loudness of a pulmonary ejection click is usually over the second and third left intercostal space.

When A1 is clicky and/or loud enough to cause a good split S1, one can further confirm it to be M1 and A1 by observing the effect of standing. Standing by reducing the venous return will tend to lower the left atrial pressure and the left ventricular end-diastolic pressure. While there may be a slight rise in heart rate secondary to sympathetic stimulation, the decreased filling pressure will lead to a slower rate of pressure rise in the left ventricle. This will imply some lengthening of the isovolumic contraction phase. The A1, which comes at onset of ejection, therefore coming after the end of the isovolumic contraction phase, will be somewhat delayed from the M1, thereby making the split somewhat wider on standing.

(For additional examples review Phono Files 0–9 and Echo Phono File 1 under Heart Sounds on the Companion CD.)

SECOND HEART SOUND (S2)

The second heart sound occurs at the end of the ejection phase of systole. It is related to the closure of the semilunar valves. Since there are two semilunar valves, aortic and pulmonary, there are also two components for the S2, namely the aortic component (A2) and the pulmonary component (P2).

Mechanism of Formation of S2

As the blood is ejected into the aorta and the pulmonary artery during systole (stroke volume), the aortic and the pulmonary pressures rise and these two vessels become

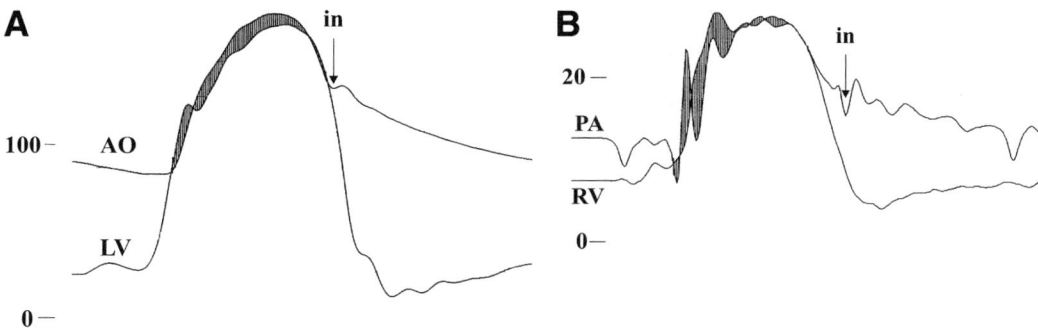

Fig. 16. Simultaneous left ventricular (LV) and aortic (AO) pressure and simultaneous right ventricular (RV) and pulmonary artery (PA) pressure are shown in **(A)** and **(B)**, respectively. The falling ventricular pressure at the end of systole leads to the development of a pressure gradient between the AO and the LV on the left side and between the PA and the RV on the right side. The aortic and the pulmonary components of the S2 occur at the time of the respective incisura (in) in the AO and PA pressures. *(Continued on next page)*

distended. At the end of systole, as the ventricular pressures begin to fall, the elastic components of the great vessels maintaining a higher pressure results in a pressure gradient, which drives the columns of blood back into the ventricles. The columns of blood in the great vessels preferably flow toward the ventricles at this time because of the lower resistance with the dropping ventricular pressures compared to the periphery. The reverse flow of the columns of blood in the aorta and the pulmonary artery parachutes the cusps of the aortic and the pulmonary valves, closing them. The sudden deceleration of the columns of blood against the closed semilunar valves causes dissipation of energy, resulting in the A2 and the P2 components of S2 (Figs. 16A–D).

NORMAL S2

The S2 is usually sharper, crisper, and shorter in duration compared to S1. This is because of the fact that the semilunar valve closures occur at much higher pressures than the A-V valves and the dissipated energy in the columns of blood is much greater. In normal young subjects one can often hear both components of S2 (A2 and P2). The S2 will therefore be heard as a split sound. The first of the two components is the A2. The higher impedance (i.e., resistance to forward flow) in the systemic circulation results in earlier acceleration of reverse flow in the aortic root, causing the aortic valve to close earlier *(29,30)*.

The pulmonary arterial bed is larger and offers markedly less resistance to forward flow. This will make the tendency to reverse flow occur later and slower compared to the left side. In addition, it is also possible that the lower pressures achieved by the right ventricle during systole may actually result in a slower rate of relaxation of the right ventricle compared to the left ventricle. For these reasons, the P2 component occurs later.

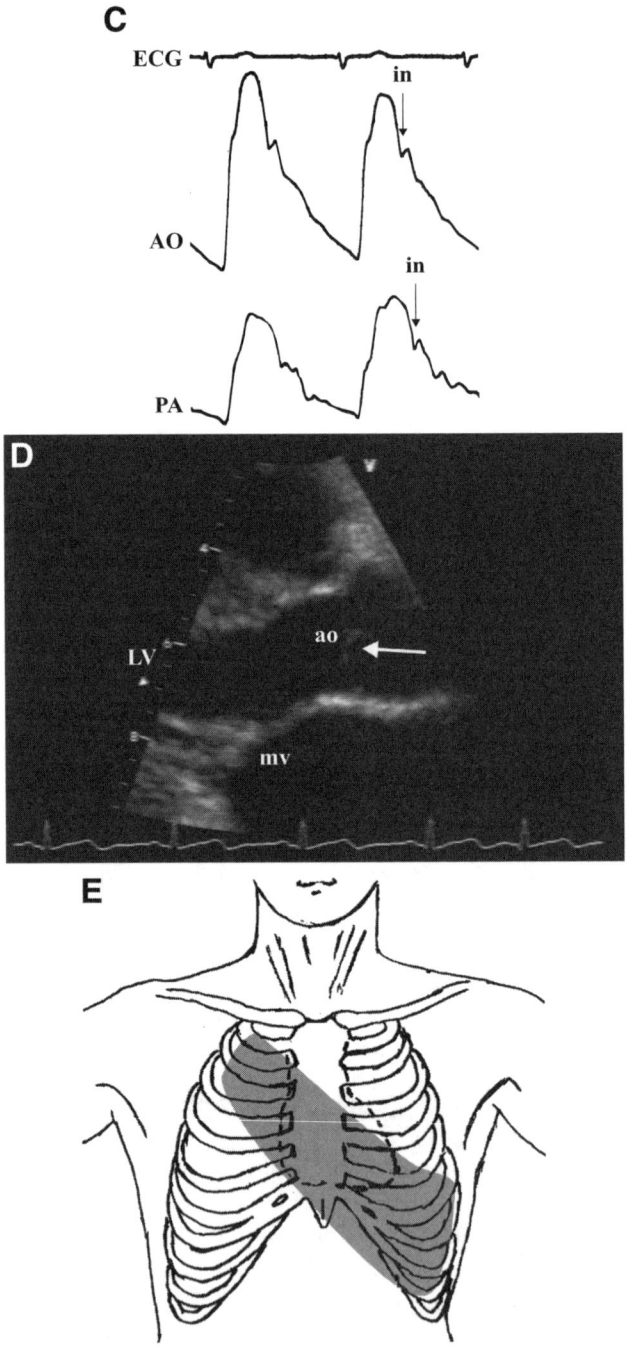

Fig. 16. *(Continued)* (**C**) Recording of the simultaneous aortic (AO) and pulmonary artery (PA) pressures show that the incisura (in) in the AO occurs earlier than in the PA. (**D**) Stop frame from a two-dimensional echocardiogram from a normal subject taken at the parasternal long axis showing the aortic valve in the closed position causing the deceleration of the column of blood, which is trying to enter the left ventricle from the aorta as a result of the pressure gradient at the end of systole between the AO and the LV. (**E**) Diagram of the chest showing the true aortic area, which is the sash area (shaded area) extending from the second right interspace to the apex.

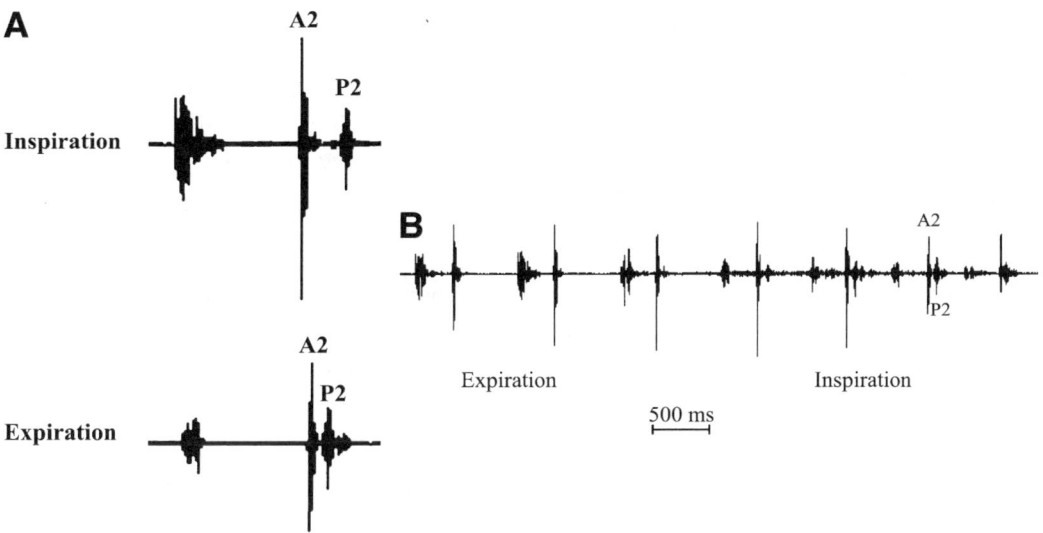

Fig. 17. (**A**) Diagram showing the two components of the S2 and their variation with respiration in normals. The normal sequence is that the aortic component (A2) occurs before the pulmonary component (P2). On inspiration, the A2 comes slightly earlier, but the P2 is significantly more delayed, widening the split. The reverse occurs on expiration, with the split becoming quite narrow. (**B**) Digital display of the magnetic audio recording from a normal young subject taken from the third left intercostal space at the left sternal border showing the normal S2 split on inspiration into A2 and P2 and essentially a single S2 on expiration.

The A2 component is normally heard over the true aortic area, which is the *sash area* (the area extending from the second right intercostal space at the sternal border to the apex) (Fig. 16E). P2, on the other hand, is heard over the second and the third left intercostal spaces near the sternal border. Therefore, the splitting of the normal S2 is best appreciated at the second and third left intercostal space. The relative loudness of the two components is such that in the normal, the A2 is always louder than the P2 mainly because the systemic arterial resistance is normally 10 times higher than the pulmonary arterial resistance *(4, 16,30)*.

Normal Respiratory Variations of A2-P2 Split

In normal subjects the splitting is often best recognized on inspiration because the two components tend to move away from each other, causing them to separate better. On expiration they tend to move closer to each other. This often results in them becoming single, or if they are still separated, the splitting is very narrow (Figs. 17A,B). During inspiration there is increased venous return to the right heart because of the fall in the intrathoracic pressures. There is also expansion of the lungs, resulting in decreased resistance in the pulmonary circulation. The expansion of the lungs also increases the pulmonary vascular capacity, leading to a slightly decreased left-sided filling. These changes affect both components of the S2 in terms of their timing, causing the A2 to come earlier and the P2 to be delayed. However, the A2 is affected to a very small degree because the systemic resistance is not affected by respiration. The P2, on the other hand, is delayed on inspiration for two reasons: the increased volume on the right side and the fall in the pulmonary resistance on inspiration. The former will result in an increase in the right ventricular ejection time. The latter will allow easier forward flow, resulting in slower tendency for reversal. On expiration, with rise in the intrathoracic pressure, the venous return to the right heart decreases and the right ventricular ejection time will shorten. The lungs collapse, the pulmonary capacity will diminish, and the resistance will rise. These changes will result in P2 occurring early on expiration *(4,16,31,32)*.

The normal respiratory variation is not as prevalent in the elderly as it is in younger patients *(32)*. This may be because of decreased compliance of the chest wall and great vessels and the relatively increased impedances in both systemic and pulmonary circulations.

ABNORMAL S2

The abnormalities of S2 may occur as a result of changes in the intensity of the individual components or changes in their timing. The latter often may lead to abnormal respiratory variations.

Intensity of S2

The loudness or intensity of the S2 can be determined by the grading system previously alluded to in relation to S1. The sounds with loudness grades IV–VI would be abnormal and increased. When S2 is either inaudible or grade I in loudness, it could be considered decreased when S1 or other sounds are normal.

Intensity of A2

The A2 intensity is dependent on the amount of energy that the column of blood in the aortic root attains in its attempt to flow toward the ventricle (assuming the integrity of the aortic valve). This in turn is dependent on the stroke volume, aortic elasticity, and most importantly the peripheral resistance. When the stroke volume is either normal or increased, the peripheral resistance becomes the major determinant of the intensity. When there is increased peripheral resistance, the diastolic pressure in the aorta remains higher than normal. When the left ventricular pressure falls because of onset of ventricular relaxation in late systole, the maintained higher pressure in the aorta provides a greater pressure head to act on the column of blood in the aortic root. The higher pressure head trying to move the column of blood in the aortic root toward the left ventricle imparts greater energy. Thus, when it decelerates it causes a louder A2. Thus, in systemic hypertension, A2 becomes louder, may be palpable, and may become musical in quality because of maintained vibrations under high tension. The sound mimics the beating on a tambour.

In patients with severe heart failure and poor stroke volume, A2 can become soft and, rarely, inaudible despite high peripheral resistance. The poor stroke volume causes poor distension of the elastic components of the aortic root, and therefore the energy in the column of blood closing the valve is very low. These patients often have low pulse pressure and low-amplitude arterial pulse.

In severe aortic stenosis, the stroke volume is ejected slowly and over a longer period and also leads to poor distension of the aortic root, leading to often a lower intensity A2, and this may be inaudible.

A2 Intensity in Aortic Regurgitation

Aortic regurgitation can occur as a result of valvular disease or aortic root pathology. Aortic regurgitation leads to increased stroke volume. The peripheral resistance is usually low because of compensatory mechanisms. The large stroke volume causes greater distension of the aortic root and therefore would cause a greater amount of energy in the column of blood in the aortic root trying to close the valve. The degree of deceleration achieved by the reversing column of blood will depend on the anatomical cause and the severity of the regurgitation. Despite significant aortic regurgitation, because of increased energy in the column of blood, the A2 intensity is often well preserved. The lower peripheral resistance will have a tendency to reduce the intensity of A2. The two effects often may balance each other. However, in very severe (wide-open) regurgitation, A2 intensity may decrease significantly because of poor deceleration. When patients with aortic regurgitation develop left ventricular failure, their stroke volume will be reduced to normal levels and their A2 may become soft or inaudible.

Sometimes A2 may be louder than normal for anatomical reasons, namely, conditions that make the aorta anterior and closer to the chest wall. These include a thin chest, straight back syndrome with decreased antero-posterior diameter, transposition of the great vessels (congenitally corrected or uncorrected), and tetralogy of Fallot where, in addition, the P2 may be attenuated because of a deformed pulmonary valve.

Intensity of P2

P2 intensity, like A2 intensity, is dependent on the stroke volume, pulmonary artery elasticity, and the pulmonary arterial resistance. When the right ventricular stroke volume is significantly increased as in left-to-right shunts through an atrial septal defect, the P2 may become louder, but not reaching the level of palpability unless significant pulmonary hypertension is also present. Along with the increased size of the right ventricle, this may also contribute to the audibility of the P2 over a wider area of the precordium. The pulmonary artery remains elastic except in severe pulmonary hypertension. The major determinant of increased P2 intensity is, in fact, the pulmonary arterial resistance. In pulmonary hypertension, whether acute or chronic, the pulmonary arterial resistance is increased because of vasospasm (increased vascular tone). Also, when the pulmonary hypertension is chronic, structural changes occur in the arterial wall with medial hypertrophy and increased intimal thickening, which make the pulmonary arterial system stiff and less elastic. The increased resistance raises the pulmonary arterial systolic and diastolic pressures. The right ventricular relaxation may be impaired, taking a longer time for the right ventricular systolic pressure to fall. In addition, the increased pulmonary pressures provide a greater pressure head. The higher pressure head, together with increased resistance to forward flow, acts to impart greater energy and velocity to the column of blood in the pulmonary root in its attempt to flow toward the right ventricle. Therefore, when it decelerates it produces a louder-intensity P2. When the P2 becomes palpable (grades IV–VI), it invariably indicates severe pulmonary hypertension.

Because of low pressures on the right side, the P2 is often soft and occasionally not audible. In significant pulmonary stenosis, the stroke volume may be quite low, and this, together with very low pulmonary arterial pressures, may lead to a very low intensity P2 that may be inaudible.

Abnormal Timing of A2 and P2 Components

The time of occurrence of the individual components A2 and P2 may be delayed if the duration of systole is lengthened either because of electrical or mechanical delays or if the onset of flow reversal in the aortic root or the pulmonary artery is delayed because of changes in impedance to forward flow *(4,32–36)*.

ELECTRICAL DELAY

When there is an electrical conduction defect such as a bundle branch block, the affected side will lengthen the electrical portion of the duration of the electromechanical systole. This in turn will result in the delayed occurrence of the individual A2 and P2 components. Left bundle branch block (LBBB) will cause A2 delay, and right bundle branch block (RBBB) will cause P2 delay (Figs. 18A,B). Similar conduction defect can also be produced artificially by pacing either ventricle, which will produce late activation of the nonpaced ventricle. In other words, right ventricular pacing will cause LBBB effect, and left ventricular pacing will cause RBBB effect. Transient bundle branch block effect can also occur during ventricular ectopic beats. The site of origin of the ectopics will determine which of the two ventricles will be delayed in excitation. Right ventricular ectopics will have LBBB and left ventricular ectopics will have RBBB morphology and effects, respectively.

MECHANICAL DELAY

The mechanical portion of systole may be delayed when there is significant outflow obstruction. This would result in high intraventricular pressure, which is required to overcome the obstruction. The time taken for the pressures to fall below the level of the pressure in the great vessel (aorta or the pulmonary artery) would be lengthened. The reversal of flow at the aortic or the pulmonary root would start later because of the delay, and this in turn would delay the occurrence of the individual component of S2 on the affected side (Fig. 19).

Similar delay may also be caused in ischemic ventricular dysfunction where the ischemic muscle fibers may lag in onset of contraction and therefore maintain the developed intraventricular pressures for a longer period preventing its fall. Because ischemia often involves primarily the left ventricle, this type of delay is more likely to affect the A2.

The A2 and the P2 components usually coincide in timing with the incisural notch on the aortic and the pulmonary artery pressure curve, respectively (Figs. 16A,B). In general, the durations of the electromechanical systole on the left side and the right side are about equal under normal circumstances if the duration of the electromechanical systole is defined as the interval from the beginning of the electrical activation (QRS onset) to the respective time when the ventricular pressures fall below the level in the great vessels (aorta and the pulmonary artery).

Right ventricular myocardial dysfunction may develop with time in pulmonary hypertension when it is severe. The rate of rise of the right ventricular systolic pressure as well as its decline during relaxation may become slower. This may selectively increase the duration of systole on the right side relative to the left side, contributing to a delayed P2 *(30)*. Similar situation tends to develop more readily in acute pulmonary hypertension.

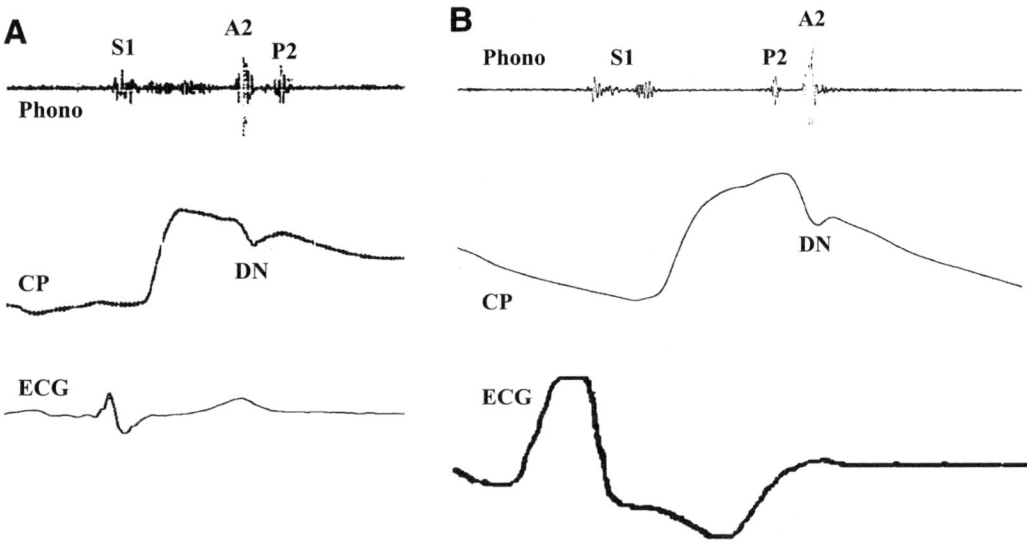

Fig. 18. **(A)** Diagram showing delayed P2 producing a wide split of the S2 in the right bundle branch block, which causes electrical delay of conduction to the right side. Note that the sequence is normal, with A2 occurring first, followed by P2. The component that is closest to the dicrotic notch (DN) on the CP is A2. The DN lags slightly behind because of the pulse transmission delay. **(B)** Diagram showing the abnormal sequence of the S2 components caused by the electrical delay because of left bundle branch block. P2 occurs before A2. The A2 is the component closest to the dicrotic notch (DN) on the CP.

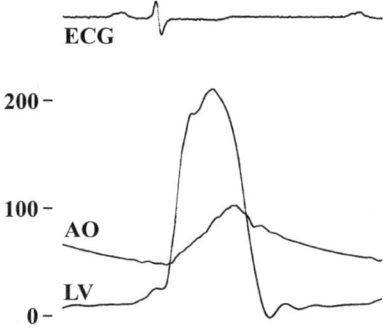

Fig. 19. Simultaneous left ventricular (LV) and aortic (AO) pressures from a patient with severe aortic valve stenosis. Note that the severe mechanical obstruction leads to high intraventricular pressure, which will take longer to fall to the level of the AO pressure, thereby delaying the A2.

DELAY SECONDARY TO EFFECTS OF IMPEDANCE

Impedance refers to resistance to forward flow of blood in the great vessels. If the impedance to forward flow is low, as the ventricular pressures begin to fall below that of the great vessels, the tendency for reversal of flow at the aortic or pulmonary root will be delayed. Therefore, the occurrence of the A2 or the P2 will be delayed depending on which circuit is affected. If the impedance is high, then the reversal tendency will be earlier, causing earlier occurrence of the affected component. This can be understood

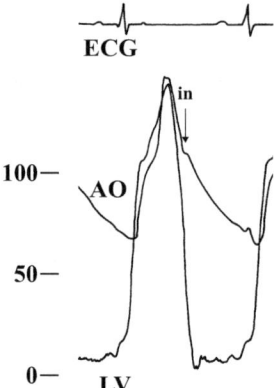

Fig. 20. Simultaneous left ventricular (LV) and aortic (AO) pressures from a patient with chronic aortic regurgitation. The A2 will occur simultaneously with the incisural notch (in) in the aortic pressure. Note the slight delay between the ventricular pressure at the leve l of the incisura (in) on the AO recording and the actual occurrence of the incisura (A2 timing). This delay has been termed by some as the *hang-out* interval, which reflects the impedance of the circuit. The hang-out interval on the pulmonary side will be greater because the pulmonary impedance is normally very low.

easily by the analogy of an automobile in motion and how far it is likely to travel after the application of the brakes. This will not only depend on the momentum of the vehicle but also on the character of the road surface: whether wet, slippery, or rough, whether there is a slope, and, if so, whether the grade is down or up as well as the resistance offered by the wind velocity and direction. The combined effects of these factors constitute the impedance to the moving automobile and will determine how far the vehicle will travel and how long before it will eventually halt. The impedance to forward flow in the great vessels is provided by the combined effects of various factors. These include the vascular capacity and how filled the system is, the vasomotor tone of the vessels (the systemic or the pulmonary vascular resistance), and the viscosity of the blood. In normal adults, the aortic or systemic impedance is approximately 10 times higher than the pulmonary impedance. This is a major factor that contributes to the earlier occurrence of A2 compared to P2. This is because the pulmonary vascular capacity is large; the pulmonary vascular resistance is low compared to that of the systemic side *(30)*.

When the ventricular pressure in late systole begins to fall below that in the aorta or the pulmonary artery, it leads to the development of a pressure gradient between the great vessel and the ventricle. The lower ventricular pressure provides a lower pressure route for the column of blood to take in the aorta or the pulmonary artery. However, the flow may still continue forward if the impedance is low. This will be reflected by the delay in the incisural notch of the aortic or the pulmonary pressure curve as measured from the point in time when the falling intraventricular pressure reaches the level of the incisural pressure (the pressure at which the aortic and the pulmonary valves close, respectively). This delay in the incisural notch has been termed by some investigators as the "*hang-out*" *interval (29)* (Figs. 16A,B and 20). This interval is quite small on the aortic side, averaging 15 ms, whereas it is usually considerably longer (between 30 and 80 ms) on the pulmonary side, almost completely accounting for the normal A2-P2 separation.

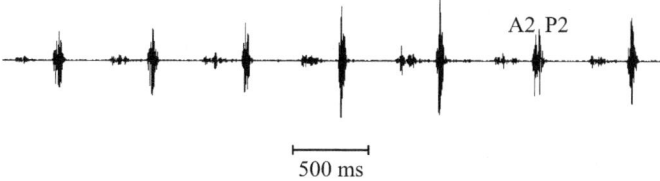

Fig. 21. Digital display of a magnetic audio recording from a patient with significant pulmonary hypertension with compensated right ventricular function, taken from the third left intercostal space at the sternal edge. P2 occurs much earlier because of high pulmonary impedance, causing a very narrow split of S2.

Because the systemic impedance is high at basal state, change in impedance must be significant to cause an appreciable effect on the A2 timing. On the other hand, small changes of the pulmonary impedance, which is usually low, may have an effect on the P2 timing because the percentage change will tend to be higher. Thus, with normal inspiration, the expansion of lungs will increase the pulmonary vascular capacity, thereby lowering the pulmonary impedance considerably in terms of percentage change. This is one of the more important contributing factors for the normal inspiratory delay of P2.

In pulmonary hypertension, the increased pulmonary impedance has the effect of shortening the delay of the incisural notch, making the P2 occur earlier because of course to the earlier occurrence of the flow reversal at the pulmonary root. This will be expected to cause a narrower split of S2 (Fig. 21).

In patients with left-to-right shunts through a ventricular septal defect who eventually develop severe pulmonary hypertension secondary to the occurrence of pulmonary vascular disease, the shunt becomes reversed, leading to cyanosis. In these patients, who are termed to have the *Eisenmenger's syndrome*, the systemic and the pulmonary impedance are about equal and would result in a single S2 *(37)*.

Effect of Delayed Occurrence of the S2 Components on the Respiratory Variation of S2 Splitting

When the A2 is delayed, however the delay is caused, if the delay is long enough then the sequence becomes altered, namely, a P2-A2 sequence is produced instead of the normal A2-P2 sequence. On inspiration when there is more volume on the right side as well as a significant drop in pulmonary impedance, the P2 will be delayed. This delayed P2 will come closer to the already delayed A2 and may actually fuse and may become a single S2. On expiration, the reverse will occur, with the P2 now coming earlier because of decreased volume being ejected by the right ventricle and a rise in the pulmonary impedance because of decreasing pulmonary vascular capacity secondary to collapsing lungs. This will then result in a split S2 on expiration *persistent or audible expiratory splitting*) *(33)*. Because the two components tend to come together on inspiration and separate from each other, causing a split S2 on expiration, it is termed *paradoxical or reversed splitting of S2 (36)* (Fig. 22A,B).

If the P2 is delayed, on the other hand, the sequence will still be normal: A2 followed by P2 *(35)*. However, the P2 will tend to be separated from A2 all the time. The separation will be greater on inspiration when the P2 is normally delayed and the separation may

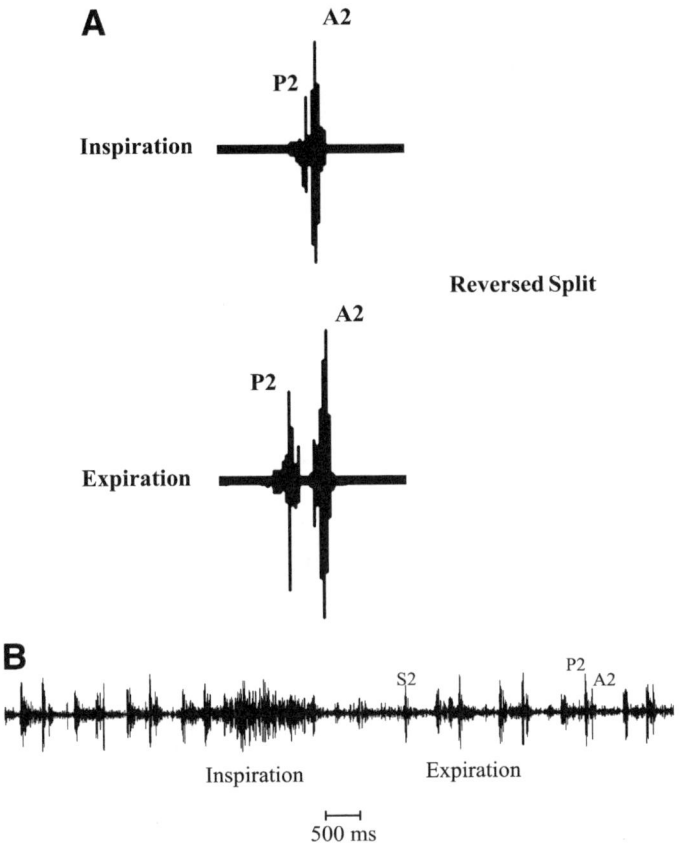

Fig. 22. (**A**) Diagram showing a reversed sequence of the S2 components caused by delayed A2, producing a paradoxical split with respiration. The normal inspiratory delay of the P2 makes the two components come together on inspiration with very little or no obvious split. On expiration the opposite occurs, with P2 coming earlier so as to make an audible split. (**B**) Digital display of a magnetic audio recording from a young patient with significant left-to-right shunt through a persistent ductus arteriosus taken from the third left interspace showing a paradoxical split of S2 caused by very low systemic impedance making a delayed A2 component. The noise in the baseline is exaggerated because of inspiration. The S2 becomes single for at least two beats after the end of inspiration. On expiration there is, on the other hand, a clear split of S2.

be narrower but maintained even on expiration. In other words, there will be a persistent expiratory split of S2 with normal physiological widening of S2 split expected because of inspiration. This can also be termed as a *wide physiological splitting of S2*.

Delayed A2

The causes of a delayed A2 component can be considered under the three general categories.

LEFT BUNDLE BRANCH BLOCK

When there is LBBB, the mechanical onset of contraction will be delayed because of the delay in electrical activation. The depolarization wave will have to reach the left ventricle through the "working-class" myocardial cells, which is a slow process as opposed to conduction through the normal His-Purkinje fibers. If the disease process in the left bundle system is focal and very proximal at its origin, then the electrical wave front may latch on to the normal Purkinje fibers of the distal divisions of the left bundle, and this may speed up the process of activation. The resulting electromechanical delay may not be severely prolonged. However, when the disease process in the left bundle branch is more extensive and involves the distal divisions, then the delay can be significant. Thus, varying degrees of electromechanical coupling may occur in different regions of the left ventricular myocardium. This will lead to delayed onset of contraction in the affected segments of the left ventricular myocardium. The QRS duration may therefore show varying degrees of prolongation of 0.12 s or more. If electromechanical coupling is variably delayed, then the rise in ventricular pressure during isovolumic phase will not be smooth and orderly. This will lead to lengthening of isovolumic contraction and a slower rate of rise of pressure. This may occur independent of the underlying myocardial function. In fact, in the majority of such patients with more extensive disease, the measurement of the individual components of the duration of the electromechanical systole will show not only lengthening of the Q-S1 interval (electrical delay), but also lengthening of the isovolumic contraction phase (the interval between S1 and the onset of ejection as assessed by aortic pressure recording) *(33,34)*.

MECHANICAL DELAY

Aortic Valvular Stenosis

When the obstruction is significant and fixed, as in severe aortic valvular stenosis, the left ventricular pressure often rises to very high levels in systole. It is necessary to overcome the obstruction for the ejection to occur. The high intraventricular systolic pressure takes a longer time to fall below that of the aorta, and the ejection continues slowly and is maintained for a longer period. This prolongation in ejection contributes to the delayed occurrence of the A2. The sequence will be reversed. The P2 may actually be buried in the end portion of the systolic ejection murmur, which is often long in significant aortic stenosis. The A2 may be soft and may be the only audible component of S2. The reversed splitting and the reversed sequence, which can be theoretically expected, may not be noticeable clinically.

Hypertrophic Obstructive Cardiomyopathy

In this disorder the interventricular septum is markedly hypertrophied. The ejection is often rapid at onset. The rapid ejection of blood has a Venturi effect on the anterior mitral leaflet, which together with the interventricular septum forms the left ventricular outflow tract. This in effect pulls the anterior mitral leaflet from its initial closed position to an open anterior position moving toward the septum (*systolic anterior motion*). This systolic anterior motion actually leads the anterior leaflet to come in contact with the interventricular septum in midsystole. This results in the outflow obstruction. This leads to near cessation of ejection and development of mitral regurgitation because of the open mitral orifice and lower left atrial pressure. The obstruction thus developed in midsystole is maintained until the later part of systole when the Venturi effect wears off and the anterior leaflet moves back to its closed posterior position. The ejection resumes during this late phase. Thus, the ejection is prolonged, causing delayed A2. The reverse sequence and the reversed splitting of S2 may in fact be clinically appreciated in this disorder when the obstruction is severe *(36)*.

Severe Hypertension

In severe hypertension, the left ventricle often has to eject blood, overcoming significant rise in peripheral resistance. Very high levels of intraventricular systolic pressure may take a longer time to fall to the level of pressure of aortic valve closure. In addition, there may often be impairment in both the onset of relaxation as well as in the rate of relaxation, resulting in slower rate of fall in the intraventricular pressure. Also, there may be coexisting ischemia aggravated by high pressures, increasing the myocardial oxygen demand. Ischemia will further aggravate the poor relaxation in addition to prolonging the mechanical systole (*see* next section). For all these reasons, the occurrence of A2 may be delayed significantly. The sequence may be reversed resulting in reversed splitting of S2. This usually requires a relatively well-preserved overall left ventricular systolic function because significant decrease in systolic function would mean decreased ejection fraction and diminished stroke volume. This will tend to shorten the duration of the mechanical systole and not lengthen it.

Ischemia

Ischemic myocardial dysfunction often involves predominantly the left ventricle. The ischemic portion of the myocardium may have delayed electrical activation and/or delayed onset of mechanical contraction contributing to prolongation of mechanical systole delaying the A2. In the presence of ischemic left ventricular dysfunction, segmental or regional variations may also come into play because coronary lesions are often nonuniform. The nonischemic areas will begin the contractile process, raising the ventricular pressure. The delayed contraction of the ischemic areas occurring after the normal segments have contracted will help to maintain the ventricular pressure preventing its fall, although the peak pressure attained may in fact be lower. This in turn will prolong the duration of mechanical systole, causing delayed A2. The same is, however, not expected in the case of completed infarction. In this instance, the infarcted area will not contract at all, causing no prolongation of the duration of mechanical systole. Therefore, in patients with acute myocardial infarction, the presence of a reversed splitting of S2 should indicate significant co-existing ischemia. Transient paradoxical splitting may occur during angina pectoris in some patients, reflecting the ischemic left ventricular dysfunction *(33)*.

DECREASED SYSTEMIC IMPEDANCE

The systemic impedance is normally high, and therefore in order for the A2 to be delayed on account of impedance change, the aortic impedance must become very low. Such situations are not common. Reversed splitting of S2 is occasionally encountered in patients with large left-to-right shunts at the aortic level through a persistent ductus arteriosus *(36,38)* (Fig. 22B). This is explainable by the fact that the aortic outflow impedance is considerably reduced in such patients because of the communication to the pulmonary artery and its branches. Decreased impedance has been considered to play a part for the delayed A2 seen in some patients with aortic stenosis and significant poststenotic dilatation as well as in some patients with chronic severe aortic regurgitation *(36)*.

Delayed P2

The causes of a delayed P2 component can also be approached using the same three categories as mentioned for delayed A2.

RIGHT BUNDLE BRANCH BLOCK

The right bundle branch is a long thin fascicle running under the endocardium on the right ventricular side of the interventricular septum. It crosses the right ventricular cavity through the muscle bundle called the moderator band and arborizes as a Purkinje network at the base of the anterior right ventricular papillary muscle. The conduction through the right bundle can be interrupted very easily even by some mechanical pressure as applied through a catheter placed in the right heart. The lesions causing RBBB need not, therefore, be extensive. The delayed electrical activation of the right ventricle in complete RBBB with QRS width of 0.12 s by itself can cause the delay in the P2. Rarely, delayed mechanical contraction with prolongation of the isovolumic contraction on the right side may also play a part.

Left ventricular pacing and left ventricular ectopics can also be associated with delayed P2 by producing late activation of the right ventricle.

MECHANICAL DELAY

Right Ventricular Outflow Obstruction

In pulmonary stenosis (infundibular or valvular), the elevated right ventricular systolic pressure will take a longer time to fall to the level of the pulmonary artery, prolonging the duration of the mechanical systole on the right side. This would result in a delayed P2. The mechanism is very similar to that described with reference to aortic stenosis. The delay, however, may vary with severity.

Pulmonary Hypertension

The effects of increased pulmonary impedance in significant pulmonary hypertension will be expected to cause an early occurrence of P2, which should result in a narrowly split S2 (Fig. 21). This is what happens in general in the early stages of chronic pulmonary hypertension. At this stage the right ventricular myocardial performance is still normal despite the high pulmonary pressures.

The mechanical effects of chronic pulmonary hypertension on the right ventricular myocardial performance may vary not only with the severity but also with the duration of the pulmonary hypertension and the development and adequacy of compensation. Right ventricular hypertrophy developing over a long period when the process is chronic may be adequate to maintain normal systolic function. However, before actual systolic dysfunction develops leading to right ventricular failure, the diastolic function will become impaired, very similar to what one finds in left ventricular dysfunction and failure. The right ventricle will manifest the diastolic dysfunction by the slower rate of relaxation in a later part of systole and during the isovolumic relaxation phase. The systolic dysfunction may also be reflected in a slower rate of rise of the systolic pressure during the isovolumic phase of contraction. The slower rate of rise and decline of right ventricular systolic pressure would lead to the prolongation of right ventricular mechanical systole relative to the left side. This often can be observed to be associated with the development of abnormal contours in the jugular venous pulsations where jugular descents show less prominence of the x' *descent* and more dominance of the *y descent* compared to the usually dominant x' *descent*. In other words, the jugular contour will show $x' = y$, $x' < y$, or *single y descent* as opposed to single x' or $x' > y$ *descent* contour, which is normally seen with the preserved right ventricular function. These changes indicate the development of right ventricular dysfunction *(39)*. In such instances, the relative lengthening of duration of right ventricular systole compared to that of the left side would result in a delayed P2. This is not uncommon when decompensation develops in chronic pulmonary hypertension *(30,40,41)*. The net effect will of course lead to a widely split S2. Rarely, the splitting may be relatively fixed as well. The latter has been attributed to the inability of the right ventricle to increase the stroke volume on inspiration *(42)*.

The right ventricle is not an efficient chamber in handling sudden rise in pulmonary artery pressures and resistance, as seen in acute pulmonary embolism. Similar myocardial dysfunction may develop in some patients with acute pulmonary embolism causing a delayed P2 *(43)*, and the effects of the delayed P2 may persist for several days and may be observed to improve and become more normal when full clinical recovery occurs.

Decreased Pulmonary Impedance

Pulmonary impedance is generally low even in the normal, as discussed earlier (*see* p. 166). However, in some instances the impedance becomes considerably lower because of increased pulmonary vascular capacity. This is the case with atrial septal defect with large pulmonary arteries and branches because of the longstanding high pulmonary flow due to the left-to-right shunt.

Persistent wide splitting of S2 in patients who have had their atrial septal defect corrected is also probably a reflection of their increased pulmonary vascular capacity with decreased pulmonary impedance. An increased pulmonary vascular capacitance can occasionally be the cause of a wider split S2, which fails to close on expiration in some normal adults *(35)*.

Idiopathic and Poststenotic Dilatation of the Pulmonary Artery

In idiopathic dilatation of the pulmonary artery as well as in poststenotic dilatation of pulmonary artery accompanying mild to moderate pulmonary valvular stenosis, there is probably some deficiency of the elastic tissue in the pulmonary artery, which may be responsible for the excessive dilatation. This may result in slower elastic recoil of the pulmonary artery, partly accounting for the delayed P2. In addition, the increased capacitance may have a lowering effect on the impedance *(30,33,44)*.

Early A2

In severe mitral regurgitation, the A2 may occur early. Mitral regurgitation offers an extra outlet for the left ventricle to empty during systole, reducing considerably the resistance to ejection. Mitral regurgitation presents a volume overload on the left ventricle because the left ventricle has to accept the regurgitant volume as well as the normal pulmonary venous return during diastole. The increased volume would increase the left ventricular contractility by its Starling effect. This, together with an extra outlet for the left ventricle, would cause more rapid and faster ejection. This will have the effect of making A2 occur early.

The effect of an early A2 is to make a relatively wide separation of A2 and P2. The splitting of S2 may be recognizable as a persistent expiratory split of S2. This often tends to occur only when the mitral regurgitation is severe and either acute or subacute, as seen, for instance, with ruptured chordae tendineae *(33)*. The clinical conditions that may result in such mitral regurgitation are usually nonrheumatic in origin.

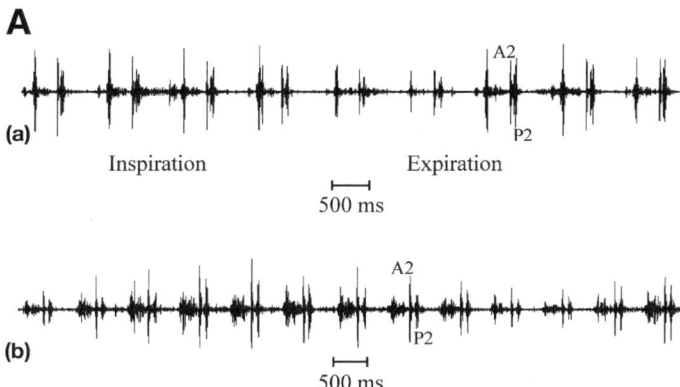

Fig. 23. **(A)** Digital display of magnetic audio recordings from two different patients with secundum atrial septal defect taken from the lower left sternal border region. Both show a relatively fixed split of S2. In **(a)** the split is somewhat narrower, whereas in **(b)** it is wider.

(Continued on next page)

Early P2

The effect of high pulmonary impedance in significant pulmonary hypertension causes the P2 to occur earlier than normal. However, this effect cannot make P2 come earlier than A2. The result of an earlier-than-normal timing of P2 will be to make a narrower split of S2 on inspiration, which will close on expiration and become a single S2.

Abnormal Respiratory Variations of A2-P2 Split

The normal respiratory variation of S2 split with A2 coming earlier and P2 occurring later on inspiration, and the reverse on expiration, depends on the inspiratory increase in venous return increasing the right ventricular volume, as well as an expanding lung increasing the pulmonary vascular capacity. The former would increase the right ventricular ejection time, and the latter would decrease the pulmonary impedance. Such a normal separation of the A2 from the P2 during inspiration is usually not noticeable in the normal adult particularly in the elderly. Even in the young adult, A2-P2 split will usually disappear and be replaced by a single S2 on expiration when the patient is examined in the standing position. If the A2-P2 split persists on expiration in the standing position but narrower than is observed on inspiration, then one has a relatively wide physiological splitting of S2. While this could be a normal variant in some, in most individuals one needs to consider the causes of a delayed P2 to account for the wide physiological splitting. Both the normal split and the relatively wide split of S2 require a normal A2-P2 sequence.

When the A2-P2 separation occurs on expiration and the S2 becomes single on inspiration, then a delayed A2 mechanism is in place, causing an abnormal sequence of P2-A2. This of course is termed the reversed or paradoxical splitting of S2.

When the A2-P2 separation remains relatively fixed and does not appreciably change with respiration, then one has a *fixed splitting of S2*, which usually occurs in atrial septal defect (Figs. 23A–C). The communication between the two atria and the flow through the defect compensates for changing venous return on both inspiration and expiration.

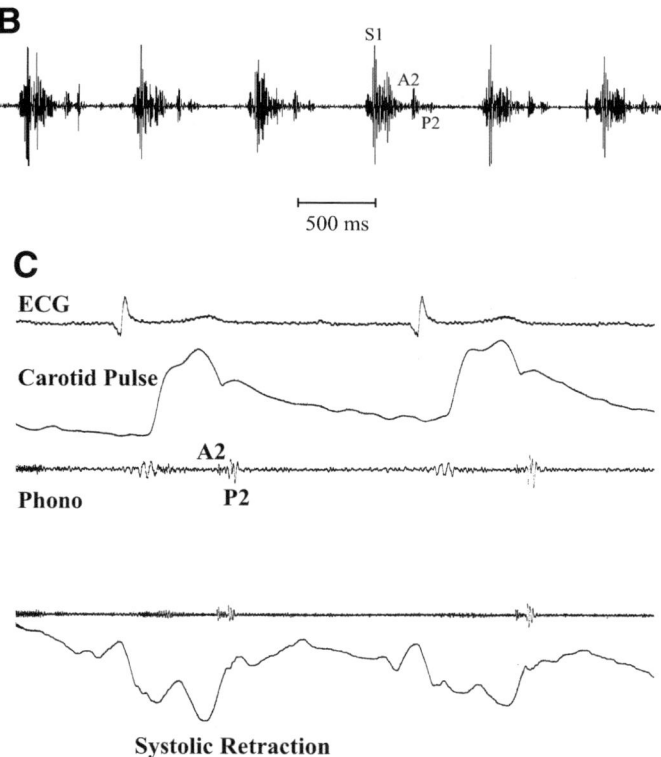

Fig. 23. *(Continued)* **(B)** Digital display of a magnetic audio recording from a patient with a secundum atrial septal defect showing a split S2 at the apex. The S1 has high amplitude because of a loud T1 component. It is followed by an ejection systolic murmur. This patient had a large right ventricle, which formed the apex beat. **(C)** Phonocardiogram (Phono) recording from a patient with atrial septal defect taken at the apex area showing a split S2. Systolic retraction is seen on the simultaneous apex recording. This area of retraction was lateral to the apical impulse caused by the enlarged right ventricle.

The inspiratory increase in right ventricular volume is associated with a decrease in the amount of shunt into the right atrium from the left side. On expiration, the venous return diminishes; this is associated with an increase in the shunt flow through the atrial septum. In other words, the right ventricular volume is more or less the same on both inspiration and expiration. Thus, the right ventricular ejection time remains the same on both inspiration and expiration, accounting for the relatively fixed S2 split. The A2-P2 sequence remains normal in atrial septal defect *(45,46)*.

CLINICAL ASSESSMENT OF S2

S2 is a sharper, crisper sound and can be mimicked by the syllable "dub." It marks the end of systole and beginning of diastole. With normal heart rates, diastole is of course longer than systole. If the jugular contour is normal and visible in the patient, then the S2 can be noted to coincide with the systolic descent or the *x′ descent* of the jugular pulse. The *x′ descent* is noted to fall onto the S2. Because the *x′ descent* can also be timed independently with the radial arterial pulse with which it coincides, it can be used to focus one's attention on the S2 at the time of auscultation. This may help the beginner, providing a visual marker for the S2 timing and appreciation of its components.

When assessing the S2, one needs to pay attention to the intensity as well as to define the nature of the individual components and their variation with respiration. Trying to pose a series of questions and answer them in a systematic manner is a useful bedside method to adapt:

1. Is the S2 single or split?
2. If split sometimes and single at other times, is the patient breathing in or out during split?
3. If split all the time, is it wider sometimes and narrower at other times or does it remain about the same all the time?
4. If wider sometimes and narrower at other times, is the patient breathing in or out when the wider split is heard?
5. If components are more or less equally separated all the time and no variation is appreciated, is it the same or does it close with patient in standing position to maximize the respiratory variation in volume on the right side?
6. When the S2 is split, over how wide an area of the precordium is the split S2 heard?
7. Is the split heard over the lower left sternal border region? Does it extend over the xiphoid area?
8. Is the split heard over the apex area?
9. If heard over the apex area, is the apical impulse palpable and, if so, is the apical impulse left or right ventricular in origin?
10. What is the grade of loudness of the S2?
11. Which is the area of maximum loudness?
12. Is it palpable?
13. Where is it best palpated?
14. If split, which component is louder, A2 or P2?
15. If split and the respiratory variation cannot be assigned clearly, is it possible to detect the sequence, whether A2-P2 or P2-A2?

Split S2

The normal A2 is heard over a sash area extending from the second right intercostal space to the apex area. The normal P2 is heard over the second and third left intercostal space. Thus, a normal split of the S2 is best heard over the second or third left intercostal space, where both components are audible. Asking the patient to take a breath in may bring in too much noise caused by the breath sounds. This may actually interfere with the assessment of the split, whether present or not, and, if present, to further assess the variation and their relationship to the phase of the respiration. Thus, it may be easier to listen to the S2 and identify its components, whether split or not, and then merely observe the relationship to normal breathing. Occasionally one may be able to direct the patient to breathe with medium effort without making too much respiratory noise. But this may be more difficult than watching the effect of the normal respirations.

The A2 is equally loud at the left ventricular apex as it is in the second right intercostal space, and it may occasionally be loudest at the apex. A2 is never palpably loud unless significant systemic hypertension is present. The intensity of the A2 does not vary with respiration.

P2, on the other hand, is never heard normally beyond the second and third left interspace, and when heard over the lower sternal border region and/or to the xiphoid region would indicate either a louder intensity P2 as in pulmonary hypertension or that the right ventricle is enlarged because of a volume-overload state such as in atrial septal defect or tricuspid or pulmonary regurgitation. For the same reason, the P2 is not usually audible at the normal apex area, which is usually formed by the left ventricle and identified as such by the presence of a medial area of retraction. On the other hand, if the apex is formed by an enlarged right ventricle, as identified by the presence of a lateral area of retraction, then the normal P2 could be audible over the apex area.

P2 often can be noted to increase in intensity with inspiration. The increased volume in the right side presumably provides a greater right ventricular stroke volume, distending the pulmonary root to a greater degree.

A palpable P2 in the second left intercostal space usually indicates pulmonary hypertension. This often correlates to a pulmonary systolic pressure of at least 75 mmHg. Grade III A2 and grade III P2 fusing on expiration may occasionally become palpable. If this happens, the S2 palpability will be restricted to expiration. But if S2 were palpable throughout inspiration and expiration in the second left intercostal space, it would definitely indicate pulmonary hypertension even if there were coexistent systemic hypertension. This stems from the fact that a palpable A2 is not felt maximally at the second left intercostal space. On the other hand, the location of maximal loudness of P2 is second left intercostal space. The exception, when an A2 may be actually palpable at the second left interspace, is transposition of the great vessels (whether congenitally corrected or not) where the aortic root is anterior, superior, and leftward.

In young, thin adults, adolescents, and children, because of the thinner chest wall the P2 may be normally audible over a larger area than in the normal adult. These patients will tend to have an easily audible split of the S2, which is sometimes wide. When examined in the erect position, the respiratory variations become maximal and can often be seen to become closer on expiration, if not actually becoming single. In patients older than 60 yr it is unusual to hear a good split of S2 because of poor chest wall compliance as well as age-related increases in the pulmonary impedance. Therefore, split S2 in the elderly is often abnormal and deserves clarification.

Sequence Identification

In the normal, A2 precedes P2. While A2 is heard over the apex, P2 is usually not heard at the normal apex, which is formed by the left ventricle. If one auscultates over the second or third left intercostal space and hears a split S2 and then quickly changes over to apex with the rhythm of the split S2 in mind, one may be able to detect which of the two components is dropped or not heard at the apex. If the first of the two components is dropped at the apex, then the sequence will have to be P2-

A2. If the second component of the split is dropped, then the sequence will be A2-P2. These conclusions stem from the fact that the normal P2 is the one that is not heard at the apex. This technique can occasionally work much more easily, particularly with practice. Sometimes it may be easier than trying to assess the relationship to respiratory phases. It is particularly useful when the split is very wide and does not close on expiration and the patient is being examined in situations where it is not possible to adapt an erect or standing position, such as in critically ill patients.

Rule of the S2 Split at the Apex

In view of the above observations, one can easily state that a split S2 at the apex is abnormal (Figs. 23B,C) and should make one consider the following possibilities:

1. P2 is loud and may indicate the presence of pulmonary hypertension.
2. If the P2 is not loud and there is no evidence of pulmonary hypertension, the right ventricle may be enlarged, as in volume overload, and one should consider lesions such as an atrial septal defect.
3. P2 is normal and probably audible at apex because of a thin chest, as in children.
4. The split S2 effect is mimicked by a normal single A2, followed by another sound such as an opening snap (OS) or S3.

Persistent or Audible Expiratory Split of S2

A split S2 that is audible on expiration is often a clue to some abnormality of the timing of the individual A2 and P2 components (Fig. 23A). It may indicate one of three possibilities:

1. Relatively wide physiological split of S2 with normal sequence and one must consider the causes of a delayed P2.
2. Reverse or paradoxical split of S2 and abnormal P2-A2 sequence and one must consider the causes of a delayed A2.
3. Relatively fixed split of S2 as in atrial septal defect.

In the normal adult, the S2 split can be made to close on expiration, particularly if assessed in the erect position with the patient either sitting or standing. This allows for maximum variation of right ventricular volume changes with inspiration and expiration. Thus, in most normal adults it would be abnormal to get a persistent S2 split on expiration when examined in this position. Therefore, one should never diagnose abnormal persistent expiratory split of S2 unless the patient has been examined in the erect and preferably standing position.

Often, applying the technique of sequence detection, particularly if the split is not heard at the apex area, one may be able to narrow down the possibilities. Even if the split is heard at the apex and the apex is formed by the left ventricle, then the concept that the P2 must be softer at the apex than at the second or third left intercostal space can be applied to detect the component that gets softer as one approaches the apex, listening and inching the stethoscope from the base to the lower left sternal border region and then to the apex. A reverse sequence is detected if the first of the two components get softer at the apex. Then causes of the A2 delay must be considered. A normal sequence is detected if the second of the two components gets softer at the apex. Then causes of delayed P2 must be considered.

These deductions are made on the basis that the apex in the given patient is left ventricular in origin.

In atrial septal defect, the persistent expiratory split may or may not be associated with a wide splitting of S2. Splitting can be fixed and yet narrow in atrial septal defect, particularly if the pulmonary flow is markedly increased and the pulmonary bed is relatively overfilled and behaves like a system with high impedance. This will tend to bring the P2 forward, causing a narrower split. The development of some degree of pulmonary hypertension may also contribute to increased impedance and a narrower split. Nevertheless, it will be relatively fixed and will not appreciably change with respiration. One must carefully assess the patient with the patient in the erect or standing position before reaching a conclusion about a fixed split. Occasionally the pulmonary systolic murmur, because of flow, may not be impressive, and often the diagnosis of atrial septal defect hinges on diagnosing a fixed split S2.

Partial anomalous pulmonary venous drainage into the right atrium may also cause a wide and sometimes relatively fixed split of S2. This lesion often coexists with an atrial septal defect and may rarely be an isolated anomaly. The clinical features often resemble atrial septal defect *(42)*. When it occurs with an intact atrial septum, fixed splitting does not occur *(47,48)*.

Patients with primary pulmonary hypertension developing some degree of decompensation may have a wide persistent split of the S2, and the variation with respiration may be minimal and therefore may mimic a relatively fixed splitting of atrial septal defect. Sometimes the effect of a *post-Valsalva strain* may help to distinguish the two. During the strain phase of the *Valsalva maneuver*, the patient attempts to breathe against a closed glottis. This leads to increased abdominal and intrathoracic pressure, which prevents normal venous return, which would lead to considerable decrease in the right heart volume. Following the release of the Valsalva strain, there is a sudden drop in intrathoracic and abdominal pressure, which leads to sudden increase in the venous return. This would markedly increase the right heart volume for a few beats, diminishing again afterwards. In the normal, the splitting may increase over 20 ms immediately following the release of strain. A few seconds later, the S2 splitting may become narrower or single *(46)*. In atrial septal defect, the flow through the septal defect from the left atrium to the right side will compensate for the changes in the venous return, more or less keeping the right ventricular volume the same. Therefore, the S2 split will remain relatively the same *(46)*. On the other hand, in primary pulmonary hypertension, the S2 split will be much wider immediately after release because of an increase in the duration of right ventricular systole due to the abnormal behavior of the right ventricle in handling the volume load, and the split will become narrower after a few beats when the venous return decreases. Exercise may also help to distinguish pulmonary hypertension from atrial septal defect. Exercise will widen the split in right ventricular failure from pulmonary hypertension and will not do so in atrial septal defect *(16)*.

(For additional examples review Phono Files 10–27 under Heart Sounds on the Companion CD.)

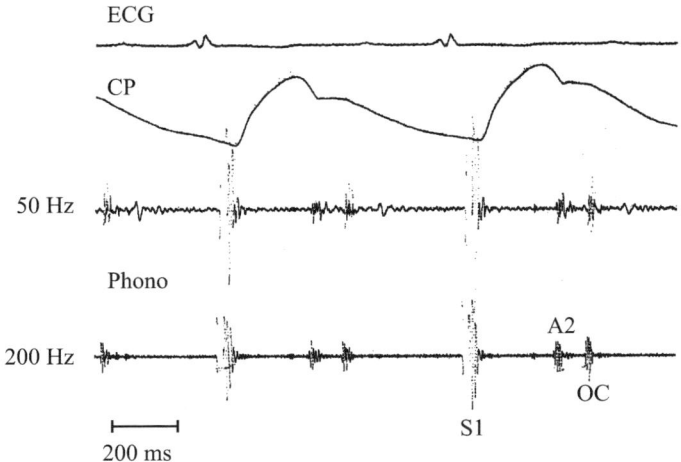

Fig. 24. Phonocardiogram (Phono) recording from a patient with a mechanical mitral valve prosthesis taken from the lower left parasternal area showing clicky sharp sounds associated with opening and closure of the mechanical valve. The closing of the valve causes a clicky sharp S1 and when it opens it produces a sharp opening click (OC) after the S2.

OPENING SNAP (OS)

After the closure of the semilunar valves, which is associated with the occurrence of the S2, the ventricles continue to relax and the ventricular pressures continue to fall. When the ventricular pressure falls below that of the atrium, the isovolumic phase of relaxation comes to an end and the A-V valves open to begin the phase of diastolic filling. If an artificial mechanical prosthetic valve has been used to replace the native valve, say the mitral valve, then one can often hear an opening click at this time of the cardiac cycle, which will follow the S2. Because such an artificial prosthetic mitral valve will also make a sharp closing click corresponding to the timing of S1 (Fig. 24), one will actually hear a cadence or rhythm made by the clicky S1 followed by S2 and an opening click. The rhythm is *Click.....Two...Click....*

Unlike the artificial mechanical prosthetic valve, when the normal mitral and tricuspid valves open, there is usually no formation of sounds. This is mainly because the valve opening causes the individual leaflets to move away from each other more or less symmetrically, resulting in no real deceleration of the moving column of blood from the atria against the leaflets themselves in their attempt to enter the ventricles. However, when the valves are stiffened and fused at the commissures, resulting in some degree of stenosis, as seen in rheumatic mitral stenosis, then one may hear a sound associated with the opening of the mitral valve. The sound is often snapping and sharp in quality and hence termed the *opening snap (49–51)*. As discussed previously in relation to S1, the M1 in mitral stenosis is loud and snapping. The OS can be considered the reverse of the closing snap, which is the loud M1 in mitral stenosis (Figs. 25A,B). The presence of a loud M1 followed by a normal S2 and a sharp OS gives rise to a recognizable cadence:

One.....Two....O.......... Lubb.....Pa...Ta..........

A similar sound can occur in rheumatic tricuspid stenosis, but the latter is very rare and therefore need not be discussed further.

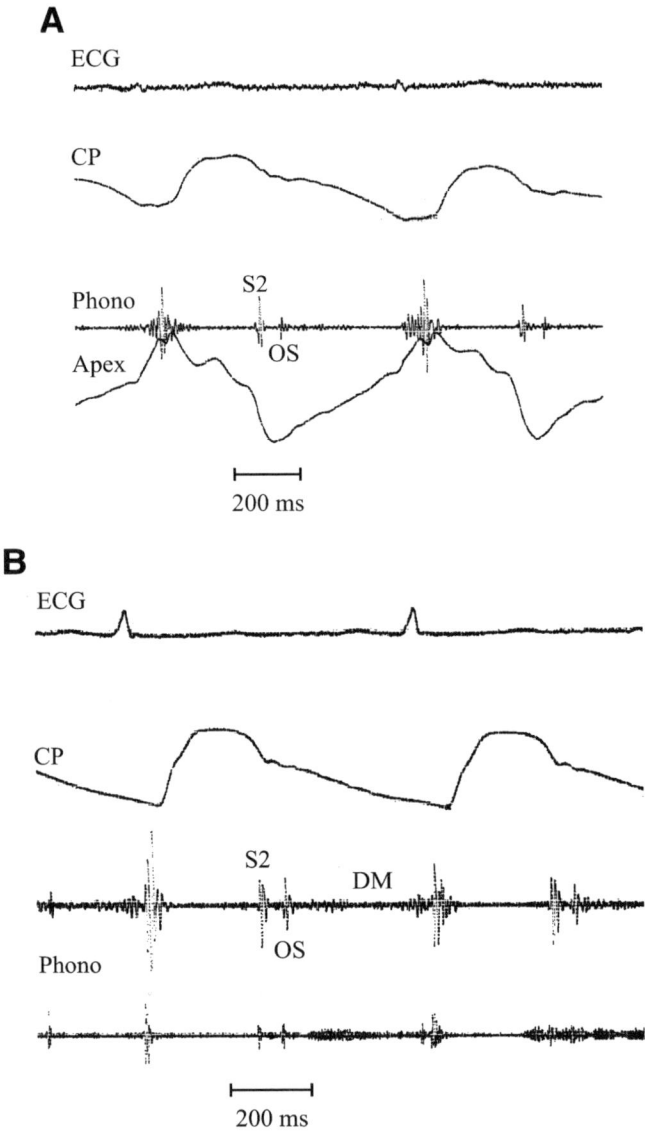

Fig. 25. **(A)** Phonocardiogram (Phono) recording taken at the apex area from a patient with rheumatic mitral stenosis who had a previous mitral valve commissurotomy for relief of the obstruction. The S1 is relatively loud. Note a sharp sound following the S2, which is the opening snap (OS). The OS occurs almost simultaneously with the most nadir point of the apex tracing, which is termed the O point. **(B)** Phonocardiogram (Phono) recording from another patient with mitral stenosis taken close to the apex area showing the loud S1 followed by the S2 and the opening snap (OS). Also seen is the diastolic murmur (DM) of the mitral stenosis.

The Mechanism of Formation of the Opening Snap

In mitral stenosis, the commissural fusion results in anatomical distortion of the mitral valve, and the valve behaves like a stiffened funnel. The tethering of the leaflets at the commissures does not allow free opening of the leaflets. Both the anterior and the pos-

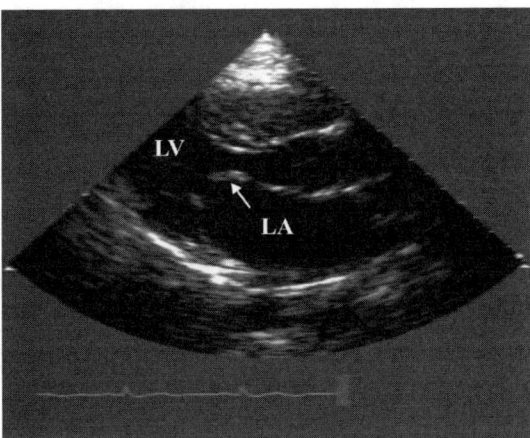

Fig. 26. Stop frame of a two-dimensional echocardiogram from a patient with mitral stenosis in the parasternal long axis at onset of diastole showing the typical bowing of the anterior mitral leaflet (arrow). Note that the leaflet tip is pointing posteriorly because of tethering caused by the stenosis making a funnel-like opening. Part of the column of blood trying to enter the left ventricle (LV) from the left atrium (LA) during diastole is oriented toward the belly of the leaflet. When the leaflet excursion reaches its anatomical limits caused by the tethering, this column of blood is suddenly decelerated. This leads to the production of the opening snap (OS).

terior leaflets tend to move together in the same direction anteriorly. If there is no excessive calcification of the main body of the anterior leaflet, it will be seen to actually bow anteriorly toward the ventricular septum with the opening motion of the valve at onset of diastole (Fig. 26). During systole, when it closes it will have a shape almost like a hockey stick, particularly when seen on a two-dimensional echocardiogram. The column of blood from the left atrium begins to enter the left ventricle when the pressure in the ventricle falls below that of the *v wave* peak in left atrial pressure, which will lead to opening of the valve. Because of the distorted orifice and incomplete separation of the leaflets, part of the column of blood will actually be oriented against the body of the anterior leaflet instead of being oriented toward the orifice. When the leaflet excursion comes to its anatomical limits because of its commissural tethering, this part of the column of blood will be decelerated suddenly, along with the leaflet. The dissipated energy at this time can be expected to produce the sound. Because in mitral stenosis the left atrial pressure is often elevated, the column of blood moving from the left atrium is under a higher pressure gradient than normal. Therefore, there is relatively greater energy in the moving column contributing to a louder sound. Characteristically, when the valve is relatively mobile, it leads to the production of the sharp snapping OS *(51–53)*.

Opening Snap in the Absence of Mitral stenosis

Rarely, excessive flow across the mitral valve in certain clinical conditions can be associated with the presence of an OS associated with the opening of the mitral valve in the absence of mitral stenosis. These include pure mitral regurgitation, ventricular septal defect, persistent ductus arteriosus, tricuspid atresia with large atrial septal defect, and thyrotoxicosis *(54–56)*. In atrial septal defect, the torrential flow across the tricuspid valve may be associated with a tricuspid OS *(56)*.

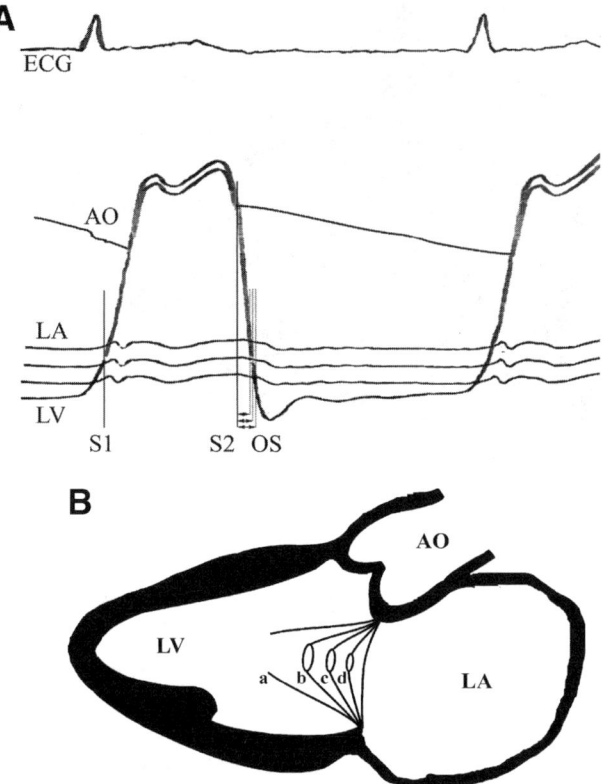

Fig. 27. **(A)** Diagram showing simultaneous left ventricular (LV) and left atrial (LA) pressures in mild, moderate, and severe degrees of mitral stenosis. The more severe the stenosis, the higher will be the left atrial pressure. The opening snap (OS) occurs at the end of the isovolumic relaxation phase of the left ventricle when the left ventricular pressure falls just below the left atrial pressure. The OS will therefore tend to occur earlier with higher LA pressure and later with lower LA pressure. Thus, the S2-OS interval is short with severe mitral stenosis and long with mild mitral stenosis. **(B)** Visual representation of the excursion of the mitral leaflets in mitral stenosis of different degrees of severity: a, normal; b, mild; c, moderate; d, severe. With milder stenosis the column of blood has to travel further before deceleration against the valve, thereby making a late OS.

Congenital mitral stenosis is not usually associated with OS because these valves are abnormal and not pliable.

Timing of the OS and the S2-OS Interval

The OS will be expected to occur at the end of the isovolumic phase of relaxation. The latter has an average duration of at least 60 ms. The S2-OS interval then must be expected to be at least 50 ms or longer. In general the OS may occur anywhere between 50 and 110 ms after S2. The OS has been reported to follow A2 by a delay ranging from 30 to 150 ms *(56)*. The interval will depend on the level of the aortic pressure, the rate of isovolumic relaxation, and the left atrial *v wave* pressure peak. Of these three, the most important determinant is the level of the peak left atrial pressure. Thus, if the left atrial *v wave* is higher, then the OS will occur earlier than when the left atrial *v wave* is lower (Fig. 27A).

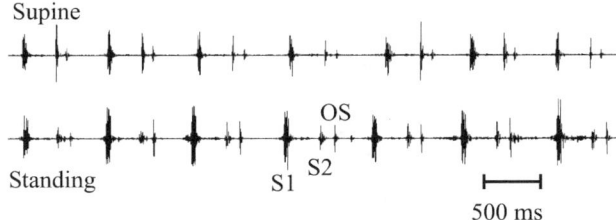

Fig. 28. Digital display of a magnetic audio recording from a patient with mitral stenosis taken at the lower left parasternal region showing the variation in the S2-OS interval between supine and standing position. The S2-OS interval is slightly longer on standing than when supine. The fall in the left atrial pressure caused by the upright posture makes the OS come later after S2. The A2-P2 split, however, will either narrow considerably or become a single S2 on assuming an upright position.

Because the height of the left atrial pressure is indirectly related to the severity of the mitral stenosis, the more severe the stenosis, the higher will be the left atrial pressure and the earlier the OS will occur after the S2 (Fig. 27A). The S2-OS interval can be either short, close to 60–70 ms; medium, close to 80–100 ms; or long, 100–120 ms.

A short S2-OS interval can be simulated by the syllables, *Lubbb...pa..da* when said as fast as one can. It can be medium and may simulate the syllables, *Lubbb...pa....ta* when said as fast as one can. When it is late it will be mimicked by *Lubbb...pa......pa*, again said as rapidly as possible.

It can also be easily visualized that the extent of the excursion of the leaflet before its sudden tensing because of the tethering will vary according to the severity of the mitral stenosis. The more severe the stenosis, the less will be the extent of the excursion and therefore the earlier will be the OS (Fig. 27B).

Because besides the left atrial pressure, the aortic pressure and the rate of isovolumic relaxation control the S2-OS interval, this interval may not always accurately predict the severity of mitral stenosis, especially in elderly patients and in the presence of hypertension. This interval will vary in atrial fibrillation because of the varying diastolic lengths. The longer cycles will be followed by lower left atrial pressure because of longer time for left atrial emptying, and the next systole will also be more likely to have a lower left atrial pressure. Thus, following long diastoles the S2-OS interval will be longer. In the presence of low cardiac output and a very large left atrium, one may have a long S2-OS interval even with significant mitral stenosis. In view of these confounding factors, a short S2–OS interval may be more helpful than a wide S2-OS interval in predicting the degree of mitral stenosis.

Maneuvers that make the left atrial pressures fall, such as making the patient stand up from a supine position, will make the OS come later (Fig. 28). The reason for this is the decreased venous return that occurs with assuming the erect posture, which will lower the left atrial pressure.

Following supine exercise, the S2-OS interval shortens because of rising left atrial pressure. Postexercise S2-OS interval of less than 60 ms will be suggestive of significant mitral stenosis *(56)*.

The Intensity of OS

In general, the presence of a good-intensity OS requires a fairly mobile valve. When the stenosis is relieved by surgical mitral valve commissurotomy, the OS will not always be abolished because there may be still enough tethering of the leaflets at the commissures with all the anatomical prerequisites for the OS production. When it is excessively restricted because of heavy calcification, the OS is unlikely to occur.

When there is severe mitral stenosis with very low cardiac output and decreased stroke volume, the OS intensity may be diminished because of the low flow. When there is significant pulmonary hypertension associated with severe mitral stenosis, the accompanying large right ventricle and low flow because of obstruction at the pulmonary arterioles will also tend to make the OS soft. When there is co-existing aortic valve disease with aortic regurgitation, the regurgitant stream is often directed toward the anterior mitral leaflet. In these patients the energy of the sudden deceleration of the mitral inflow against the anterior mitral leaflet is somewhat cushioned by the regurgitant stream and the resulting sound is often soft and may be even absent.

Clinical Assessment of the OS

The OS is generally maximally loud somewhere between the lower left sternal border and the apex. When it is very loud it can be heard over a wide area, including the base. At the apex, it coincides with the onset of the diastolic murmur of the mitral stenosis. The presence of OS following the S2 almost always simulates a widely split S2. In addition, a good-intensity OS tends to be associated with a loud S1. Thus, when one hears a loud S1 and what sounds like a widely split S2, one should always suspect an OS, and attempts should be made to confirm or rule out its presence. This essentially consists in looking for the following specific features of the OS:

1. It is maximally loud between the left sternal border and the apex.
2. It is sharp and generally high in frequency
3. Its intensity may vary slightly, with respiration becoming slightly softer on inspiration because of less blood flowing through the left side and slightly louder on expiration because of increase in flow through the left heart. It behaves similar to A2 in this regard. It is different from P2, which will become louder on inspiration.
4. The S2-OS interval tends to remain relatively the same with inspiration and expiration. Sometimes the P2 coming earlier on expiration may give one the impression that the S2-OS interval is widening. A wide paradoxical split of LBBB may sometimes be confused with S2-OS. In the absence of LBBB, however, if the second component of a wide split should increase in loudness at the apex or the split should become wider on expiration, it is unlikely to be a delayed P2, and an OS should then be suspected as the cause of the split.
5. When the patient's posture is changed from supine to sitting with feet dangling or, better still, to a standing position, the OS will be found to come later. In other words, the fall in the left atrial pressure that accompanies the erect position because of the decreased venous return will make the OS occur later, and this will make the split wider than when supine. The A2-P2 split will do the opposite because any decrease in venous return will make the P2 come earlier. This simple observation will often help in distinguishing between the two. Occasionally, however, the OS may become

>   too soft altogether on standing because of a significant drop in output and flow across the mitral valve, particularly in severe mitral stenosis.
> 6. The most definite way of recognizing the presence of OS is the ability to appreciate all three components on inspiration, namely, A2, P2, and the OS. This tends to happen in most patients when it is specifically looked for. The effect of such a triple sound on auscultation is unique, and once heard anyone can appreciate it. The tripling or trilling on inspiration with a simple split on expiration can be picked up over the second to fourth left sternal border area, depending on the width of the area where the P2 is audible in a given patient (Fig. 29). The *trill* usually sounds like beating on a snare drum. It can also be mimicked by triple-clicking on the commonly used mouse attachment on any modern computer.
>
> A late OS, when soft, may mimic an early S3. The distinctions will be discussed under S3.

(For additional examples review Phono Files 28–34 under Heart Sounds on the Companion CD.)

THIRD HEART SOUND (S3)

After the opening of the mitral and the tricuspid valves, blood flows into the ventricles from the atria during diastole. Diastolic filling of the ventricle is divisible into three phases, an early rapid filling phase followed by a slow filling phase or diastasis and at the end by the atrial contraction phase. The early phase of the ventricular filling is characterized by sudden vigorous expansion associated with rapid inflow of blood. The peak of this filling period may be accompanied by a sound, which is termed the third heart sound, or S3.

Diastolic Function

The rapid filling phase of diastole is a very dynamic process, which begins with the active ventricular relaxation. Henderson wrote in 1923, "in the heart, diastolic relaxation is a vital factor and not merely a mechanical stretching like that of a rubber bag" *(57)*. It begins at the later half of systole and involves the isovolumic relaxation phase and the early rapid filling phase. It involves actin–myosin cross-bridge dissociation by the reuptake of Ca^{2+}. Relaxation is an active process because it is energy dependent and requires ATP and phosphorylation of phospholamban (one of the proteins involved in the modification of sarcoplasmic calcium ATPase function) for uptake of calcium into the sarcoplasmic reticulum. Metabolic control of this complex process is through coronary perfusion and neurohumoral and cardiac endothelial activation. For instance, cyclical release of nitric oxide has been noted to be most marked subendocardially, peaking at the time of relaxation and diastolic filling. In addition, the intrinsic viscoelastic properties of the myocardium are also important. Fibrosis that accompanies hypertrophy probably plays a role in the impairment of relaxation *(58–60)*.

Just as force of contraction is alterable because of variation in filling or preload and afterload (the systolic load that the left ventricle has to face after it starts to contract), mechanical factors can also alter the rate of relaxation *(61)*. Five types of loading affecting relaxation are recognized. One slows the rate of relaxation, and four tend to increase the rate of relaxation *(62–64)* (Fig. 30).

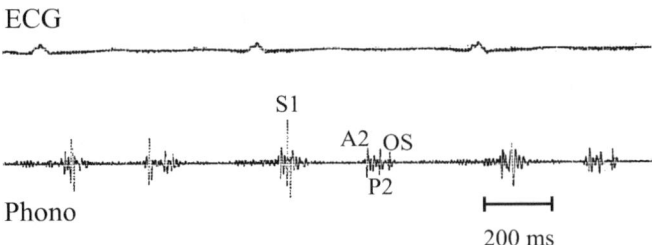

Fig. 29. Phonocardiogram (Phono) recording from a patient with mitral stenosis taken from the third left interspace showing the split S2 with A2 and P2 as well as the opening snap (OS) making a triple sound (trill), which is easily recognized.

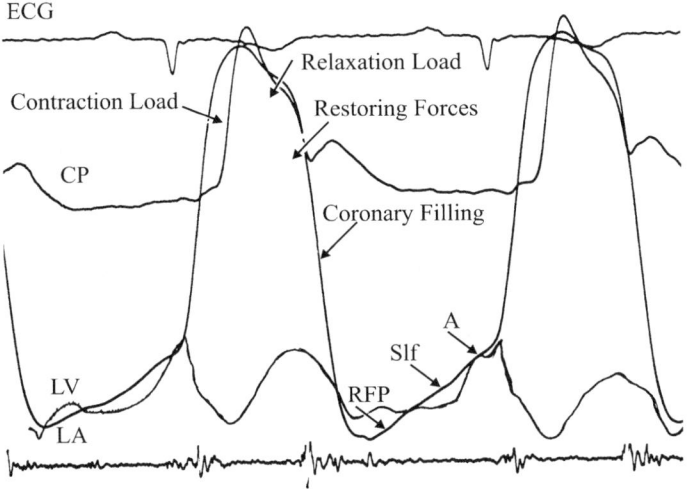

Fig. 30. Diagram of simultaneous left ventricular (LV) and left atrial (LA) pressures and the carotid pulse (CP), indicating the various mechanical forces affecting the relaxation of the left ventricle operating at different phases of the cardiac cycle. While an increase in volume or pressure in early systole (contraction load) slows relaxation, the same in later systole (relaxation load) hastens it. Restoring force resulting from the deformation of contraction and the coronary filling during isovolumic relaxation improves relaxation. When the LV pressure falls below that of the LA, diastolic filling begins. Diastole consists of three phases: the early rapid filling phase (RFP), followed by the slow filling phase (Slf), and finally the atrial contraction (A) phase. Active expansion during RFP is favored by increasing wall stress (*see* the text).

1. Increase in volume or pressure in the early phase of systole tends to slow relaxation.
2. Increase in volume or pressure in late systole hasten relaxation.
3. The deformation caused by contraction itself provides a stored potential energy, which contributes to the restoring forces.
4. During the period of isovolumic phase of relaxation, coronary filling begins and acts to improve relaxation.
5. The prevailing wall stress affects the rate of relaxation during the early rapid filling phase of diastole.

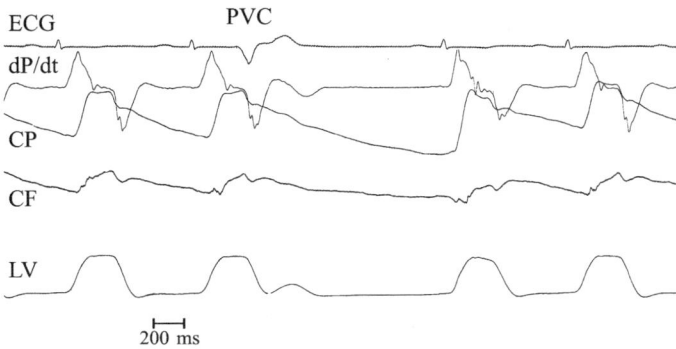

Fig. 31. Simultaneous left ventricular (LV) pressure and its first derivative (*dP/dt*) shown along with the carotid pulse (CP) and electrocardiogram (ECG). Note that the first beat following the premature ventricular beat (PVC) has a significant decrease in the rate of relaxation, as shown by the depth of the negative *dP/dt*.

The load effect on the rate of relaxation has been studied in isolated muscle-clamp experiments as well as in canine hearts studied with microcomputer-assisted pumps. In these studies volume increments in specific portions of systole have demonstrated the same phenomenon *(63,65)*. The potential energy gained by contraction is thought to act through cytoskeletal proteins, such as titin, which are compressed. During diastole they expand like springs, expending this stored energy, and provide a recoiling force for the myocardial filament to regain its length *(59)*.

Three clinical examples will be considered.

HYPERTROPHIC CARDIOMYOPATHY WITH OBSTRUCTION

The nature of this condition is such that it is accompanied by impairment of relaxation. The fibrosis that accompanies the hypertrophy may be expected to contribute to this *(60)*. One can expect some load-dependent alteration in relaxation as well. In hypertrophic cardiomyopathy with obstruction, the midsystolic obstruction will lead to increased pressure in the left ventricle, which will act as an increased "contraction-phase" load. In addition, these patients have a very high ejection fraction and low end-systolic volume. This leads to poor late systolic relaxation load. Both of these factors could also contribute to poor relaxation.

POSTEXTRASYSTOLIC BEAT

It is common knowledge that the beat following an extrasystole is strong and forceful, but it is usually not recognized that this postectopic beat has slower relaxation. If one records the rate of ventricular pressure rise and fall (*dP/dt*), it will be seen that the peak negative *dP/dt* reflecting the rate of relaxation is smaller in the postectopic beat compared to the normal beat (Fig. 31). The reasons for this are probably twofold. An excess of calcium is made available to the myocardial cells from the extrasystole, and the cells are somewhat calcium overloaded, which would be expected to slow relaxation. The second reason is the poor relaxation phase load in the postectopic beat because of near-complete ejection.

MILD LEFT VENTRICULAR DYSFUNCTION

In a study of left ventricular function using characteristics of the apical impulse as measured by apexcardiography *(66)*, we observed that the rate of isovolumic relaxation slope was slower in patients with mild left ventricular systolic dysfunction, whereas this slope was not abnormally slow when the ventricular systolic function was moderately or severely depressed. In the presence of significant systolic dysfunction, the ejection fraction is reduced. This leads to an increased end-systolic volume. It is conceivable that this may act as a "relaxation-phase" load, which could indirectly help in improving relaxation. It is known that the rate of left ventricular relaxation as measured by peak negative dP/dt is impaired in patients with ischemic heart disease and known systolic dysfunction and decreased ejection fraction *(67)*. The diastolic time intervals, like the isovolumic relaxation time and other noninvasive measurements, however, are affected by many factors, and they do not consistently gauge left ventricular relaxation *(68)*. This may be the reason that this noninvasive measurement by apexcardiography failed to pick up the abnormality in the presence of significant left ventricular dysfunction.

Finally, both the process of calcium inactivation and the load effects on the rate of relaxation could be variable and not uniform through the entire myocardium, depending on the pathological process *(62)*. This is best exemplified by ischemic heart disease, which is often segmental.

Early Rapid-Filling Phase

The *rapid filling phase* of diastole is part of this active phase of relaxation. The S3, when present, occurs at the end of this period. The rate of expansion of the ventricle during this phase is conditioned by the prevailing load or wall stress, increasing with the increasing wall stress. The latter can be defined by Lamé's modification of the *Laplace relationship*, where the wall stress or the wall tension is directly proportional to the pressure and the dimension or the radius and inversely related to the wall thickness. This phase begins at the onset of mitral and tricuspid valve opening. The peak pressure head driving the filling of the ventricle is the peak *v wave* pressure in the atrium because the ventricular pressure is close to zero at the beginning of this phase. During this phase of filling, the ventricle receives volume and expands, and its walls continue to thin. This means that there is an increasing wall stress from the beginning of this phase (at the mitral opening) to the end of this period. Thus, this period of filling accelerates under increasing rate of active expansion favored by the increasing wall stress, which characterizes this period. If the *v wave* height is increased for any reason, then this will add to the wall stress achieved, further hastening relaxation and expansion *(62)* (Fig. 30).

Slow Filling Phase and Atrial Contraction Phase

As opposed to the early rapid filling phase of diastole, the period of *slow filling or diastasis* and the *atrial contraction phase* are influenced by compliance, which is mainly secondary to the passive elastic properties of the myocardium (Fig. 30). Compliance can be expressed for the whole ventricle in terms of volume–pressure relationship (dV/dP) or the converse, expressing it as unit pressure change for unit increase in volume (dP/dV). The latter is termed *chamber stiffness*. When the same is expressed for an individual muscle fiber, it is called *muscle stiffness* (measured by stress–strain relationship, force per unit area/fractional change in dimension) *(69–73)*.

Factors that affect the compliance of the ventricle are:

1. *Completeness of relaxation*
2. *Chamber size*
3. *Thickness of the wall*
4. *Composition of the wall (inflammation, infiltrate, ischemia or infarction, scars, etc.)*
5. *Pericardium*
6. *Right ventricular volume/pressure and effects on the left ventricular compliance*

The ventricle can become stiff and offer more resistance to expansion when the overall size is small, as in children. It also is stiffer when the process of relaxation is impaired for any of the reasons mentioned previously (e.g., hypertrophic cardiomyopathy with obstruction, ischemic heart disease because of ischemia). The degree of decrease in compliance when there is hypertrophy of the myocardium depends on the cause of hypertrophy. When there is physiological hypertrophy, as seen in athletes, the decrease in compliance is slight. When the hypertrophy is a result of pressure load, as in significant hypertension or outflow obstruction (e.g., aortic stenosis), the decrease in compliance is more marked. Profound decrease in compliance tends to occur in hypertrophic cardiomyopathy. In addition, any pathological process (ischemia, scars, inflammation, infiltrative process, etc.) that affects the myocardium can alter the compliance of the ventricle by making the affected segments stiff. Ischemia is particularly of interest. It makes the ischemic segments relax poorly. The segments become stiff because of incomplete relaxation *(74)*. This affects the overall distensibility of the ventricle when the ischemia is significant. The decreased compliance leads to increased diastolic filling pressure when the ventricle fills during diastole. The increased diastolic pressure is transmitted to the atrium because the mitral valve is open during diastole and the increased left atrial pressure is in turn transmitted to the pulmonary capillary bed. This increased pulmonary alveolar capillary pressure leads to the production of symptoms of dyspnea during an episode of angina. The increased diastolic pressure in the ventricle, however, causes greater stretch of the nonschemic segments and increases their contractility, thereby preserving the forward cardiac output.

If for any reason the ventricle becomes stiff or less compliant, then the expansion during the slow filling period becomes difficult and slower. The compensation for this inadequate ventricular filling is provided by a stronger-than-normal contraction of the atrium during the atrial contraction phase, assuming that the atrium is healthy.

Mechanism of Formation of S3

S3 occurs at the end of the rapid filling phase of diastole *(75,76)*. The column of blood entering the ventricle during this phase is under the pressure head provided by the *v wave* pressure in the atrium. This phase of diastolic expansion is generally rapid and vigorous for reasons discussed earlier. But in almost all hearts this rapid expansion suddenly changes to a period of slower expansion. Thus, there is a tendency almost in all hearts for the moving column of blood entering the ventricle during the rapid-filling phase to decelerate somewhat toward the end of this period (Fig. 32). When the transition becomes more abrupt, this will be expected to affect the moving column of blood, causing it to decelerate more abruptly. The factors that are likely to make the transition more abrupt in general are those that decrease the compliance of the ventricle *(77–80)*.

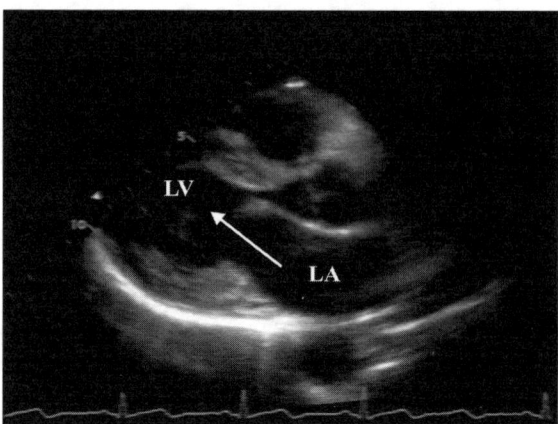

Fig. 32. Stop frame of a two-dimensional echocardiogram taken from a normal subject in the parasternal long axis at the end of the rapid filling phase of diastole when the moving column of blood (arrow) entering the left ventricle (LV) from the left atrium (LA) is suddenly decelerated because of the fact that the rapid expansion suddenly changes to a period of slower expansion. Factors that make the transition more abrupt tend to produce an S3 (*see* the text).

The energy achieved by the moving column of blood during the active rapid filling phase of diastole is related to the rate of relaxation, the velocity, and the volume of blood entering the ventricle and the pressure head provided by the *v wave* peak in the atrium. When the momentum achieved by the moving column of blood is significant and the transition from the early rapid filling phase to the slow filling phase more abrupt because of decreased ventricular compliance, however brought about, then the deceleration will occur more suddenly and the dissipation of energy will result in the production of an audible sound within the ventricle. The sound will obviously occur at the peak of the rapid filling wave, which is the S3. Intraventricular pressure and transmitral flow studies in dogs have demonstrated a small but consistent reverse transmitral gradient to always accompany this deceleration *(81)*. In addition, the sounds accompanying the flow deceleration could be recorded inside the ventricles as well as over the epicardial surface of the exposed ventricles, ruling out the external origin theory of S3 *(82)*. The whole hemic mass, including the blood, as well as the ventricular wall and the papillary muscles probably participate in the vibration.

Physiological S3

This occurs in children and in pregnant women and in other conditions associated with rapid circulation such as anemia and thyrotoxicosis. In children, the rapid inflow and the small size of their hearts together contribute to the development of S3 (Fig. 33). The small size offers increased resistance to expansion initially, like when one tries to blow up a balloon. Once expanded, there is not much resistance to further filling. Physiological S3, however, is rare after the age of 35. In pregnant women, the blood volume is increased and there is a relatively rapid circulation and increased sympathetic tone. The compliance need not be decreased. In the presence of a rapidly moving large volume of inflow, the transition from the rapid expansion to slow expansion may be sufficient to cause enough deceleration to produce the S3.

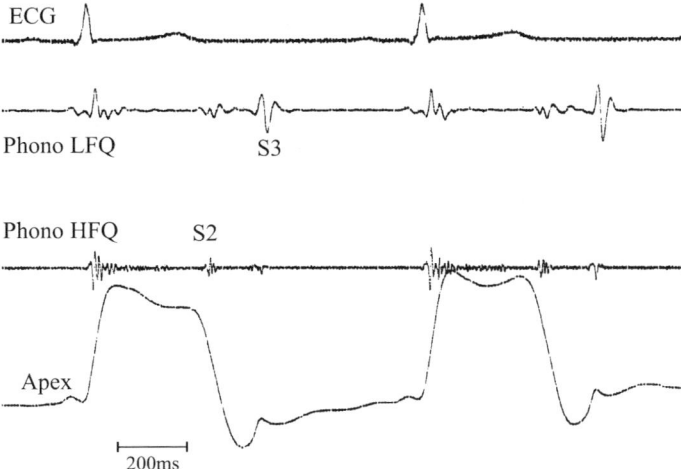

Fig. 33. Phonocardiogram (Phono) recording from a young subject taken at the apex area along with an apexcardiogram (Apex) showing a physiological S3. The S3 is well seen in the low-frequency (LFQ) range of 25–50 Hz. It is not as prominent in the high-frequency (HFQ) range of 200 Hz. The S3 is seen to coincide with the peak of the rapid filling wave (arrow) in diastole.

S3 in Ventricular Volume Overload

In volume overload states such as mitral and tricuspid regurgitations, the inflow volume during diastole into the ventricle is larger because the regurgitant blood into the atrium as well as the usual venous (systemic or pulmonary) return will enter the ventricle during diastole. The ventricle is also hyperdynamic in its contraction in these states because of the Starling effect caused by the large volume of diastolic filling. The relaxation following such stronger contraction will also be expected to be very rapid because of better restoring forces. In addition, the *v wave* peak pressure in the atrium will be higher because of the regurgitation (through the mitral and the tricuspid valves). For these reasons, the inflow into the ventricle not only will be large in volume but will also move with greater velocity, achieving greater energy. In fact, an apexcardiogram obtained in patients with volume-overloaded left ventricle will often show an exaggerated large rapid filling wave with an overshoot (Figs. 34A,B). The response of the ventricles to chronic volume overload is to dilate and enlarge. This is accompanied by increased compliance. Therefore, the deceleration is mainly brought about from the rapid expansion to slow expansion alone. The S3 in these states may in fact have enough duration and sound like a short murmur. In late stages when the ventricles have developed secondary hypertrophy and focal fibrosis, particularly in the subendocardial regions, the resulting decrease in compliance will also play a part in the production of the S3. Similar situations are also likely to occur and result in left-sided S3 in large left-to-right shunts through persistent ductus arteriosus and ventricular septal defects. In these conditions, the increased pulmonary flow received through the communication has to exit through the pulmonary veins into the left atrium.

In atrial septal defect with large shunts, the increased flow from the left atrium into the right atrium causes a right ventricular volume overload. Similar considerations apply.

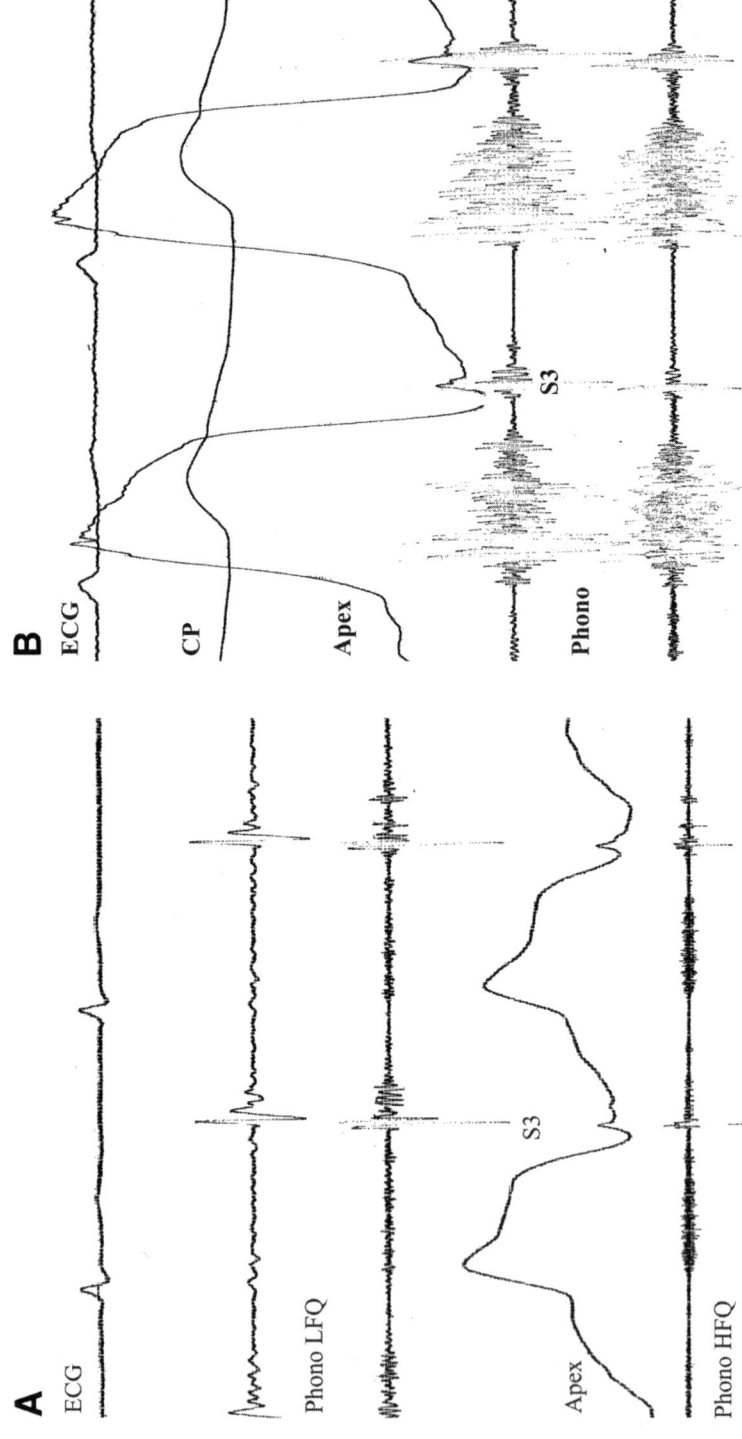

Fig. 34. Phonocardiogram (Phono) recordings taken from the apex area along with apexcardiogram (Apex) from two patients, both with significant mitral regurgitation causing left ventricular volume overloads. In both, overshoot of the rapid filling phase can be seen on the Apex coinciding with the S3 on the Phono.

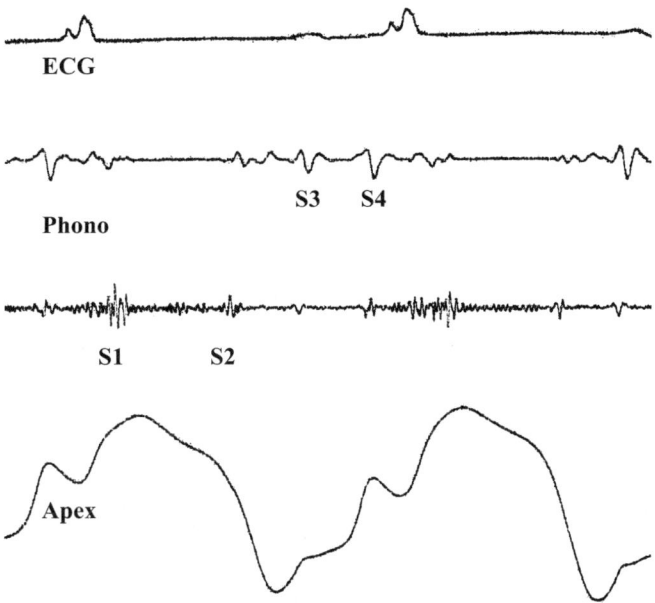

Fig. 35. Phonocardiogram (Phono) recording from a patient with severe aortic stenosis and left ventricular failure taken from the apex area along with the recoding of the apexcardiogram (Apex). The Phono shows both the fourth (S4) and third heart (S3) sounds.

However, because the right ventricle is more compliant than the left ventricle, increased flow through the tricuspid valve alone will not be sufficient to produce a right-sided S3. One can expect to hear a tricuspid inflow murmur in diastole instead *(83)*.

S3 in Ventricular Dysfunction

In patients with significant left ventricular dysfunction of whatever etiology, the left ventricular diastolic pressure will rise because of decreased ventricular compliance. Because during diastole the mitral valve is open, the rise in the left ventricular *pre-a wave* pressure will raise the baseline left atrial pressure. This will indirectly raise the level of both the *a* and *v waves* in the left atrium. The increased left atrial *v wave* pressure (in heart failure, cardiomyopathy, or in the postmyocardial infarction state) will aid in the development of greater energy acquired by the moving column of blood during the rapid filling phase. The ventricular compliance is generally decreased in these conditions because of the pathological processes involving the myocardium. Thus, the setup is there for the production of S3 in these states (Fig. 35). When the symptoms and signs of heart failure improve with therapy, there will be an associated fall in the left ventricular diastolic and the left atrial pressures. Often at this time the S3 will become soft or inaudible. If S3 remains relatively loud after the symptoms of dyspnea and edema have improved with associated radiological clearance of signs of failure, it indicates marked decrease in left ventricular compliance. This is usually not a good prognostic sign.

S3 in acute myocardial infarction usually occurs when there is a large infarct associated with left ventricular failure. If improvement in symptoms and signs of failure is accompanied by the disappearance of S3, it usually is a good prognostic sign. A loud persistent S3 in the postinfarction state may result either from significant mitral regurgitation or a marked decrease in compliance because of extensive myocardial damage. Occasionally both of these may play a role.

In patients with ventricular aneurysm, S3 is not usually seen in the absence of heart failure. Also, S3 is uncommon in acute ischemia unless it is severe enough to produce hemodynamic deterioration with or without mitral regurgitation secondary to papillary muscle dysfunction *(76)*.

In significant pulmonary hypertension when the right ventricle begins to fail, a right-sided S3 is likely to develop. The mechanism involves essentially the same principles as discussed for left ventricular dysfunction. The rise in right ventricular *pre-a wave* pressure leads to raised baseline pressure in the right atrium. This will add to the *v wave* pressure in the right atrium. With right ventricular dilatation, the tricuspid ring will eventually be stretched, leading to the development of tricuspid regurgitation. This adds further to the *v wave* pressure height in the right atrium. This is slightly different from the left side, where the mitral valve does not become fully stretched by left ventricular dilatation because only the posterior annulus, which is attached to the ventricle, becomes stretched. Anteriorly the mitral valve is attached to the aortic root. The latter does not stretch with left ventricular dilatation. Thus, mitral regurgitation does not usually arise from left ventricular dilatation alone. The increased right atrial *v wave* pressure head, together with significant decrease in compliance of the right ventricle brought about by the hypertrophy caused by the pulmonary hypertension, provides the setup for the right-sided S3. Right-sided S3 in general requires not only increased flow across the tricuspid valve, but also significant elevation of right atrial pressure, usually seen in the context of pulmonary hypertension during the stage of decompensation.

The right ventricle does not tolerate acute rises in pulmonary artery pressure, however. Thus, in acute pulmonary thromboembolism, the right ventricle will dilate acutely, and this may not only produce tricuspid regurgitation but also cause steep rises in the systolic and the diastolic pressures in the right ventricle. The latter, by raising the right atrial pressure, will provide the necessary conditions for the right-sided S3.

S3 in Constrictive Pericarditis (Pericardial Knock)

In chronic constrictive pericarditis, the thickened and fibrosed, sometimes even calcified pericardium surrounds the ventricles like steel armor, not allowing their full expansion. The ventricles generally are able to expand only during the phase of rapid inflow. Once the peak of this expansion is reached, further expansion is often impossible because of the thickened and unyielding pericardium. The diastolic pressure in the ventricles will abruptly rise to high levels and plateau thereafter until the end of diastole, giving the classic *square-root sign* to the ventricular pressure curves. In classic constrictive pericarditis, both the left and right ventricular diastolic pressures will in fact be equal under resting conditions (Fig. 36). The raised diastolic ventricular pressures will be transmitted to the respective atria. This, of course, is the reason for the raised *v wave* pressure head for the rapid filling period. The rapid inflows will be abruptly decelerated by the decreased compliance of the ventricles caused by the abnormal pericardium producing the S3 *(84)*.

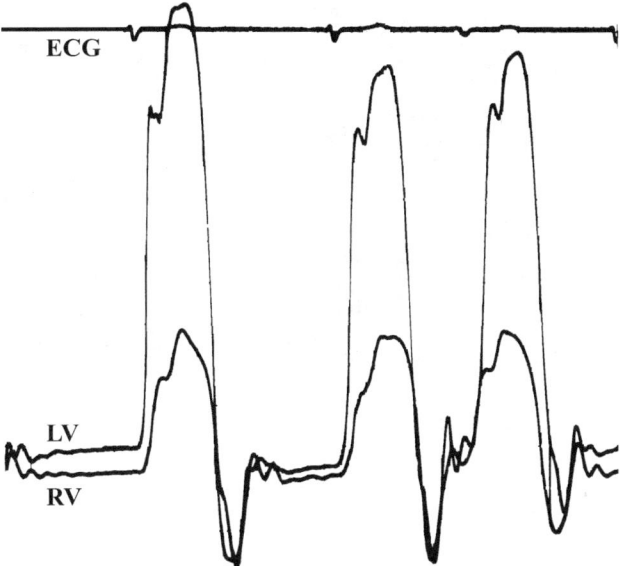

Fig. 36. Simultaneous recording of left ventricular (LV) and right ventricular (RV) pressures from a patient with severe chronic constrictive pericarditis showing the raised diastolic pressures with equalization between the two sides along with the typical dip and plateau pattern (the square-root sign).

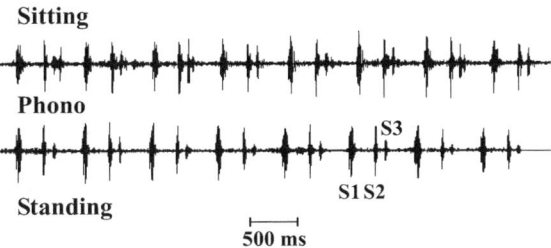

Fig. 37. Digital display of a magnetic audio recording from a patient with chronic constrictive pericarditis taken from the left lower parasternal area showing an early S3, which persists even in the erect position (standing) because of high atrial pressures.

The degree of cardiac compression may vary slightly in different patients. The rapid-filling phase may also be slightly shortened. The S3, therefore, may occur slightly earlier than usual. The sound may also be somewhat sharper *(84)* (Fig. 37). It is sometimes called a *pericardial knock*. However, in the majority the S3 is quite similar in character to the usual S3, most likely because the constriction does not shorten the rapid filling phase and begins to impede filling only at the end of the rapid filling phase.

S3 in Atrial Myxoma (Tumor Plop Sound)

In atrial myxoma, one may hear an S3-like sound termed the *tumor plop*. The sound is actually produced when the tumor plops into the ventricle in diastole. The tumor is usually attached by a stalk to the interatrial septum. For instance, in the case of a left atrial myxoma, the tumor may in fact protrude and get in the way of the mitral inflow, causing

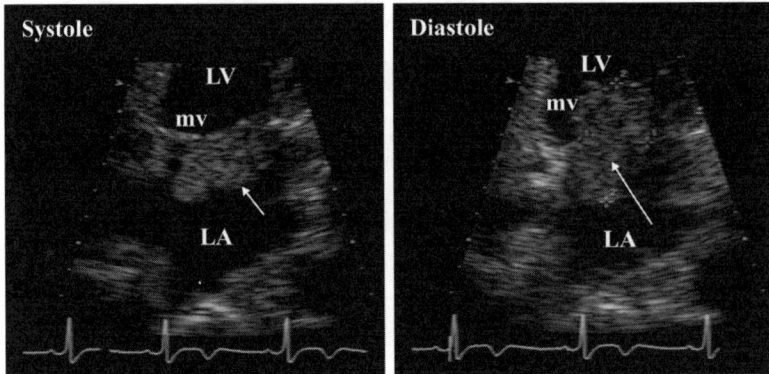

Fig. 38. Stop frames from two-dimensional echocardiogram taken from a patient with left atrial myxoma. During systole the dense echogenic mass representing the tumor in the left atrium (LA) is seen just at the edge of the closed mitral valve (mv). The tumor mass is seen to protrude into the left ventricle (LV) in diastole when the mv opens.

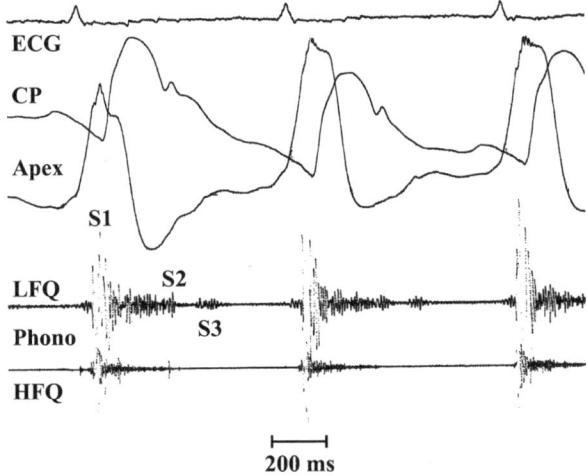

Fig. 39. Phonocardiogram (Phono) recording taken at the lower left sternal border area from a patient with left atrial myxoma along with the apexcardiogram (Apex) and carotid pulse (CP) recordings. The tumor plop sound (S3) is seen in the low-frequency (LFQ) range. Also seen in the Phono are the loud S1 and the systolic mitral regurgitation murmur.

mitral orifice obstruction. This, of course, also leads to elevation of the left atrial pressure, as in mitral stenosis. The elevated left atrial *v wave* pressure initiates a vigorous expansion during the rapid filling phase. When the opening of the mitral valve occurs, the tumor tends to move along with the anterior mitral leaflet and enters the left ventricle. When it reaches its maximum excursion, its further movement is suddenly stopped. This results in a sound that has characteristics similar to the S3 *(85)* (Fig. 38). The sound tends to occur slightly after the rapid filling wave peak. It often is followed by a low- to medium-frequency diastolic murmur because of the mitral obstruction. In addition, the elevated left atrial pressure produces a loud banging M1, which may be palpable (Fig. 39). Also, one will be able to note the presence of a systolic murmur of mitral regurgitation.

Summation Gallop

When the atrial contraction happens to occur during the rapid filling phase for any reason, then the energy acquired by the moving column of blood becomes augmented. In such situations, the deceleration that follows, because of the normal transition from the period of rapid expansion to the slow expansion, may be sufficient to generate an S3. This requires a normal atrial contraction and abnormal timing of the atrial depolarization in relationship to the ventricular depolarization. This can occur in the presence of mild sinus tachycardia with shortening of diastole, resulting in atrial contraction at the time of the rapid filling phase. This can also occur when the PR interval is long enough (first-degree A-V block) that the atrial contraction occurs early in diastole. It can also occur if the atrial contraction and the ventricular contraction are dissociated, as in A-V dissociation caused, for instance, by complete A-V block, or in patients whose ventricles are paced by an electronic pacemaker and who have an underlying undisturbed regular atrial rhythm. The augmentation can occur only when the atrial contraction occurs during the rapid filling phase. Therefore, in A-V dissociation this is likely to occur only intermittently.

When an S3 is made louder by the fortuitous occurrence of atrial contraction at the time of the rapid filling phase, it is termed a *summation sound or gallop*. When this occurs in the presence of mild sinus tachycardia, application of carotid sinus pressure by slowing the sinus rate may be able to prevent the atrial contraction from occurring at the rapid filling phase, thereby abolishing the summation effect.

Summation gallop itself may not signify a pathological state, particularly if seen only during mild sinus tachycardia. The significance of the summation gallop sound will depend on the clinical circumstance under which it develops *(76)*.

If either the S3 or S4 is pathological and the sound is made louder by the timing of the atrial contraction at the time of the rapid filling phase, the resulting sound is sometimes termed "*augmented gallops*" *(86)*.

Clinical Features of S3

S3 is a sound that occurs at the end of the rapid filling phase of diastole at pressures that are generally low. Therefore, the S3 is a low-frequency sound or a thud similar to the sound caused by a small lead ball falling on a cushioned floor. It occurs at the peak of the rapid filling phase and is therefore separated from the S2 by the combined duration of the isovolumic relaxation and the period of rapid inflow. The former is approximately between 60 and 100 ms. The latter lasts an average of 100 ms. The S3 occurs, therefore, a fair distance after S2. This creates a cadence:

Lubb ....dup....bum.

The left-sided S3 is obviously best audible over the apex area, which is usually formed by the left ventricle. It is best elicited by auscultation with the bell, which picks up the low frequencies. S3 is also somewhat affected by proximity. Often S3 may be best heard only when the patient is turned to the left lateral position and auscultated over the area of the apical impulse. It is usually uncommon to have S3 when the apex beat is not palpable. Rarely it may be audible in the absence of a palpable apex beat, e.g., in acute myocardial infarction, in severe cardiomyopathy with severe reduction in the left ventricular ejection fraction, and in constrictive pericarditis.

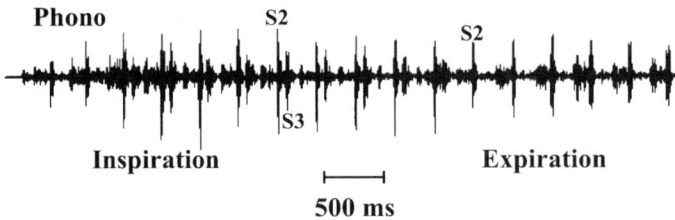

Fig. 40. Digital display of a magnetic audio recording taken at the xiphoid area of the sternum from a patient with severe pulmonary hypertension secondary to scleroderma with right ventricular decompensation. During inspiration (identified by the noise in the baseline) an S3 is seen clearly, which is not seen during expiration, confirming the right-sided origin of the sound.

If the apex beat were to hide behind the ribs during a certain phase of respiration, the S3 may also become soft or inaudible at that time. It may become audible only when the apex beat becomes palpable between the ribs, namely in the intercostal space. The phase of respiration during which this may happen may vary from patient to patient. Although the left ventricular filling becomes relatively greater on expiration, the usual left-sided S3 does not always increase on expiration. If the proximity effect is better on inspiration, it may become more audible only on inspiration. When loud, S3 may be audible even at the base. S3 generally will tend to disappear or become softer in the standing position because of decreased venous return.

Right-sided S3 generally is best heard over the xiphoid area and over the lower sternal region. It usually will increase in intensity or loudness on inspiration (Fig. 40).

Physiological S3 and pathological S3 are very similar in all respects with regard to the auscultatory features. Therefore, the distinction is only made by the associated features. Generally, S1 intensity is good in physiological S3, and the apical impulse will be normal and not sustained on palpation.

CLINICAL ASSESSMENT OF S3

S3 should be looked for in situations where it is expected to be heard, such as in children, pregnant women, rapid circulatory states, patients in whom the apical impulse is felt to be abnormal and sustained or hyperdynamic as in ventricular volume overload, or patients with signs and symptoms of peripheral or systemic congestion with elevated jugular venous pressure. Because it is a low-frequency sound, it must be searched for with the bell of the stethoscope. The patient should be turned to the left lateral position and the apical impulse located, and the area of the palpable apex beat must be auscultated. The presence of S3 is identified by its typical cadence, namely:

One...two.....bum
Lubb......dup.....bum.

In mitral regurgitation and other similar ventricular volume overload states, if S3 is heard it will often have some duration and sound more like a short low- to medium-frequency murmur. The presence of S3 in these conditions often indicates that the lesion causing the volume overload is significant. In mitral regurgitation, for instance, the presence of S3 would only be heard when the degree of regurgitation is moderately severe or severe. If the degree of regurgitation is not significant and a definite S3 is present, then it must mean coexisting left ventricular dysfunction. If tricuspid regurgitation is considered, either on the basis of an elevated venous pressure with jugular contour showing a large prominently rising *v wave* with a *y descent* or by detecting the murmur, then a right-sided S3 should be looked for. A right-sided S3 is classically heard maximally over the xiphoid and the lower sternal area and increases typically on inspiration.

S3 Persisting on Standing

S3 generally disappears or becomes softer on standing. Most physiological S3, S3 associated with ventricular volume overload, and even the usual heart failure S3 generally follow this rule. However, if it persists and continues to be well heard, it must indicate an unusual situation in which a high *v wave* pressure in the atrium is associated with significant decrease in compliance. This may occur, for instance, in constrictive pericarditis and/or severe cardiomyopathy (Fig. 37).

S2-S3 Vs Wide-Split S2

1. S3 is separated far enough from the S2; therefore, it is unusual for it to be mistaken for a wide-split S2. In addition, when the S2 is widely split, both components of S2 are sharper and of higher frequencies. They also tend to be similar to each other. This is unlike the S3, which has a much lower frequency and is often better heard with the bell.
2. The maximum loudness of left-sided S3 is over the area of a palpable left ventricular apex beat. Split S2 when wide is often better heard over the second, third, and sometimes fourth left intercostal space at the left sternal border.
3. S3 tends to get softer and usually tends to disappear on standing.

S3 Differentiation From OS

A late-occurring OS may sometimes be mistaken for an S3. Distinguishing features are:

1. S3 is of low frequency and heard best over the apex, whereas the OS is of high frequency and often best heard between the apex and the lower left sternal border.
2. The S1 is often loud and may be palpable in the presence of a good OS. It is unusual to have a palpable S1 with an S3.
3. If a clear-cut "triple sound" or "trill" is identified, then the presence of OS is confirmed.
4. On standing, S3 will become softer or often disappear, whereas the OS, if still audible, will be found to come later.
5. If the sound in question is audible on standing and does not change much in timing, consider unusual S3 such as a pericardial knock or that caused by a severe cardiomyopathy.

Very rarely, one may encounter the presence of both an S3 and an OS. This may occur in the presence of significant mitral regurgitation in rheumatic mitral disease, which is characterized by a shortened and severely restricted posterior mitral leaflet together with a freely mobile anterior leaflet. The severe mitral regurgitation may bring out the S3, and the freely mobile anterior leaflet may be part of the causation of the OS *(87)*.

S3 Differentiation From Tumor Plop

Tumor plop sounds like an S3. However, it is associated with a loud banging M1, which may be palpable. In addition, there often will be low- to medium-frequency diastolic murmur following the sound because of the mitral obstruction.

Intermittent S3

When heard, S3 is often intermittent and occasionally varies with different phases of respiration. The most common cause for this is proximity. The location of the apex beat and whether it hides intermittently behind the ribs may determine when it may be heard best.

When there is A-V dissociation as in complete A-V block or a patient with a permanent ventricular demand single-chamber electronic pacemaker, one may hear an S3 whenever the dissociated atrial contraction occurs during the rapid-filling phase of diastole. Such A-V dissociation will also be expected to affect the intensity of S1 and will produce variable softer and louder intensity of M1. If atrial contraction were to occur in the rapid filling phase and produce an S3 effect, the S1 immediately following the S3 would be soft. This unique situation with varying S1 intensity and intermittent S3 is likely to occur only with the presence of A-V dissociation.

(For additional examples review Phono Files 35–44 under Heart Sounds on the Companion CD.)

FOURTH HEART SOUND (S4)

Mechanism of Formation of S4

The atrium normally contracts at the end of diastole and gives an extra stretch to the ventricles. When the ventricular compliance is significantly reduced because of factors such as hypertrophy, ischemia, infarction, fibrosis, or infiltrates, then this evokes a more vigorous contraction from the atrium. This augments ventricular filling at the end of diastole and helps in its expansion *(88)*. The increased force of atrial contraction also raises the atrial *a wave* pressure peak. This augmented pressure head tends to accelerate the diastolic inflow at the end of diastole. Because the ventricular compliance is reduced, the accelerated inflow at this phase of diastole is decelerated fairly rapidly. This will depend, of course, on the extent of reduction in the compliance. This sudden deceleration of the column of blood entering the ventricle at end-diastole leads to dissipation of energy, which results in the production of the sound (Fig. 41). The sound forms inside the ventricle, and the entire hemic mass, the papillary muscles, and the underlying ventricular myocardium probably participate in its production. The sound is sometimes referred to as *atrial gallop* and can be simply called S4. The sound, being generated at

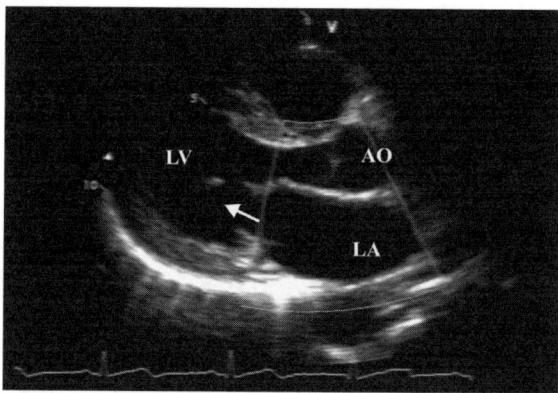

Fig. 41. Stop frame during end diastole from a two-dimensional echocardiogram of a patient taken in the parasternal long axis. The moving column of blood (arrow) from the left atrium (LA) into the left ventricle (LV) is shown. Strong atrial contraction during this phase augments the ventricular filling, which could be decelerated abruptly if the ventricular compliance is reduced for any reason, producing an S4.

low pressures of diastole, has a low frequency very similar to the S3. However, the timing is different; it is closer to S1.

The cadence therefore is different:

$$S4..S1.....S2........Ha..ha.....tu........$$

The prerequisites for S4 formation are:
1. *Reduced ventricular compliance*
2. *Healthy atrium*
3. *Regular sinus rhythm*
4. *Absence of A-V valve obstruction*

The causes of reduced compliance have been discussed in relation to S3. These are completeness of relaxation, chamber size, thickness of the wall, composition of the wall (inflammation, infiltrate, ischemia or infarction, scars, etc.), pericardium, and right ventricular volume/pressure in the case of the left ventricle.

While the small size of the ventricle in children offers resistance to rapid inflow in early diastole, once the ventricle has begun to expand because of the onrushing flow, by the end of diastole the size may no longer be restrictive to filling. This explains the usual absence of S4 in children. This is best appreciated by the analogy of blowing into a balloon to expand it. The resistance is maximal when the size is smallest, namely, when one first begins to blow. Once the balloon is partially expanded it is easier to inflate it further.

On the other hand, with increasing age, the ventricle does become more stiff because of various factors, including age-related hypertrophy as well as acquired diseases including ischemic heart disease, even if asymptomatic. Thus, S4 is often heard in older subjects (>60 yr) even in the absence of clear clinical heart disease *(89)*. Hypertension is the most common cause of hypertrophy in the elderly. However, there could also be atrial disease as well as sinus node dysfunction with development of atrial arrhythmias, such as atrial fibrillation. Therefore, S4 may not be always present in everyone in this age group. Calcific aortic stenosis is more common in people over the age of 65, and yet

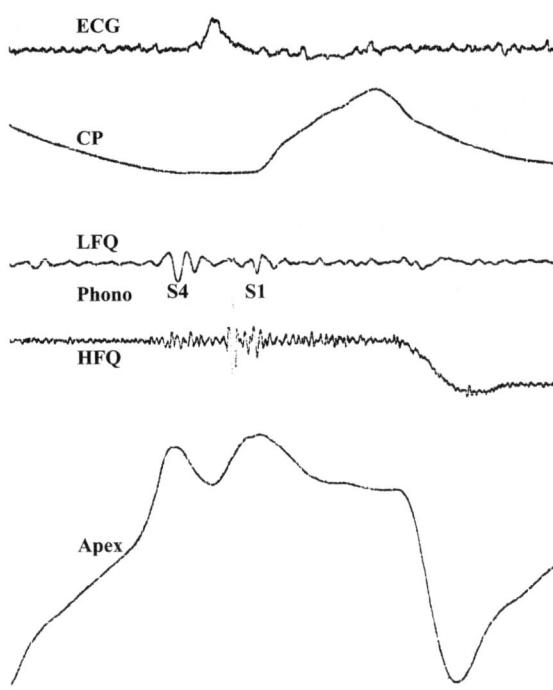

Fig. 42. Phonocardiogram (Phono) recording from a patient with significant aortic valvular stenosis taken from the apex area along with the apexcardiogram (Apex) and carotid pulse (CP) tracings. The Phono shows a low-frequency sound (S4) at the time of the augmented A wave in the Apex recording.

not everyone with significant stenosis (outflow gradient >74 mmHg) with resultant marked hypertrophy will have a definite S4.

Significant aortic stenosis in the younger age group, on the other hand, will have a loud S4 because the hypertrophy associated with such outflow obstruction not only will result in marked decrease in compliance of the ventricle, but also the left atrium is more than likely to be healthy and normal enough to help generate a strong contraction. When a vigorous left atrial contraction occurs in such a situation, the expansion of the ventricle at that time will raise its wall tension enough to become palpable at the apex. The palpable expansion of the apical impulse resulting from such a strong atrial contraction is referred to as the *atrial kick (88)* (Fig. 42). It must be understood that the sound itself never becomes loud enough to be palpable. The atrial kick has the same significance as the S4.

The presence of S4 in a hypertrophic ventricle with outflow tract obstruction usually indicates significant stenosis or obstruction whether right-sided or left-sided (pulmonary or aortic stenosis) *(90)*. S4 in the presence of systemic hypertension would imply a significant decrease in compliance because of hypertensive heart disease. The associated pathological changes may be significant hypertrophy, focal fibrosis, and/or associated coronary heart disease. In the absence of significant left ventricular outflow obstruction, such as aortic stenosis or significant hypertension, a loud S4 at the left ventricular apex area may be indicative of a cardiomyopathy (e.g., hypertrophic cardiomyopathy *[91]*, occasionally other myocardial diseases) or ischemic heart disease *(66,92–94)* (Figs. 43 and 44).

Chapter 6 / Heart Sounds

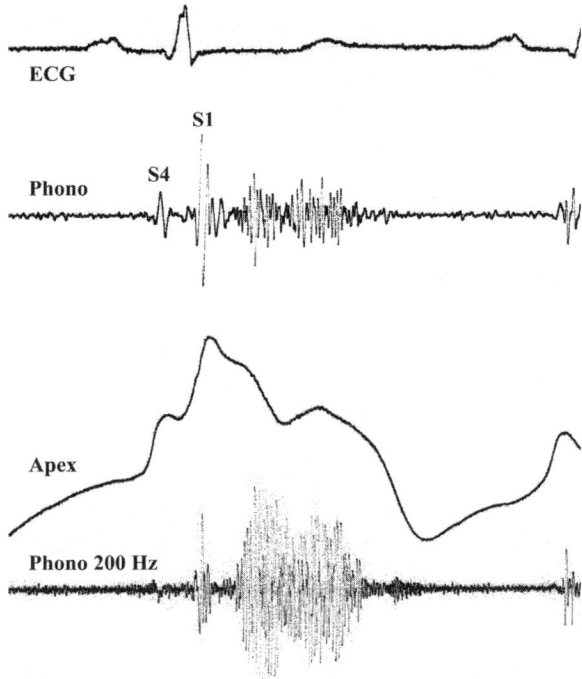

Fig. 43. Phonocardiogram recording from a patient with hypertrophic cardiomyopathy with significant left ventricular outflow tract obstruction taken from the apex area along with the apexcardiogram (Apex) tracing. The Phono shows a low-frequency sound (S4) at the time of the atrial kick in the Apex recording. Note also the systolic ejection murmur of the subaortic stenosis.

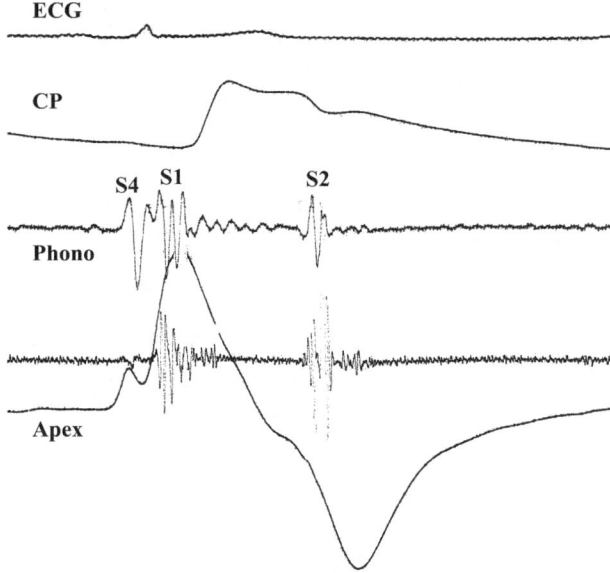

Fig. 44. Phonocardiogram (Phono) recording from a patient with ischemic heart disease taken from the apex area along with the apexcardiogram (Apex) and carotid pulse (CP) tracings. The Phono shows a low-frequency sound (S4) at the time of the augmented A wave in the Apex recording.

Ventricular volume overload usually causes dilatation of the ventricle and therefore is accompanied by better ventricular compliance. Thus, S4 is not a feature of volume-overload states such as mitral regurgitation. Acute mitral regurgitation because of ruptured chordae tendineae, either spontaneous or secondary to infective endocarditis, is, however, an exception in which an S4 may be heard *(95)*. In acute mitral regurgitation both the left atrium and the left ventricle are often presented with significant volume because of the regurgitation, and yet they have not had time to develop secondary dilatation. The lack of significant dilatation of the left ventricle means relatively decreased left ventricular compliance and raised left ventricular diastolic pressures. Sometimes the levels of the left ventricular diastolic pressures and the left atrial pressures are very high and may produce pulmonary edema. When left atrial pressure is elevated but not to the degree of causing pulmonary edema, then the extra stretch provided by the volume may evoke a powerful Starling effect from the left atrium. This in the presence of a relatively less compliant left ventricle produces an S4.

Constrictive pericarditis does not allow expansion of the ventricle beyond the early rapid filling phase, and therefore S4 is not a feature of this condition.

CLINICAL ASSESSMENT OF S4

Left-sided S4 is best audible close to the left ventricular apex area. Often when the S4 is loud, it may be heard over a wide area of the precordium. Right-sided S4 is best audible over the xiphoid area and the lower sternal region. It is detected by an increase in intensity on inspiration or audibility only on inspiration. The jugular contour is also likely to show a prominent rise before the usual systolic x' *descent*. Left-sided S4 may also be somewhat better heard with the patient in the left lateral decubitus position, although when loud enough it does become audible in the usual supine position and medial to the apex. Occasionally, left-sided S4 may be accompanied by a palpable atrial kick of the apical impulse *(93)*. Rarely, with significant right ventricular hypertrophy, as in pulmonary hypertension, the right-sided S4 may be accompanied by similar right atrial kick, which may be palpated by the subxiphoid palpation of the right ventricle on deep inspiration.

S4, being a low frequency sound, is best elicited by listening with the bell of the stethoscope with just enough pressure to make an air seal. Firm pressure with the chest piece of the stethoscope may sometimes eliminate the transmission of such low frequencies by tightening the skin, thus making the S4 soft or altogether disappear. S4 is also affected by venous return and atrial filling. Thus, on standing, when the venous return falls and the atrial filling diminishes, S4 will either become soft or disappear. The increased sympathetic activity associated with diminished venous return may speed up the heart rate and shorten the PR interval and thus may also make the S4 come closer to S1 and actually merge with the latter.

In hypertrophic cardiomyopathy, the compliance is markedly decreased, and this often evokes a loud S4 *(91)*. When there is significant associated left ventricular outflow obstruction in this disorder, the strong atrial contraction may also generate a palpable atrial kick. These patients are generally younger and often have hypertrophied but otherwise healthy left atria early in the course of their disease process.

S4 also is usually sensitive to changes in venous return and filling of the heart. Maneuvers that reduce venous return, such as standing posture, will tend to decrease the intensity or abolish the S4 all together. Rapid volume expansion, cold pressor test, and isometric hand grip will accentuate the S4 *(93)*. Isometric hand grip tends to raise heart rate, cardiac output, and the blood pressure *(96,97)*. It can also raise the peripheral resistance.

If S4 does not disappear on standing, one must consider the presence of significant decrease in compliance as seen in patients with markedly hypertrophied hearts. The S4-S1 interval is not only determined by the PR interval but also to a certain extent by the degree of decrease in compliance or the severity of the underlying disease. When the decreased compliance is significant, as in markedly hypertrophied ventricle, the resultant S4 tends to be well separated from S1 *(93,98)*. Thus, in patients with significant decrease in compliance, S4 may still be heard on standing.

S4 Differentiation from Split S1

S4 sounds different from the M1 component that follows it because it contains more lower-frequency ranges and therefore is heard better with the bell. This is unlike the M1-A1 split, where both components are more or less similar in frequency and more often in the higher ranges. Thus, the split S1 is heard just as well with the diaphragm.

The lower-frequency S4 may be abolished or made softer by firm pressure with the chest piece (the bell), whereas the split S1 is not likely to be affected by such pressure.

Decreasing venous return by standing the patient will only lengthen the isovolumic contraction phase that separates the M1 from A1 by decreasing the rate of rise of ventricular pressure that will accompany reduced ventricular filling. Thus, the split is usually better separated on standing. On the other hand, the decreased atrial filling because of reduced venous return and the slight shortening of PR associated with increase in heart rate secondary to sympathetic stimulation will make the S4 softer and make it come closer to M1, making the separation less distinct.

(For additional examples review Phono Files 45–51 under Heart Sounds on the Companion CD.)

Gallop Rhythm

In the presence of tachycardia, diastole is somewhat shortened, and when an S3 is heard, it is often called the *protodiastolic gallop*, the *S3 gallop* or sometimes the *ventricular diastolic gallop*. The cadence or the rhythm of the S1 and S2 followed by S3 simulates the sounds of a galloping horse:

one ….tu…..bum…..one ….tu….bum….one….tu….bum

This is usually heard in patients with significant heart failure and decreased cardiac output. Occasionally in some patients with left ventricular dysfunction, the pathophysiological changes may provide the prerequisites for both an S3 and an S4. If the heart rate is fast, then both sounds may in fact merge with each other, causing a summation or summation gallop. It will be difficult to distinguish this as such at these fast heart rates and may be simply detected as a gallop rhythm. However, when the heart rate is only mildly fast and both sounds are easily audible in diastole, this is called the *double gallop or the quadruple rhythm or gallop*. This will have a cadence of both S4 and S3 together, namely:

ha…ha …..tu……bum…ha…ha…..tu……bum.

Treatment of the heart failure and clearance of the symptoms and signs of failure may be accompanied by an S3 becoming either softer or totally inaudible. This usually indicates falling left atrial pressure as well as improvement in left ventricular function. At this time an S4 may become audible even if it was not present initially. This means that the left atrium is no longer overstretched or dilated, but the left ventricular compliance is still abnormal, thereby evoking a good atrial contraction. Such a sequence usually indicates good prognosis.

S3 and S4 and Left Ventricular Dysfunction

One recent study evaluating the sensitivity and the specificity of the presence of phonocardiographically detected S3 and/or S4 for detecting left ventricular dysfunction as measured by left ventricular diastolic pressures, left ventricular ejection fraction, and the B-type natriuretic peptide concluded, as expected, that the phonocardiographic S3 and S4 are not sensitive markers of left ventricular dysfunction and that the phonocardiographic S3 was more specific for left ventricular dysfunction than the phonocardiographic S4 *(99)*. Over the years, significant clinical experience has been accumulated as to the significance of these sounds when they are audible. When one takes proper account of the mechanisms behind the production of these sounds, it becomes obvious what their significance is when they are detected at the bedside. Thus, S4, when clinically audible, is relatable only to a strong atrial contraction of a healthy atrium in the presence of decreased left ventricular compliance. The latter could result from a variety of pathological processes, not all of which would necessarily entail left ventricular systolic dysfunction. Thus, it is not expected to be very specific for left ventricular systolic dysfunction. Because an S3 can be physiological as well as pathological, the clinical group of patients being evaluated is another important determinant of whether it is going to correlate clinically to significant left ventricular dysfunction. Therefore, the presence or otherwise of these sounds on auscultation will become relevant only when taken in conjunction with the clinical context. Finally, it is important to realize that studies based merely on phonocardiographic recordings of low-frequency vibrations could lead to misleading information, because they may not be audible.

REFERENCES

1. Dock W. The forces needed to evoke sounds from cardiac tissues and the attenuation of heart sounds. Circulation 1959;19:376.
2. Rushmer RF. Cardiovascular Dynamics, 3rd Ed. Philadelphia, PA: W.B. Saunders, 1970.
3. Leon DF, Shaver JA. Physiologic principles of heart sounds and murmurs. American Heart Association Monograph 46, 1975:1.
4. Leatham A. Splitting of the first and second heart sounds. Lancet 1954;267:607–614.
5. Shah PM, Mori M, Maccanon DM, Luisada AA. Hemodynamic correlates of the various components of the first hear sound. Circ Res 1963; 2:386–392.
6. Sakamoto T, Kusukawa R, Maccanon DM, Luisada AA. Hemodynamic determinants of the amplitude of the first heart sound. Circ Res 1965;16:45–57.

7. Luisada AA, Shah PM. Controversial and changing aspects of ausculation. I. Areas of ausculation: a new concept. II. Normal and abnormal first and second sounds. Am J Cardiol 1963;11:774–789.
8. Piemme TE, Barnett GO, Dexter L. Relationship of heart sounds to acceleration of blood flow. Circ Res 1966;18:303–315.
9. Thompson ME, Shaver JA, Heidenreich FP, Leon DF, Leonard JJ. Sound, pressure and motion correlates in mitral stenosis. Am J Med 1970;49:436–450.
10. Laniado S, Yellin EL, Miller H, Frater RW. Temporal relation of the first heart sound to closure of the mitral valve. Circulation 1973;47:1006–1014.
11. Lakier JB, Fritz VU, Pocock WA, Barlow JB. Mitral components of the first heart sound. Br Heart J 1972;34:160–166.
12. Shah PM. Hemodynamic determinants of the first heart sound. American Heart Association Monograph 46, 1975:2.
13. O'Toole JD, Reddy SP, Curtiss EI, Griff FW, Shaver JA. The contribution of tricuspid valve closure to the first heart sound. An intracardiac micromanometer study. Circulation 1976;53:752–758.
14. Kincaid-Smith P, Barlow J. The atrial sound and the atrial component of the first heart sound. Br Heart J 1959;21:470–478.
15. Waider W, Craige E. First heart sound and ejection sounds. Echocardiographic and phonocardiographic correlation with valvular events. Am J Cardiol 1975;35:346.
16. Constant J. Bedside Cardiology, 2nd ed. Boston: Little Brown and Company, 1976.
17. Luisada AA. "Tricuspid" component of the first heart sound. American Heart Association Monograph 46, 1975:9–26.
18. Shaver JA, Griff W, Leonard JJ. Ejection sounds of left sided origin. American Heart Association Monograph 46, 1975:27–34.
19. Shah PM, Kramer DH, Gramiak R. Influence of the timing of atrial systole on mitral valve closure and on the first heart sound in man. Am J Cardiol 1970;26:231–237.
20. Thompson ME, Shaver JA, Leon DF, Reddy SP, Leonard JJ. Pathodynamics of the first heart sound. American Heart Association Monograph 46, 1975:8–18.
21. Reddy PS, Leon DF, Krishnaswami.V, O'Toole JD, Salerni R, Shaver JA. Syndrome of acute aortic regurgitation. American Heart Association Monograph 46, 1975:166–174.
22. Wigle ED, Labrosse CJ. Sudden, severe aortic insufficiency. Circulation 1965;32:708–720.
23. Meadows WR, Vanpraagh S, Indreika M, Sharp JT. Premature mitral valve closure: a hemodynamic explanation for absence of the first sound in aortic insufficiency. Circulation 1963;28:251–258.
24. Fontana ME, Wooley CF. Sail sound in Ebstein's anomaly of the tricuspid valve. Circulation 1972;46:155–164.
25. Mills PG, Brodie B, McLaurin L, Schall S, Craige E. Echocardiographic and hemodynamic relationships of ejection sounds. Circulation 1977;56:430–436.
26. Hancock.E.W. The ejection sound in aortic stenosis. Am J Med 1966; 40:569.
27. Martin. C.E, Shaver JA, O'Toole JD, Leon DF, Reddy SP. Ejection sounds of right sided origin. American Heart Association Monograph 46, 1975:35–44.
28. Hultgren HN, Reeve R, Cohn K, McLeod R. The ejection click of valvular pulmonic stenosis. Circulation 1969;40:631–640.
29. Shaver JA, Nadolny RA, O'Toole JD, et al. Sound pressure correlates of the second heart sound. An intracardiac sound study. Circulation 1974;49:316–325.
30. Shaver JA, O'Toole JD, Curtiss EI, Thompson ME, Reddy PS, Leon DF. Second heart sound: the role of altered greater and lesser circulation. American Heart Association Monograph 46, 1975:58–67.
31. Curtiss EI, Matthews RG, Shaver JA. Mechanism of normal splitting of the second heart sound. Circulation 1975;51:157–164.
32. Curtiss EI, Shaver JA, Reddy PS, O'Toole JD. Newer concepts in physiologic splitting of the second heart sound. American Heart Association Monograph 46, 1975:68–73.
33. Adolf RJ. Second heart sound. The role of altered electromechanical events. American Heart Association Monograph 46, 1975:45–57.
34. Hultgren HN, Craige E, Fujii J, Nakamura T, Bilisoly J. Left bundle branch block and mechanical events of the cardiac cycle. Am J Cardiol 1983;52:755–762.
35. Shaver JA, O'Toole JD. The second heart sound: newer concepts. Part I: normal and wide physiological splitting. Mod Concepts Cardiovasc Dis 1977;46:7–12.
36. Shaver JA, O'Toole JD. The second heart sound: newer concepts. Part II: Paradoxical splitting and narrow physiological splitting. Mod Concepts Cardiovasc Dis 1977;46:13–16.

37. Wood P. The Eisenmenger syndrome or pulmonary hypertension with reversed central shunt. Br. Heart J 1963;2:701.
38. Luisada AA. The second heart sound in normal and abnormal conditions. Am J Cardiol 1971;28:150–161.
39. Ranganathan N, Sivaciyan V. Abnormalities in jugular venous flow velocity in pulmonary hypertension. Am J Cardiol 1989;63:719–724.
40. Shapiro S, Clark TJ, Goodwin JF. Delayed closure of the pulmonary valve in obliterative pulmonary hypertension. Lancet 1965;2:1207–1211.
41. Perloff JK. Auscultatory and phonocardiographic manifestations of pulmonary hypertension. Prog cardiovasc Dis 1967;9:303.
42. Perloff JK. The Clinical Recognition of Congenital Heart Disease. Philadelphia, PA: W.B. Saunders, 1979–81:279.
43. Logue RB, Woodfin B, Cobbs BW, Dorney ER. The second heart sound in pulmonary embolism and pulmonary hypertension. Trans Am Clin Climatol Assoc 1967;78:38–50.
44. Schrire V, Vogelpoel L. The role of the dilated pulmonary artery in abnormal splitting of the second heart sound. Am Heart J 1962;63:501–507.
45. Perloff JK, Harvey WP. Mechanisms of fixed splitting of the second heart sound. Circulation 1958;18:998–1009.
46. Aygen MM, Braunwald E. The splitting of the second heart sound in normal subjects and in patients with congenital heart disease. Circulation 1962;25:328–345.
47. Kalke BR, Carlson RG, Ferlic RM, Sellers RD, Lillehei CW. Partial anomalous pulmonary venous connections. Am J Cardiol 1967;20:91–101.
48. Frye RL, Marshall HW, Kincaid OW, Burchell HB. Anomalous pulmonary venous drainage of the right lung into the inferior vena cava. Br Heart J 1962;24:696–702.
49. Wood.P. An appreciation of mitral stenosis I. Clinical features. BMJ 1954;1:1051.
50. Wood.P. An appreciation of mitral stenosis. II. Investigations and results. BMJ 1954;1:1113–1124.
51. Margolies A, Wolferth.CC. The OS (claquement d'ouverture de la mitrale) in mitral stenosis. Its characteristics, mechanism of production and diagnostic importance. Am Heart J 1932;7:443.
52. Perloff JK. The physiological mechanisms of cardiac and vascular physical signs. J Am Coll Cardiol 1983;1:184–198.
53. Wooley CF, Klassen KP, Leighton RF, Goodwin RS, Ryan.J.M. Left atrial and left ventricular sound and pressure in mitral stenosis. Circulation 1968;38:295.
54. Perloff JK, Harvey WP. Auscultatory and phonocardiographic manifestations of pure mitral regurgitation. Prog Cardiovasc Dis 1962;5:172–194.
55. Neil P, Mounsey P. Auscultation in patent ductus arteriosus with description of two fistulae simulating patent ductus. Br Heart J 1958;20:51.
56. Tavel.ME. Opening snaps: mitral and tricuspid. American Heart Association Monograph 46, 1975;85–91.
57. Henderson Y. Diastolic relaxation. Physiol Rev 1923;3:165–208.
58. Zile MR, Brutsaert DL. New concepts in diastolic dysfunction and diastolic heart failure: Part I: diagnosis, prognosis, and measurements of diastolic function. Circulation 2002;105:1387–1393.
59. Zile MR, Brutsaert DL. New concepts in diastolic dysfunction and diastolic heart failure: Part II: causal mechanisms and treatment. Circulation 2002;105:1503–1508.
60. Hein S, Arnon E, Kostin S, et al. Progression from compensated hypertrophy to failure in the pressure-overloaded human heart: structural deterioration and compensatory mechanisms. Circulation 2003;107:984–991.
61. Leite-Moreira AF, Correia-Pinto J, Gillebert TC. Afterload induced changes in myocardial relaxation: a mechanism for diastolic dysfunction. Cardiovasc Res 1999;43:344–353.
62. Brutsaert DL, Rademakers FE, Sys SU. Triple control of relaxation: implications in cardiac disease. Circulation 1984;69:190–196.
63. Zile MR, Gaasch WH. Load-dependent left ventricular relaxation in conscious dogs. Am J Physiol 1991;261:H691–H699.
64. Zile MR, Blaustein AS, Gaasch WH. The effect of acute alterations in left ventricular afterload and beta-adrenergic tone on indices of early diastolic filling rate. Circ Res 1989;65:406–416.
65. Ariel Y, Gaasch W.H, Bogen DK, McMahon.TA. Load-dependent relaxation with late systolic volume steps: servo-pump studies in the intact canine heart. Circulation, 1987;75:1287–1294.

66. Ranganathan N, Juma Z, Sivaciyan V. The apical impulse in coronary heart disease. Clin Cardiol 1985;8:20–33.
67. Papapietro SE, Coghlan HC, Zissermann D, Russell RO, Jr., Rackley CE, Rogers WJ. Impaired maximal rate of left ventricular relaxation in patients with coronary artery disease and left ventricular dysfunction. Circulation 1979;59:984–991.
68. Gamble WH, Shaver JA, Alvares RF, Salerni R, Reddy PS. A critical appraisal of diastolic time intervals as a measure of relaxation in left ventricular hypertrophy. Circulation 1983;68:76–87.
69. Gaasch WH, Levine HJ, Quinones MA, Alexander JK. Left ventricular compliance: mechanisms and clinical implications. Am J Cardiol 1976;38:645–653.
70. Levine HJ, Gaasch WH. Diastolic compliance of the left ventricle. I: causes of a noncompliant ventricular chamber. Mod Concepts Cardiovasc Dis 1978;47:95–98.
71. Levine HJ, Gaasch WH. Diastolic compliance of the left ventricle. II: chamber and muscle stiffness, the volume/mass ratio and clinical implications. Mod Concepts Cardiovasc Dis 1978;47:99–102.
72. Zile MR, Baicu CF, Gaasch WH. Diastolic heart failure—abnormalities in active relaxation and passive stiffness of the left ventricle. N Engl J Med 2004;350:1953–1959.
73. Grossman W, McLaurin LP. Diastolic properties of the left ventricle. Ann Intern Med 1976;84: 316–326.
74. McLaurin LP, Rolett EL, Grossman W. Impaired left ventricular relaxation during pacing-induced ischemia. Am J Cardiol 1973;32:751–757.
75. Van de Werf F, Boel A, Geboers J, et al. Diastolic properties of the left ventricle in normal adults and in patients with third heart sounds. Circulation 1984;69:1070.
76. Shah PM, Jackson.D. Third heart sound and summation gallop. American Heart Association Monograph 46, 1975:79.
77. Drzewiecki GM, Wasicko MJ, Li JK. Diastolic mechanics and the origin of the third heart sound. Ann Biomed Eng 1991;19:651–667.
78. Glower DD, Murrah RL, Olsen CO, Davis JW, Rankin JS. Mechanical correlates of the third heart sound. J Am Coll Cardiol 1992;19:450–457.
79. Downes TR, Dunson W, Stewart K, Nomeir AM, Little WC. Mechanism of physiological and pathological S3 gallop sounds. J Am Soc Echocardiogr 1992;5:211–218.
80. Tribouilloy CM, Enriquez-Sarano M, Mohty D, et al. Pathophysiological determinants of third heart sounds: a prospective clinical and Doppler echocardiographic study. Am J Med 2001;111:96–102.
81. Van de Werf.F, Minten. J, Carmiliet.P, De Geest. H, Kesteloot.H. The genesis of the third and fourth heart sounds. A pressure flow study in dogs. J Clin Invest 1984;73:1400–1407.
82. Reddy PS, Meno F, Curtiss EI, O'Toole JD. The genesis of gallop sounds: investigation by quantitative phono- and apexcardiography. Circulation 1981;63:922–933.
83. Feruglio GA, Sreenivasan A. Intracardiac phonocardiogram in thirty cases of atrial septal defect. Circulation 1959;20:1087–1094.
84. Tyberg TI, Goodyer AV, Langou RA. Genesis of pericardial knock in constrictive pericarditis. Am J Cardiol 1980;46:570–575.
85. Bass NM, Sharratt GP. Left atrial myxoma diagnosed by echocardiography, with observations on tumour movement. Br Heart J 1973;35:1332–1335.
86. Grayzel J. Gallop rhythm of the heart. I. Atrial gallop, ventricular gallop and systolic sounds. Am J Med 1960;28:578–592.
87. Nixon PG, Wooler GH, Radigan LR. Mitral incompetence caused by disease of the mural cusp. Circulation 1959;19:839–844.
88. Gibson TC, Madry R, Grossman W, McLaurin LP, Craige E. The A wave of the apexcardiogram and left ventricular diastolic stiffness. Circulation 1974;49:441–446.
89. Spodick DH, Quarry VM. Prevalence of the fourth heart sound by phonocardiography in the absence of cardiac disease. Am Heart J 1974;87:11–14.
90. Goldblatt A, Aygen MM, Braunwald E. Hemodynamic-phonocardiographic correlations of the fourth heart sound in aortic stenosis. Circulation 1962;26:92–98.
91. Braunwald E, Morrow AG, Cornell.W.P, Aygem. M.M, Hilbish.T.F. Idiopathic hypertrophic subaortic stenosis. Clinical, hemodynamic and angiographic manifestations. Am J Med 1960;29:924.
92. Benchimol A, Dimond EG. The apex cardiogram in ischaemic heart disease. Br Heart J 1962;24: 581–594.
93. Craige.E. The fourth heart sound. American Heart Association Monograph 46, 1975:74.
94. Adolph RJ. The fourth heart sound. Chest 1999;115:1480–1481.

95. Cohen LS, Mason DT, Braunwald E. Significance of an atrial gallop sound in mitral regurgitation. A clue to the diagnosis of ruptured chordae tendineae. Circulation 1967;35:112–118.
96. Cohn PF, Thompson P, Strauss W, Todd J, Gorlin R. Diastolic heart sounds during static (handgrip) exercise in patients with chest pain. Circulation 1973;47:1217–1221.
97. Grossman W, McLaurin LP, Saltz SB, Paraskos JA, Dalen JE, Dexter L. Changes in the inotropic state of the left ventricle during isometric exercise. Br Heart J 1973;35:697–704.
98. Duchosal.P. A study of gallop rhythm by a combination of phonocardiographic and electrocardiographic methods. Am Heart J 1932;7:613.
99. Marcus GM, Gerber IL, McKeown BH, et al. Association between phonocardiographic third and fourth heart sounds and objective measures of left ventricular function. JAMA 2005;293:2238–2244.

7

Heart Murmurs
Part I

CONTENTS

> PRINCIPLES GOVERNING MURMUR FORMATION
> HEMODYNAMIC FACTORS AND CARDIAC MURMURS
> FREQUENCIES OF MURMURS
> GRADING OF MURMURS
> SYSTOLIC MURMURS
> EJECTION MURMURS
> REGURGITANT SYSTOLIC MURMURS
> MITRAL REGURGITATION
> TRICUSPID REGURGITATION
> VENTRICULAR SEPTAL DEFECT (VSD)
> CLINICAL ASSESSMENT OF SYSTOLIC MURMURS
> REFERENCES

PRINCIPLES GOVERNING MURMUR FORMATION

In the cardiovascular system, the blood essentially flows through cylindrical tubes (blood vessels) and the cardiac chambers. It is a common experience that water flow through a normal garden hose that is unkinked or uncoiled with an open end (without a constricting nozzle at the end) is essentially noiseless. The flow through such a garden hose can be described as "laminar" and is defined by determinants of Poiseuille's law. The head of pressure is directly proportional to the length of the pipe, the velocity of flow, and the viscosity of the liquid and is inversely related to the fourth power of the radius *(1)*. The term "laminar" comes from the fact that if you inject dye to observe the nature of the stream in a transparent tube it will have a parabolic shape; the particles in the central axis of the tube move faster than those near the wall, with each succeeding layer distributing itself as a series of laminae. Closest to the wall, the particles may almost be motionless. If the garden hose is suddenly partially kinked or its open end is partially pinched, the pressure proximal to the end will rise and the flow coming out will be under this higher pressure head with greater velocity and will also lead to production of noise. The flow at the point of this constriction is no longer laminar and is turbulent. When turbulent flow is observed by injection of dye, the particles will be seen to have many different randomly distributed directions in addition to the general direction of flow.

With the advent of two-dimensional echocardiography and the application of Doppler techniques together with color-coded flow mapping, one can easily appreciate the

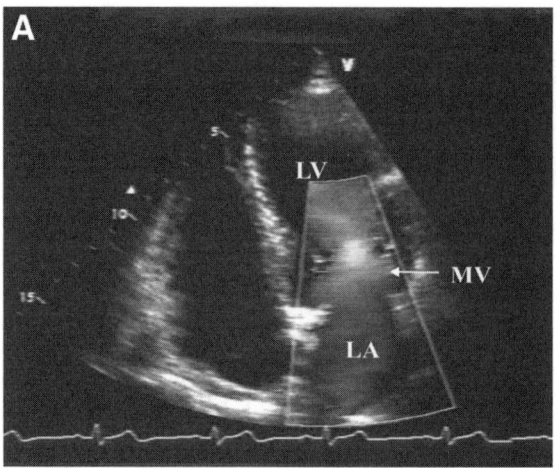

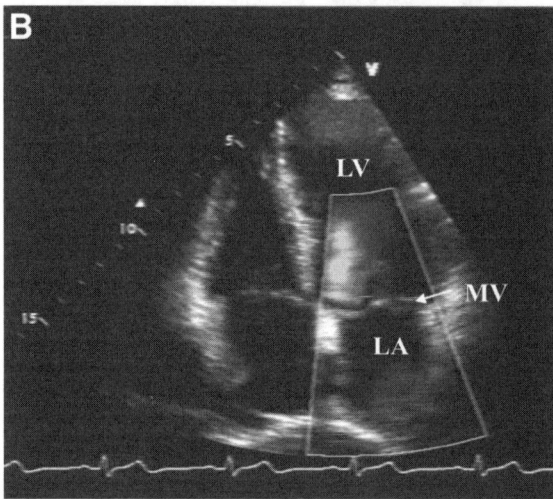

Fig. 1. (Color Plate 1, following p. 270) Two-dimensional echocardiographic images with Doppler color flow mapping from a normal subject in the apical four-chamber view taken in diastole (**A**) and systole (**B**). The normal mitral inflow in diastole from the left atrium (LA) into the left ventricle (LV) through the open mitral valve (MV) is laminar and appears smooth shown in red, indicating the direction of flow, which is toward the probe facing the apex of the left ventricle located at the top of the screen. The systolic flow out through the left ventricular outflow tract is in a smooth blue color, indicating that it is laminar but with a direction away from the probe (apex).

difference between the normal smooth undisturbed laminar flow through the heart vs a disturbed and abnormal turbulent flow. In this technique of color coding of flow, the smooth laminar flow toward the interrogating ultrasound probe is usually depicted by the color red, whereas similar flow but opposite in direction to the probe is depicted by the color blue. On the monitoring screen, the probe location is usually displayed at the top of the screen. Looking at the image of the heart's chambers and their anatomy as revealed through the various views, one can easily appreciate the directional flow through the chambers, as depicted by the simultaneous color display (Fig. 1A,B).

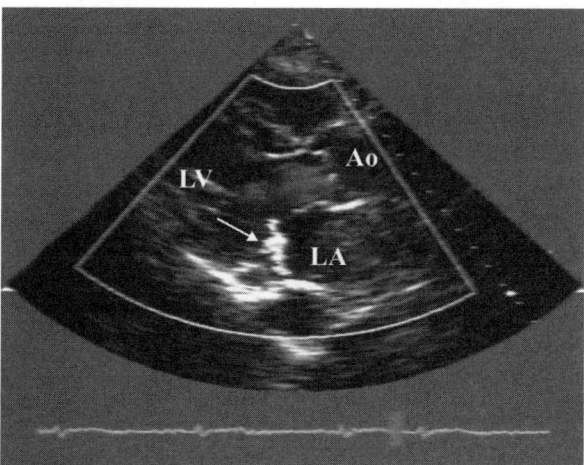

Fig. 2. (Color Plate 2, following p. 270) Two-dimensional echocardiographic image and Doppler color flow mapping from a patient with mitral regurgitation taken in the parasternal long axis. The arrow points to the regurgitation jet in the left atrium (LA), which is seen to have a mosaic appearance because of a mixture of colors depicting that the red cells are moving in different directions with varying velocities secondary to a turbulent flow.

However, whenever the color flow depicts a mixture of colors or a mosaic pattern, we know that the flow is no longer the normal laminar flow but turbulent, implying that the red cells that are bouncing off the ultrasound beam are moving in various random directions. If a patient with mitral regurgitation is observed by this technique, the regurgitant stream will appear in the left atrium during systole and will have a mixture of colors (Fig. 2). Similarly, the aortic outflow jet in a patient with aortic stenosis will demonstrate the characteristic pattern of turbulence. In fact, whenever a significant cardiac murmur is noted, one can always demonstrate turbulent flow associated with it by color flow mapping. The amount and extent of turbulence may vary according to the underlying abnormality and its severity. Thus, turbulent flow is an important cause of cardiovascular murmurs *(1–4)*.

The factors governing turbulent flow were described by Osborne Reynolds (1883). The critical point where laminar flow turns into turbulent flow seems to be dependent on the diameter of the tube, mean velocity of flow, the density of the liquid, and its viscosity *(1)*. The greater the velocity of flow, the greater will be the resulting turbulence. Cardiac lesions such as narrowed outflow tracts from the ventricles, as seen in aortic or pulmonary stenosis, will be expected to have a high velocity of flow under high systolic pressures and therefore will be expected to produce turbulence. Similarly, obstructive lesions to inflow, such as mitral stenosis, will cause turbulent flow through the mitral valve. The velocity of flow will be greater than is normally seen through normal mitral valves because of the elevated left atrial pressures caused by the mitral stenosis. In addition, the entire systemic venous return flows through the mitral valve in diastole. This also means that a large volume of flow is subjected to turbulence. In regurgitant lesions, by virtue of the fact that the flow occurs in a reverse direction and from a high-pressure chamber to a low-pressure chamber (e.g., mitral regurgitation, flow occurring from the left ventricle to the left atrium), the velocity will also be high because of a higher-pressure head and will contribute to the resulting turbulence.

Given all the necessary conditions, turbulence is more likely to occur in a larger than in a smaller vessel. Turbulence is also related to the density of the liquid, being directly related to it, whereas it is inversely related to its viscosity. It is well known that in anemia the viscosity of blood is low, and therefore the resulting Reynolds number from the Reynolds formula will be high. The Reynolds formula is as follows:

$$Re = VD/v$$

where V is the mean velocity of flow, D is the diameter of the tube, and v is the fraction expressing the density of liquid over viscosity of the liquid (1). The volume of flow usually does not enter into the Reynolds formula; increased volume of flow is often associated also with increased velocity in general. Tortuosity and irregularities of vessels will also be expected to cause more turbulence.

Although turbulence is an important cause of cardiovascular murmurs, sometimes turbulent flow within the heart or the blood vessels may be noted and yet there may be no associated murmur. This has become more and more evident because color flow mapping techniques have become available. This should be evidence of the fact that perhaps other factors are needed besides turbulence, such as production of eddies or vortices or resonance of structures. Eddies most certainly must occur around the edge of the cardiac valves. In addition, in situations where blood flows at high velocity but through narrow vessels, e.g., arteriovenous fistula or persistent ductus, large eddies are likely to be created as the jet from the narrowed orifice enters a wider area of vessel. These may also contribute to the murmurs in these conditions (1,4).

In addition, the sounds generated by turbulence need to be in the audible range of frequencies and also have enough energy to overcome the muffling effect of the surrounding anatomical structures and body tissues as well as loss from conduction through the body surface before they can become audible (2). The latter may be an important reason why in a number of instances valvular regurgitation and associated turbulent flow could be demonstrated by color flow mapping and yet auscultation may not reveal a corresponding murmur.

HEMODYNAMIC FACTORS AND CARDIAC MURMURS

The timing and the character or the quality of murmurs as determined by the predominant frequencies will depend on the underlying abnormality and the resulting turbulence and hemodynamic factors associated with the turbulence. The loudness or intensity is also to a certain extent determined by the degree of underlying disturbance in flow. The timing of the murmurs can thus be related to systole, diastole, or both. This will obviously depend on the lesion (e.g., aortic stenosis, which will cause turbulent flow in systole and therefore a systolic murmur, whereas mitral stenosis will cause a diastolic turbulence and diastolic murmur). The character of the resulting murmur, as determined by its predominant frequencies, depends to a large extent on the pressure gradients as well as the volume of flow involved in the resulting turbulence.

FREQUENCIES OF MURMURS

Most cardiovascular murmurs show a frequency range extending from almost zero to 700 Hz (cycles/s). The louder the murmur, the wider will be the spectrum of recordable frequencies. The musical term "pitch" refers to what one hears. High pitch, as when a soprano in an opera makes a note, usually reflects high frequency, whereas the low pitch of a man's voice in an opera indicates lower frequency. The frequencies of murmurs that are clinically important generally relate to both the pressure gradients involved in the production of the turbulent flow as well as the actual volume or amount of flow involved. Turbulent flow differs from laminar flow in the relationship between the pressure gradient and velocity of flow. Turbulent flow requires a larger pressure gradient than the equivalent laminar flow. Because of random directions, more energy is also required to maintain flow, necessitating a higher pressure gradient *(1)*.

It is generally observed that when the pressure gradients are high and produce turbulence, the resulting murmur often tends to be predominantly high in frequency, e.g., mitral regurgitation, where the turbulence because of the regurgitation occurs under a high-pressure difference between the left ventricle and the left atrium. In a normotensive patient this may be as high as 100 mmHg. The murmur of mitral regurgitation is often blowing in character like the noise caused by blowing through a hollow reed. When the regurgitation is mild, it often is almost all high in frequency. When the mitral regurgitation is severe and large in volume, then the murmur may assume lower and medium frequencies and begins to sound harsher. In mitral stenosis, the narrowed mitral orifice causes a turbulent mitral inflow into the left ventricle. The flow occurs under a higher diastolic pressure gradient between the left atrium and the left ventricle. Normally the left atrial pressure *v wave* (~12–15 mmHg) provides the pressure difference during the beginning of diastole, i.e., during the rapid filling phase. In mitral stenosis, the left atrial pressure may be elevated to twice the normal level or more (25–35 mmHg.) The pressure gradient may also tend to persist throughout diastole. The pressure gradient, although persistent, is still in the lower ranges (10–20 mmHg). Thus, the turbulent flow occurs under low-pressure gradients. However, the entire stroke volume of the left ventricle must go through the mitral orifice in diastole. Therefore, there is a large volume of flow associated with the turbulence. Because of these two factors, the mitral stenosis murmur tends to be low and medium in frequency and is described as resembling the rumble of distant thundering clouds. In aortic stenosis, the outflow obstruction will raise the left ventricular systolic pressure in order to maintain forward stroke output. This pressure gradient between the left ventricle and the aorta will depend on the severity of the obstruction. In addition, the entire systemic output must go through the aortic valve. Thus, the murmur of aortic stenosis must have mixed frequencies (low and high) because of both flow and pressure gradients contributing to the turbulence.

Thus, the general relationship between the murmur frequencies and the pressure gradients and flow can be stated as follows: (1) the greater the pressure gradient, the higher the frequency of the murmur; (2) the greater the flow, the lower the frequency. The two heads of the stethoscope are selectively designed to capture the higher- and lower-frequency ranges of sounds and murmurs. The high-frequency and blowing-type murmurs are better brought out by the use of the diaphragm, and the lower-frequency murmurs are better defined by the use of the bell. An experienced auscultator may define the characteristics of the murmur irrespective of the chest piece used, as long as the murmur is loud enough. Faint low-frequency rumbles are best identified by the use of the bell.

GRADING OF MURMURS

The murmurs are also graded as to their loudness using the same system as described in relation to the heart sounds *(5)*. Palpable murmurs are described as having a *thrill*. Thrills, like murmurs, have duration as opposed to sounds, which are transients. Thrills give a feeling to the hand, as when one feels the purring of a cat. When a murmur is not immediately audible, the moment one begins to auscultate and has to tune in to detect the presence of the murmur by eliminating mentally the room noise, then the grade of the murmur is grade I. Grade I murmurs are not generally appreciated by the beginners in auscultation. Grade II murmur does not require this tuning in process. It is immediately audible the moment one begins to listen. Grade III murmur is the loudest murmur audible, but is not associated with a palpable thrill. When a murmur is audible and associated with a thrill, it must be between grades IV and VI. Grade IV murmur requires full contact of the chest wall with the chest piece of the stethoscope for its detection. Grade V murmur requires only partial contact, like the edge of the chest piece, for its detection. Grade VI murmur, on the other hand, is audible even when the chest piece is held slightly but completely off the chest.

SYSTOLIC MURMURS

Cardiac murmurs heard during systole (systolic murmurs) have been traditionally classified in different ways by terms descriptive of some features of the murmurs. Some are defined by the timing of the murmurs in relation to the duration of systole from the first to the second heart sound, some are defined by their quality or character, and some are defined according to their assumed shape. When it is confined to part of the duration of systole, it has been called early systolic, midsystolic, or late systolic, depending on which part of systole it is heard. When it lasts throughout systole, it is described as holosystolic or pansystolic *(6,7)*. Whereas pansystolic murmurs are often caused by regurgitation, regurgitant lesion can also produce murmurs confined to only part of systole, for instance, late systole. When described according to quality or character, terms such as harsh or blowing are used. These terms in general describe the predominant pitch or frequency of the murmur whether medium or high. The character or the predominant frequency of the murmur relates to the pressure gradients and the flow involved in the turbulence. However, it does not help to define the origin of the murmur. Terms such as diamond-shaped or kite-shaped systolic murmur, when used, assume a certain shape of the murmur, which is hardly definable by auscultation. It would require a phonocardiogram to confirm. Even when defined as such on a phonocardiogram, it does not relate to the origin or the cause of the murmur.

Systolic murmurs arise generally because of turbulent flow across the ventricular outflow tract during ejection or from regurgitation of blood (i.e., flow in reverse direction) from the ventricle into a low-pressure chamber like the atrium, as in mitral or tricuspid regurgitation, or through a communication in the ventricular septum from the left ventricle into the right heart. Ejection of blood through the ventricular outflow tract is a normal function of the heart. On the other hand, the occurrence of regurgitation of blood from the ventricle in a reverse direction is always abnormal. The factors governing ejection of blood across the ventricular outflow tract and the abnormalities that may lead to turbulent flow and cause systolic murmurs of ejection origin are, therefore, different from those that are associated with regurgitation *(8)*.

Murmurs of ejection origin have certain characteristic features that are not shared by murmurs of regurgitant origin. Because this distinction has direct practical clinical application, the two types will be discussed separately.

EJECTION MURMURS

Normal Physiology of Ventricular Ejection

In addition to the inherent contractility of the ventricular myocardium and the heart rate at which the ventricle performs its pumping function, the major determinant of its stroke output is the end-diastolic volume, which is essentially the preload. The end-diastolic pressure achieved prior to the onset of systolic contraction will primarily depend on the diastolic function reflecting both ventricular relaxation and compliance. These have been discussed in relation to the heart sounds S3 and S4. Once systole is set in motion by electrical depolarization of the ventricular myocardium, the excitation–contraction coupling leads to actin–myosin bridge formation. As the ventricular contraction proceeds, more and more of the myofibrils are recruited into contraction, resulting in rise of the ventricular pressure. The force exerted by the contracting ventricle on the blood mass it contains imparts energy to it. Once the inertial resistance offered by the blood mass is overcome, the blood mass begins to accelerate and move toward the low-pressure area of the mitral region where it gets decelerated because of the closure of the mitral valve. The energy dissipated when deceleration occurs results in the production of the M1. After this event, continued ventricular contraction during the isovolumic phase (extending from the time of mitral valve closure to the time when the aortic valve opens) produces further rise in the ventricular pressure. When the ventricular pressure exceeds the aortic pressure, the aortic valve opens and ejection begins. Similar events occur on the right side as well. By this time the blood mass has gained significant momentum, which aids its forward movement. The forces that operate to oppose this forward flow have been called impedance (*see* Chapter 6). These include the vascular capacity, the viscosity of the blood, and the resistance of the systemic arterial and the pulmonary vascular beds. To this one can also add the proximal aortic and pulmonary artery distensibility or compliance. The momentum gained by the blood mass will keep it moving forward into the aorta and the pulmonary artery, even during the later part of systole when the ventricular pressure begins to fall below that of the aorta and the pulmonary artery, respectively *(9)*. However, with the falling ventricular pressure, the opposing impedance will prevent further forward flow. The blood mass close to the aortic and the pulmonary valves will suddenly tend to reverse its flow direction toward the ventricle, which presents a low-pressure area because of the falling ventricular pressure. This will close the aortic and the pulmonary valves. Deceleration of the column of blood in the aorta against the closed aortic valve generates the A2, and similar deceleration against the pulmonary valve results in P2. Because the impedance in the pulmonary circuit is lower, this deceleration occurs later. These have been discussed previously under S2.

During the ejection phase, the left ventricular pressure remains slightly higher than the aortic pressure in the early to mid part of systole. This pressure gradient, which has been measured by catheter-tip microsensors, has been termed the *impulse gradient* (Fig. 3). The peak flow acceleration and peak impulse gradients occur very early in systole *(9)*. The aortic flow velocity peaks slightly later, with a slow return to zero flow at the end of

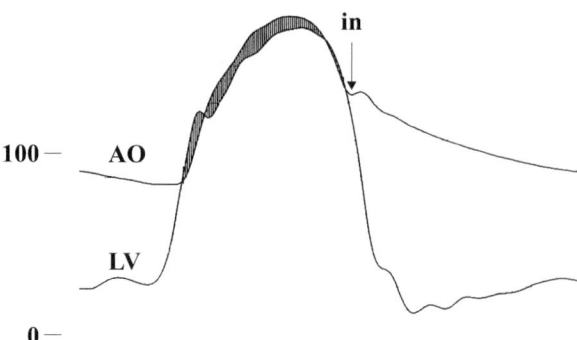

Fig. 3. Simultaneous recording of the left ventricular (LV) and the aortic (AO) pressures through catheters placed in the LV and AO, respectively, showing a small but discernible pressure gradient, "the impulse gradient" between the LV and the AO.

ejection. A smaller right-sided impulse gradient has also been shown between the right ventricle and the pulmonary artery *(9)*.

With exercise the cardiac output is increased because of the increased venous return. There is a significant increase in heart rate in untrained individuals, and the stroke output may or may not be increased. With trained athletes, the heart rate increases slowly. The increased cardiac output is achieved by the increased stroke volume. With exercise, the ejection time shortens, particularly when the heart rate increases. The stroke output, whether increased or normal, is accomplished over a shorter ejection time. This has been shown to be accompanied by an increase in the impulse gradient and an increase in flow acceleration *(9)*.

The flow through normal ventricular outflow tracts and the semilunar valves is still smooth and laminar in most instances. Conditions that lead to an increase in the velocity of flow or actual increase in volume of flow, particularly in the presence of anatomical abnormalities of the outflow tract, are all likely to result in turbulent flow.

Formation of Ejection Murmurs

Turbulent flow during ejection leading to the formation of ejection murmurs can be expected to occur under the following circumstances:

1. Increased velocity of ejection of either normal or increased stroke volume of blood across normal aortic and/or pulmonary valves and the respective outflow tracts
2. Ejection of a large stroke volume of blood across a normal aortic and/or the pulmonary valves and the respective outflow tracts
3. Ejection of blood across roughened or stenosed aortic and/or pulmonary valves or their respective outflow tracts

Characteristics of Ejection Murmurs

1. *Ejection murmurs are often harsh and have predominant medium and low frequencies.*
   Because the entire stroke output of the ventricle flows through the outflow tract and will be involved in any turbulence during ejection, ejection murmurs will tend to have many medium- and low-frequency components caused primarily by flow. If the stroke volume is actually increased for some reason, then this effect will be enhanced. The pre-

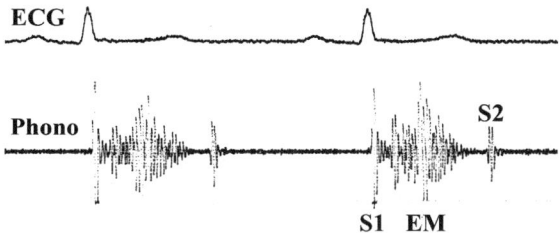

Fig. 4. Phonocardiographic (Phono) recording from the apex area of a patient with an ejection murmur. Note that the murmur starts with the S1 and reaches a peak in mid-systole and gradually tapers and ends before the S2, thus showing a crescendo and decrescendo effect.

dominant low and medium frequency will make the ejection murmurs sound harsh in quality.

2. *Ejection murmurs have a characteristic cadence or rhythm.*

   The ejection phase begins as soon as the isovolumic phase of contraction ends. The S1 with its M1 and A1 components, just precede ejection and ejection murmurs, therefore begin with the S1 *(10)*. The physiology of ejection is such that there is an initial phase of acceleration with buildup of momentum. When there is no fixed outflow obstruction or stenosis, this reaches a peak in early to mid-systole and begins to decline thereafter. The flow velocity also reaches a peak in early to mid-systole and gradually returns to zero flow in late systole. Reflecting this, the ejection murmur also increases in intensity to reach a peak and thereafter declines in late systole and ends before the S2 (Fig. 4). The murmur thus has a crescendo–decrescendo character *(8)*. Depending on the side of origin, whether it is left-sided or right-sided, the murmur will end before the A2 or the P2. The S1, the peak of the crescendo followed by a pause before S2, makes a cadence or rhythm:

   S1…. peak …S2
   Da…..Ha ….Da

   When there is significant fixed obstruction or stenosis in the outflow tract, the ventricular pressure will be increased to overcome the stenosis. The systolic pressure gradient between the ventricle and the aorta or the pulmonary artery, depending on the side involved in the obstruction, will reflect its severity. The pressure gradient will rise with onset of ejection, becoming maximal in midsystole. It will decrease later in systole with falling ventricular pressure. The more severe the stenosis, the greater is this pressure gradient. In severe stenosis, the pressure gradient may be in excess of 75 mmHg. The stroke volume in the presence of outflow tract obstruction is ejected over a longer period. The flow velocity increases gradually and reaches a peak in midsystole, and the murmur also becomes somewhat longer and achieves peak intensity in mid-systole. Following the peak it decreases in intensity, still retaining the crescendo–decrescendo character, and eventually fades out before the S2. Thus, a pause is often recognizable between the end of the murmur and the S2. In addition to the low and medium frequencies produced by the flow, the higher-pressure gradient in severe stenosis will contribute to some of the higher frequencies of the murmur.

3. *Ejection murmur tends to increase in intensity or loudness after long diastolic intervals.*

   A long diastolic period occurs following premature ventricular beat because of the compensatory pause. The ejection murmur during the beat after the compensatory pause has a louder intensity than the regular sinus beat before it (Fig. 5). The reason for

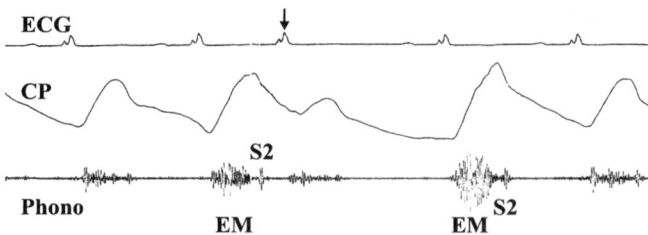

Fig. 5. Simultaneous recordings of phonocardiogram (Phono), electrocardiogram (ECG), and carotid pulse (CP) from a patient with a systolic murmur. The ECG shows the presence of a premature beat (arrow). Note the murmur has greater amplitude in the beat following the ectopic (premature) beat compared to the sinus beat before it. This confirms that the systolic murmur is an ejection murmur.

this is that the postectopic beat has a stronger contraction and increased stroke output. The compensatory pause allows longer diastolic filling time, thus increasing the volume and providing a Starling effect on contractility. This helps in enhancing the stroke output of the postectopic beat. In addition, during the long pause the aortic diastolic pressure continues to fall and the postectopic beat thus has less afterload or impedance to ejection. The third reason for the augmented contractility is the postextrasystolic potentiation that a premature depolarization provides. This is probably because of the availability of extra calcium within the myocardium for the contractile process. Any early or premature depolarization will cause this (see Chapter 2). A similar phenomenon can be observed during atrial fibrillation, where the diastolic intervals naturally vary. The ejection murmur will vary in intensity and will be noted to be louder following long diastoles *(11)*.

Anatomical Differences Between the Left and Right Ventricular Outflow Tract

Because ejection murmurs are caused by turbulent flow accompanying ejection of blood through the ventricular outflow tract, the anatomy of the outflow tracts needs to be understood. The outflow tract of both ventricles is formed not only by the respective semilunar valve (the aortic and the pulmonary valves), but also by the structures just above and below the valve itself. The supravalvular portion of the outflow tract consists of the aortic root on the left side and the pulmonary artery on the right side.

The left ventricular outflow tract below the semilunar aortic valve has essentially two boundaries. The subaortic ventricular septum is on the antero-medial side, whereas on the lateral side is the anterior mitral leaflet. This is because the anterior mitral leaflet shares its attachment to the aortic root with the aortic valve (Fig. 6A). The anatomical organization is different on the right side where the pulmonary valve shares no such common attachment with the tricuspid valve ring. The latter fully occupies the entire circumference of the right atrioventricular ring. The pulmonary valve is separated from the inflow tract by the infundibular chamber or tract. The infundibulum is separated from the main body of the right ventricle by the crista supraventricularis muscle (Fig. 6B).

These anatomical differences are important with regard to abnormalities or lesions, which may contribute to the turbulent flow and the production of ejection murmurs from the left and right sides of the heart.

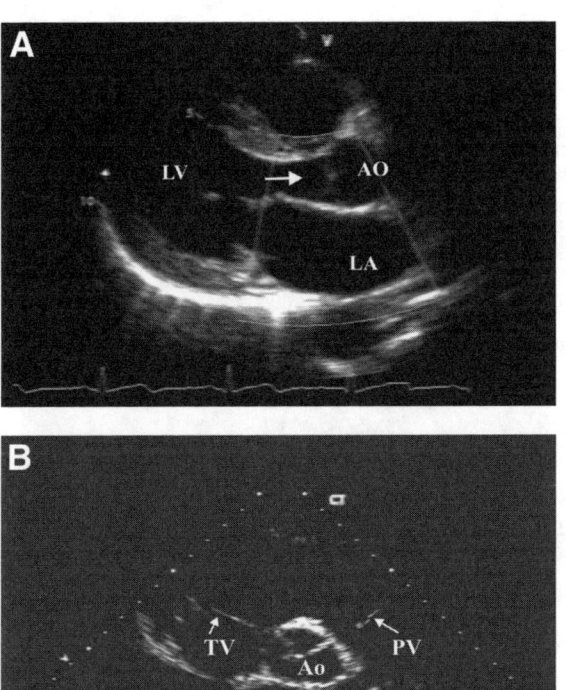

Fig. 6. Two-dimensional echocardiographic images in the parasternal view. (**A**) The long axis of the left ventricle (LV). The transducer on the anterior chest wall is shown at the top of the image. The LV outflow tract (arrow) is between the interventricular septum anteriorly and the anterior mitral leaflet posteriorly, which has a common attachment to the aortic root. (**B**) The short axis view at the aortic level. The pulmonary valve (PV) is separated from the tricuspid valve (TV) by the right ventricular outflow tract anterior to the aortic root.

Causes of Ejection Murmurs

RAPID CIRCULATORY STATES

Rapid circulatory states such as in young children, anemia, and thyrotoxicosis are often associated with systolic ejection murmurs, although the aortic and the pulmonary valves and the outflow tracts are often entirely normal. In these conditions the increased velocity of flow contributes to the increased turbulence. The murmur will often have peaks in early to mid-systole. Occasionally, the normal flow through a normal pulmonary outflow tract in children may be associated with some turbulence, which may be shown to be associated with an ejection murmur, which may be recordable in the pulmonary outflow tract with intracardiac phonocatheters. These pulmonary ejection murmurs may be more easily audible in some subjects than in others because of either thin body build or decreased antero-posterior diameter of the chest, which may help to bring the heart to a closer proximity of the chest wall. In some adults, with loss of the normal thoracic kyphosis and with a straight back, similarly closer proximity of the heart to the chest wall may contribute to the audible ejection murmurs, which are presumably pulmonary in origin because they are often of maximal loudness in the second left interspace *(12)*.

In some young children, the ejection murmur may be somewhat vibratory in quality like twanging a string. This is often because of pure or uniform frequencies in the medium range. It has been called *Still's murmur* after Still, who described it first *(13)*. The mechanism may actually involve some structures in the heart, such as congenital longitudinal intracardiac bands in the ventricle actually vibrating. The rapid circulatory state may be a contributory factor *(14,15)*.

EJECTION OF A LARGE STROKE VOLUME

Ejection of a large stroke volume as may be found in bradycardia, complete atrioventricular block, and secondary to conditions such as aortic regurgitation (where the blood flowing backward into the left ventricle from the aorta as well as the normal mitral inflow are received by the ventricle in diastole and ejected during systole) are all known to cause ejection systolic murmurs of left-sided origin. In atrial septal defect, the right ventricle receives an extra volume of blood because of the left-to-right shunt across the interatrial septum in addition to the usual systemic venous return. This increases the right ventricular stroke volume. Often the main pulmonary artery is also dilated because of the large volume of blood that it receives. Both of these factors contribute to the pulmonary ejection murmur in this condition *(16)*.

ABNORMALITIES OF THE OUTFLOW TRACT STRUCTURES OR THE SEMILUNAR VALVES WITHOUT STENOSIS

Aortic valve may be bicuspid congenitally. This may lead to ejection of an eccentric jet into the proximal aorta. Because the bicuspid valves are structurally inadequate for perfect competence of the valve, it may be accompanied by aortic regurgitation. The bicuspid aortic valve may also become calcific in the elderly. Even the normal aortic valve may also become thickened and sclerosed and occasionally even calcified in the elderly. But the cusp opening may be still good with very little stenosis, if any. The intima of the aortic root may also be abnormally thickened or roughened with atherosclerotic plaques. In addition, the aorta or the proximal aortic root may be dilated or aneurysmal, particularly in the presence of hypertensive and/or atherosclerotic disease. The orientation of the normal interventricular septum is usually along the axis of left ventricular cavity. This can sometimes be easily visualized on a two-dimensional echocardiographic image. Occasionally, the interventricular septum may be somewhat angulated, and the proximal portion of the septum may be hypertrophied focally. In some of these patients the septum may be *sigmoid* in shape *(17)*. The outflow tract is, therefore, oriented slightly off in axis to the direction of the longitudinal axis of the left ventricular cavity (Fig. 7A,B). This often would result in turbulence in flow, which can be seen on the color Doppler mapping of the aortic outflow in such patients. Under all these circumstances, aortic ejection murmurs are often common. In fact, for these various reasons, ejection murmur is fairly common above the age of 50 years (Fig. 8).

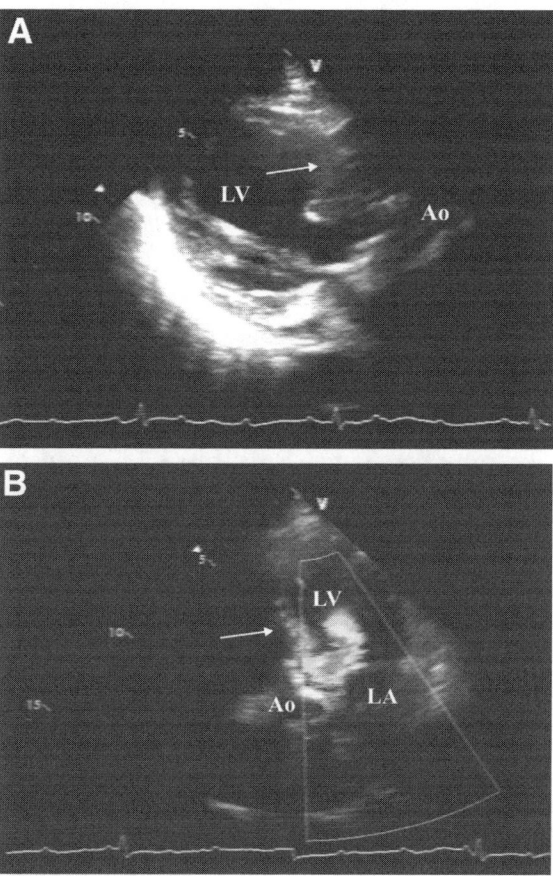

Fig. 7. (A) Two-dimensional echocardiographic image in the parasternal long axis showing the interventricular septum (arrow) to be sigmoid in shape. (B) (Color Plate 3, following p. 270) The color flow image shows turbulent flow across the left ventricular outflow in the apical four-chamber view.

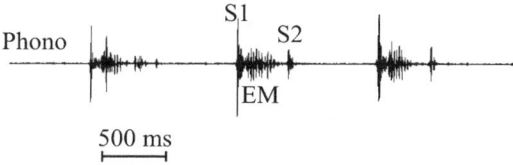

Fig. 8. Digital display of a magnetic audio recording from an elderly patient taken at the apex area showing a typical ejection systolic murmur beginning with the first heart sound (S1) and ending with a pause before the second heart sound (S2).

LEFT VENTRICULAR OUTFLOW TRACT OBSTRUCTION

Aortic Valve Stenosis

Isolated aortic valve stenosis is often congenital in origin, even in the elderly, because of calcification of an abnormal often bicuspid aortic valve. This may typically lead to symptoms in the sixth or the seventh decade in men. Bicuspid aortic valve may be

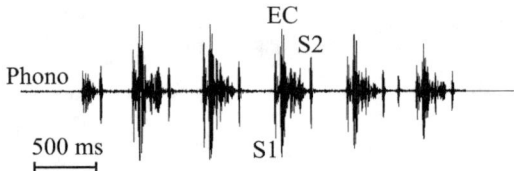

Fig. 9. Digital display of a magnetic audio recording from a patient with congenital aortic stenosis taken at the apex area showing a high frequency sharp ejection click (EC) closely following the first heart sound (S1) at the onset of the ejection murmur.

associated with stenosis or obstruction even in the younger age group. Aortic stenosis may result occasionally from rheumatic heart disease. In this instance it often is associated with aortic regurgitation and/or mitral valve disease *(18,19)*. Rarely, degenerative changes of the cusps occurring with old age may eventually lead to stenosis in the eighth decade.

The ejection murmur of aortic valve stenosis is no different in quality or even loudness from those in which there is no structural abnormality of the outflow tract. When the valve is still mobile, one may hear an aortic ejection click before the onset of the murmur (Fig. 9). The presence of the aortic ejection click may sometimes be surmised by the presence of a clicking S1 with the onset of the murmur.

The murmur may be audible all along the true aortic sash area extending from the second right interspace along the left sternal border to the left ventricular apex. The murmur may also be transmitted to the neck. However, the murmur is usually loudest at the second right interspace but may be equally loud at the apex. In some elderly patients, the murmur may be loudest only at the apex. If the stenosis is severe, the murmur will be often longer and will have a delayed peak. The murmur of aortic stenosis is occasionally quite high in frequency and even musical and cooing in quality at the apex, while it retains the harshness at the base. This may be partly because of the fact that the higher frequencies of the turbulence tend to be transmitted upstream more selectively (*Gallavardin phenomenon*) *(20)*.

In severe stenosis, the left ventricular pressure is very high and takes a long time to fall below that of the aorta (Fig.10). The A2 will be significantly delayed, and there will be a reversed sequence. The P2 will be buried in the end of the murmur, and the only component that may be audible will be A2. The latter, however, will be soft. If in the presence of a long and loud systolic murmur a soft S2, which is softer than the murmur, is heard, it would mean that the murmur has ended before the S2. This will be a clue to the fact that the murmur is in fact ejection in type (Fig. 11). Occasionally, one may also hear an S4 just before the onset of the murmur. This will reflect the severity as well, because S4 will only occur when the stenosis is severe enough to evoke significant left ventricular hypertrophy, thereby causing decreased ventricular compliance *(18,21,22)*.

Subvalvular Aortic Obstruction

Subvalvular aortic stenosis can be of two types: fixed (membranous) and dynamic (hypertrophic).

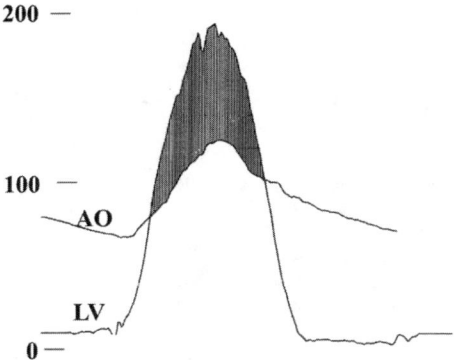

Fig. 10. Recording of simultaneous left ventricular (LV) and aortic (AO) pressure curves from a patient with severe aortic stenosis. It can be seen that the significantly high peak LV systolic pressure will necessarily take a long time to fall below that of the aorta, thereby delaying the occurrence of the A2.

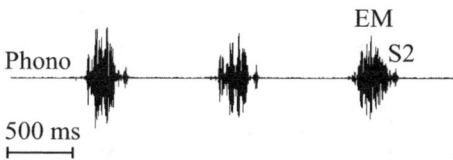

Fig. 11. Digital display of a magnetic audio recording from a patient with severe aortic stenosis taken from the apex area showing a large-amplitude (loud) systolic murmur followed by a distinct but significantly lower amplitude (soft) S2. Because the S2 is still clearly audible, it must mean that the murmur ends before S2 and therefore must be an ejection murmur.

Membranous. The subvalvular aortic outflow may be the seat of obstruction congenitally because of a membrane stretching from the anterior mitral leaflet to the interventricular septum. Rarely, there could be abnormal attachments of parts of the anterior mitral leaflet or its chordae, leading to narrowing of the outflow tract *(19)*. The membrane is usually made of a thick fibrous structure with a stenosed or narrow orifice. Often the aortic outflow jet from the subvalvular obstruction will over time cause structural damage to the aortic cusps, resulting in some degree of aortic regurgitation. The abnormal tissue from the anterior mitral leaflet rarely can encroach into the mitral orifice, leading to some interference with mitral inflow in diastole.

Hypertrophic. The second cause of subaortic obstruction is usually associated with *hypertrophic cardiomyopathy*. In this condition, there is often severe hypertrophy of the left ventricle, particularly involving the interventricular septum. The cavity is small, and the ventricle contracts powerfully and ejects blood very rapidly. The obstruction is dynamic *(23)* and is because of the sudden anterior movement of the anterior mitral leaflet from its closed posterior position. This systolic anterior motion (SAM) of the mitral leaflet causes abnormal apposition of the anterior mitral leaflet with the hypertrophic and bulging interventricular septum in the middle of systole causing the outflow obstruction. The reason for this sudden anterior movement of the anterior mitral leaflet

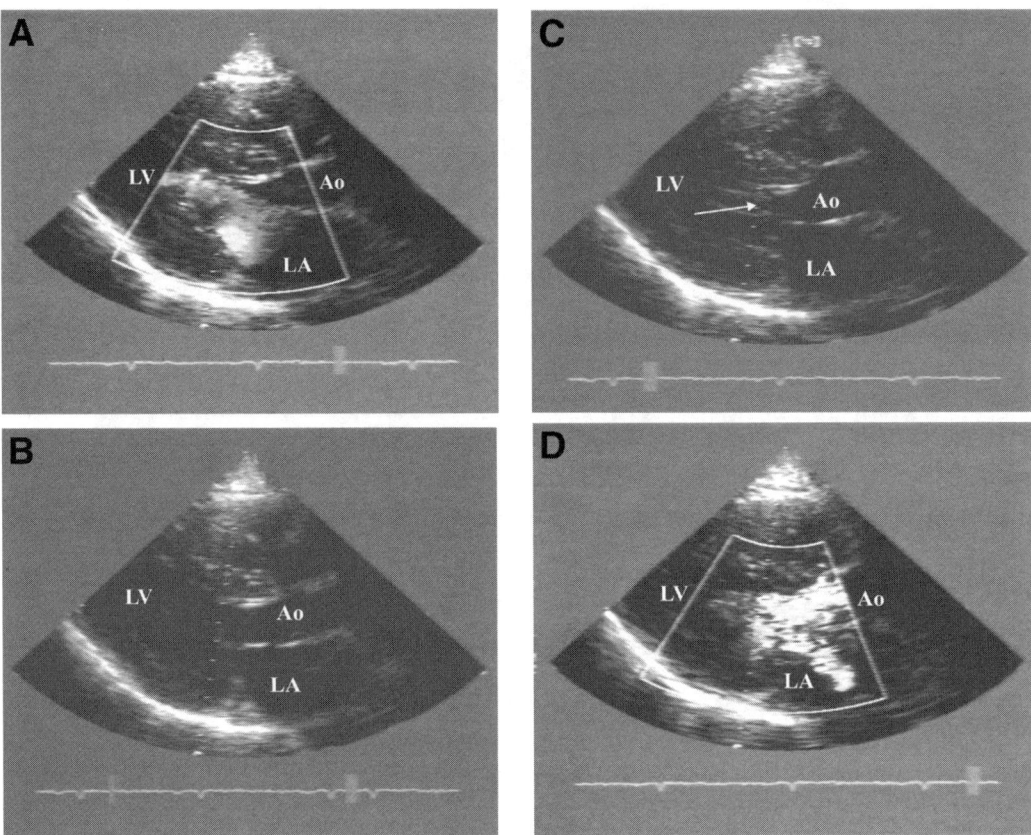

Fig. 12. Two-dimensional echocardiographic images in the parasternal view from a patient with hypertrophic obstructive cardiomyopathy with severe subaortic obstruction. **(A)** The diastolic frame shows the open mitral valve allowing the inflow from the left atrium (LA) into the left ventricle (LV). The interventricular septum in continuity with the anterior wall of the aorta (AO) as well as the posterior left ventricular free wall are markedly hypertrophied. **(B)** Stop frame at the onset of systole showing the mitral valve in the closed position. **(C)** The left ventricle contracts powerfully and causes rapid ejection. This rapid ejection out of the left ventricle causes a suction-like effect on the anterior leaflet, leading to it being pulled forward and anteriorly (arrow). This systolic anterior motion of the anterior mitral leaflet and the resulting contact with the interventricular septum causes obstruction to the left ventricular outflow in midsystole. This leads to turbulent outflow as well as some mitral regurgitation seen in the Doppler color flow **(D)**. (*See* Color Plate 4, following p. 270.)

is the rapid and powerful ejection that is characteristic of this disorder. This leads to the development of a negative pressure or suction like effect (Venturi effect) on the mitral leaflet as the blood is being ejected very rapidly out of the left ventricle (Fig. 12A–D) *(23–30)*. The latter mechanism has been questioned by some. and the SAM has been attributed to pushing or pulling of the mitral valve by the anatomical distortion aggravated by vigorous contraction in these patients with marked hypertrophy of the left ventricular walls associated with small cavity *(28)*.

If the septal hypertrophy is severe, the obstruction may be present at rest. Occasionally the obstruction may not be evident at rest and may only be brought out under certain conditions. These include interventions or maneuvers that decrease the ventricular size,

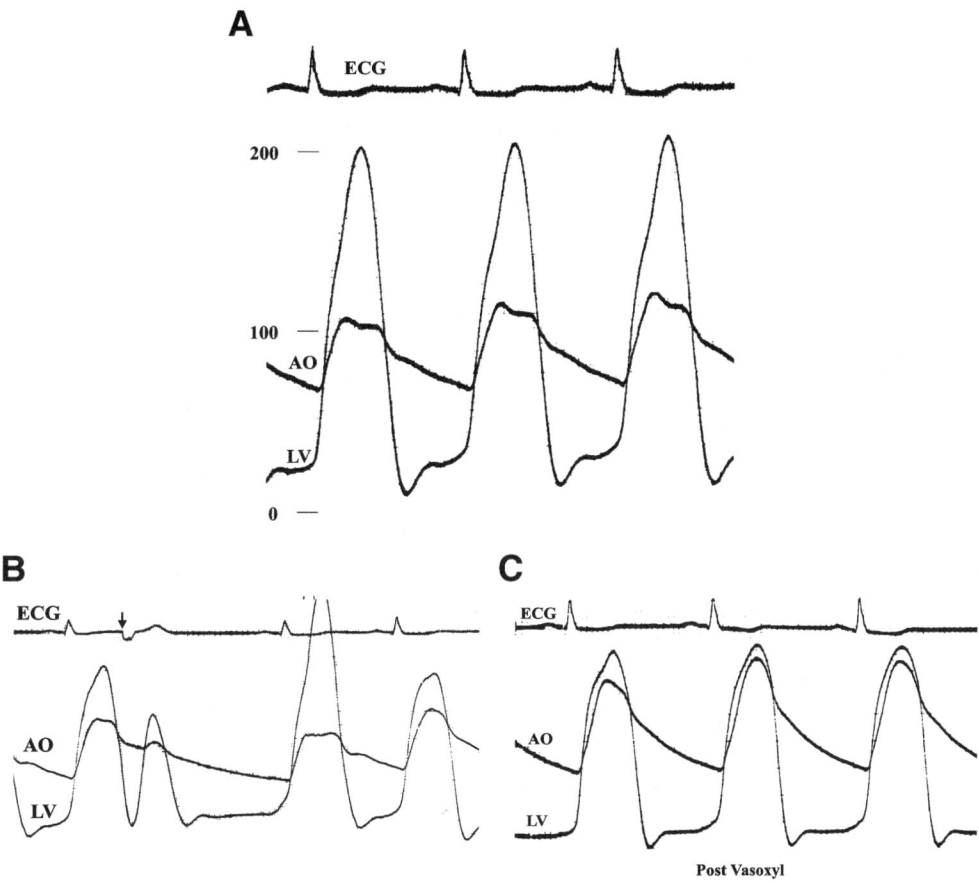

Fig. 13. Simultaneous recordings of the electrocardiogram (ECG) and the left ventricular (LV) and aortic (AO) pressure curves obtained at cardiac catheterization from a patient with hypertrophic obstructive cardiomyopathy. **(A)** The measurements at rest, indicating the presence of a systolic pressure gradient across the left ventricular outflow tract. The rise of the aortic pressure curve is relatively rapid, distinguishing this from the valvular form of aortic stenosis. **(B)** Recordings made during mechanically induced premature ventricular contractions. The systolic pressure gradient between the LV and the AO at rest is accentuated in the beat following the premature ventricular contraction (arrow). This is because of the effect of the postextrasystolic potentiation of the ventricular contractility. **(C)** The abolition of the resting systolic pressure gradient after the administration of a peripheral arterial vasoconstricting agent, vasoxyl.

thus increasing the septal–mitral contact. This can be achieved by assumption of a standing position, which will decrease the venous return. The smaller ventricular size aids in the septal–mitral apposition or contact during systole. Obstruction can also be augmented by inotropic stimuli (including pharmacological agents such as isoproterenol or digoxin), which increase the contractile force. The increased inotropic effect caused by exercise can also augment the obstruction. When there is inotropic stimulation, the increased contractile force favors the development of the Venturi effect on the mitral leaflet more readily (Fig. 13A,B). Finally, the obstruction can also be made worse by lowering the peripheral resistance, as caused by peripheral arterial dilatation.

This includes pharmacological agents that lower the blood pressure by dilating the peripheral vessels. The pressure distending the aortic root acts on the mitral leaflet, opposing the Venturi effect of the rapidly moving outflow. When the aortic pressure is lowered by peripheral arterial dilatation, the mitral–septal contact becomes more pronounced. The pressure gradient across the left ventricular outflow tract will thus be increased by amyl nitrite inhalation, which causes peripheral arterial dilatation. Raising the blood pressure by peripheral vasoconstriction will do the opposite and help to prevent the systolic anterior motion of the anterior mitral leaflet (Fig. 13C) *(18,23,31)*.

When the subaortic obstruction develops in mid-systole because of the systolic anterior motion of the anterior mitral leaflet, the mitral valve does become incompetent *(29)*. The outflow obstruction at this point favors mitral regurgitation as well. The degree of mitral regurgitation is variable. Generally it is mild and does not contribute much to the characteristics of the murmur.

The murmur of hypertrophic subaortic stenosis shares all the features of the ejection murmur described previously (p. 218). The murmur is generally maximally loud at the apex. The murmur also tends to be somewhat longer, but nevertheless ends before A2. The murmur intensity or loudness is variable, and this usually depends to a large extent on the degree and severity of the obstruction. The murmur may be absent at rest and may be only brought out by maneuvers that produce one or more of the following: decrease in ventricular size, increase in contractility, or decrease in the peripheral resistance. The simplest maneuver that will bring on the murmur or accentuate the loudness of the murmur is making the patient stand suddenly from a supine position. This will decrease the venous return, thereby decreasing the left ventricular volume. Standing also causes a slight fall in arterial pressure, causing sympathetic stimulation and increase in heart rate. The subaortic obstruction will get worse, and this will accentuate the murmur intensity. An opposite maneuver is to make the patient squat. During squatting, the venous return increases from the periphery because of increased abdominal pressure and compression of the veins in the lower extremities. This will help to increase the ventricular size. In addition, the arteries in the lower extremities are compressed, increasing the arterial resistance and the blood pressure. This will also cause a decrease in heart rate. The combined effects of these changes will reduce the intensity of the ejection murmur (Fig. 14A). Similarly, other maneuvers can also be used to change the hemodynamic status to either augment or decrease the obstruction *(18,23,31,32)*. During the strain phase of the Valsalva maneuver, the decreased venous return and increase in heart rate will accentuate the murmur *(33)*. The Müller maneuver will produce the opposite effect. Inhalation of amyl nitrite will increase the murmur intensity because the powerful arterial dilatation it causes will drop the aortic pressure and increase the degree of obstruction. The tachycardia and the sympathetic stimulation, which accompany the drop in blood pressure, will also help augment the obstruction.

When the obstruction is severe at rest, the A2 will be significantly delayed, resulting in a reversed sequence of S2. The P2 may be buried in the end of the murmur, and the only component audible will then be a delayed A2. Occasionally the reversed sequence with a paradoxical split on expiration may also be audible. The decreased left ventricular compliance because of abnormal hypertrophy will often evoke an S4, which may be heard and will precede the onset of the ejection murmur *(18)* (Fig. 14B).

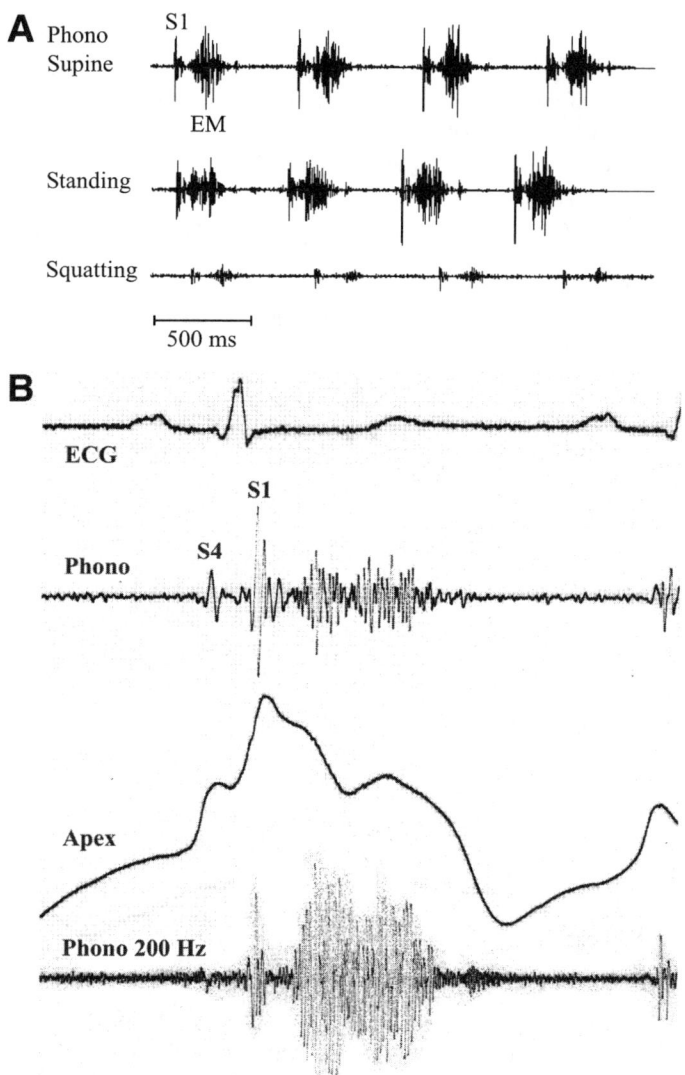

Fig. 14. **(A)** Digital display of a magnetic audio recording from a patient with hypertrophic subaortic stenosis taken from the apex area demonstrating the effects of the changing postures on the intensity of the ejection murmur. The murmur is slightly accentuated on standing and significantly diminished in intensity on squatting compared to the supine position. **(B)** Simultaneous recordings of electrocardiogram (ECG), phonocardiogram (Phono), and apexcardiogram (Apex) from a patient with hypertrophic cardiomyopathy with obstruction taken from the apex area demonstrating the typical long ejection murmur. There is an S4 with a corresponding atrial kick on the apexcardiogram.

Proximal Septal Hypertrophy With Angulated Septum Causing Mild Outflow Obstruction

Occasionally in patients with an angulated septum or when the septum is somewhat sigmoid in shape, the most proximal portion of the septum may be hypertrophied because of co-existing hypertension or co-existing mild to moderate aortic valvular stenosis.

This may actually cause some mild degrees of outflow obstruction in the subaortic region and generate pressure gradients, which on Doppler flow mapping may be late peaked as in hypertrophic cardiomyopathy *(17)*. The two-dimensional images, however, will be marked by the absence of any systolic anterior motion of the anterior mitral leaflet *(34)*. The murmur will be typically ejection and behave more like the murmur of aortic valvular stenosis. The features of classic hypertrophic obstructive cardiomyopathy mentioned above will be absent because the underlying pathology is totally different.

Supravalvular Stenosis

Supravalvular aortic stenosis is often congenital and affects the aorta above the sinuses of Valsalva. The obstruction may be caused by focal stenosis by a membrane or because of diffuse hypoplasia of the ascending aorta. Occasionally the supravalvular aortic stenosis is associated with hypercalcemia, mental retardation, and typical facial features, as well as abnormal dentition. Rarely, stenosis of the pulmonary arteries may coexist. The poststenotic segment of the aorta is not usually dilated.

In supravalvular stenosis, the murmur is often maximal at the suprasternal notch. The high velocity jet from the supravalvular stenosis tends to be preferentially directed to the right innominate artery, making the murmur more prominent over the right side. In many of these patients, the right carotid and the right arm vessels are more prominent than the left. Often the arterial pressure in the right arm is higher than in the left *(35–38)*. The preferential direction of the high velocity jet toward the right innominate artery has been attributed to a *Coanda effect (39)*.

RIGHT VENTRICULAR OUTFLOW TRACT OBSTRUCTION

Pulmonary Valvular Stenosis

Pulmonary valvular stenosis is often congenital, the cusps are often fused and shaped like a fish mouth, and the valve may become domed during ejection. There is often some poststenotic dilatation of the main pulmonary artery as well as the left pulmonary artery. Rarely, the cusps may be thickened and fused and show abnormal myxomatous degeneration. Because of low pressures on the right side, pulmonary valve stenosis never becomes progressively worse or calcified, even with increasing age. The pulmonary stenosis can be associated with other congenital defects, in particular a ventricular septal defect (VSD).

When the ventricular septum is intact, the ejection murmur of pulmonary stenosis is no different in quality or loudness from other ejection murmurs. The murmur is generally audible over the second and third left interspace close to the sternal border, and when louder it may be heard over the lower sternal border region as well. The location of maximal loudness, however, is usually the second left interspace. The murmur may be equally loud in the third left interspace, particularly if there has been secondary infundibular hypertrophy (Fig. 15A,B). The murmur also tends to become louder on inspiration, although this may be difficult to appreciate. Often one can hear the characteristic pulmonary ejection click at onset of the murmur. The pulmonary ejection click typically becomes softer on inspiration and louder on expiration. Occasionally the click may actually be the predominant feature and may be heard as a clicking S1.

When pulmonary stenosis is mild or moderate in severity, the murmur will be noted to be followed by a widely split S2. When the pulmonary stenosis is significant or severe, the murmur becomes quite long and has a late peak and may then go past the A2, which may be buried in the end of the murmur. The soft S2 heard after the long murmur will be the delayed P2 *(40)*.

Chapter 7 / Heart Murmurs: *Part I*

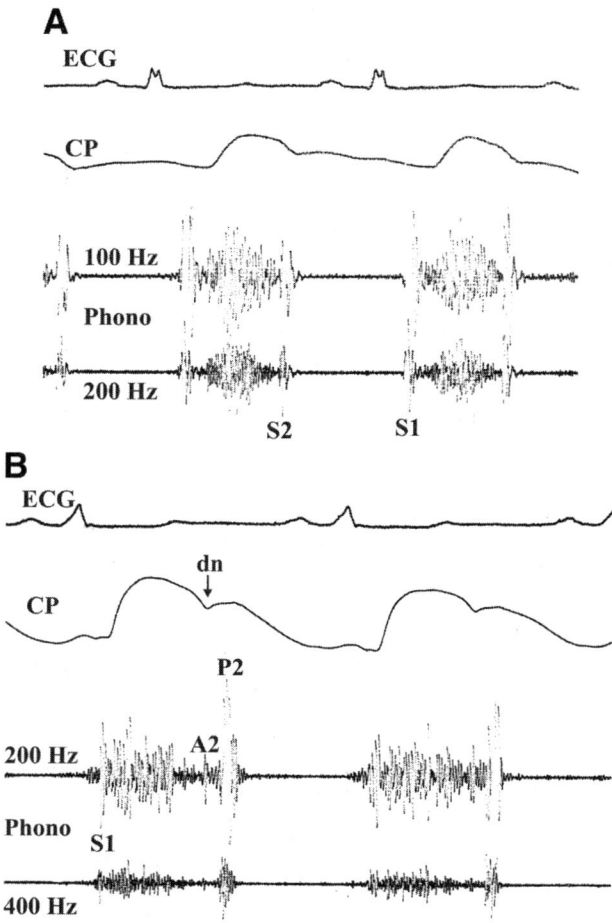

Fig. 15. **(A)** Simultaneous recordings of electrocardiogram (ECG), carotid pulse (CP), and phonocardiogram (Phono) from a patient with pulmonary stenosis taken from the second left interspace close to the sternal border, showing the ejection systolic murmur. The murmur appears to go all the way to the S2, which is essentially the aortic component (A2), but it ends before the pulmonary component (P2). The P2, being soft and not easily audible, is not seen on the Phono tracing. **(B)** Simultaneous recordings of ECG, CP, and Phono from a patient with atrial septal defect secundum taken at the second and third left interspace. A split S2 follows the ejection murmur. The A2, which usually occurs at the time of the incisura of the aortic pressure curve, is seen to occur slightly before the dicrotic notch (dn) because of the transmission delay of the CP. The P2 has greater intensity and is well separated from the A2.

When the ventricular septum is intact, severe pulmonary stenosis will evoke a strong right atrial contraction. The decreased compliance caused by the hypertrophied right ventricle is the cause of this strong atrial contraction, which may produce a right-sided S4, which is usually accentuated with inspiration. The effect of this may be visible in the jugular of *a wave* as well, which may become prominent (Fig. 16). These signs will tend to be absent in the presence of a ventricular septal defect despite severe pulmonary stenosis *(40,41)*.

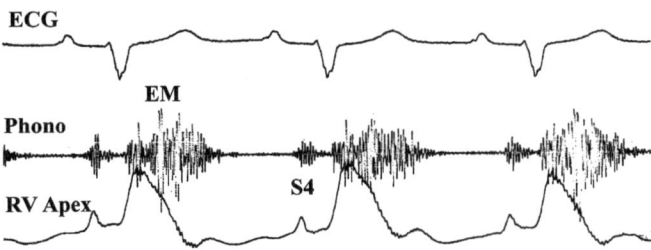

Fig. 16. Simultaneous recordings of electrocardiogram (ECG), phonocardiogram (Phono), and the right ventricular impulse (RV apex) from a patient with severe pulmonary stenosis with intact interventricular septum taken at the third left interspace at the left sternal border. The prominent fourth heart sound (S4) on the Phono corresponds to the A wave of the RV apex recording, indicating it is probably right-sided in origin. The ejection systolic murmur (EM) is quite long in duration.

Pulmonary stenosis in the presence of a ventricular septal defect is the important component of the tetralogy of Fallot.

Subvalvular Pulmonary Stenosis

The subvalvular area on the pulmonary side is the infundibulum. This may be the seat of a congenital localized narrowing at the entrance of the outflow tract, beyond which the infundibulum may be dilated. Occasionally the stenosis may result from the hypertrophied crista supraventricularis muscle. In rare instances the stenosis can be subinfundibular. Subvalvular stenosis is often associated with a ventricular septal defect *(40)*. The maximal loudness of the murmur in infundibular stenosis is often found at the third left interspace, although occasionally it can be the fourth left interspace. Pulmonary ejection click will be absent in infundibular stenosis. The lesion may be associated with a ventricular septal defect, as seen in Fallot's tetralogy.

Supravalvular Pulmonary Stenosis

The site of stenosis is either in the pulmonary trunk, its bifurcation, or the branches. Rarely, a supravalvular membrane may be the site of stenosis. The murmur is often systolic ejection in type. The obstruction is usually associated with a systolic gradient across the stenotic segment and will be expected to cause a rise in the systolic pressure in the proximal segment. The murmurs may be at the base but may also be heard peripherally over the chest. Rarely, there may be a gradient even in diastole, and this may be associated with some turbulent flow persisting into diastole. This will be accompanied by a longer duration of the systolic murmur, which may spill into diastole, making the murmur continuous *(40)*. Neither the intensity nor the timing of the pulmonary component of S2 is affected in supravalvular pulmonary artery stenosis. The S2 split is often entirely normal.

(For additional examples review Phono Files 1–13 and Echo Phono File 6 under Heart Murmurs Part 1 on the Companion CD.)

REGURGITANT SYSTOLIC MURMURS

Regurgitation usually implies blood flow in the reverse direction across the cardiac chambers, usually from a high-pressure chamber into a low-pressure chamber.

Regurgitation during systole can occur under the following conditions:
1. When the mitral valve is incompetent, reverse flow can occur from the high-pressure left ventricle into the low-pressure left atrium.
2. When the tricuspid valve is incompetent, reverse flow can occur from the high-pressure right ventricle into the low-pressure right atrium.
3. In ventricular septal defect, the reverse flow can occur from the high-pressure left ventricle into the low-pressure right ventricle across the septal defect.
4. In persistent ductus arteriosus, the reverse flow can occur form the high-pressure aorta into the low-pressure pulmonary artery through the ductus. In this condition, however, the reverse flow in systole can also continue into the diastole as long as the pulmonary resistance is lower than the systemic resistance

Characteristics of Regurgitant Systolic Murmurs

1. The high-pressure gradient that is usually present in most regurgitant lesions mentioned above will imply that regurgitant systolic murmurs will have predominantly high frequency, and this will make the murmurs sound more blowing in quality *(42)*. They can be imitated by long whispering "hoo," "haaa," or saying a long "shoo."
2. The regurgitant murmur could acquire lower and medium frequencies and sound harsher if the degree of regurgitation is severe, resulting in a large amount of backward flow.
3. Since the pressure gradient often persists between the chambers well into the isovolumic relaxation phase and beyond, the murmur often will not end before the S2 and will often spill over into the very early part of diastole. Thus, there is generally no pause between the end of the murmur and the S2. The audibility of S2 with a regurgitant murmur, however, is mainly related to the relative loudness of the murmur and the S2. The S2 may be audible if the grade of the murmur is softer than the grade of the S2. If the murmur is louder than the S2, then the murmur lasting all the way to the S2 will engulf the S2. This will result in S2 not being heard separately.
4. Regurgitant murmurs, unlike ejection murmurs, usually do not change in intensity significantly following sudden long diastole, as may happen following the compensatory pause after a premature or ectopic beat or during varying cycle lengths in atrial fibrillation *(43)*. The mechanisms involved in postextrasystolic potentiation were discussed under ejection murmurs. Regurgitant lesions imply that there are two outlets for the blood to flow during systole. For instance, in the case of mitral regurgitation, one outlet is the aorta and the other is through the regurgitant or incompetent mitral valve into the left atrium. The extra volume of blood received by the ventricle during the long diastolic interval by the Starling mechanism will increase the contractility of the ventricle. This will be further aided by the extrasystolic potentiation from the premature depolarization. During the long diastolic pause the aortic pressure will continue to fall, and this will result in decrease in afterload when the ventricle will begin to eject. The more complete emptying of the ventricle will result in a larger amount of forward flow into the aorta because of the fall in afterload accompanying the falling aortic pressure during the pause. This usually means that the volume of blood going in the reverse direction would remain relatively the same, keeping the regurgitant flow and the resulting murmur the same.

MITRAL REGURGITATION

Normal Mitral Valve and Function

The mitral valve apparatus is a complex unit consisting of the annulus, the anterior and the posterior mitral leaflets, the chordae tendineae, the papillary muscles, and the under-

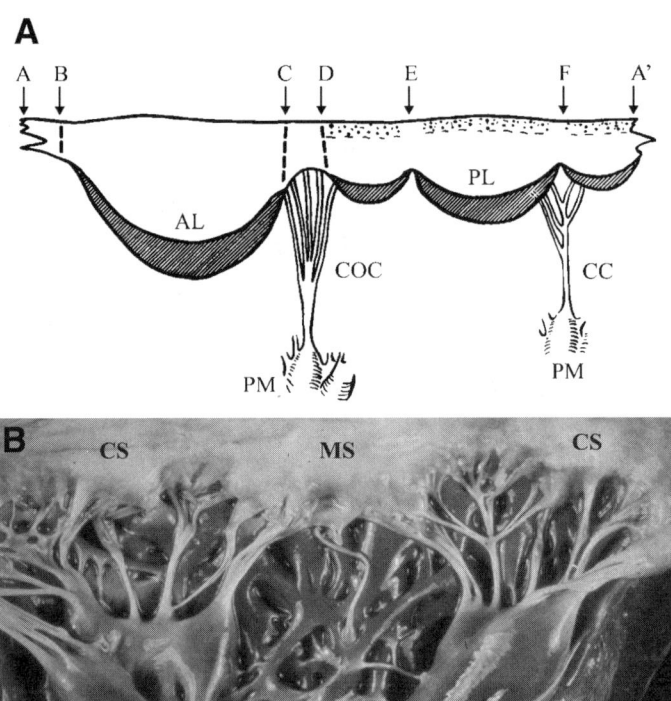

Fig. 17. **(A)** Diagrammatic representation of the mitral valve cut open to show the atrial surface of the anterior leaflet (AL) on the right and the posterior leaflet (PL) on the left side. The commissural chordae (COC), which are fan-shaped charade, insert and define the commissural areas between the AL and the PL. C–D is the posteromedial commissural area, whereas A–B is the anterolateral commissural area. The distal third of the leaflets is thick and rough and receives insertion of chordae on the ventricular surfaces. The proximal two-thirds of the leaflet are clear and membranous. The PL is usually a tri-scalloped structure. Fan-shaped chords called the cleft chordae (CC) insert and define the clefts between the individual scallops of the PL. (Modified and reproduced from ref. *44*, with kind permission from Lippincott Williams and Wilkins.) **(B)** The mitral valve cut open to show the atrial surface of the normal triscalloped posterior leaflet. The middle scallop (MS) is usually the largest, with the two respective commissural scallops (CS) on either side of it. The fan-shaped chordae insert into the clefts between the individual scallops. *(Continued on next page)*

lying left ventricular wall *(44–47)*. The annulus shares a common attachment to the aortic root anteriorly. The posterior annulus is a large fibromuscular structure. The commissural areas can be easily defined by the recognition of the fan-shaped chordae— *the commissural chordae*. These arise as single stems and branch like the struts of a fan to insert into the free margins of the leaflet tissue at the commissures (Fig. 17A). Although both commissural areas have an equal amount of valvular tissue, the posteromedial commissural chordae have a wider spread, making this region more vulnerable for mitral regurgitation. The posterior leaflet, which covers a larger annular circumference, is usually divided into three scallops, the middle one being the largest, with two smaller scallops on either side near the commissures. Fan-shaped chords also insert into the clefts in between the scallops of the posterior leaflet (Fig. 17B). The anterior leaflet

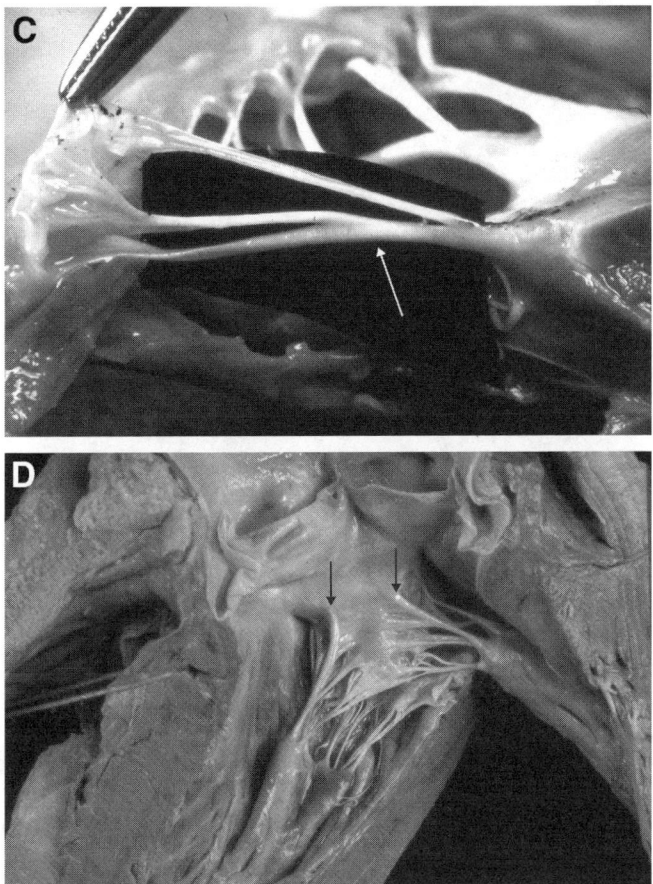

Fig. 17. *(Continued)* **(C)** A typical rough zone chordae with its three branches (arrow), one inserting into the free margin of the leaflet, one inserting into the proximal edge of the rough zone, and the third in between the two on the ventricular aspect of the mitral leaflet. **(D)** The anterior mitral leaflet and its attachment to the aortic root. The arrows indicate the two strut chordae arising from the tips of the papillary muscles and inserting on the rough zone of the ventricular surface of the anterior mitral leaflet. *(Continued on next page)*

is generally larger than the middle scallop of the posterior leaflet. The distal third of the leaflet surface is rough to palpation and receives the insertion of chordae on the ventricular aspect. The rough zones of both the anterior and the posterior leaflets receive insertion of chordae. Typically each rough zone chord divides into three branches: one inserts into the free margin, one branch inserts beyond the free margin at the line of closure (the proximal edge of the rough zone), and one branch inserts in between the two (Fig. 17C). Two of the rough zone chordae to the anterior leaflet are by far the thickest, and these arise from the tips of the papillary muscles and insert between the four and five o'clock positions on the posteromedial side and between the seven and eight o'clock positions on the anterolateral side. These are the *strut chordae* (Fig. 17D). *Avulsion* or rupture of these would result in severe mitral regurgitation.

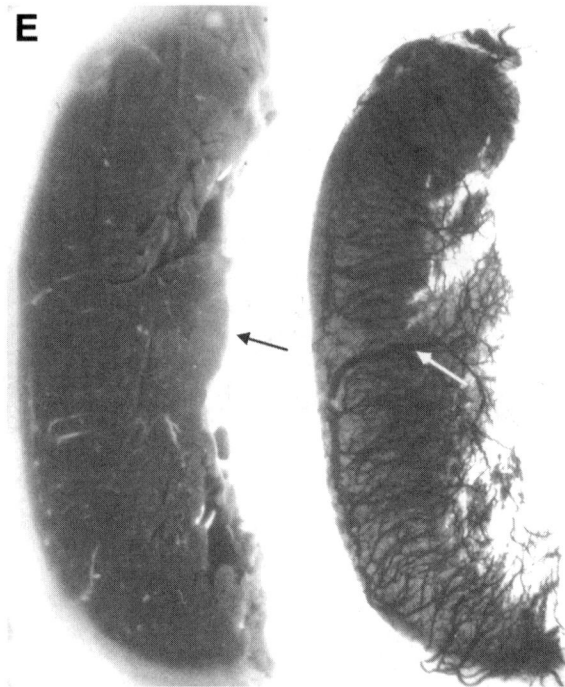

Fig. 17. *(Continued)* **(E)** The excised left ventricular wall obtained at necropsy demonstrating a free finger-like morphology of the papillary muscle (first picture) and its arterial supply (second picture) demonstrated by contrast injection into the coronary vessels with stereo-radiography prior to the section. The finger-like papillary muscle has arterial supply through a central artery with very few vascular connections to the extrapapillary subendocardial network.

The chordae passing to the anterolateral commissure and the adjoining half of the anterior and the posterior leaflets arise from the anterolateral papillary muscle group. The chordae passing to the posteromedial commissure and the adjoining half of the anterior and the posterior leaflets arise from the posteromedial papillary muscle group. In all there are 25 chordae, which insert into the mitral valve: 9 into the anterior leaflet, 14 into the posterior leaflet, and 2 to the commissures *(47)*.

There are two groups of papillary muscles in the left ventricle: the anterolateral and the posteromedial. Each group supplies one-half of the chordae to half of both leaflets. Each group of papillary muscle may have one or two distinct "bellies" of muscle—occasionally more than two, especially in the posteromedial group. The left ventricular papillary muscle groups may have varying morphological features. They may be free and finger-like, very much tethered to the underlying subendocardium of the ventricular wall, or have an intermediate morphology. The arterial supply for the anterolateral papillary muscle arises from the anterior descending, one of the diagonal branches or the marginal branches of the circumflex. The posteromedial group derives its blood supply from the right coronary or the circumflex branch of the left coronary artery. The arterial vasculature of the papillary muscles is often related to the morphological feature. The finger-like papillary muscle has a central artery, which arises at its base from one of the

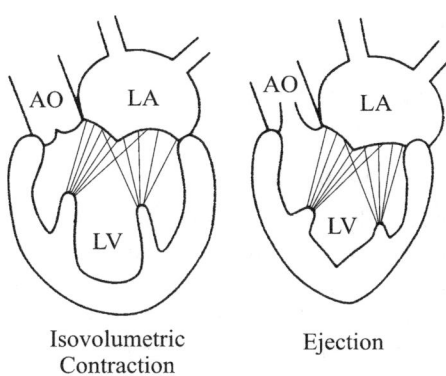

Fig. 18. Diagrammatic representation of the normal spatial relationship between the mitral valve and the left ventricular cavity. This relationship, seen at the onset of systole at the isovolumic phase, is maintained during the remainder of systole during the ejection phase despite the rising intraventricular pressure and decreasing size of the left ventricular cavity, by the contracting papillary muscles and the underlying left ventricular wall, which prevent eversion of the mitral leaflets into the left atrium, keeping the mitral valve competent.

epicardial arteries. This vessel is often terminal and has very few vascular connections to the extrapapillary subendocardial network (Fig. 17E). The tethered type of papillary muscle often has a segmental type of distribution of the long penetrating intramyocardial vessels. The mixed or intermediate type has a mixed-type arterial vasculature *(46)*. The arterial vasculature has a bearing on the incidence of papillary muscle dysfunction in ischemic heart disease.

When the left ventricle contracts and raises the pressure during systole above that of the left atrium, the mitral valve leaflets come together and close the orifice. After the valve closure the continued rise in pressure from the ventricular contraction will open the aortic valve once the pressure exceeds the aortic pressure. With onset of ejection, the ventricle will begin to decrease in volume and size. During most of ejection the ventricular pressure remains fairly high. The chordae tendineae have fixed lengths, and they cannot shorten to keep the leaflets together. The closed mitral valve leaflets would evert and prolapse into the left atrium under the high pressure but for the synchronous and effective contraction of the papillary muscles and the underlying left ventricular myocardium. The muscular fibers in the annulus do contract to help reduce the annular width toward the end of systole as well, thereby maintaining a competent valve (Fig. 18).

Causes of Mitral Regurgitation

Mitral regurgitation, therefore, can arise from anatomical and/or functional defect from any one of the components of its complex anatomy *(48)*. The lesion may result from a congenital or an acquired cause. The process may be genetic, inflammatory, infective, traumatic, ischemic, degenerative, or neoplastic in nature. As often is the case, more than one component of the structures may be involved. Rarely, mitral regurgitation may also be induced iatrogenically during surgical commissurotomy or balloon techniques of mitral valvuloplasty for relief of mitral stenosis.

ANNULAR ABNORMALITIES

The annulus may become idiopathically dilated or calcified and therefore may not function normally. Dilated annulus, making the orifice larger, allows poor apposition of the leaflets. This is compounded by the fact that it also contracts poorly. Calcification, on the other hand, interferes with the normal annular contraction.

LEAFLET AND CHORDAL ABNORMALITIES

The leaflet may be congenitally cleft, and this abnormality may be seen in association with *ostium primum atrial septal defect (40)*. The leaflets may also be congenitally large and redundant and may show overhanging hooded or prolapsed appearance because of myxomatous degeneration *(49,50)*. The chordae may also be excessively lengthened as well as showing some thickening. The chordae could rupture spontaneously if the elastic fibers are significantly destroyed because of myxomatoaus degeneration. The leaflets, on the other hand, may be contracted and scarred because of repeated inflammation, as may happen with rheumatic involvement. They may eventually show areas of calcification. The chordae that are scarred and shortened will prevent proper leaflet closure. In addition, the commissures may be fused, resulting in varying degrees of stenosis. In infective endocarditis, the infective process could cause destructive lesions in the leaflets or the chordae besides formation of vegetation. The latter may interfere with proper leaflet apposition, particularly when large. The chordae could rupture as a result of the infective process *(51)*. In congenitally corrected transposition of the great vessels, which is a rare congenital defect, the left atrioventricular valve, which has a morphology similar to that of the tricuspid valve of the normal heart, may show downward displacement, as in Ebstein's anomaly. With this malformation, part of the arterial ventricle becomes atrialized and thin and the valve is often incompetent, resulting in "mitral regurgitation" *(52)*.

PAPILLARY MUSCLE AND LEFT VENTRICULAR WALL PATHOLOGY

In ischemic heart disease, the papillary muscles may not contract properly because of ischemia with or without concurrent necrosis, which may also involve the underlying myocardium *(53–56)*. The papillary muscles may show scarring because of ischemic damage. When ischemic necrosis occurs involving the papillary muscles, it may sometimes lead to avulsion of the chordal origin from the necrotic muscle *(57,58)*. The papillary muscle could also rupture because of its involvement in the acute infarction *(59)*. In late stages of infarction with development of aneurysm of the underlying myocardium, the papillary muscles may be displaced and the distortion may make the valve incompetent *(55)*. A similar disturbance in function could occur in other myocardial diseases, such as dilated cardiomyopathy.

ATRIAL MYXOMA

Rarely, a left atrial myxoma, which is usually considered a benign tumor, attached to the atrial septum by a stalk could be large enough to prolapse into the left ventricle during diastole. With the onset of systole the tumor may move back into the left atrium but in the process may obstruct proper leaflet apposition and cause mitral regurgitation *(60)*.

The severity of the mitral regurgitation may depend on the extent of the lesions and the functional derangement as well as the acuteness of the process. Long-standing mitral regurgitation would result in left atrial and left ventricular dilatation, which will cause further stretching of the annulus, making the mitral regurgitation worse. Thus, "*mitral regurgitation begets more mitral regurgitation.*"

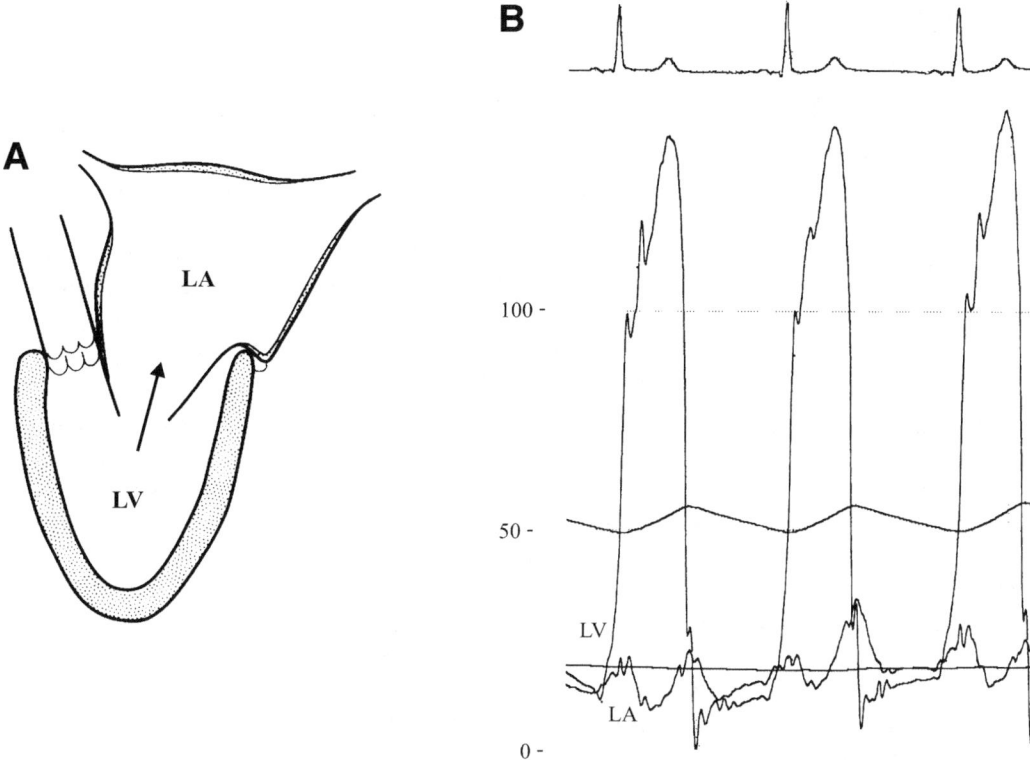

Fig. 19. **(A)** Diagrammatic representation of the left atrium (LA) and the left ventricle (LV) in chronic severe mitral regurgitation. The volume overload leads to enlargement and dilatation of the LV and the LA. The LV, however, has a systolic advantage because it has two outlets. **(B)** Simultaneous recordings of the electrocardiogram (ECG) and the left ventricular (LV) and left atrial (LA) pressure curves from a patient with chronic severe mitral regurgitation showing only a mild elevation of the left atrial *v wave*. The pressure difference between the LV and the LA is seen to persist throughout systole.

Pathophysiology of Mitral Regurgitation

CHRONIC MITRAL REGURGITATION

Mitral regurgitation is a volume-overload state for the left ventricle because during diastole the ventricle receives not only the normal pulmonary venous return but also the extra volume of blood that went into the left atrium during systole. This volume overload, when significant, would result in left ventricular dilatation and enlargement. The left ventricular dilatation is accompanied initially by a better compliance of the left ventricle, which helps to maintain relatively normal left ventricular diastolic pressures (*pre-a wave*) despite the large volume of blood, which enters the left ventricle during diastole. The left atrium will also become enlarged when the regurgitation is significant and chronic in duration. The left atrial enlargement is accompanied by increased compliance of the left atrium, which helps to maintain a low *v wave* pressure in the left atrium during systole despite the increased volume it receives because of the regurgitation (Fig. 19A,B).

In addition, the left ventricle has an advantage during systole because it has two outlets for emptying, namely, the aorta as well as the left atrium. The two outlet system allows supernormal emptying (ejection fraction) when the ventricular function is normal and preserved and a near-normal ejection fraction when the left ventricle actually develops some dysfunction *(61–63)*.

In late stages, however, the increased size of the left ventricle will lead to increased wall tension, stimulating hypertrophy. The hypertrophy is often *eccentric* rather than *concentric (64)*. This will reduce the left ventricular compliance. In addition, subendocardial ischemia and fibrosis may develop, which will further depress the compliance and begin to raise the "*pre-a wave* pressure". Because the latter forms the baseline filling pressure over which the *a* and *v wave* buildup occurs (very similar to what has been shown and discussed in relation to the right-sided pressures in Chapter 4), the raised *pre-a wave* pressure will further raise the *v wave* pressure height in the left atrium. The upper normal left ventricular diastolic pressure for the end of diastole (*post- a wave*) is usually between 12 and 15 mmHg, whereas the upper normal left ventricular *pre-a wave* pressure is between 5 and 8 mmHg. The normal *v wave* in the left atrium may be 12–18 mmHg. In chronic mitral regurgitation, even when the regurgitation is severe, the left atrial *v wave* height may only be mildly to moderately elevated (20–35 mmHg.) This would mean a persistent pressure difference between the left ventricle and the left atrium throughout systole, making the regurgitant flow last until the very end of systole and well into the isovolumic relaxation phase (Fig. 19B). The murmur, therefore, usually lasts for the whole of systole (thus termed *pansystolic*) and thus all the way to the S2. In addition, the gradient remains relatively large and constant from the beginning of systole to its end, giving rise to a plateau high-frequency murmur.

ACUTE MITRAL REGURGITATION

If the mitral regurgitation is severe and acute in onset, as with ruptured chordae, then there may not be enough time to develop compensatory dilatation of either the left atrium or the left ventricle (Fig. 20A). The large volume of regurgitant blood entering a relatively stiff and nondilated left atrium will result in a steep rise in the *v wave* pressure in the left atrium (sometimes as high as 50–70 mmHg) (Fig. 20B) *(65,66)*. The entry of a large volume of blood during diastole into a nondilated left ventricle will tend to raise the diastolic filling pressures in the left ventricle. The raised *pre-a wave* pressure may further add to the *v wave* height. The high *v wave* buildup in the left atrium during systole would mean a decreased and rapidly falling pressure difference between the left ventricle and the left atrium toward the later part of systole. This will in turn limit the regurgitant flow during the later part of systole, making the regurgitant flow and the murmur decrescendo. In addition, the excess flow would cause lower and medium frequencies, making the murmur sound harsher.

Characteristics of Mitral Regurgitation Murmurs

1. Mitral regurgitation murmur shares all the features listed previously for all regurgitation murmurs. In general, it is high in frequency and blowing in quality, will usually last all the way to S2, and may even spill slightly beyond S2 (Fig. 21).
2. It may be harsh and have low and medium frequencies if the regurgitation is severe.
3. Mitral regurgitation murmurs will be expected to change very little in loudness following sudden long diastole, as may happen in atrial fibrillation or following an ectopic beat (Fig. 22).

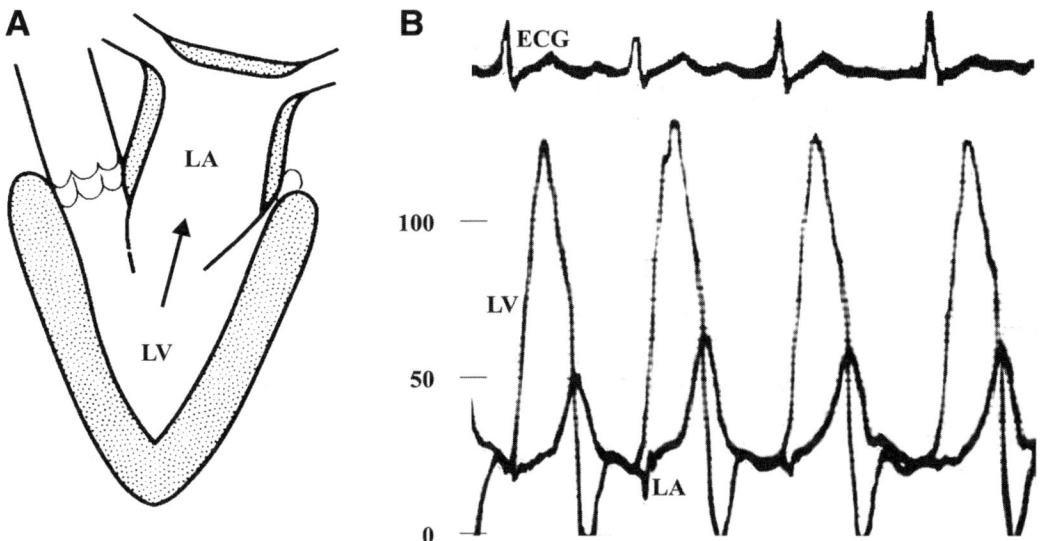

Fig. 20. (**A**) Diagrammatic representation of the left atrium (LA) and the left ventricle (LV) in acute severe mitral regurgitation. The LV and the LA do not have time to develop compensatory dilatation. The relatively normal-sized LA, receiving a large regurgitant volume in systole, builds up a high pressure. (**B**) Simultaneous recordings of the electrocardiogram (ECG) and left ventricular (LV) and left atrial (LA) pressure curves from a patient with acute severe mitral regurgitation showing a high *v wave* measuring up to 50 mmHg. The pressure difference between the LV and the LA is seen to fall toward the later part of systole, which will in turn limit the regurgitation during this phase.

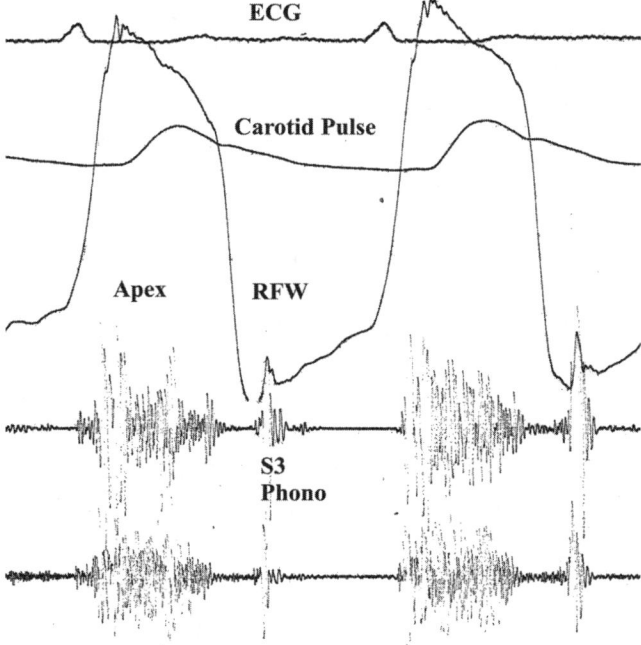

Fig. 21. Simultaneous recordings of electrocardiogram (ECG), carotid pulse (CP), apexcardiogram (Apex), and phonocardiogram (Phono) from a patient with severe mitral regurgitation taken at the apex area. The systolic murmur is seen to last all the way to the S2. The Apex shows an exaggerated rapid filling wave (RFW) with a corresponding third heard sound (S3) on the Phono.

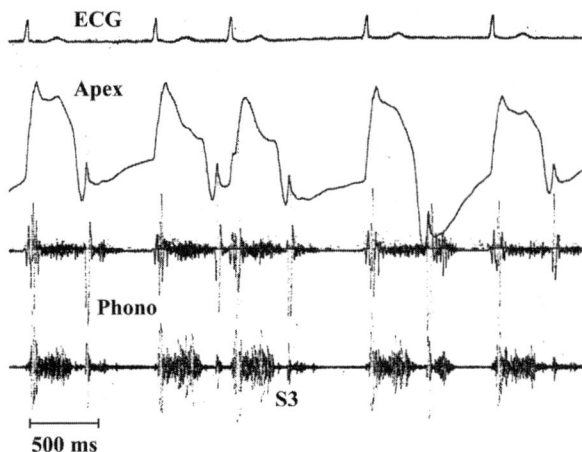

Fig. 22. Simultaneous recordings of electrocardiogram (ECG), apexcardiogram (Apex), and phonocardiogram (Phono) from a patient with mitral regurgitation and atrial fibrillation. Note that the changing diastolic durations and the varying filling do not affect the intensity of the systolic regurgitant murmur. The presence of S3 would indicate that the regurgitation must be significant.

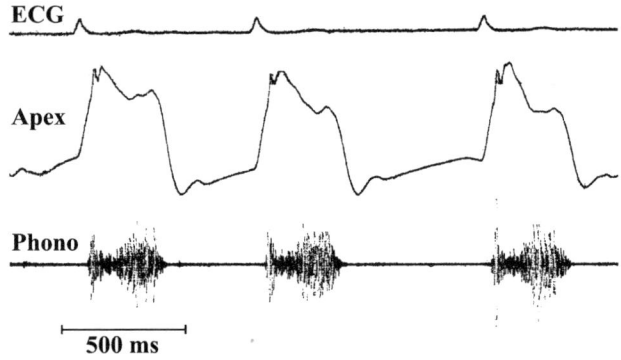

Fig. 23. Simultaneous recordings of electrocardiogram (ECG), apexcardiogram (Apex), and phonocardiogram (Phono) from a patient with mitral regurgitation secondary to prolapsed myxomatous mitral valves taken from the apex area showing accentuation in intensity of the murmur in late systole.

4. Mitral regurgitation murmurs may have different shapes depending on the etiology (Fig. 23). It is often pansystolic in relatively fixed orifice regurgitation, as with rheumatic involvement. It may be confined to mid- and late systole when caused by papillary muscle dysfunction or prolapsed myxomatous mitral leaflets and chordae (Fig. 24). In these conditions it may also increase in intensity toward the end of systole, i.e., crescendo to the S2. With prolapsed myxomatous mitral leaflets and chordae the mid- to late systolic murmur may start with a mid-systolic click or clicks. In addition in this disorder, the murmur may be shown to start earlier in systole and also increase in intensity with maneuvers that decrease the ventricular size, such as standing. With squatting, which will cause increased venous return and therefore increase the ventricular size, the click will start later, and the murmur may either disappear or decrease in intensity *(49,67–69)*.

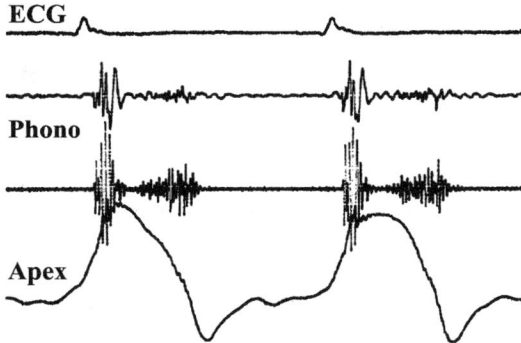

Fig. 24. Simultaneous recordings of electrocardiogram (ECG), apexcardiogram (Apex), and phonocardiogram (Phono) from a patient with ischemic heart disease and papillary muscle dysfunction. The regurgitant murmur is late systolic in timing and appears to peak toward the end of systole.

Rarely, mitral regurgitation may be confined to early and mid-systole, start with S1, and become decrescendo. This is characteristically associated with acute and severe mitral regurgitation caused by ruptured chordae. Because of the excess flow the murmur will also be harsh due to many low and medium frequencies *(65)*.

5. Irrespective of the etiology, the mitral regurgitation murmur is maximal in loudness at the apex. The murmur may be equally loud slightly lateral to the apex.

Severity of Mitral Regurgitation

1. The loudness of the mitral regurgitation murmur does not always correlate with the severity of the regurgitation. If the murmur is harsher and has a lot of low and medium frequencies, it usually indicates a lot of flow and therefore will imply significant regurgitation.
2. If the murmur, on the other hand, is all pure high frequency and confined only to late systole, then it must indicate a high pressure difference between the left ventricle and the left atrium and therefore only mild regurgitation.
3. When the mitral regurgitation is severe, the volume overload on the left ventricle will be high, resulting in an enlarged left ventricle. This may be reflected in a displaced hyperdynamic wide-area left ventricular apical impulse. In addition, the hyperdynamic left ventricle will have rapid ejection. This will make the A2 occur early, resulting in a wide-split S2. Thus, a wide-split S2 in the presence of mitral regurgitation is a sign of severe regurgitation if the wide split is not caused by P2 delay.
4. In addition, severe regurgitation because of the volume load effect will have a torrential inflow through the mitral valve during diastole. This will set up the necessary conditions for the production of an S3 or a mid-diastolic inflow rumble. The presence of an S3 or an inflow rumble at the apex will, therefore, be a sign of significant mitral regurgitation as well.
5. As mentioned previously, a harsh decrescendo mitral regurgitation murmur is usually indicative of severe regurgitation because the decrescendo effect is caused by early buildup of a very high *v wave* pressure in the left atrium resulting from a severe degree of regurgitation, thus decreasing the gradient in late systole (Fig. 25).

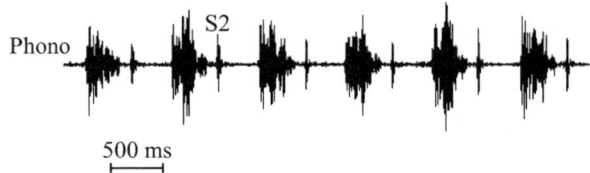

Fig. 25. Digital display of a magnetic audio recording from a patient with acute severe mitral regurgitation secondary to ruptured chordae taken from the apex area. The murmur diminishes in intensity toward the later part of systole (decrescendo shape).

6. Severe mitral regurgitation may also cause symptoms and signs of high left atrial pressure, such as nocturnal dyspnea, orthopnea, and pulmonary congestion, both clinically and radiologically.
7. The elevated left atrial pressure may also indirectly raise the pulmonary artery pressures, causing signs of pulmonary hypertension. The latter may be evidenced by the presence of elevated venous pressure with or without abnormal jugular contours, loud and/or palpable P2, and sustained right ventricular impulse as judged by subxiphoid palpation.

Specific Etiological Types of Mitral Regurgitation

RHEUMATIC MITRAL REGURGITATION

In acute rheumatic fever the inflammatory process may affect the leaflets or the chordae and the valve may become incompetent with somewhat rolled-up edges of the leaflets without any significant stenosis. With chronic rheumatic involvement, the mitral valve becomes predominantly stenotic because of commissural fusion. When the leaflets are significantly tethered and in particular contracted, mitral regurgitation could result. The pathological changes will often be such that the orifice is not only stenosed but also fails to close completely, causing regurgitation. Calcification of the leaflets may occur but is not a prerequisite for regurgitation. Rarely, the posterior leaflet may be more involved and significantly retracted and contracted, resulting in predominant or pure regurgitation alone. Occasionally after mitral stenosis is either surgically corrected by open or closed commissurotomy or by modern balloon valvuloplasty, one may have some iatrogenic mitral regurgitation. This may be caused by unintended noncommissural tears. In long-standing cases, marked left atrial enlargement will eventually result in the development of atrial fibrillation. The underlying rheumatic process may also involve the atrium and the conduction system, including the sino-atrial node, which also predisposes partly to the development of atrial fibrillation.

Mitral regurgitation, because of rheumatic process, has pathophysiological changes described under chronic mitral regurgitation. The murmur is often high in frequency and blowing with maximal loudness at the apex. It often begins with S1 and will generally last all the way to S2. The S1 intensity may be normal if the ventricular function is not impaired and the mitral regurgitation is not severe. If diminished, it indicates that one or both factors may be operative. The associated findings of stenosis, such as a loud S1, an opening snap, or mitral diastolic murmur, may or may not be present. If the regurgitation is severe, however, a short mid-diastolic rumble may be heard, indicative of the large volume load causing excess mitral inflow.

MITRAL REGURGITATION SECONDARY TO PROLAPSED MITRAL LEAFLETS

The most common cause of isolated mitral regurgitation (i.e., without mitral stenosis), particularly in the developed countries, would appear to be nonrheumatic in etiology. Myxomatous degeneration leads the list under the nonrheumatic causes *(51,63,70)*. Myxomatous degeneration of the mitral leaflets and chordae may be isolated and idiopathic, and rarely familial. It can also occur as part of other inherited connective tissue defect, such as Marfan's syndrome. The disorder may be associated with mitral regurgitation in all age groups and is often somewhat more common in the female gender *(49, 69,71–77)*. The posterior mitral leaflet is more commonly affected. The involved scallops of the posterior leaflet become markedly hooded and redundant. The chordae often are thickened and elongated as well. Often the annulus is also involved in the process and shows dilatation. The condition results in prolapse of the hooded and redundant leaflets during systole. This may be identified on two-dimensional echocardiographic imaging or a left ventricular angiogram easily.

The onset of prolapse typically is quite early in systole in the excessively redundant valves. This is clearly different from some bulging of the normal mitral leaflets at end-systole, which may be seen in any two-dimensional echo imaging. The maximal prolapse with the abnormal redundant leaflets and chordae will occur at a critical ventricular dimension *(77)*. The critical dimension is relatable to the leaflet and chordal redundancy or length because chordae have fixed lengths and they cannot shorten during systole. When the ventricular dimension diminishes during systole, the chordal length may become disproportionately longer during systole when the leaflets can no longer be maintained together and the involved leaflet or parts of the leaflet bulge or prolapse into the left atrium (Fig. 26A). The S1 intensity is often well preserved because the mitral leaflet coaptation is intact initially and the column of blood will be able to decelerate against the closed valve, as in normals. However, as systole proceeds the leaflets may become prolapsed once the critical dimension is reached, which is dependent on the redundancy of the leaflet and chordae. The column of blood will not only be ejected through the aorta, but part of the blood mass will also continue to move behind the bulging leaflets toward the low-pressure left atrium. When the prolapse reaches the maximum limit, as determined by the ventricular dimension achieved, there will be a sudden deceleration of the column of blood against the prolapsed leaflet or scallops. This may be associated with an audible clicking sound during middle of systole, termed the *nonejection click* (Fig. 26B). Sometimes there may be multiple clicks. The latter may represent minute variations in time of maximal prolapse of the different portions of the leaflet (Fig. 26C). The timing of the clicks may vary in systole. They can also be made to come earlier or later by maneuvers that alter the venous return and thereby the ventricular size. For instance, standing the patient suddenly, decreasing the venous return, will make the heart small and bring the maximal prolapse early and thereby make the click come earlier. Squatting, by increasing the venous return and the ventricular size, will make the click occur later. Mitral leaflets may lose coaptation once prolapse begins to occur, and this will result in onset of mitral regurgitation in early or mid-systole. The regurgitation may appear more in late systole when the ventricle reaches the maximum shortening and causes maximal prolapse. Thus, the click in mid-systole may be followed by a late-systolic, regurgitant, high-frequency murmur (Figs. 26D and 27). The auscultatory features associated with the prolapsed mitral valve leaflets may vary.

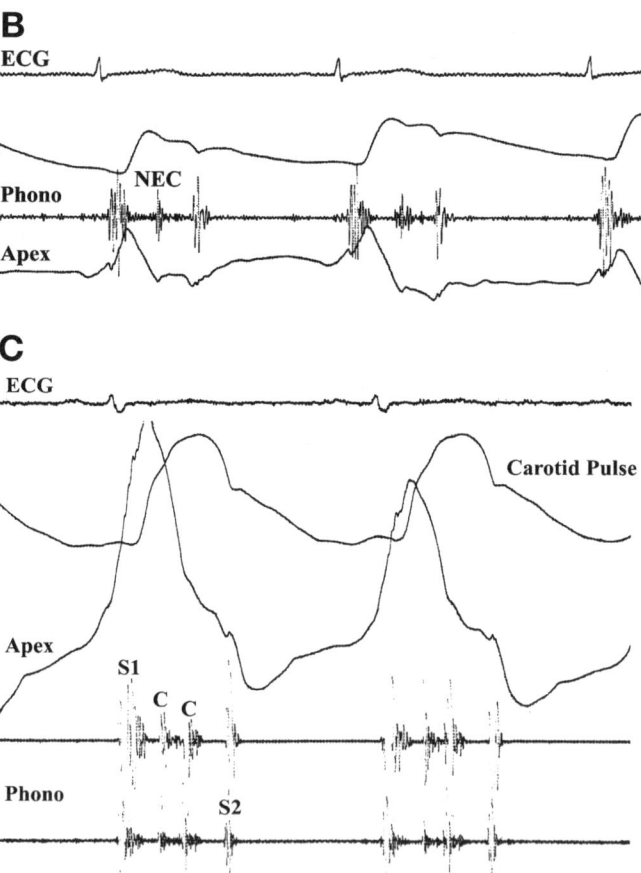

Fig. 26. (**A**) Two-dimensional echocardiographic image of the left ventricle (LV), the aorta (AO), and the left atrium (LA) in the parasternal long axis from a patient with redundant myxomatous posterior mitral leaflet scallops with prolapse and mitral regurgitation. Stop frame taken relatively early in systole shows the bulging posterior mitral leaflet (arrow) prolapsing into the LA. (**B**) Simultaneous recordings of electrocardiogram (ECG), carotid pulse (CP), apexcardiogram (Apex), and phonocardiogram (Phono) from a patient with prolapsed mitral valve syndrome taken from the apex area showing a mid-systolic nonejection click (NEC). (**C**) Simultaneous recordings of ECG, CP, Apex, and Phono from a patient with prolapsed mitral valve syndrome taken from the apex area showing two clicks (C) in systole. *(Continued on next page)*

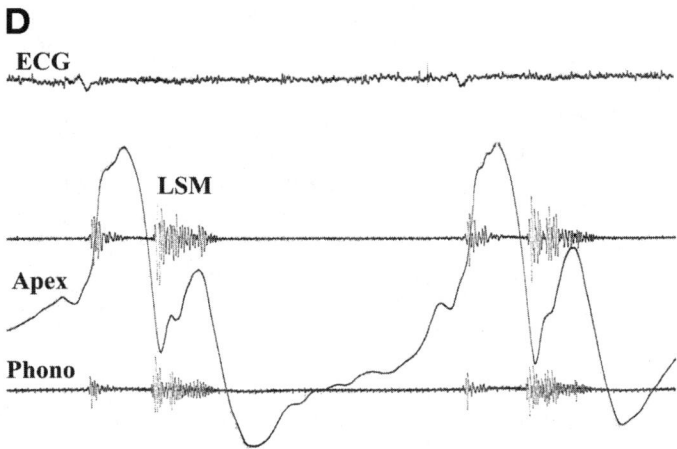

Fig. 26. *(Continued)* **(D)** Simultaneous recordings of ECG, Apex, and Phono from a patient with prolapsed mitral valve syndrome taken from the apex area showing a systolic murmur confined to late systole.

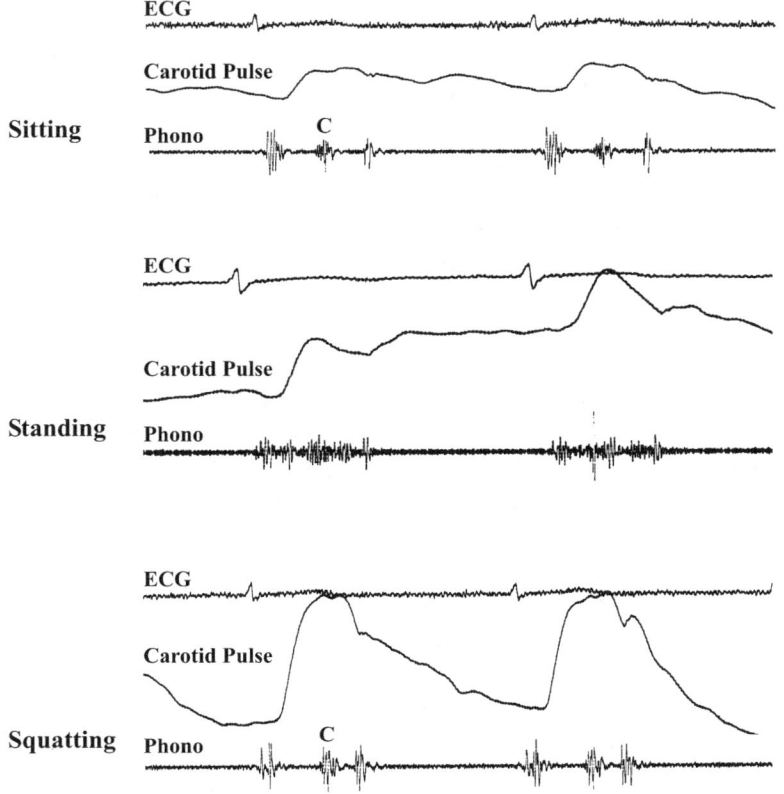

Fig. 27. Simultaneous recordings of electrocardiogram (ECG), carotid pulse (CP), and phonocardiogram (Phono) from a patient with prolapsed mitral valve syndrome taken from the apex area demonstrating the effect of changing postures on the auscultatory findings. The systolic click (C) is seen to occur earlier in systole in the sitting position compared to the squatting position. On standing the click is replaced by a pansystolic mitral regurgitation murmur.

Occasionally the patient may only have a nonejection click. The murmur of mitral regurgitation may be intermittent. In some the click is followed by the typical late systolic murmur. In others the regurgitation may start quite early in systole and last throughout systole and cause a pansystolic murmur. The nonejection click may then be conspicuously absent. In some patients the mitral regurgitation murmur associated with the prolapsed leaflets may have a peculiar loud *honking or whooping* quality. Occasionally the patients themselves may be aware of the loud systolic honk or the whoop. Sometimes they may be audible from a distance.

The disorder, when it occurs in the idiopathic form, may be characterized by symptoms that have no particular relationship to the degree or severity of the mitral regurgitation. The patients may present for reason of chest pains, palpitations, or abnormal T waves on the electrocardiogram, arrhythmias, or simply because of the characteristic auscultatory features. They may exhibit certain skeletal abnormalities, such as scoliosis, significant laxity of joints, and a high-arched palate. In some patients with chest pain in this condition, abnormal lactate uptake has been demonstrated, and in some coronary spasm has also been shown. Some patients may have transient embolic symptoms because of platelet thrombi forming between the hooded leaflets and the left atrial wall underneath it. Rarely, infective endocarditis may develop. In view of the variety of symptoms that they may present with, the disorder is often described as *idiopathic prolapsed mitral leaflet syndrome*. The mitral regurgitation is usually mild or mild to moderate in most patients. However, it can become more severe and cause acute symptoms of high left atrial pressure, such as sudden pulmonary edema, orthopnea, or paroxysmal nocturnal dyspnea. The reason for such deterioration is usually ruptured chordae, either because of spontaneous rupture or secondary to infective endocarditis.

Occasionally papillary muscle dysfunction can be associated with prolapse of the leaflets, but careful assessment of the leaflet and chordal morphology on the two-dimensional echo image as well as the assessment of the mitral annular dimension will help to identify secondary prolapse as a result of papillary muscle dysfunction as opposed to prolapse resulting from chordal leaflet pathology. Rarely, coronary disease can exist with the prolapsed and abnormal mitral leaflets in the same patient. Coexistence with hypertrophic obstructive cardiomyopathy has also been described. In some rare patients with hypertrophic obstructive cardiomyopathy, loud midsystolic nonejection clicks may be heard *(78)*. Our observation in one such patient revealed the coexistence of abnormal prolapsed and redundant mitral leaflet at surgery for relief of the severe outflow obstruction.

MITRAL REGURGITATION SECONDARY TO PAPILLARY MUSCLE DYSFUNCTION

In ischemic heart disease, mitral regurgitation may be noted to develop during an active episode of angina, and the murmur may be noted to be typically late systolic and often crescendo to the S2. It is often high in frequency *(79)*. The murmur may actually disappear when the angina is relieved by nitroglycerin or rest. However, if one were to selectively damage the papillary muscle belly alone without affecting the underlying left ventricular myocardium, as can be done in experimental animal models, mitral regurgitation does not always develop *(53)*. The reason for this is that a scarred or fibrosed papillary muscle alone may not lead to failure in maintaining mitral leaflet coaptation as long as the left ventricular contraction is preserved at the base of the papillary muscles. The contraction at the base pulling on the scarred papillary muscles can effectively keep the mitral leaflets together. This observation has, therefore, led to the concept that mitral regurgitation, because of papillary muscle dysfunction, usually implies that the left ventricular myocardium underneath the papillary muscles must also be involved in the dysfunction *(54)*. This does not exclude the possibility of mitral regurgitation from a markedly contracted and scarred papillary muscle, which can effectively keep the leaflets retracted or pulled down on the affected side, thereby preventing proper coaptation of the two leaflets during systole *(55,56)*.

The arterial vasculature of the papillary muscles has been shown to be related to the morphology of the papillary muscle itself. The free and finger-like papillary muscles would appear to be more vulnerable in ischemic disease because of the less prominent collateral connection to the extrapapillary subendocardial network in this morphological type. It is reasonable to expect that acute coronary occlusion can result in necrosis of the papillary muscle and the underlying left ventricular wall *(46)*. Because of the fact that the posteromedial commissural area is wider than the anterolateral commissural area, ischemia and/or infarction involving the posteromedial group of the papillary muscles would likely produce mitral regurgitation more easily than those involving the anterolateral group. In fact, mitral regurgitation is more often clinically encountered in inferior and posterior infarction than the anterior infarction *(80,81)*. Acute necrosis of the papillary muscles may leave the origins of the main stems of the rough zone chordae quite vulnerable to avulsion. Papillary muscles, being the most terminal regions of the subendocardial circulation, may suffer necrosis even though the clinical picture of the patient may be interpreted as simply acute coronary insufficiency and not necessarily acute myocardial infarction. Depending on the location and number of chords avulsed, one may develop a fair degree of mitral regurgitation. For instance the mitral regurgitation can be very severe when the anterior leaflet strut chord is avulsed because of necrosis of the papillary muscle *(45,50)*. In addition, in acute myocardial infarction, rarely the papillary muscle head could actually rupture, causing wide open and severe mitral regurgitation and pulmonary edema *(59)*.

In the late stages of myocardial infarction, the underlying myocardium may become aneurysmal and the left ventricle may become dilated. This may displace the papillary muscle base downward and produce distortion of the mitral apparatus. This will effectively interfere with proper leaflet apposition and result in mitral regurgitation.

Papillary muscle dysfunction may occur in anomalous origin of the left coronary artery from the pulmonary artery. This congenital lesion can result in ischemia and infarction of the anterolateral wall and the anterolateral papillary muscle *(40)*. When the high pulmonary artery pressures of the newborn fall after a few weeks after birth, the low-pressure left coronary artery offers a path of least resistance through intercoronary anastomotic connections for the blood from the aorta to reach the pulmonary artery. Once this retrograde flow is established, the capillary bed of the left coronary artery is bypassed and the myocardium supplied by it becomes ischemic. The symptoms characteristically start a few months after birth, reflecting the lag period before retrograde flow will become established.

Papillary muscle dysfunction can also occur in myocardial diseases of other etiology besides the ischemic heart disease *(80)*. It can, for instance, occur in dilated cardiomyopathy.

Clinical Features of Papillary Muscle Dysfunction

The degree or severity of mitral regurgitation in papillary muscle dysfunction is somewhat variable *(55,56,82)*. It can vary in severity from mild to severe, depending on the underlying pathology. The murmur more typically is late systolic and crescendo to the S2. Such is the case with active ischemia. If pathological alterations cause disruption of chordal support, then the regurgitation will more than likely be pansystolic and severe, depending on the extent and location of such disruption. If the pathology is such as to cause distortion of the mitral apparatus, as in ventricular aneurysm, then the regurgitation murmur will also be pansystolic and the severity may be variable. Mitral regurgitation with a severely scarred and retracted papillary muscle may begin early in systole and could be pansystolic or may decrease toward the end of systole.

Mitral regurgitation murmurs of papillary muscle dysfunction are like other mitral regurgitation murmurs: maximal in intensity or loudness at the apex. Papillary muscle dysfunction, because of active ischemia, often results in a soft blowing, high-frequency, late systolic murmur (Fig. 24). Occasionally, the papillary muscle dysfunction, because of ischemia, may be associated with midsystolic or nonejection click or sound. The nonejection sound or click probably arises from a mechanism similar to that described with prolapsed leaflet. The ischemic papillary muscle by failure of its contraction may allow the leaflets to bulge into the left atrium because of rising ventricular pressure during systole. The column of blood may move with the bulging leaflets or scallops as well. When the anatomical length of the chordal-leaflet unit is maximally taut during midsystole, the moving column of blood underneath will suddenly become decelerated, resulting in dissipation of energy and production of the midsystolic sound or click. The latter may occur without any significant mitral regurgitation. This click may not be as sharp and high in frequency as heard in mitral leaflet prolapse.

When acute chordal avulsion has taken place because of necrosis of the papillary muscles, the resulting regurgitation murmur could be quite loud and have a fair amount of medium and low frequencies secondary to the large flow. On the other hand, when acute rupture of the papillary muscle head complicates myocardial infarction, the mitral regurgitation could be quite severe, and yet in some of these patients the regurgitation murmur may not be very loud and sometimes even very faint or silent. This may be because of a wide-open mitral valve with coexisting left ventricular dysfunction resulting from the myocardial infarction *(81,83,84)*.

MITRAL REGURGITATION SECONDARY TO RUPTURED CHORDAE

There are approximately 25 chordae in the human mitral valve. Except for the fan-shaped chordae that insert into the commissures between the leaflets and into the clefts between the scallops of the posterior leaflet, the remaining chords are primarily those that insert into the distal rough zone of the leaflets. These arise as main stems from the papillary muscles, and each main stem divides into three branches, with one branch inserting into the line of leaflet closure, one into the free edge of the leaflets, and the third in between the two. Two of the rough zone chords of the anterior leaflet are particularly large and thick and are termed the "*strut chordae*" *(47)*. Chordae tendineae may rupture either spontaneously or because of trauma or infective endocarditis *(81)*. While infective endocarditis may affect any part of the leaflet and therefore cause rupture of any part of the chordae and their branches, spontaneous rupture will generally affect the main stem of the chordae. Spontaneous rupture could occur if the tensile strength of the chordae is weakened because of elastic tissue loss, as may happen in myxomatous degeneration or for idiopathic reasons *(85)*. In fact, in patients with prolapsed mitral leaflet, chronic mild mitral regurgitation may suddenly become severe because of the development of rup-

Table 1
Severe Mitral Regurgitation Secondary to Ruptured Chordae

Etiology	Acute 9 pts	Acute on chronic 18 pts
Idiopathic	4	2
Avulsion secondary to papillary muscle necrosis	2	1
Myxomatous degeneration	3	12
Infective endocarditis	0	3

pts, Patients.

tured chordae. Rarely, chordal origins from the papillary muscle may avulse because of necrosis of the papillary muscle. This may happen with underlying ischemic heart disease. This may also lead to sudden severe mitral regurgitation.

In a series of 27 consecutive patients with ruptured chordae studied by us over a period of 10 years, 9 presented with acute onset of severe mitral regurgitation with no known previous mitral regurgitation (acute group), whereas 18 had sudden deterioration of chronic mild mitral regurgitation(acute on chronic group) (Table 1). The majority of patients (23 of 27) were male, and they varied in age between 37 and 75 yr. Both groups of patients had symptoms secondary to high left atrial pressures causing orthopnea, pulmonary congestion, and/or pulmonary edema as well as nocturnal dyspnea. The majority of the patients had mitral regurgitation murmurs, grade IV or more in intensity. S3 gallop was noted in most of them, while an S4 gallop was noted in about 7 patients (3 in the acute group and 4 of the acute-on-chronic group). Accentuated and loud P2 was noted in half of all patients, indicating pulmonary hypertension. Hemodynamic measurements confirmed evidence of pulmonary hypertension as well as very high *v wave* pressures in the pulmonary capillary wedge reflecting high left atrial pressures. The presence of pulmonary edema was, however, uncommon in isolated posterior leaflet rough zone chordal rupture (1 of 17 patients). It was more common with anterior leaflet strut chordal rupture and or when both leaflets had rough zone chordae rupture. Atrial fibrillation was noted in a few of the patients. Despite similarities in clinical symptoms and signs, the pathology of the ruptured chordae in the two groups was somewhat different. Myxomatous degeneration was the most common cause in those with acute-on-chronic mitral regurgitation, but rare in acute mitral regurgitation. In the acute group the etiology was idiopathic in 4, avulsion of chordae secondary to papillary muscle necrosis in 2, and myxomatous degeneration in 3. In those with acute-on-chronic mitral regurgitation, the cause was myxomatous degeneration in 12, infective endocarditis in 3, papillary muscle necrosis in 1, and idiopathic in 2 (Fig. 28A,B) *(58)*.

The location and type of chordal rupture also had a bearing on the etiology of the rupture. The anterior leaflet chordal rupture was mostly idiopathic or a result of papillary muscle necrosis, whereas the majority of posterior leaflet chordal ruptures appeared to be secondary to myxomatous degeneration (13 of 17 patients) *(58)*.

Clinical Features of Mitral Regurgitation Secondary to Ruptured Chordae
1. Typically the pathophysiology is alluded to under acute mitral regurgitation. The excess flow into the left atrium gives rise to a harsh murmur because of a lot of low and medium frequencies. The murmur also tends to become decrescendo due to high *v wave* buildup in the left atrium, which would limit the regurgitation in late systole (Fig. 25).

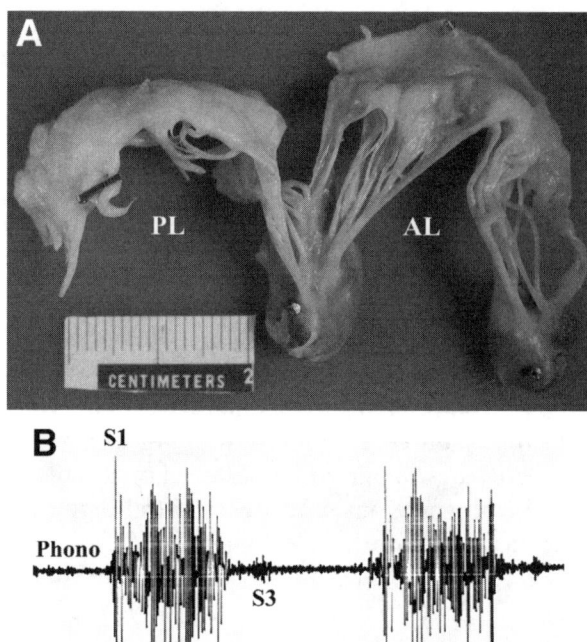

Fig. 28. (**A**) Excised mitral valve from a patient with myxomatous prolapsed posterior leaflet (PL), who had acute on chronic mitral regurgitation secondary to ruptured chordae. The clip around it shows the ruptured rough zone chordae of the PL. AL, Anterior leaflet. (**B**) Phonocardiographic (Phono) recording taken at the apex area from the patient with acute on chronic mitral regurgitation whose excised mitral valve is shown in (A). The regurgitation murmur is followed by a third heart sound (S3).

2. The maximal intensity of the murmur is at the apex. In addition, the murmur may be transmitted either to the base or to the back. The posterior leaflet chordal rupture has been considered to cause radiation of the murmur to the base more readily than toward the back. The anteriorly directed jet of mitral regurgitation is presumed to be conducted toward the aorta and therefore to the base. The reverse is postulated for anterior leaflet chordal rupture with radiation of the murmur toward the back *(80)*. This was not always the case in our experience.
3. Because of severe mitral regurgitation, the apex may become more hyperdynamic. The P2 may become loud secondary to the development of pulmonary hypertension.
4. The S2 may be widely split because of the early occurrence of A2.
5. In addition, there will often be an S3 because of excess mitral inflow that the volume overload state produces. The S3 may sound like a short mid-diastolic murmur.
6. If the patient remains in sinus rhythm, which is often the case because of the shorter duration of severe mitral regurgitation, an S4 may also be heard (Fig. 29) *(86)*. This is due to the fact that the left atrium is still healthy and the relatively less dilated left ventricle will be somewhat noncompliant, offering resistance to filling in diastole.
7. Unlike papillary muscle rupture, the murmurs of ruptured chordae are never silent and they are often fairly loud: grade III–IV or more. Because they are harsh and decrescendo,

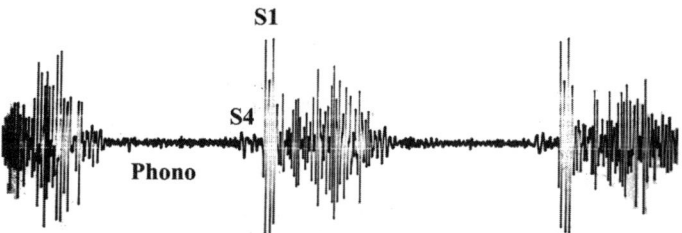

Fig. 29. Phonocardiographic (Phono) recording taken at the apex area from a patient with acute severe mitral regurgitation showing a fourth heart sound (S4) indicating that the left ventricle, which is not very dilated offers resistance to filling.

they are likely mistaken for ejection murmurs. Occasionally, the fact that they do not intensify following long diastoles may have to be used for their differentiation and recognition.

(For additional examples review Phono files 14–24 and Echo Phono Files 8 and 005-MVP under Heart Murmurs Part 1 on the Companion CD.)

TRICUSPID REGURGITATION

Tricuspid Valve Anatomy and Function

Tricuspid valve anatomy differs from that of the mitral valve in some respects. It has three leaflets, namely, the anterior, the posterior, and the septal leaflet. The leaflets vary in size, and in most normals the anterior leaflet is the largest. All three leaflets and the commissures in between them are inserted into the tricuspid valve ring or the annulus, which forms part of the entire circumference of the right atrioventricular groove *(87)*. Medially it is attached to the central cardiac skeleton. Thus, the tricuspid valve has no common attachment to the pulmonary valve like the mitral valve does to the aortic root. The pulmonary valve is separated from the inflow by an outflow tract or the infundibulum. This arrangement has a bearing on the function of the tricuspid valve. This means that any degree of right ventricular dilatation can lead to stretching of the tricuspid annulus, resulting in valvular incompetence. The chordal arrangement of the tricuspid valve is similar to the mitral valve, except that in general the chordae are often somewhat thinner and one does not find chordae similar to the strut chordae of the mitral anterior leaflet.

The competence of the tricuspid valve is maintained during ventricular systole by the contracting papillary muscles and the underlying right ventricular myocardium pulling on the chordae to keep the leaflets together in apposition, very similar to the mitral valve.

Causes of Tricuspid Regurgitation

Tricuspid regurgitation can arise from an anatomical and/or functional defect of any of the components of its complex anatomy. The etiological factors may be congenital or acquired. The pathological process can be genetic, inflammatory, infective, traumatic, degenerative, or neoplastic. Sometimes more than one component of the valve structures may be involved *(88,89)*.

ANNULAR ABNORMALITIES

The annulus may become idiopathically dilated or calcified and therefore may not function normally. Dilated annulus with voluminous leaflets may be part of cardiac involvement of connective tissue diseases such as Marfan's and Ehlers–Danlos syndromes. Dilatation of the annulus secondary to right ventricular dilatation is another important cause, which can either induce tricuspid regurgitation or worsen the degree of pre-existing tricuspid regurgitation. The ventricle will generally dilate secondary to volume overload, especially when it is significant and longstanding. This can occur, for instance, in atrial septal defect, which brings in an extra volume of blood because of the left-to-right shunt at the atrial level. The right ventricle will also dilate in the late stages of chronic pressure overload, as in pulmonary hypertension or significant pulmonary stenosis. Acute dilatation of the right ventricle may also occur when there is a sudden and significant rise in pulmonary artery pressures, as may happen with acute pulmonary embolism. Under all these circumstances annular dilatation will eventually lead to the development of tricuspid regurgitation. No matter how tricuspid regurgitation is produced initially, the resulting right ventricular dilatation will only lead to an increase in the degree of regurgitation because of annular stretch. This will be particularly the case in the presence of pulmonary hypertension since right ventricle does not usually tolerate raised pulmonary pressures.

LEAFLET AND CHORDAL ABNORMALITIES

The leaflet may be congenitally cleft, and this may be an associated feature of endocardial cushion defect. One or more of the leaflets may be large; in particular, the anterior leaflet and the whole leaflet insertion may be displaced downward, resulting in atrialization of part of the base of the right ventricle. This congenital abnormality of the tricuspid valve is called *Ebstein's anomaly (40,90)*. The tricuspid valve in this disorder is often incompetent.

The tricuspid leaflets and chordae may also be large and redundant, hooded, and prolapsed because of myxomatous degeneration. This may occur in association with similar mitral valve abnormality. The disorder may also occur as part of other connective tissue defects as in Marfan's syndrome. Leaflets and chordae may be scarred and contracted, with some commisssural fusion in rheumatic involvement. This is quite rare and usually will occur only with associated mitral and aortic valve involvement. The leaflets may also be involved in *carcinoid syndrome* with fibrous carcinoid plaques deposited on the ventricular surfaces of the leaflets, making them adhere to the underlying right ventricular wall, thereby making the valve incompetent *(91)*. Infective endocarditis can also cause destructive lesions of leaflet and chordae as well as vegetations. Tricuspid valve endocarditis and pulmonary valve endocarditis are well-recognized complications of intravenous drug abuse. Whereas chordal rupture can occur as a result of endocarditis, spontaneous rupture of tricuspid valve chordae is extremely rare.

PAPILLARY MUSCLE AND RIGHT VENTRICULAR WALL PATHOLOGY

Infarction of the right ventricle is less common than that of the left ventricle. It may occur in about 10% of patients with acute inferior myocardial infarction. In that setting, acute right ventricular dysfunction may compromise cardiac output and contribute to low-output state or cardiogenic shock. Some patients who have recovered from this may have residual chronic right ventricular dysfunction contributing to tricuspid regurgitation *(89)*. Ischemia of the right ventricle is extremely rare and not usually a cause of tricuspid regurgitation.

ATRIAL MYXOMA

Right atrial myxoma is even more uncommon than left atrial myxoma. When it does occur, it can present with tricuspid obstruction as well as interfere with proper leaflet closure and therefore produce tricuspid regurgitation.

OTHERS

Transvenous pacemaker wires inserted across the tricuspid valve will often interfere with proper valve closure and invariably will produce tricuspid regurgitation. However, the degree of tricuspid regurgitation is generally no more than mild to moderate in most instances.

Pathophysiology of Tricuspid Regurgitation

TRICUSPID REGURGITATION SECONDARY TO PULMONARY HYPERTENSION

From the foregoing consideration, it will be apparent that tricuspid regurgitation may occur with either normal right ventricular systolic pressures or elevated right ventricular systolic pressures. Chronic pulmonary hypertension, regardless of etiology, will have an element of reactive vasospasm initially in the pulmonary arterial bed. With persistence of high pressures, intimal damage will ensue and lead to obstructive changes resulting from thrombosis. In addition, there will be smooth muscle proliferation in the media and replacement fibrosis. These secondary changes lead to reduction of the total cross-sectional area of the pulmonary vascular bed. This will aggravate the pulmonary hypertension and make this more irreversible *(92–98)*. The etiological factors that can cause pulmonary hypertension are:

1. Left-sided pathology, which raises the left atrial pressures as with mitral obstruction (e.g., mitral stenosis, left atrial myxoma, or *cor-triatriatum*) mitral regurgitation or left ventricular failure. In these situations the raised left atrial pressure is passively transmitted to the pulmonary arteries through the pulmonary capillary bed. Rarely, the problem may be one of obstruction to pulmonary venous drainage as in pulmonary veno-occlusive disease.
2. Large intracardiac left-to-right shunts such as through a ventricular septal defect, atrial septal defect,or persistent ductus. Initially the high pulmonary pressures may be secondary to large flow alone (*hyperkinetic pulmonary hypertension*). When reactive and obstructive changes develop in the pulmonary arterial bed, the pulmonary pressures will rise significantly and may reach systemic levels. This will lead to reversal of the left-to-right shunt causing, right-to-left shunt. This will result in central cyanosis and the clinical disorder *Eisenmenger's syndrome (97)*.
3. Pulmonary arterial obstruction in particular pulmonary thromboembolism.
4. Pulmonary disease: Pulmonary hypertension may develop in certain longstanding diseases of the lungs, particularly those that lead to reduction of the total cross-sectional area of the pulmonary bed because of structural changes in the parenchyma that involve the vessels as well. The ensuing pulmonary hypertension and its effects on the right heart constitute the condition *cor pulmonale*. The hypoxia may trigger pulmonary vasospasm and directly raise the pulmonary pressures. This may be an important mechanism of pulmonary hypertension in chronic obstructive pulmonary disease, restrictive lung disease, and various forms of interstitial pulmonary fibrosis. In addition, a direct effect of

tobacco smoke on the intrapulmonary vessels has also been implicated, causing abnormal production of mediators that control vasoconstriction, vasodilatation, and vascular cell proliferation, leading to abnormal vascular remodeling and aberrant vascular physiology. These changes are similar to those seen in other forms of pulmonary hypertension. The vessels themselves may become distorted, occluded, and entrapped in replacement fibrosis, as may occur with various forms of interstitial pulmonary fibrosis. In addition, the vessels may be involved in a vasculitis. This may be an important mechanism in some disorders, such as collagen vascular disease (e.g., progressive systemic sclerosis, lupus erythematosus, and rheumatoid arthritis).

5. Hypoventilatory disorders: When hypoxia is associated with respiratory acidosis, as may happen with alveolar hypoventilation, pulmonary artery pressures tend to rise significantly. This situation may occur in various hypoventilatory disorders (e.g., Pickwickian syndrome in which marked obesity plays a prominent role, sleep apnea, neuromuscular disorders such as myasthenia, chest wall abnormalities as in kyphoscoliosis).

6. Primary pulmonary hypertension: This is rare but tends to be seen in women of childbearing age. In this disorder pathological changes develop in the pulmonary arterial bed for unknown reasons. The intimal fibrosis may have an onion-skin appearance. The medial hypertrophy may be accompanied by fibrinoid necrosis and formation of plexiform lesions, which are not usually seen in other forms of pulmonary hypertension.

In all these situations, the tricuspid valve itself is anatomically normal and the regurgitation is caused by right ventricular dilatation. The latter will stretch the tricuspid annulus and cause tricuspid regurgitation. The latter occurs in late stages when right ventricular hypertrophy is no longer able to compensate for the pressure load. The high-pressure tricuspid regurgitation is often less well tolerated by the right ventricle. The right ventricular hypertrophy would usually precede the development of the tricuspid regurgitation, and the right ventricular diastolic pressures, in particular the *pre-a wave* pressure, would be elevated. This will lead to significant elevation of the right atrial and jugular venous pressures. The raised venous pressure would cause systemic venous congestion, resulting in abdominal distension, hepatomegaly, pulsatile liver, and peripheral edema. The jugular venous contour will be abnormal, reflecting the tricuspid regurgitation showing large-amplitude *v wave* with a *y descent*. The normal dominant *x' descent* will be absent because of the regurgitation raising the right atrial pressure during systole. The contour is often visible from a distance. The right ventricular dysfunction will often cause low-output symptoms such as fatigue and tiredness.

TRICUSPID REGURGITATION WITH NORMAL PULMONARY ARTERY PRESSURES

In contrast to tricuspid regurgitation in the presence of pulmonary hypertension, tricuspid regurgitation with normal right ventricular systolic pressure usually occurs because of some primary tricuspid valve abnormality. In addition, the tricuspid regurgitation associated with normal pulmonary pressures may be well tolerated. Because the problem is primarily valvular in origin, the right ventricle will have a primary volume load. The resulting compensatory dilatation will help maintain good right ventricular compliance for a long time, especially when the lesion producing the tricuspid regurgitation is chronic. This will maintain relatively normal right ventricular diastolic pressures. The resulting venous pressure elevation will therefore be somewhat minimized. Finally, secondary right ventricular hypertrophy will develop in late stages, which may reduce the compliance, leading to elevation of the right ventricular diastolic pressures.

The latter may cause further rise in the venous pressures. The signs of systemic congestion may therefore be less pronounced and appear later in the course.

ACUTE TRICUSPID REGURGITATION

This may be seen as part of the clinical presentation of patients with acute pulmonary embolism, post-right-ventricular infarction, or secondary to tricuspid valve endocarditis *(99)*. In acute pulmonary embolism alone the tricuspid regurgitation will be associated with pulmonary hypertension. The right ventricular diastolic pressures will be elevated because of right ventricular dysfunction as well as because of the acuteness of the disorder, which does not allow time for compensatory right ventricular dilatation. The clinical picture, however, will be dominated by the underlying condition and not by the tricuspid regurgitation.

Characteristics of Tricuspid Regurgitation Murmurs

1. Tricuspid regurgitation murmur shares all the features listed under the general characteristics of regurgitant murmurs. In general it is high in frequency and blowing in quality and usually lasts all the way to S2.
2. The frequency will tend to be higher in the presence of pulmonary hypertension. In the initial stages of decompensation the murmur may be intermittent and audible only on inspiration. In some patients the murmur may have a whoop or honking character. When decompensation becomes more pronounced, the regurgitation murmur may be audible throughout the phases of respiration. The co-existent right ventricular dysfunction and consequent decrease in cardiac output will lead to some decrease in the right ventricular systolic pressures (to about 50 mmHg), but the pressure is still high enough to contribute to the high frequencies.
3. Tricuspid regurgitation murmurs may have some low and medium frequencies when the regurgitation is severe.
4. Tricuspid regurgitation murmurs will also not change in intensity or loudness following sudden long diastoles as in atrial fibrillation or following an ectopic beat.
5. Irrespective of the etiology, tricuspid regurgitation murmurs are maximal in loudness over the xiphoid area and over the lower sternal region. In addition, tricuspid regurgitation murmur will typically increase in intensity or loudness on inspiration (*Carvallo's sign*) *(6)*. It may be heard over the apex area if the right ventricle is enlarged or dilated and has taken over the apex area.
6. Tricuspid regurgitation murmurs may have different shapes depending on the etiology. In general it will be pansystolic when there is annular dilatation primary or secondary as well as when the orifice is fixed, as in rheumatic involvement. It may be late systolic if caused by prolapsed myxomatous leaflets and chordae. The murmur may also begin with a midsystolic click in some of these patients. However, the findings may be compounded by the coexistence of mitral prolapse. In the presence of Ebstein's anomaly, the murmur may be preceded by a somewhat delayed and loud T1.

   The murmur may vary in length, early systolic to being holo- or pansystolic. When the regurgitation is associated with normal right ventricular pressures, the murmur is often soft and short with low to medium frequencies and confined to the early half of systole *(99)*. The intensity often diminishes toward the end of systole because the right atrial *v wave* and the rising right ventricular systolic pressures tend to equalize toward the end of ejection. This will cause the regurgitant flow to diminish in later systole. The inadequacy of the right ventricular function may also produce a poor inspiratory increase in its stroke volume. This may, therefore, result in a poor inspiratory increase in the intensity of the murmur.

In rheumatic involvement of the tricuspid valve, which is quite rare, there may be associated features of loud T1 and even tricuspid opening snap. Right atrial myxoma producing tricuspid regurgitation will be associated with loud tricuspid component of S1, which may accentuate with inspiration. In addition, there may be a loud sound in diastole mimicking an S3 resulting from *tumor plop*. This would be followed by a diastolic rumble because of the tricuspid obstruction that often would occur with the right atrial myxoma. Transvenous pacemakers may cause squeaky tricuspid regurgitation murmur, which may accentuate with inspiration.

7. If the regurgitation is significant and severe, then the excess diastolic inflow from the right atrium may result in a right-sided S3 or short mid-diastolic low-frequency murmur or rumble. Both of these will be most audible over the xiphoid area or the lower sternal region and will accentuate in intensity on inspiration.

8. The audibility of tricuspid regurgitation murmur is often variable. Sometimes significant tricuspid regurgitation may be present on the Doppler, and yet the associated murmur may be absent. This is more likely when the right ventricular systolic pressures are normal. Jugular venous pulse contour may sometimes be characteristic of tricuspid regurgitation, and yet the murmur may be inconspicuous. While the *x′ descent* may be visible with mild and occasionally mild-to-moderate tricuspid regurgitation on the Doppler, significant tricuspid regurgitation will usually lead to the loss of the normal *x′ descent* in the jugulars. In addition, the typical fast-rising large-amplitude *v wave* followed by the *y descent* will reveal the tricuspid regurgitation. In Ebstein's anomaly, the huge right atrium, because of partial atrialization of the right ventricle and the resultant high capacitance effect of the right atrium, may sometimes hide the presence of tricuspid regurgitation in the jugulars, and the jugular pulsations may in fact be quite unimpressive in such patients.

VENTRICULAR SEPTAL DEFECT (VSD)

Defect in the interventricular septum can be either congenital or acquired. Congenital defects may involve either the membranous or the muscular portion of the interventricular septum. The defect in the membranous ventricular septum is by far the most common *(40,100–105)*. It is usually located below the aortic valve close to the commissure between the right coronary and the noncoronary cusps. The outer edge of the defect may involve the adjoining portion of the muscular septum. For this reason the defect is usually termed *perimembranous*. Occasionally the membranous portion of the septum can be aneurysmal, and the defect may be located in the wall of the aneurysmal bulge. The aneurysm can cause some obstruction to the right ventricular outflow as well.

The muscular septum consists of three portions as viewed from the right ventricular side, namely, *the inlet, the trabecular*, and *the outlet portions (105)*. The defects in the muscular septum, in turn, may involve the inlet, the trabecular, or the outlet portion of the septum, respectively. The defect can be either single or multiple. In addition, the size of these defects may also vary. Doubly committed subarterial VSDs are located in the outlet portion of the septum and they are bordered by a fibrous continuity of the aortic and the pulmonary valves. These defects are more common in Asian patients.

The acquired form of VSD usually occurs as a result of septal rupture complicating acute myocardial infarction *(106–109)*. Septal rupture complicating anterior myocardial infarction usually involves the apical region of the muscular septum, whereas those that complicate infero-posterior infarction usually involve the posterobasal portion of the muscular septum. The latter is less common.

Congenital Ventricular Septal Defects

The degree of left-to-right shunt through a congenital VSD is dependent on the size of the defect and on the pulmonary vascular resistance *(101,103,104)*. The larger the size, the larger the flow, as long as the pulmonary vascular resistance is not high. The pulmonary vascular resistance is initially high in the newborn because of the muscular nature of the pulmonary vasculature. This usually takes a few weeks to regress. Thus, the murmur of the VSD may not be apparent at birth and may become audible only a few weeks after birth.

If the defect is large enough, then there could be a large left-to-right shunt causing excess pulmonary flow. Contrary to what may seem logical to a beginner, despite the fact that the shunt through a VSD occurs from the left ventricle to the right ventricle, the volume overload is presented to the left atrium and the left ventricle and not to the right ventricle. The shunt occurs during systole because of the higher left ventricular pressure. The contracting right ventricle is in no position to accept the shunted volume because the right ventricle is also contracting and emptying at the same time. Therefore, the left-to-right shunt goes through the defect and directly into the pulmonary artery. The excess pulmonary flow, because of the shunt, is eventually returned through the pulmonary veins to the left atrium. This will lead to left atrial and left ventricular enlargement because these two chambers receive the extra volume of blood. The volume overload of the left ventricle may result in congestive heart failure during the first year of life. However, spontaneous improvement may often occur because of reduction in size of the defects with the normal growth of the heart or the development of increased pulmonary vascular resistance or occasionally because of development of infundibular hypertrophy, which may also reduce the left-to-right shunt because of the acquired infundibular stenosis.

Spontaneous closure of VSDs is fairly common during infancy and early childhood years (up to 45% of cases) *(40)*. Occasionally spontaneous closure may occur, even in older children and young adults. Even large defects causing excess pulmonary flow with flow-related pulmonary hypertension are known to undergo spontaneous closure. Several factors may play a role in spontaneous closure. These include appositions of the margins of defects, endocardial proliferation, adherence of the septal leaflet of tricuspid valve, or prolapse of the aortic cusp through the defect. The prolapsed aortic cusp may be associated, however, with varying degrees of aortic regurgitation.

Large VSDs causing excess left-to-right shunt in early childhood may either decrease in size, undergo spontaneous closure, or develop increased pulmonary vascular resistance because of intrinsic changes in the vascular bed brought about by the excess flow and pressure (*Eisenmenger's reaction*) *(97)*. When the pulmonary vascular resistance is high, this not only will limit the left-to-right shunt but eventually can lead to reversal of shunt and development of cyanosis. The fact that the process can be prevented by timely surgical closure of large VSDs with increasing pulmonary vascular resistance at a stage when there is still significant left-to-right shunt would suggest that the pulmonary vascular damage is, to an extent, dependent on the excess flow.

VSDs, which are small or medium in size and associated with normal pulmonary vascular resistance and do not undergo spontaneous closure, will persist through the adult years. These will produce typical VSD murmurs because of flow through the defect. However, they often will not cause large enough left-to-right shunt to either produce left ventricular volume load or raise the pulmonary pressures. However, the normal left-sided pressures together with normal pulmonary pressures will give a large pressure gradient, driving the left-to-right flow through the defect. These will, therefore, result in a high-velocity flow jet, which can be picked up by using Doppler echocardiography. The only important risk, however, is that of infective endocarditis. The high-velocity jet may damage the endocardium on the right ventricular side of the defect near the septal leaflet of the tricuspid valve, which may become the nidus of infection when there is a bacteremia. The risk of endocarditis is always a possibility in all VSDs.

The clinical spectrum of small, moderate, and large isolated VSDs had been classified based on physiology into two types: *restrictive and nonrestrictive*. The term restrictive is applied when the resistance that limits the left-to-right shunt is at the site of the defect alone. It means, therefore, that the right ventricular pressure is either normal or, if elevated, it is still less than that of the left ventricle in the absence of right ventricular outflow obstruction. When the left-to-right shunt is not limited at the site of the defect, the term nonrestrictive is applied. This means equal right and left ventricular systolic pressures in the absence of right ventricular outflow obstruction. It implies, therefore, equal pulmonary and aortic systolic pressures, and the amount of left-to-right shunt is determined essentially by the pulmonary vascular resistance *(110)*.

Hemodynamic severity has been classified into four grades based on the ratio of right ventricular to left ventricular systolic pressures and the ratio of pulmonary flow (QP) to systemic flow (QS) determined at cardiac catheterization *(111)*:

1. Small: when the ratio of pulmonary to aortic systolic pressure is <0.3 and the QP:QS ratio is <1.4.
2. Moderate: when the ratio of pulmonary to aortic systolic pressures is >0.3 and the QP:QS ratio is 1.4–2.2.
3. Large: when the systolic pressure ratio is >0.3 and the QP:QS ratio is >2.2.
4. Eisenmenger: when the systolic pressure ratio is close to 1 and the QP:QS ratio is <1.5 and the net intracardiac shunt is right to left.

Septal Rupture Secondary to Myocardial Infarction

This complication used to occur before the thrombolytic era in approx 1–2% of patients with myocardial infarction. In the current era of routine thrombolytic therapy, its frequency has fallen to about 0.2% *(107)*. It accounts for about 5% of all deaths from myocardial infarction. The septal rupture is usually associated with the first myocardial infarction and will generally occur within the first week after the infarct. It is more common with anterior myocardial infarction than with inferior infarct. Rupture may be simple or complex and serpigenous. The electrocardiogram may show right bundle branch block or complete atrioventricular block. The onset is recognizable with the detection of a new murmur. The left ventricular volume load, because of the shunt, will not be well tolerated by the already compromised left ventricle secondary to the myocardial infarction. Eventually this may lead to the development of congestive cardiac failure within a few hours to a few days. The outcome is poor when associated with cardiogenic shock (usually in the context of a large infarct), when there is significant right ventricular dysfunction, or when the rupture involves the posterior septum.

General Characteristics of the Ventricular Septal Defect Murmur

1. VSD is a regurgitant lesion because the blood flows through the defect from the high-pressure left ventricle into the low-pressure right ventricle. The flow through the defect

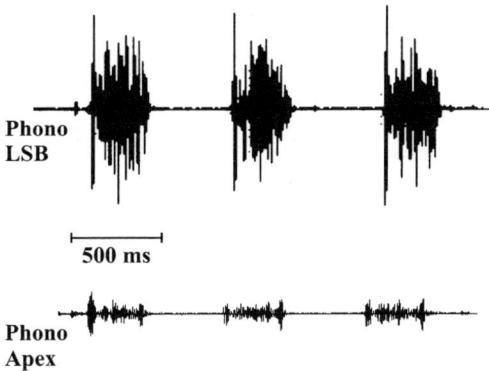

Fig. 30. Digital display of magnetic audio recordings from a patient with congenital ventricular septal defect showing the maximal loudness of the murmur at the lower left sternal border area (top) and not at the apex area (bottom).

is turbulent because of the high pressure difference. The high pressure gradient would produce a high-frequency systolic murmur, which is plateau, and will last throughout systole *(112,113)*. The murmur will last until the S2. The holo- or pansystolic murmur will sound very much like a mitral regurgitation murmur because of the predominant high frequencies.

2. The VSD murmur also will not be expected to change significantly in intensity during sudden long diastoles such as following a postextrasystolic pause or during atrial fibrillation. The left ventricle has two outlets for systole when there is a VSD, namely, the normal aorta and the right heart through the septal defect. Although the long diastole allows greater filling of the left ventricle and increases the force of contraction both by a Starling's mechanism as well as through postextrasystolic potentiation, the larger volume is ejected more easily through the aorta because of a fall in the aortic diastolic pressures during the pause. Thus, the flow through the defect will not increase and the murmur will remain essentially unchanged.

The maximal loudness of the murmur in most VSDs is the lower left sternal border area in the third and the fourth left interspace (Fig. 30).

Variations in Clinical and Auscultatory Features in Ventricular Septal Defects

SUBPULMONIC VENTRICULAR SEPTAL DEFECT

When the defect is subpulmonic, the left ventricle ejects blood directly into the pulmonary artery through the defect. The resulting murmur will, therefore, be maximally heard at the second left interspace. The murmur may have some crescendo character because of decrease in size of the defect by the late contraction of the infundibulum causing an increased velocity of flow *(114)*. Often the S2 will also be widely split. Aortic regurgitation also tends to develop in these patients because of prolapse of the right coronary cusp of the aortic valve. The latter might help to reduce the size of the defect. The long systolic murmur, which is crescendo to the A2, followed by diastolic murmur of aortic regurgitation heard over the second left interspace may be mistaken for a continuous murmur of persistent ductus arteriosus.

Large Ventricular Septal Defect

When the VSD is large and allows significant left-to-right shunt, the resulting left ventricular volume load will produce an enlarged left ventricle. The apical impulse may demonstrate a wide-area hyperdynamic impulse with good medial retraction. The excess pulmonary flow received by the left atrium will have to go through the mitral valve in diastole, and the rapid and large volume inflow may cause a short mid-diastolic flow rumble (like an S3 with a duration) at the apex.

Small Muscular Ventricular Septal Defect

When the VSD is small and affects the muscular portion of the septum, the murmur may be predominantly early systolic because during end systole the defect itself may be fully closed secondary to the ventricular contraction. Similarly, when the defect begins to undergo spontaneous closure in early childhood, the murmur may become shorter and predominantly early systolic because in the later part of systole the defect may be in fact closed. In both these instances, however, the murmur will retain the high frequencies because of the high-pressure gradient between the left ventricle and the right side *(40)*.

Ventricular Septal Defect Murmurs and Vasoactive Agents

VSD murmurs can be influenced by vasoactive agents as well as by other maneuvers, which alter the systemic pressures. Vasopressor agents, by increasing the systemic arterial pressures, will increase the left-to-right pressure difference and cause the murmur to become loud. If the VSD is small and/or in the process of closing and has a short early systolic high-frequency murmur, the murmur may be noted to become longer and pansystolic and louder, indicating that the defect is not fully anatomically closed. Squatting, by raising the aortic pressure, could cause a similar change in the intensity of the murmur. Amyl nitrite inhalation, by reducing the systemic arterial pressure, will reduce the left-to-right shunt through the defect and therefore diminish the loudness of a VSD murmur. In the presence of a vasoreactive pulmonary hypertension, amyl nitrite inhalation could cause a more significant fall in the pulmonary artery pressures, and the intensity of the murmur may remain unchanged or increase somewhat.

Ventricular Septal Defect Eisenmenger

When the VSD develops *Eisenmenger reaction* (pulmonary vascular disease) and increased pulmonary vascular resistance, the murmur will become shorter with increasing right ventricular systolic pressures *(97)*. Eventually when the pulmonary pressures are equal to systemic levels, there is no pressure difference, as such, between the left and the right ventricle. The VSD murmur is no longer heard and is replaced by an ejection murmur because of ejection of blood into a dilated pulmonary artery. The right-to-left shunt occurs predominantly during the isovolumic relaxation phase of the cardiac cycle. Simultaneous left and right ventricular pressure recordings would demonstrate that the pulmonary hypertensive right ventricle has a slower rate of fall of pressure during the phase of isovolumic relaxation. This presumably reflects the presence of diastolic dysfunction in the right ventricle. As a result of this, the pressure on the right ventricular side falls more slowly, compared to the left side. This creates enough pressure difference to cause a right-to-left shunt. Injection of agitated saline containing microbubbles of air into a systemic vein during Doppler echocardiography can be shown to cross over to the left heart only during the phase of isovolumic relaxation. It must also be pointed out that right-to-left shunt never produces turbulence to cause murmurs.

The other signs of pulmonary hypertension may also be present, such as a subxiphoid right ventricular impulse. The P2 may be loud and palpable. The S2 split at this stage is not present, resulting in a single S2. There may also be a pulmonary ejection sound. Rarely, the pulmonary valve may be regurgitant secondary to the high pulmonary artery pressures. This may cause an early diastolic blowing murmur, which starts with a loud P2. This murmur termed, the *Graham Steell murmur*, is often loudest at the second left interspace *(115)*.

VENTRICULAR SEPTAL DEFECT WITH PULMONARY STENOSIS

The combination of a VSD with pulmonary stenosis is an important feature of classic Fallot's tetralogy, where these two components are the major determinants of the clinical features and presentation. The other two components of the tetralogy, namely the straddling or overriding aorta and right ventricular hypertrophy, have very little bearing on the clinical features. The spectrum of clinical findings that can occur will depend on the size of the VSD and the severity of the pulmonary stenosis and the specific combinations of the two lesions *(116,117)*.

Large VSD With Severe Pulmonary Stenosis

With a large VSD in the presence of severe pulmonary stenosis, the right ventricular pressures will rise secondary to the obstruction to systemic levels but no higher because of the large size of the VSD. Less blood will be ejected into the pulmonary artery because of the obstruction, and the venous blood from the right ventricle may be directly ejected into the aorta. This is the case with *classic cyanotic forms of tetralogy*. The pulmonary stenosis can be either at the valve or, as is more often the case, at the infundibular level. The aorta would receive a large volume of blood from the right ventricle and may become dilated. The VSD will not have significant left-to-right shunt because of the raised right ventricular pressures, and the VSD murmur will be replaced by a pulmonary ejection murmur. The murmur, however, may be shorter and softer when the obstruction is severe because pulmonary blood flow will be significantly diminished. The dilated aorta may be associated with an aortic ejection sound. The S2 is usually single because the P2 is often inaudible. The right ventricle of the newborn is usually able to withstand the systemic pressures and will seldom show dilatation or failure with secondary tricuspid regurgitation. The jugular venous pulse will also show a relatively normal contour for the same reason. When the obstruction is very severe, as in pulmonary atresia, then there will be no blood reaching through to the pulmonary trunk. There will be compensatory bronchial collaterals, which may supply the lungs. They may produce continuous murmurs. The cyanosis may be present at birth, unlike classic tetralogy, where the cyanosis may be noted only weeks or months after birth.

Large VSD With Mild Pulmonary Stenosis

When the VSD is large but the pulmonary stenosis is mild, then the clinical features may be like those of an isolated large VSD (sometimes called the *acyanotic form of tetralogy*). The large left-to-right shunt through the defect will cause predominant left ventricular volume load. The systolic murmurs may be a result of both the VSD and the pulmonary stenosis. The ejection murmur of pulmonary stenosis may be audible over the third left interspace because the stenosis may be infundibular. The S2 split may be somewhat wide; this is not usually the case in isolated VSD. The pulmonary stenosis may increase because of hypertrophy of the crista supraventricularis, causing some infundibular stenosis as well. As the degree of resistance at the site of stenosis keeps increasing, then the left-to-right shunt will diminish and the VSD murmur may shorten and eventually be replaced by an ejection murmur of pulmonary stenosis.

Small VSD With Severe Pulmonary Stenosis

The VSD may be small initially, or a large VSD may have been partially closed by the septal leaflet of the tricuspid valve. In the presence of a small defect and severe pulmonary stenosis, the right ventricular pressures can rise above the systemic level because the right ventricle will not have direct access to the aorta. The clinical features will therefore more closely resemble pulmonary stenosis with an intact ventricular septum. The murmur will be essentially that of pulmonary stenosis, namely ejection in type, because the high right ventricular pressure will not allow any left-to-right shunt. The stenosis is generally infundibular in the presence of a VSD, and the murmur will be maximal in loudness in the third and fourth left interspace.

Small VSD With Mild Pulmonary Stenosis

The defect will allow very little volume overload of the left ventricle, and the right-sided pressures will be only minimally elevated. The murmur is, however, predominantly a result of the VSD and will be pansystolic and regurgitant in type.

TOTAL ABSENCE OF VENTRICULAR SEPTUM

This congenital anomaly implies that there is a *single ventricle*. The most common type is morphologically a left ventricle with a small remnant of the right ventricular infundibulum forming the outflow into the aorta. The great vessels are invariably transposed, meaning that the aorta is anterior and somewhat to the right of the posterior pulmonary artery. The anomaly may or may not be associated with pulmonary stenosis. Both atrioventricular valves are present generally and properly related.

When there is no pulmonary stenosis, the blood from both atria stream through the ventricle without too much mixing. Pulmonary blood flow is increased and the cyanosis is minimal. The increased pulmonary flow would cause volume load on the left atrium and the single ventricle. Sometimes there may be an element of subaortic obstruction at the level of the infundibulum. Ejection murmurs may be best heard at the lower left sternal border and the apex. The S2 is usually loud and single from both components. A2 is accentuated because of the anterior position of the aorta. Pulmonary hypertension, which is usually present, would increase the P2. The increased flow through the mitral valve may cause a short mid-diastolic flow murmur.

When there is pulmonary stenosis or when the pulmonary vascular resistance is increased, there will be greater mixing and the pulmonary flow will be reduced with increased cyanosis. The loudness and length of the ejection murmur of the pulmonary stenosis will vary inversely with the severity of the stenosis. The S2 will be single because of the A2 component.

POST-MYOCARDIAL-INFARCTION SEPTAL RUPTURE

In the acquired septal rupture secondary to acute myocardial infarction, the murmur may be audible near the apex, particularly when the septal rupture is in the apical por-

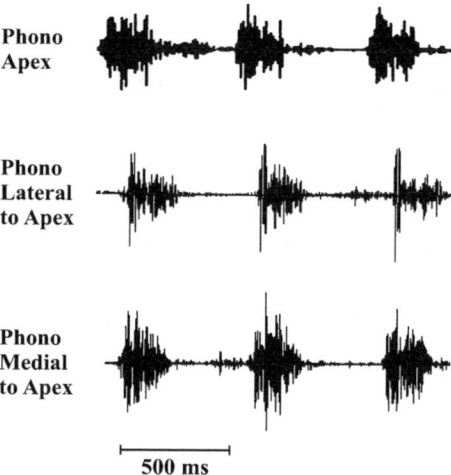

Fig. 31. Digital display of magnetic audio recordings taken at the apex (top), lateral to the apex (middle), and medial to the apex (bottom) from a patient with septal rupture complicating acute myocardial infarction. The maximal loudness of the murmur is at the apex and medial to the apex. The murmur is less intense lateral to the apex.

tion of the septum. However, the maximal loudness may be demonstrated to be medial to the apex. This is different from papillary muscle rupture causing mitral regurgitation murmur, which has maximal loudness at the apex and immediately lateral to the apex (Fig. 31).

(For additional examples review Phono Files 25–29 under Heart Murmurs (Part 1) on the Companion CD)

CLINICAL ASSESSMENT OF SYSTOLIC MURMURS

Clinical history, when obtained and properly interpreted, will often give direction as to what possibilities need to be considered in the differential diagnosis. Then a more focused physical examination can be performed, taking into account all of the possibilities that are being considered, paying careful attention to the features of the venous pulse, the arterial pulse, and the precordial pulsations, including the apical impulse. Each one of these must be evaluated in relation to the possible diagnoses entertained. If one trains oneself to do such a focused examination, often by the time one is ready to auscultate the diagnosis is generally obvious. Auscultation then becomes confirmatory of what one suspects the diagnosis to be. For instance, in the case of a 65- year-old man presenting with exertional dyspnea and angina, differential diagnosis must include, among other things, aortic valve disease. A slow rate of rise of the carotid pulse with normal or low amplitude will point to aortic stenosis, whereas a large-amplitude carotid pulse with normal or fast rate of rise together with bounding peripheral pulses and a hyperdynamic wide area left ventricular apical impulse will suggest the presence of aortic regurgitation. On the other hand, a fast-rising carotid pulse with normal amplitude and normal peripheral pulses and a wide-area hyperdynamic left ventricular impulse would suggest a lesion such as mitral regurgitation. In such a situation one looks for the murmur of mitral regurgitation on auscultation, and one also will look for the auscultatory signs to assess its severity.

Sometimes, however, asymptomatic patients may be referred for evaluation of heart murmurs. Often when a patient is referred for heart murmur evaluation, it will be for a systolic murmur because they are generally more easily detected. The clinical assessment of systolic murmurs, even in asymptomatic patients, still includes the careful assessment of the venous pulse, the arterial pulses and the precordial pulsations, and the evaluation of the clues that these can provide in terms of the cause of the systolic murmurs. The auscultatory assessment comes next.

The Auscultatory Assessment of Systolic Murmurs

Auscultatory assessment of systolic murmurs presupposes that the heart sounds have been auscultated, identified, and characterized, including the normal S1 and S2 as well as any extra sounds that may be recognized such as the S4, S3, opening snap, ejection clicks, as well as nonejection click or clicks. Next, the systolic murmur itself is auscultated, noting its character, its predominant frequencies, whether low, medium (harsh), or high (blowing), its length, the location of its maximal loudness, as well as all the locations where it is heard. The following points will be of help in its analysis:

1. An attempt should be made to determine whether the murmur is ejection or regurgitant in type. If the S2 is present, one should listen for the cadence of the ejection murmur, namely:

    da ...ha.. da.

    formed by the S1, the peak of the crescendo of the ejection murmur, and then the S2. If a typical cadence of an ejection murmur is recognized, then the problem becomes easy.

2. Mere audibility of S2 does not mean a murmur is ejection in type, indicating a pause between the end of the murmur and the S2. This sign is only helpful when the relative grade of loudness of the murmur and that of the S2 are considered together. When the murmur is louder than the S2, then audibility of S2 will mean that there is a distinct pause between the end of the murmur and the S2; therefore, the murmur must be ejection in type. In the converse situation, where the murmur is softer than the S2, the S2 may be audible and the murmur could be regurgitant. In such a situation more importance needs to be paid to the predominant frequencies of the murmur, namely, whether it is harsh and low, medium or blowing and high in frequency. The former, of course, is more characteristic of an ejection murmur, while the latter favors a regurgitant murmur. In general, radiation of the murmurs has no diagnostic value in terms of its origins. While mitral regurgitation murmurs generally may be transmitted to the axilla and posteriorly and the aortic ejection murmurs may be transmitted to the carotids, exceptions to these occur more often than not to make this a useful distinguishing feature.

3. When S2 is not heard, then the cadence of the ejection murmur will not exist and this method of recognition will no longer be possible. When ejection murmurs are

long and have delayed peak, it may cause some confusion. This may happen, for instance, with significant pulmonary valvular or infundibular stenosis murmurs. These murmurs may go past the A2, and if the P2 is soft, the S2 may not be clearly audible. Then other methods such as the effect of sudden long diastole may have to be looked for. One should attempt to look for any sudden change in rhythm of the heart, such as may be caused by a premature beat. Sometimes turning the patient to the left lateral decubitus position may bring out a premature beat. Occasionally patients may have spontaneous extrasystoles or could be in atrial fibrillation with changing RR intervals and therefore changing durations of diastoles. If any of these is present, one needs to pay attention to the effect of the long diastolic pause on the loudness of the murmur. Sometimes this may occur even before one is ready to look for it. It is important to make use of the situation as and when it presents when listening to a systolic murmur. A sudden long diastolic pause accentuates the intensity of the ejection murmurs for reasons that have been dealt with at length in the previous sections.

4. Once the murmur is characterized as ejection in type, then all causes of ejection murmurs need to be considered. These include increased ejection velocity of either normal or increased stroke volume, ejection of increased stroke volume through normal outflow tracts, as well as ejection through roughened or stenosed outflow tracts. The length of the murmur often helps because short-ejection murmurs are not usually associated with significant stenosis. The next location of maximal loudness, whether it is second left interspace, third left interspace, lower left sternal border area, apex area, or second right interspace, becomes an important consideration. Pulmonary ejection murmurs are often maximally loud at the second left interspace, whereas aortic ejection murmurs are best heard at the apex and occasionally at the apex and the second right interspace. Hypertrophic obstructive cardiomyopathy usually has maximal murmur intensity at the left sternal border and the apex. The infundibular pulmonary stenosis murmurs usually have maximal intensity over the third left interspace.

5. When right-sided ejection murmurs are considered, the effect of inspiration on the intensity of the murmur also needs to be assessed because these murmurs typically get louder on inspiration. In addition, one needs to pay attention to whether or not an ejection click is present. If an ejection click is detected, then an attempt should be made to decide whether it has the characteristics of a pulmonary ejection click, which typically softens or disappears on inspiration. If a left-sided ejection murmur is detected, one needs to look for aortic ejection click. When outflow tract obstruction is being considered, the presence of ejection click would indicate stenosis at the valvular level of the outflow tract.

6. In addition, evaluation of left-sided ejection murmurs requires assessment of the effects of changing posture such as standing and squatting on the intensity of the murmurs. These are obviously important in confirming or ruling out hypertrophic obstructive cardiomyopathy, which is an important cause of left-sided ejection murmur. The dynamic obstruction in this disorder gets worse on standing because of a decrease in heart size caused by decreased venous return. The murmur, therefore, gets louder. On squatting the reverse will happen. The murmur will get softer or disappear. Aortic ejection murmurs of all other causes will either not change or actually diminish in intensity because of the decreased stroke output caused by the decreased venous return caused by standing.

7. If the murmur is considered regurgitant and is pansystolic, then the location of maximal loudness becomes important in the differential diagnosis. Mitral regurgitation murmurs are typically maximal in intensity at the apex and slightly lateral to the apex, whereas the maximal loudness of a VSD murmur is at the lower left sternal border area and medial to the apex. The tricuspid regurgitation murmur is maximally loud over the lower sternum and the xiphoid area. In addition, tricuspid regurgitation murmur may be noted to increase on inspiration. Abnormal jugular contours (large-amplitude *v wave* with a *y descent*) characteristic of tricuspid regurgitation and a subxiphoid right ventricular impulse are additional features that will favor tricuspid regurgitation. Sometimes an enlarged right ventricle may take over the normal apex area, and the murmur of tricuspid regurgitation may be heard fairly well at the apex. The character of the apical impulse may reveal this to be right ventricular with a lateral retraction. Both mitral regurgitation as well as VSD, when significant, will cause left ventricular volume overload and therefore would be associated with a wide-area hyperdynamic left ventricular impulse. Both may produce an S3 or a short mid-diastolic flow rumble at the apex, reflecting the increased mitral inflow. A wide-split S2, if present, may reflect severe mitral regurgitation. This is not a feature in VSD. Loud M1 and an opening snap, when detected, will point to a rheumatic etiology for the mitral regurgitation. If the murmur is mid- to late systolic and crescendo to S2 or preceded by the presence of nonejection mid- to late systolic click or clicks, it will suggest the presence of mitral prolapse as a cause of the mitral regurgitation murmur.

8. The effect of change in posture becomes important because mitral regurgitation murmurs from prolapsed and redundant mitral valve leaflets become longer and louder on standing with decrease in venous return and decreased heart size. The opposite will happen with squatting. The papillary muscle dysfunction murmurs usually do not behave this way. In fact, they may increase in intensity with squatting if there is significant blood pressure rise. Ventricular septal defect murmurs may also tend to increase in intensity on squatting if there is a significant rise in blood pressure.

9. Occasionally both an ejection murmur and a regurgitant murmur may be present in the same patient as in some instances of aortic stenosis and mitral regurgitation. The recognition of the presence of both murmurs may be easy. The aortic stenosis ejection murmur may be maximally loud at the second right interspace and may have all the characteristics of an ejection murmur and its typical cadence. The mitral regurgitation murmur may be maximally loud at the apex and may have all the features of the mitral regurgitation murmur, with typical blowing quality and high frequency, lasting all the way to S2. At other times, however, the recognition may not be so easy because of the well-known *Gallavardin phenomenon*, whereby the high-frequency components of an aortic ejection murmur may be selectively transmitted upstream and therefore to the apex. If this should happen, there may be only one lesion, for instance, aortic stenosis, and yet one may mistake it for two lesions, namely both aortic stenosis and mitral regurgitation. The best way to be sure of the presence of both lesions and two different murmurs is identification of two different responses of the murmurs to sudden change in rhythm producing a long diastole. If the patient is in atrial fibrillation, it will be easier. Then one can assess the effect of the long pause on the intensity of the murmur in both locations, namely, the second right interspace and the apex area. If they behave differently,

namely, if the murmur at the second right interspace becomes louder and the one at the apex does not change much, then one can be certain of the presence of both the ejection and the regurgitant murmurs.

10. A similar problem may arise with acute severe mitral regurgitation. In this instance the murmur will have often a lot of low and medium frequencies and may sound harsher in quality. The murmur may end before S2, being decrescendo secondary to early buildup of a high left atrial *v wave* pressure. In addition, the murmur may be heard over a wide area, including the base of the heart. A hyperdynamic left ventricular apical impulse and a fast-rising carotid pulse with normal amplitude and an S3 (or its equivalent short mid-diastolic flow murmur) may bear clues to the presence of significant mitral regurgitation. If the patient has premature beats, the behavior of the murmur following the postectopic pause will show that it is not an ejection murmur.

11. If the murmur cannot be categorized accurately as to whether it is ejection or regurgitant in type, then it is best described by its predominant frequencies as to whether it is harsh and low to medium in frequency (meaning ejection in quality) or it is high in frequency and blowing (meaning regurgitant in quality). It gives a reference point to work with in trying to arrive at its cause. It needs to be considered obviously in relation to all the findings on examination. Again, the length of the murmur, the location of maximal loudness, the effect of inspiration, and the effect of changing postures, namely, the effect of standing and squatting, all need to be determined and used in a similar fashion, as described previously.

REFERENCES

1. McDonald DA. Blood Flow in Arteries. London: Edward Arnold Publishers Ltd, 1960.
2. McKusick VA. Cardiovascular Sound in Health and Disease. Baltimore, MD: Williams and Wilkins, 1958.
3. Rushmer RF. Cardiovascular Dynamics. Philadelphia, PA: W.B. Saunders, Co., 1970.
4. Bruns DL. A general theory of the causes of murmurs in the cardiovascular system. Am J Med. 1959; 27:360–374.
5. Constant J, Lippschutz EJ. Diagramming and grading heart sounds and murmurs. Am Heart J 1965; 70:326–332.
6. Perloff JK. The physiologic mechanisms of cardiac and vascular physical signs. J Am Coll Cardiol 1983;1:184–198.
7. Lembo NJ, Dell'Italia LJ, Crawford MH, O'Rourke RA. Bedside diagnosis of systolic murmurs. N Engl J Med 1988;318:1572–1578.
8. Leatham A. Systolic murmurs. Circulation 1958;17:601–611.
9. Murgo JP, Altobelli SA, Dorethy JF, et al. Normal ventricular ejection dynamics in man during rest and exercise. In: Leon DF, Shaver JA, eds. Physiologic Principles of Heart Sounds and Murmurs, Vol. 92. New York, NY: American Heart Association, 1975.
10. Constant J. Bedside Cardiology. Boston, MA: Little, Brown and Company, 1976.
11. Henke RP, March HW, Hultgren HN. An aid to identification of the murmur of aortic stenosis with atypical localization. Am Heart J 1960;60:354–363.
12. Deleon AC, Jr., Perloff JK, Twigg H, Majd M. The straight back syndrome: clinical cardiovascular manifestations. Circulation 1965;32:193–203.
13. Still GF. Common Disorders and Diseases of Childhood. London, UK: Frowde, Hodder and Stoughton, 1909.
14. Joffe HS. Genesis of Still's innocent systolic murmur. Br Heart J 1992;67:206.
15. Donnerstein R, Thomsen VS. Hemodynamic and anatomical factors affecting the frequency content of Still's innocent murmur. Am J Cardiol 1994;74:508–510.

16. Leatham A, Gray I. Auscultatory and phonocardiographic signs of atrial septal defect. Br Heart J 1956;18:193–208.
17. Dalldorf FG, Willis PW, 4th. Angled aorta ("sigmoid septum") as a cause of hypertrophic subaortic stenosis. Hum Pathol 1985;16:457–462.
18. Paley HW. Left ventricular outflow tract obstruction heart sounds and murmurs. American Heart Association Monograph 1975;46:107–117.
19. Edwards JE. Pathology of left ventricular outflow tract obstruction. Circulation 1965;31:586.
20. Gallavardin L, Pauper-Ravault. Le souffle' duretrecissement aortique puet changer de timbre et devenir dans sa propagation apexienne. Lyon Med 1925:523.
21. Bonner AJ, Jr., Sacks HN, Tavel ME. Assessing the severity of aortic stenosis by phonocardiography and external carotid pulse recordings. Circulation 1973;48:247–252.
22. Braunwald E, Roberts WC, Goldblatt A, Aygen MM, Rockoff SD, Gilbert JW. Aortic stenosis: physiological, pathological, and clinical concepts. Combined Clinical Staff Conference at the National Institutes of Health. Ann Intern Med 1963;58:494–522.
23. Glancy DL, Shepherd RL, Beiser D, Epstein SE. The dynamic nature of left ventricular outflow obstruction in idiopathic hypertrophic subaortic stenosis. Ann Intern Med 1971;75:589–593.
24. Ross J, Jr, Braunwald E, Gault JH, Mason DT, Morrow AC. The mechanism of intraventricular pressure gradient in idiopathic hypertrophic subaortic stenosis. Circulation 1966;34:558.
25. Murgo JP, Alter BR, Dorethy JF, Altobelli SA, McGranahan GM, Jr. Dynamics of left ventricular ejection in obstructive and nonobstructive hypertrophic cardiomyopathy. J Clin Invest 1980;66:1369–1382.
26. Braunwald E, Morrow AG, Cornell WP, Aygem MM, Hilbish .TF. Idiopathic hypertrophic subaortic stenosis. Clinical, hemodynamic and angiographic manifestations. Am J Med 1960;29:924.
27. Shah PM, Gramiak R, Adelman AG, Wigle ED. Role of echocardiography in diagnostic and hemodynamic assessment of hypertrophic subaortic stenosis. Circulation 1971;44:891–898.
28. Sherrid MV, Gunsburg DZ, Moldenhauer S, Pearle G. Systolic anterior motion begins at low left ventricular outflow tract velocity in obstructive hypertrophic cardiomyopathy. J Am Coll Cardiol 2000;36:1344–1354.
29. Wigle ED, Adelman AG, Auger P, Marquis Y. Mitral regurgitation in muscular subaortic stenosis. Am J Cardiol 1969;24:698–706.
30. Braunwald E, Seidman CE, Sigwart U. Contemporary evaluation and management of hypertrophic cardiomyopathy. Circulation 2002;106:1312–1316.
31. Mason DT, Braunwald E, Ross J, Jr. Effects of changes in body position on the severity of obstruction to left ventricular outflow in idiopathic hypertrophic subaortic stenosis. Circulation 1966;33:374–382.
32. Grewe K, Crawford MH, O'Rourke RA. Differentiation of cardiac murmurs by dynamic auscultation. Curr Probl Cardiol 1988;13:669–721.
33. Nishimura RA, Tajik AJ. The Valsalva maneuver and response revisited. Mayo Clin Proc 1986;61:211–217.
34. Iida K, Sugishita Y, Ajisaka R, et al. Sigmoid septum causing left ventricular outflow tract obstruction: a case report. J Cardiogr 1986;16:237–247.
35. Logan WF, Jones EW, Walker E, Coulshed N, Epstein EJ. Familial supravalvar aortic stenosis. Br Heart J 1965;27:547–559.
36. Beuren AJ, Schulze C, Eberle P, Harmjanz D, Apitz J. The syndrome of supravalvular aortic stenosis, peripheral pulmonary stenosis, mental retardation and similar facial appearance. Am J Cardiol 1964;13:471–483.
37. Wooley CF, Hosier DM, Booth RW, Molnar W, Sirak HD, Ryan JM. Supravalvular aortic stenosis. Clinical experiences with four patients including familial occurrence. Am J Med 1961;31:717–725.
38. Goldstein RE, Epstein SE. Mechanism of elevated innominate artery pressures in supravalvular aortic stenosis. Circulation 1970;42:23–29.
39. French JW, Guntheroth WG. An explanation of asymmetric upper extremity blood pressures in supravalvular aortic stenosis: the Coanda effect. Circulation 1970;42:31–36.
40. Perloff JK. The Clinical Recognition of Congenital Heart Disease. Philadelphia, PA: W.B. Saunders, 1979–1981:279,312.
41. Perloff JK. Recognition and differential diagnosis of pulmonary stenosis. In: Segal BL, ed. The Theory and Practice of Auscultation. Philadelphia, PA: F.A. Davis Co., 1963.

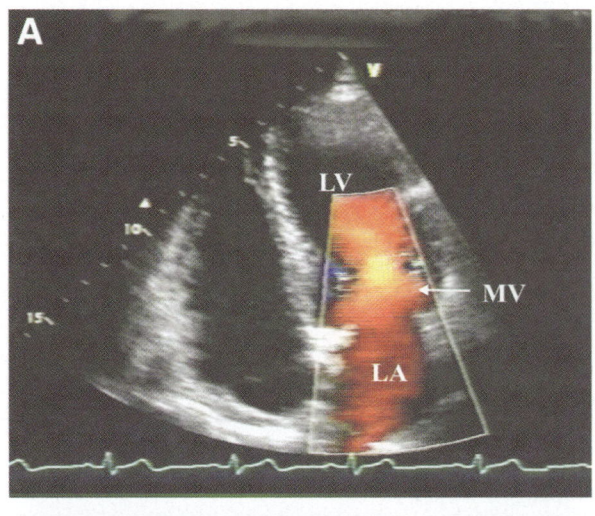

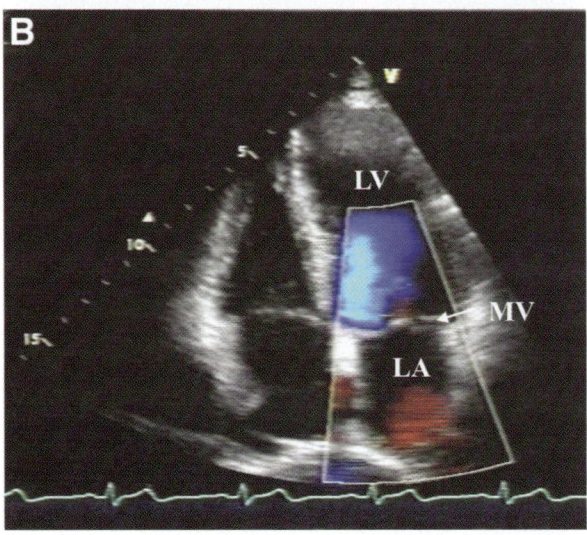

Color Plate 1, Fig. 1A,B. Two-dimensional echocardiographic images with Doppler color flow mapping from a normal subject in the apical four-chamber view taken in diastole (**A**) and systole (**B**). (*See* complete caption and discussion on p. 212 in Chapter 7.)

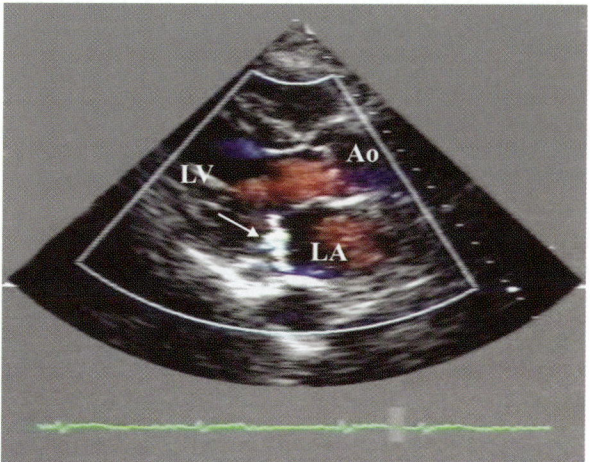

Color Plate 2, Fig. 2. Two-dimensional echocardiographic images and Doppler color flow mapping from a patient with mitral regurgitation taken in the parasternal long axis. (*See* complete caption and discussion on p. 213 in Chapter 7.)

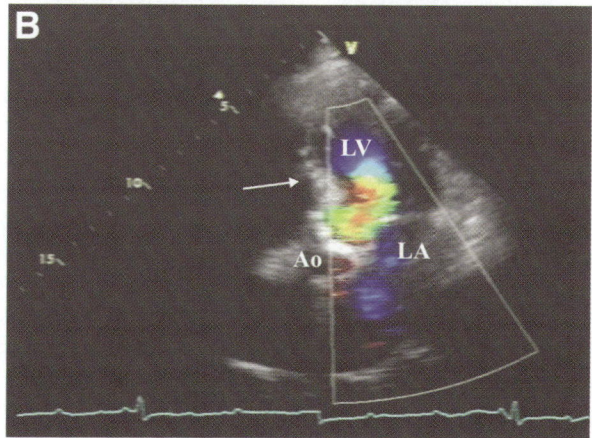

Color Plate 3, Fig. 7B. Doppler color flow image showing turbulent flow across the left ventricular outflow, in apical four-chamber view. (*See* complete caption on p. 223 and discussion on p. 222 in Chapter 7.)

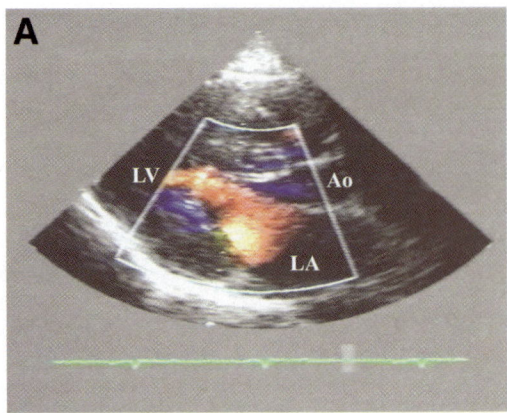

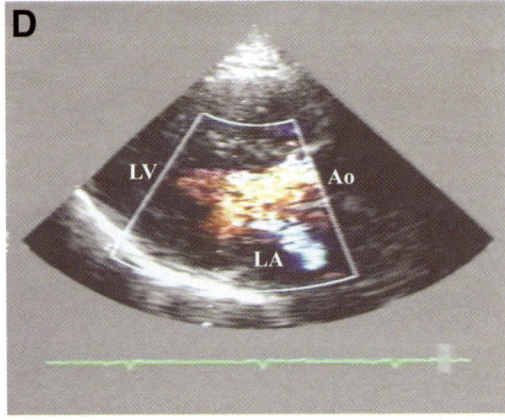

Color Plate 4, Fig. 12A,D. Two-dimensional echocardiographic images in the parasternal view from a patient with hypertrophic obstructive cardiomyopathy with severe subaortic obstruction. The diastolic frame (**A**) shows the open mitral valve allowing the inflow from the left atrium (LA) into the left ventricle (LV). In (**D**), turbulent outflow as well as some mitral regurgitation. (*See* complete caption and discussion on p. 226 in Chapter 7.)

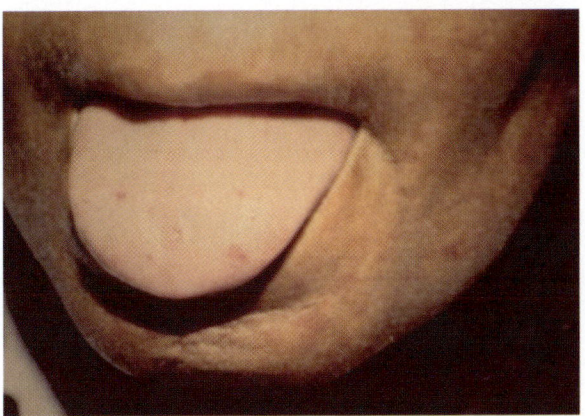

Color Plate 5, Fig. 3. Osler–Weber–Rendu syndrome. (*See* complete caption on p. 367 and discussion on p. 365 in Chapter 11.)

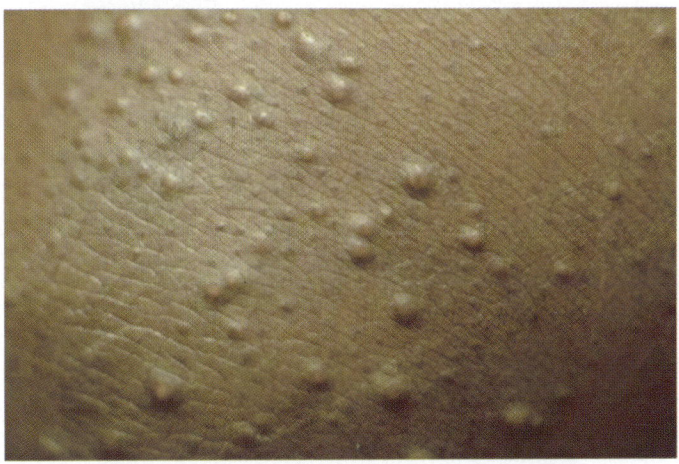

Color Plate 6, Fig. 6. Eruptive xanthoma. Skin lesions over back and chest resemble acne. (*See* complete caption on p. 370 and discussion on p. 369 in Chapter 11.)

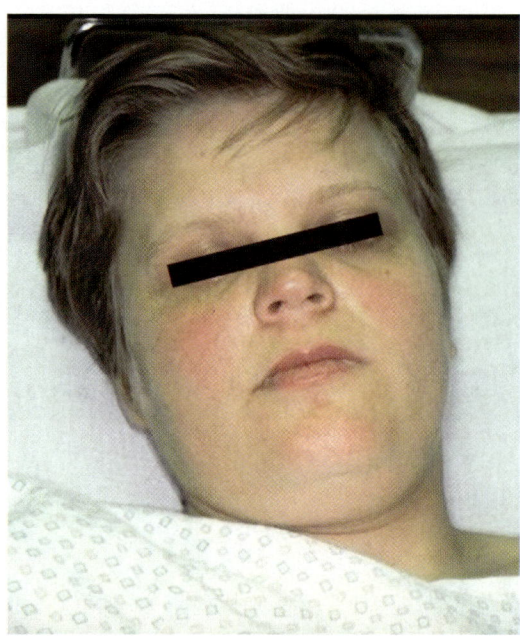

Color Plate 7, Fig. 7. Mitral facies and malar flush in 35-yr-old woman with mitral stenosis and mitral regurgitation. (*See* complete caption and discussion on p. 373 in Chapter 11.)

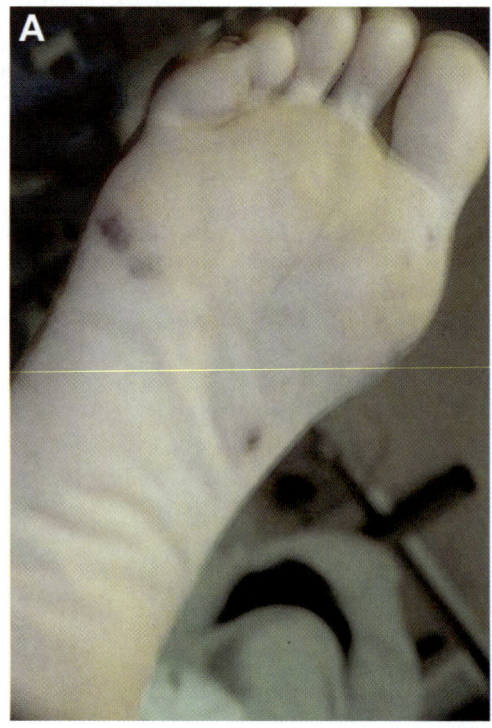

Color Plate 8, Fig. 12A. Janeway lesions in infective endocarditis in 50-yr-old drug addict. (*See* complete caption on p. 378 and discussion on p. 377 in Chapter 11.)

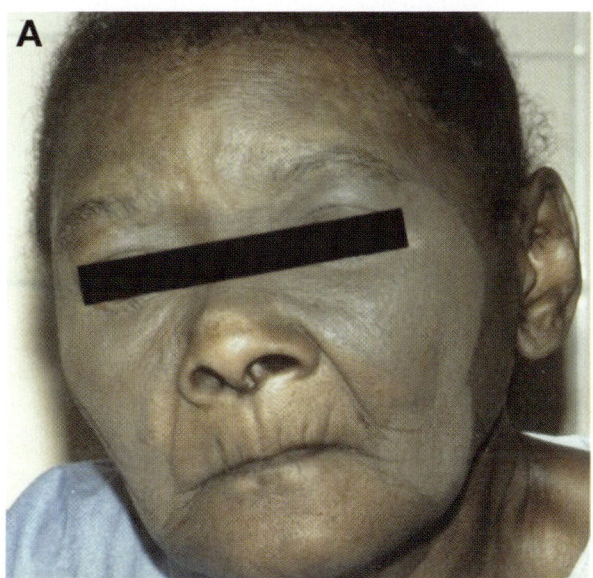

Color Plate 9, Fig. 13A. Mixed connective tissue diseases: patient with mask facies with puckering of skin around lips and malar depigmentation. (*See* complete caption and discussion on p. 379 in Chapter 11.)

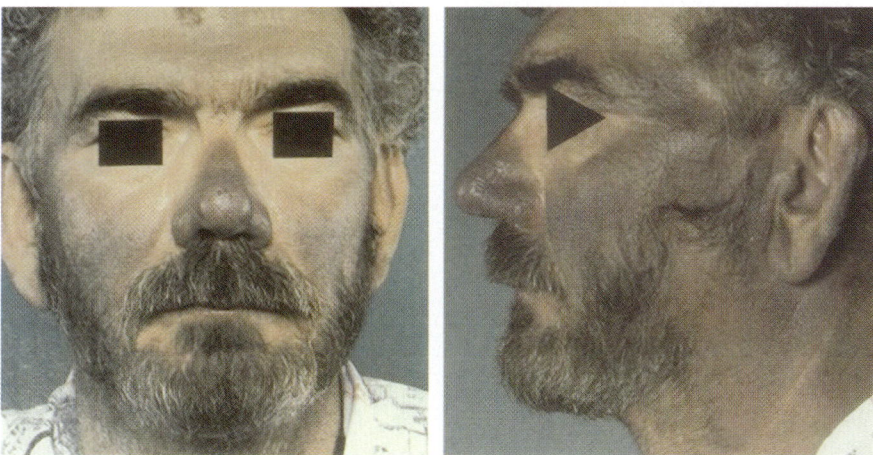

Color Plate 10, Fig. 17. Amiodarone skin toxicity. (*See* complete caption and discussion on p. 383 in Chapter 11.)

42. Perloff JK, Harvey WP. Auscultatory and phonocardiographic manifestations of pure mitral regurgitation. Prog Cardiovasc Dis 1962;5:172–194.
43. Karliner JS, O'Rourke RA, Kearney DJ, Shabetai R. Haemodynamic explanation of why the murmur of mitral regurgitation in independent of cycle length. Br Heart J 1973;35:397–401.
44. Ranganathan N, Lam JH, Wigle ED, Silver MD. Morphology of the human mitral valve. II. The value leaflets. Circulation 1970;41:459–467.
45. Ranganathan N, Silver MD, Wigle ED. Recent advances in the knowledge of the anatomy of the mitral valve. In: Kalmanson D, ed. The Mitral Valve—A Pluridisciplinary Approach. Acton, MA: Publishing Sciences Group Inc., 1976:3–13.
46. Ranganathan N, Burch GE. Gross morphology and arterial supply of the papillary muscles of the left ventricle of man. Am Heart J 1969;77:506–516.
47. Lam JH, Ranganathan N, Wigle ED, Silver MD. Morphology of the human mitral valve. I. Chordae tendineae: a new classification. Circulation 1970;41:449–458.
48. Perloff JK, Roberts WC. The mitral apparatus. Functional anatomy of mitral regurgitation. Circulation 1972;46:227–239.
49. Fontana ME, Sparks EA, Boudoulas H, Wooley CF. Mitral valve prolapse and the mitral valve prolapse syndrome. Curr Probl Cardiol 1991;16:309–375.
50. Ranganathan N, Silver MD, Robinson TI, et al. Angiographic-morphologic correlation in patients with severe mitral regurgitation due to prolapse of the posterior mitral valve leaflet. Circulation 1973;48:514–518.
51. Selzer A, Katayama F. Mitral regurgitation: clinical patterns, pathophysiology and natural history. Medicine (Baltimore) 1972;51:337–366.
52. Rotem CE, Hultgren HN. Corrected transposition of the great vessels without associated defects. Am Heart J 1965;70:305–318.
53. Tsakiris AG, Rastelli GC, Amorim Dde S, Titus JL, Wood EH. Effect of experimental papillary muscle damage on mitral valve closure in intact anesthetized dogs. Mayo Clin Proc 1970;45: 275–285.
54. Mittal AK, Langston M, Jr., Cohn KE, Selzer A, Kerth WJ. Combined papillary muscle and left ventricular wall dysfunction as a cause of mitral regurgitation. An experimental study. Circulation 1971;44:174–180.
55. Phillips JH, Burch GE, Depasquale NP. The syndrome of papillary muscle dysfunction. Its clinical recognition. Ann Intern Med 1963;59:508–520.
56. Shelburne JC, Rubinstein D, Gorlin R. A reappraisal of papillary muscle dysfunction; correlative clinical and angiographic study. Am J Med 1969;46:862–871.
57. Cuasay RS, Morse DP, Spagna P, Fernandez J, Lemole GM. Massive mitral regrgitation from chordal rupture and coronary artery disease. Ann Thorac Surg 1978;25:438–443.
58. Ranganathan N, Silver MD, Freeman.M, Wilson.J.K. Clinico-pathological correlations in acute and acute on chronic mitral regurgitation. XII Inter-American Congress of Cardiology, Vancouver, June 16–21, 1985.
59. Clements SD, Jr., Story WE, Hurst JW, Craver JM, Jones EL. Ruptured papillary muscle, a complication of myocardial infarction: clinical presentation, diagnosis, and treatment. Clin Cardiol 1985; 8:93–103.
60. Bass NM, Sharratt GP. Left atrial myxoma diagnosed by echocardiography, with observations on tumor movement. Br Heart J 1973;35:1332–1335.
61. Carabello BA. Progress in mitral and aortic regurgitation. Prog Cardiovasc Dis 2001;43:457–475.
62. Bonow RO, Carabello B, de Leon AC, et al. ACC/AHA guidelines for the management of patients with valvular heart disease. A report of the American College of Cardiology/American Heart Association. Task Force on Practice Guidelines (Committee on Management of Patients with Valvular Heart Disease). J Am Coll Cardiol 1998;32:1486–1588.
63. Carabello BA. Mitral valve regurgitation. Curr Probl Cardiol 1998;23:202–241.
64. Carabello BA. Concentric versus eccentric remodeling. J Card Fail 2002;8:S258–263.
65. Ronan JA, Jr., Steelman RB, DeLeon AC, Jr., Waters TJ, Perloff JK, Harvey WP. The clinical diagnosis of acute severe mitral insufficiency. Am J Cardiol 1971;27:284–290.
66. Sutton GC, Craige E. Clinical signs of severe acute mitral regurgitation. Am J Cardiol 1967; 20:141–144.
67. Barlow JB, Pocock WA. The significance of late systolic murmurs and mid-late systolic clicks. Md State Med J 1963;12:76–77.

68. Fontana ME, Pence HL, Leighton RF, Wooley CF. The varying clinical spectrum of the systolic click-late systolic murmur syndrome. Circulation 1970;41:807–816.
69. Ranganathan N, Silver MD, Robinson TI., Wilson JK. Idiopathic prolapsed mitral leaflet sysndrome Angiographic clinical correlations. Circulation 1976;54:707–715.
70. Waller BF, Morrow AG, Maron BJ, et al. Etiology of clinically isolated, severe, chronic, pure mitral regurgitation: analysis of 97 patients over 30 years of age having mitral valve replacement. Am Heart J 1982;104:276–288.
71. Barlow J, Pocock WA, Marchand.P, Denny M. The significance of late systolic murmurs. Am Heart J 1963;66:443–452.
72. Ronan JA, Perloff JK, Harvey WP. Systolic clicks and the late systolic murmur; intracardiac phonocardiographic fvidence of their mitral valve origin. Am Heart J 1965;70:319–325.
73. Wigle ED, Rakowski H, Ranganathan N, Silver MC. Mitral valve prolapse. Annu Rev Med 1976; 27:165–180.
74. Criley JM, Lewis KB, Humphries JO, Ross RS. Prolapse of the mitral valve: clinical and cineangiocardiographic findings. Br Heart J 1966;28:488–496.
75. Leon DF, Leonard JJ, Kroetz FW, Page WL, Shaver JA, Lancaster JF. Late systolic murmurs, clicks, and whoops arising from the mitral valve. A transseptal intracardiac phonocardiographic analysis. Am Heart J 1966;72:325–336.
76. Hancock EW, Cohn K. The syndrome associated with midsystolic click and late systolic murmur. Am J Med 1966;41:183–196.
77. Fontana ME, Kissel GL, Criley M. Functional anatomy of mitral valve prolapse. American Heart Association Monograph 1975;46:126.
78. Luisada AA, Leon F, Singhal A, Nunez A. Various types of systolic clicks in patients with muscular subaortic stenosis. Jpn Heart J 1985;26:133–143.
79. Holmes AM, Logan WF, Winterbottom T. Transient systolic murmurs in angina pectoris. Am Heart J 1968;76:680–684.
80. Sanders CA, Armstrong PW, Willerson JT, Dinsmore RE. Etiology and differential diagnosis of acute mitral regurgitation. Prog Cardiovasc Dis 1971;14:129–152.
81. DePace NL, Nestico PF, Morganroth J. Acute severe mitral regurgitation. Pathophysiology, clinical recognition, and management. Am J Med 1985;78:293–306.
82. Tavel ME, Campbell RW, Zimmer JF. Late systolic murmurs and mitral regurgitation. Am J Cardiol 1965;15:719–725.
83. Forrester JS, Diamond G, Freedman S, et al. Silent mitral insufficiency in acute myocardial infarction. Circulation 1971;44:877–883.
84. Nishimura RA, Schaff HV, Shub C, Gersh BJ, Edwards WD, Tajik AJ. Papillary muscle rupture complicating acute myocardial infarction: analysis of 17 patients. Am J Cardiol 1983;51:373–377.
85. Caulfield JB, Page DL, Kastor JA, Sanders CA. Connective tissue abnormalities in spontaneous rupture of chordae tendineae. Arch Pathol 1971;91:537–541.
86. Cohen LS. Atypical and acute mitral regurgitation. American Heart Association Monograph 1975;46:122–125.
87. Silver MD, Lam JH, Ranganathan N, Wigle ED. Morphology of the human tricuspid valve. Circulation 1971;43:333–348.
88. Wooley CF. The spectrum of tricuspid regurgitation. American Heart Association Monograph 1975;46:139–148.
89. Ewy GA. Tricuspid valve disease. In: Alpert JS, Dalen .JE, Rahimtoola SH, eds. Valvular Heart Disease. Philadelphia, PA: Lippincott Williams and Wilkins, 2000:377–392.
90. Gotzsche H, Falholt W. Ebstein's anomaly of the tricuspid valve; a review of the literature and report of 6 new cases. Am Heart J 1954;47:587–603.
91. Roberts WC. A unique heart disesae associated with a unique cancer: carcinoid heart disease. Am J Cardiol 1997;80:251–256.
92. Rubin LJ. Primary pulmonary hypertesnion. N Engl J Med 1997;336:111–117.
93. Dartevelle P, Fadel E, Mussot S, et al. Chronic thromboembolic pulmonary hypertension. Eur Respir J 2004;23:637–648.
94. Wright JL, Levy RD, Churg A. Pulmonary hypertension in chronic obstructive pulmonary disease: current theories of pathogenesis and their implications for treatment. Thorax 2005;60:605–609.
95. Keogh AM, McNeil KD, Williams T, Gabbay E, Cleland LG. Pulmonary arterial hypertension: a new era in management. Med J Aust 2003;178:564–567.

96. Palevsky HI, Fishman AP. Chronic cor pulmonale. Etiology and management. JAMA 1990;263: 2347–2353.
97. Wood P. The Eisenmenger syndrome or pulmonary hypertension with reversed central shunt. Br Heart J 1963;2:701.
98. Wood P. Pulmonary hypertension. Br Med Bull 1952;8:348.
99. Rios JC, Massumi RA, Breesmen WT, Sarin RK. Auscultatory features of acute tricuspid regurgitation. Am J Cardiol 1969;23:4–11.
100. Becu LM, Burchell HB, Dushane JW, Edwards JE, Fontana RS, Kirklin JW. Anatomical and pathological studies in VSD. Circulation 1956;14:349–364.
101. Blount SG, Jr, Mueller H, McCord MC. Ventricular septal defect clinical and hemodynamic patterns. Am J Med 1955;18:871.
102. Beck W, Schrire V, Vogelpoel L, Nellen M, Swanepoel A. Hemodynamic effects of amyl nitrite and phenylephrine on the normal human circulation and their relation to changes in cardiac murmurs. Am J Cardiol 1961;8:341–349.
103. Bloomfield DK. The natural history of VSD in patients surviving infancy. Circulation 1964;29:914–955.
104. Schrire V, Vogelpoel L, Beck W, Nellen M, Swanepoel A. Ventricular septal defect: the clinical spectrum. Br Heart J 1965;27:813–828.
105. Anderson RH, Becker AE, Lucchese E. Morphology of Congenital Heart Disease. Baltimore, MD: University Park Press, 1983.
106. Topaz. O, Taylor AL. Interventricular septal rupture complicating acute myocardial infarction: from pathophysiologic features to the role of invasive and noninvasive diagnostic modalities in current management. Am J Med. 1992;93:683–688.
107. Birnbaum Y, Fishbein MC, Blanche C, Siegel RJ. Ventricular septal rupture after acute myocardial infarction. N Engl J Med 2002;347:1426–1432.
108. Crenshaw BS, Granger CB, Birnbaum Y, et al. Risk factors, angiographic patterns, and outcomes in patients with VSD complicating acute myocardial infarction. GUSTO-I (Global Utilization of Streptokinase and TPA for Occluded Coronary Arteries) Trial Investigators. Circulation 2000;101:27–32.
109. Figueras J, Cortadellas J, Soler-Soler J. Comparison of ventricular septal and left ventricular free wall rupture in acute myocardial infarction. Am J Cardiol 1998;81:495–497.
110. Perloff JK. The Clinical Recognition of Congenital Heart Disease. Philadelphia, PA: W.B. Saunders, 2001: 315.
111. Therrien J, Dore A, Gersony W, et al. CCS Consensus Conference 2001 update: recommendations for the management of adults with congenital heart disease. Part I. Can J Cardiol 2001;17:940–959.
112. Leatham A, Segal B. Auscultatory and phonocardiographic signs of VSD with left to-right shunt. Circulation 1962;25:318–327.
113. Hollman A, Morgan JJ, Goodwin JF, Fields H. Auscultatory and phonocardiographic findings in VSD. A study of 93 surgically treated patients. Circulation 1963;28:94–100.
114. Farru O, Duffau G, Rodriguez R. Auscultatory and phonocardiographic characteristics of supracristal VSD. Br Heart J 1971;33:238–245.
115. Perloff JK. Auscultatory and phonocardiographic manifestations of pulmonary hypertension. Prog Cardiovasc Dis 1967;9:303.
116. Perloff JK. Ventricular septal defect with pulmonary stenosis. In: The Clinical Recognition of Congenital Heart Disease. Philadelphia, PA: W.B. Saunders Co, 1970:349–391.
117. McCord MC, Van Elk J, Blount SG, Jr. Tetralogy of Fallot. Clinical and hemodynamic spectrum of combined pulmonary stenosis and VSD. Circulation 1957;16:736.

8 Heart Murmurs
Part II

CONTENTS

- DIASTOLIC MURMURS
- DIASTOLIC MURMURS OF MITRAL ORIGIN
- DIASTOLIC MURMURS OF TRICUSPID ORIGIN
- SEMILUNAR VALVE REGURGITATION
- AORTIC REGURGITATION
- PULMONARY REGURGITATION
- CLINICAL ASSESSMENT OF DIASTOLIC MURMURS
- CONTINUOUS MURMURS
- PERSISTENT DUCTUS ARTERIOSUS
- AORTO-PULMONARY WINDOW
- SINUS OF VALSALVA ANEURYSM
- CORONARY ARTERIOVENOUS FISTULAE
- VENOUS HUM
- MAMMARY SOUFFLE
- CLINICAL ASSESSMENT OF CONTINUOUS MURMURS
- PERICARDIAL FRICTION RUB
- INNOCENT MURMURS
- REFERENCES

DIASTOLIC MURMURS

Diastolic murmurs can be caused by turbulent flow through the atrioventricular valves (the mitral and tricuspid valves) or turbulence caused by regurgitation of blood through the semilunar valves (the aortic and pulmonary valves). We will first discuss diastolic murmurs arising from turbulent flow through the atrioventricular valves.

DIASTOLIC MURMURS OF MITRAL ORIGIN

Turbulent flow across the mitral valve capable of producing a diastolic murmur can occur under the following conditions:
- When there is increased pressure in the left atrium because of obstruction at the valve
- When there is excessive volume of flow during diastole through the mitral valve with or without elevated left atrial pressure
- Normal or increased mitral inflow velocity through a somewhat abnormal mitral valve
- Normal mitral inflow through a functionally stenotic mitral orifice in the absence of organic valvular disease

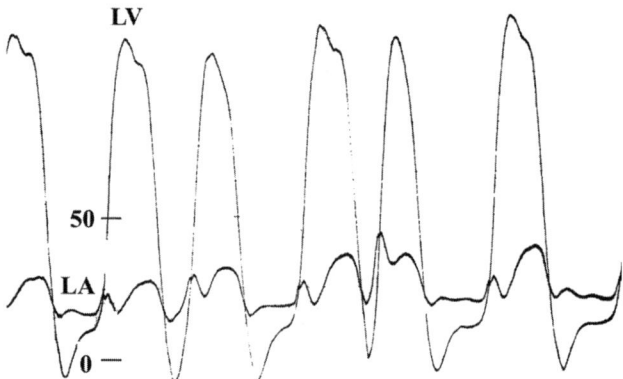

Fig. 1. Simultaneous recording of the left ventricular (LV) and the left atrial (LA) pressure curves obtained at cardiac catheterization from a patient with significant mitral stenosis. The rhythm is atrial fibrillation with varying diastolic intervals. A significant and persistent gradient throughout diastole is noted between the LA and the LV pressures even when the diastole is relatively long (e.g., following the fifth beat).

Mitral Obstruction Secondary to Mitral Valvular Stenosis

Mitral valvular obstruction may result from a congenitally stenosed valve or acquired stenosis such as caused by rheumatic heart disease where the leaflets are tethered and the commissures become fused because of the rheumatic process *(1–4)*. Congenital mitral stenosis is rare, and when it occurs in combination with an atrial septal defect, the condition goes by the name of *Lutembacher syndrome (5–7)*. Rarely, the obstruction may be caused by a left atrial tumor such as an *atrial myxoma (8,9)*. An atrial myxoma is a benign tumor with a myxoid matrix of gelatinous consistency. It may be associated with constitutional symptoms, such as fever, and systemic inflammatory signs, such as elevated sedimentation rate. The myxoma is usually attached by a stalk to the interatrial septum and may prolapse into the ventricle in early diastole when the valve opens and cause obstruction to the mitral inflow.

In the normal heart, the *v wave* pressure that is built up in the left atrium at the end of systole provides the gradient in early diastole for the diastolic flow to occur through the mitral valve. At this time the left ventricular pressure is close to zero. During the rapid filling phase of diastole, there is a fall in the left atrial pressure and a rise in the left ventricular diastolic pressure because of emptying of the left atrium and filling of the left ventricle, respectively. When there is any significant obstruction to flow at the mitral valve, the left atrial pressure will be elevated due to the obstruction, and the flow through the valve in diastole will occur under a higher *v wave* pressure gradient. The more severe the obstruction or the stenosis, the more persistent will be the elevation in the left atrial pressure. The pressure gradient between the left atrium and the left ventricle will tend to persist throughout diastole. The diastolic flow occurring under a higher and persistent pressure gradient will contribute to a turbulent flow, which may persist throughout diastole. The normal left atrial *v wave* pressure is usually about 12–15 mmHg. When there is significant mitral stenosis, the *v wave* pressure may be elevated up to 25–30 mmHg (Fig. 1). However, the pressure gradient noted even with severe mitral stenosis is still fairly low in terms of the absolute mmHg elevation.

On the other hand, the volume of flow through the mitral valve is always significant since the entire stroke volume of the heart will have to go through the mitral valve in diastole. Thus, a large volume going through the mitral valve under relatively low levels of pressure will be expected to give rise to turbulence, which will produce predominantly low-frequency murmur. In fact, the low pitch of the mitral stenosis murmur gives its characteristic rumbling quality on auscultation. The loudness of the murmur produced by the turbulence will depend to a certain extent on the adequacy of the cardiac output, whereas the length will depend more on the length of time the pressure gradient persists in diastole. The latter will tend to last throughout diastole when the stenosis is severe *(1,3,10–13)*.

CHARACTERISTICS OF MITRAL STENOSIS MURMURS

The diastolic murmur of mitral stenosis will be expected to begin in diastole after the mitral valve opens and the rapid filling phase of diastole begins. The murmur is low pitched and often very well localized to the apex. The murmur may be so localized that unless one auscultates at the apex it may be missed. The best way to hear the murmur is to have the patient turn to the left lateral decubitus position and locate the left ventricular apex and use the bell to listen. The murmur has a rumbling quality and sounds like a distant roar of a thunder. The loud S1 and the opening snap following the S2, which are invariably present in classical mitral stenosis, give the background for auscultation. Together they make a cadence:

One .....Two ...ta r r r r r r r r

The loudness of the murmur has no relationship to the severity of the stenosis. The loudness of the murmur may be related to the adequacy of the cardiac output.

In severe pulmonary hypertension secondary to the mitral stenosis, the high pulmonary vascular resistance is usually associated with decreased cardiac output. In such patients with severe mitral stenosis and low-output symptoms the murmur may be soft and may even be inaudible. Occasionally in overdiuresed patients and decreased intravascular volume, the murmur may be soft despite significant stenosis. When the cardiac output is increased by slight exercise, such as walking for a few minutes, the murmur may be brought out more clearly.

The length of the murmur has an important relationship to the severity of the mitral stenosis. If the stenosis is severe and is associated with a persistent diastolic gradient, the murmur will last throughout diastole until the beginning of next systole (Fig. 2). In atrial fibrillation the varying diastolic pauses provide a good opportunity to assess the length of the murmur in relation to the long pauses of diastole.

The diastolic murmur of mitral stenosis will often have a presystolic crescendo to the loud M1 (Fig. 2) *(14,15)*. Occasionally one may hear only the presystolic murmur (Fig. 3). If this is the case, it usually means that the mitral stenosis is mild. The presystolic murmur tends to have some higher frequencies in that one can easily hear this with the chest piece of the stethoscope, unlike the diastolic rumble. Generally the presystolic murmur is not heard when the valve is heavily calcified and rigid.

The left ventricle begins to contract at the end of diastole. When the left ventricular pressure exceeds the left atrial pressure, the mitral valve will close. The column of blood contained in the left ventricle, being moved by the contracting left ventricle, will be suddenly decelerated against the closed mitral valve, causing the loud M1. The loudness of M1 stems from the high *dP/dt* of the left ventricle at the time of closure of the

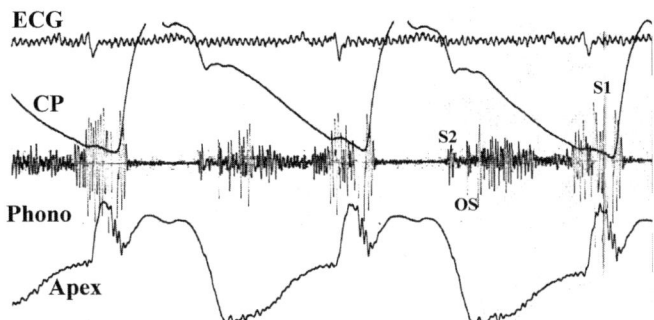

Fig. 2. Simultaneous recording of eclectrocardiogram (ECG), carotid pulse (CP), apexcardiogram (Apex), and phonocardiogram (Phono) taken at the apex area from a patient with severe mitral stenosis. The Phono recording shows the full-length diastolic murmur, which begins immediately following the opening snap (OS). The low-frequency murmur is initially loud and diminishes slightly later to become accentuated with a crescendo shape ending with a loud intensity first heart sound (S1). The systole is free of murmur.

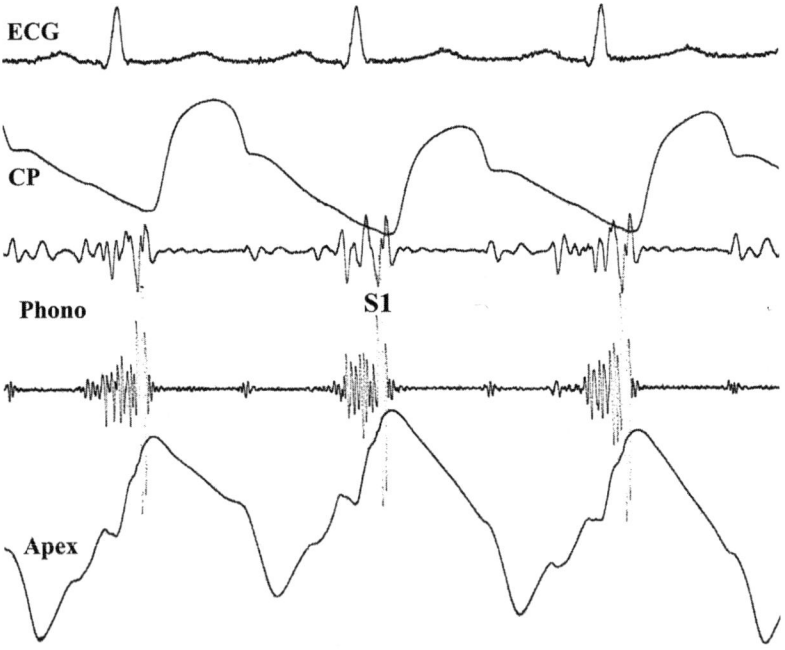

Fig. 3. Simultaneous recording of electrocardiogram (ECG), carotid pulse (CP), apexcardiogram (Apex), and phonocardiogram (Phono) taken at the apex area from a patient with mild mitral stenosis. The Phono shows predominantly a presystolic murmur increasing in intensity ending with a large-amplitude first heart sound (S1). Note that the murmur has predominantly high frequency.

mitral valve as a result of the elevated left atrial pressure. This has been discussed previously in relation to the S1.

Although with sinus rhythm and preserved atrial contraction and relaxation one should expect a crescendo–decrescendo murmur with the increasing flow velocity associated with atrial contraction and decreasing flow velocity during atrial relaxation, only the crescendo presystolic murmur is characteristic of mitral stenosis. Very rarely, when the PR interval is prolonged, one may observe and record a crescendo–decrescendo murmur. Simultaneous recording of the left ventricular and left atrial pressures will show that the presystolic crescendo effect actually occurs at a time when the gradient is diminishing with the rising left ventricular pressure because of its contraction just before the crossover point of the pressures *(4)*. In addition, the presystolic crescendo of the diastolic murmur can be recognized in shorter diastoles during atrial fibrillation *(15)*. This would suggest that the increased volume and velocity of flow during the *a wave* rise in the left atrial pressure because of atrial systole in sinus rhythm alone is not adequate to explain its mechanism. Doppler measurements of mitral flow velocity at the time of diminishing pressure gradient at the end of diastole show that the flow velocity decreases and the slope of deceleration appears to be more steep with the crescendo effect seen on the murmur. It is conceivable that the rising left ventricular pressure caused by its contraction and its increasing *dP/dt* not only decelerates the mitral flow but also produces increased turbulence, resulting in the increased intensity of the murmur *(16)*.

Mitral Obstruction Secondary to Left Atrial Myxoma

This benign tumor is usually attached by a stalk to the interatrial septum. If it is large enough it will obstruct mitral inflow during diastole and cause turbulence of mitral inflow, giving rise to the diastolic murmur *(8,9)*. It has been previously discussed in the context of the tumor plop sound how the tumor, by elevating the left atrial *v wave*, helps to initiate a rapid expansion in the rapid filling phase. The tumor prolapses into the left ventricle when the mitral valve opens. When it reaches its maximum excursion, its further movement is suddenly stopped. This gives rise to a filling sound, which is a loud S3-like sound called the *tumor plop*. The tumor plop sound occurs shortly after the rapid-filling wave peak. It is followed by a low-pitched diastolic rumble. The length of the murmur again will correspond to the duration of the diastolic gradient. Because the tumor will prevent proper leaflet apposition, there will always be some mitral regurgitation. This is usually not severe. The elevated left atrial pressure increases the M1 intensity. The loud S1, the S2, and the tumor plop sound followed by the low-pitched diastolic murmur as well as the high-frequency blowing systolic regurgitation murmur are very characteristic of this condition (Fig. 4).

Excess Diastolic Mitral Inflow

The entire stroke volume of the heart usually goes through the mitral valve during diastole except when there is an atrial septal defect. In certain conditions, however, there may not be increased forward output through the aorta but there may be more than normal pulmonary venous inflow, which may go through the mitral valve in diastole. These conditions are associated with volume overload of the left atrium and the left ventricle, as may be seen in mitral regurgitation, ventricular septal defect, and persistent ductus arteriosus *(10,17,18)*. In mitral regurgitation, the mitral inflow will have to include not only the volume that went back into the left atrium because of the systolic regurgitation but also the normal pulmonary venous return. In ventricular septal defect and persistent ductus arteriosus, the excess pulmonary flow due to the left-to-right shunt is added onto the normal pulmonary venous return. In these two conditions with left-to-right shunt, the left atrial *v wave* pressure may still be normal as long as the left ventricular diastolic function is preserved and its *pre-a wave* pressure remains normal (approximately 5 mmHg).

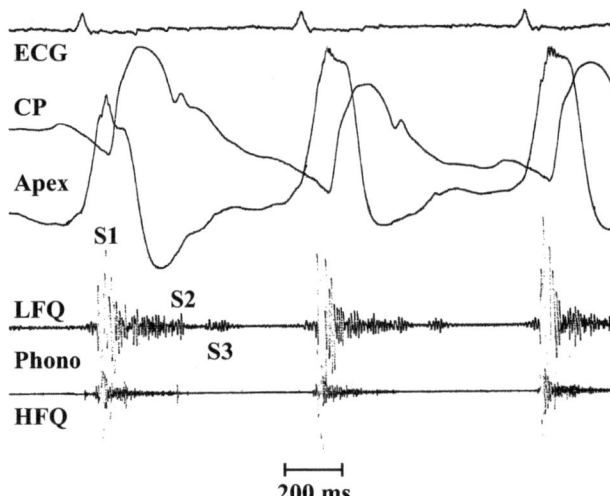

Fig. 4. Simultaneous recording of electrocardiogram (ECG), carotid pulse (CP), apexcardiogram (Apex), and phonocardiogram (Phono) taken from the apex area from a patient with a left atrial myxoma. The Phono shows the characteristic features of a loud first heart sound (S1), a regurgitant systolic murmur followed by a tumor plop sound at the time of a third heart sound (S3).

In mitral regurgitation, however, the *v wave* pressure in the left atrium may be somewhat elevated secondary to the systolic regurgitation. The degree of elevation of the left atrial *v wave* pressure will depend not only on the severity of the mitral regurgitation but also its duration and the left atrial compliance or distensibility. Thus, the increased mitral inflow during diastole in the above conditions may or may not be accompanied by increased *v wave* pressure gradient during early diastole. Nevertheless, the excess flow in diastole through the mitral valve will produce enough turbulence to generate mid-diastolic low-frequency murmurs *(17)*. The normal semiclosure movement of the mitral valve leaflets, after the full opening in early diastole, which can be easily appreciated in two-dimensional echocardiographic images, further helps to increase the turbulence by slightly narrowing the functional orifice.

When there is high cardiac output, as may occur in anemia, thyrotoxicosis, pregnancy, etc., there will be an obligatory increase in mitral inflow along with increased velocity of flow. In children the increased sympathetic tone will also be accompanied by increased velocity of flow through the heart. In children, pregnant women, anemia, and other high-output states, it is not uncommon to have physiological S3. Occasionally there may be some turbulence caused by the excessive and/or rapid inflow to produce short mid-diastolic flow murmurs in these states.

In patients with complete atrioventricular block (where atrial depolarizations of sinus nodal origin fail to conduct to the ventricle), when the independent atrial contraction happens to occur during the rapid filling phase of diastole, a short mid-diastolic flow murmur may also be noted to occur. The mechanism of origin of these intermittent mid-diastolic flow murmurs (sometimes called the *Rytand murmur*) is also similar *(19, 20)*.

Flow Through Abnormal But Nonstenotic Mitral Valve

In acute rheumatic fever, the mitral valve structures may be acutely inflamed with some thickening and edema. The involvement of the mitral structures in the acute rheumatic process may be accompanied by mid-diastolic murmurs presumably caused by some turbulence of flow during the rapid filling phase. These murmurs are typically low pitched and of short duration in mid-diastole. At this stage of the rheumatic process the mitral valve is far from being stenosed. Often there may be at least a moderate degree of mitral regurgitation. The latter will also contribute to the increased mitral inflow during diastole. The presence of this murmur is good evidence of active carditis in rheumatic fever. It is called the *Carey Coombs murmur (21)*.

Flow Through Functionally Stenotic Mitral Valve

In aortic regurgitation, often the regurgitant jet is directed toward the anterior mitral leaflet. In fact, the anterior mitral leaflet may be shown to exhibit some fine fluttering in diastole because of this jet hitting it. This can be seen particularly well on the M-mode of the echocardiogram. When the aortic regurgitation is significant and directed toward the anterior mitral leaflet, it may actually prevent the latter from opening well during diastole. The semi-closed mitral valve can also be well seen on the two-dimensional echocardiogram well separated from the ventricular septum. In such patients, the diastolic inflow through the mitral valve will be accompanied by turbulence. The left atrial *v wave* pressure may not be elevated, however. The turbulent mitral inflow, because of the functional stenosis caused by the aortic regurgitation, may be accompanied by a low-frequency diastolic murmur. The murmur will sound quite similar to the diastolic rumble of mitral stenosis and is best heard at the apex. This is called the *Austin Flint murmur (4,22–26)*. That the Austin Flint murmur is a sign of severe aortic regurgitation can in fact be proven by improving forward flow through the aorta by an arterial dilator, such as amyl nitrite, thereby diminishing the degree of aortic regurgitation. Amyl nitrite is usually administered as a vapor through inhalation. It causes profound arterial and arteriolar dilatation. It has a very short half-life in the body and is usually eliminated by the lungs. The profound arterial and arteriolar dilatation causes the systemic arterial pressure to fall. This leads to sympathetic stimulation and tachycardia. The sympathetic stimulation often will cause veno-constriction and increase the venous return. This will lead to increased cardiac output. Amyl nitrite differs from nitroglycerin in this respect. The latter causes a less dramatic fall in blood pressure, and the sympathetic stimulation is less profound. In addition, nitroglycerin lasts slightly longer in the body, which leads to significant veno-dilatation. This results in decreased venous return and decreased cardiac output. The decreased venous return is an important hemodynamic effect, which helps to reduce the heart size, and by diminishing the size of the heart it reduces the wall tension, thereby reducing the oxygen demand. This is one of the important effects of nitroglycerin for the improvement of ischemia in addition to its effect on direct coronary vasodilatation and peripheral arterial bed. When amyl nitrite is administered in aortic regurgitation, the resulting peripheral arterial and arteriolar dilatation improve forward runoff, thereby decreasing the degree of aortic regurgitation. When the aortic regurgitation is reduced, there will be less restriction on the mitral anterior leaflet. Austin Flint murmur will disappear on amyl nitrite inhalation despite the fact that the actual volume of flow through the mitral valve is increased because of the increased venous return and cardiac output. Amyl nitrite will have an opposite effect on organic mitral stenosis murmur since the increased flow through the mitral valve will actually increase the intensity of the murmur. This method was often used at the bedside to distinguish between Austin Flint murmur and true mitral stenosis before the advent of two-dimensional echocardiography. It is still a useful bedside method *(27)*.

DIASTOLIC MURMURS OF TRICUSPID ORIGIN

Turbulent flow across the tricuspid valve capable of producing a diastolic murmur can occur under the following conditions:

1. When there is increased pressure in the right atrium because of obstruction at the valve
2. When there is normal or increased tricuspid inflow velocity through abnormal nonstenotic tricuspid valve
3. When there is excessive volume of flow during diastole through the tricuspid valve with or without elevated right atrial pressure

Tricuspid Obstruction Secondary to Tricuspid Valve Stenosis

Tricuspid stenosis resulting from rheumatic heart disease is quite rare, and it is usually associated with mitral stenosis and aortic valve disease. The right atrial and jugular venous pressures will be elevated. The latter may show a large-amplitude *a wave* followed by an *x' descent* in patients with sinus rhythm. Generally the pressure gradient in patients with sinus rhythm is noted at the end of diastole (presystole). In patients with atrial fibrillation, the gradient may be observed in mid-diastole. The entire stroke volume of the heart goes through the tricuspid valve as well, similar to the mitral valve at fairly low-pressure gradients. The murmur, therefore, is low pitched and generally reflects the diastolic gradient *(28–33)*.

CHARACTERISTICS OF TRICUSPID STENOSIS MURMUR

In patients with sinus rhythm, the murmur is only presystolic but with a crescendo–decrescendo effect because of atrial contraction augmenting flow velocity followed by atrial relaxation diminishing the velocity. In patients with atrial fibrillation, the murmur will tend to be more mid-diastolic and low pitched.

The tricuspid component of S1 may be loud, and there may be a tricuspid opening snap, but both may be difficult to recognize because of a loud M1 and mitral opening snap secondary to associated mitral stenosis.

The maximal loudness of the murmur will be at the lower sternal region, and the murmur may be shown to augment in intensity on inspiration and also by turning the patient to the right lateral decubitus *(29)*.

Tricuspid Obstruction Secondary to Right Atrial Myxoma

The mechanism of tricuspid valve obstruction secondary to a right atrial myxoma is similar to what has been described under mitral obstruction secondary to a left atrial myxoma. The right atrial pressure will be elevated, raising the jugular venous pressure. The myxoma will cause obstruction to the tricuspid inflow and also interfere with the apposition of the leaflets and therefore cause tricuspid regurgitation. The elevated right atrial pressure will cause a diastolic gradient and contribute to the diastolic turbulence and murmur. The jugular venous pulse may show both *x'* and *y descents*. The loud T1 will be the reason for a loud S1 and will be shown to increase in intensity on inspiration. There may be a loud tumor plop sound corresponding to the timing of an S3, which will be followed by a low-pitched diastolic murmur. The latter again will be best heard over the lower left sternal area and may also increase in intensity on inspiration *(34,35)*.

Flow Through Abnormal But Nonstenotic Tricuspid Valve

The tricuspid valve may be congenitally abnormal as in Ebstein's anomaly. In certain acquired disorders, such as the carcinoid syndrome, the tricuspid valve leaflets may show abnormal thickening and fibrosis. The tricuspid valve will often be regurgitant in these conditions. The tricuspid inflow under these conditions will often be associated with a low-pitched diastolic murmur as well *(36,37)*.

Excess Diastolic Tricuspid Inflow

Excess volume of tricuspid inflow will be expected in certain situations where there is right atrial and right ventricular volume overload. These include atrial septal defect with a left-to-right shunt and tricuspid regurgitation. In atrial septal defect when there is a significant left-to-right shunt, the shunt flow added onto the normal venous return will cause both right atrial and right ventricular volume overload. In significant tricuspid regurgitation of whatever etiology, tricuspid inflow will be increased in the same way in which mitral regurgitation increases mitral inflow. In both conditions the right atrial pressure may or may not be elevated. Nevertheless, one can expect a tricuspid inflow rumble. In fact, the presence of such a rumble in atrial septal defect is a sign of a significant left-to-right shunt. In tricuspid regurgitation there may be a right-sided S3, and occasionally it may have enough duration to it simulating a low-pitched diastolic murmur *(38–40)*.

SEMILUNAR VALVE REGURGITATION

Regurgitation of blood (backward flow) through the semilunar valves, namely, the aortic and the pulmonary valves, during diastole can cause turbulence and lead to the production of diastolic murmurs.

AORTIC REGURGITATION

Causes of Aortic Regurgitation

Aortic regurgitation can result either from intrinsic valvular pathology or from aortic root dilatation *(31,41–43)*.

VALVULAR CAUSES

Valvular abnormalities that result in aortic regurgitation can either be congenital or acquired. Congenitally the aortic valve cusps may have fenestrations, which may result in regurgitation, particularly when there is associated systemic hypertension. Occasionally the aortic valve may be bicuspid. In fact, this abnormality is often the most common congenital anomaly of the heart, occurring in about 1% of the population. The bicuspid valve is often eccentric with unequal cusps and generally tends to be insufficient *(44)*. Aortic valve cusps sometimes develop prolapse in the presence of a congenital perimembranous ventricular septal defect. While this may help in the spontaneous closure of the defect, it can result in varying degrees of aortic regurgitation *(38)*.

The aortic valve may be involved in rheumatic heart disease, and the valve can become both stenotic and regurgitant because of commissural fusion and thickening and scarring of the cusps. In the elderly the aortic valve may become calcific, and these will be more commonly associated with some degree of regurgitation. Rarely, the aortic valve cusps may have myxomatous infiltration, which may make the cusps somewhat large and allow them to prolapse into the left ventricle. These changes generally occur in individuals with Marfan's syndrome, who may also have aortic root disease and dilatation. Infective endocarditis can occur on the aortic valve, and this may cause aortic regurgitation to become clinically evident for the first time. Formations of vegetations may interfere with apposition of the cusps. In addition, infective destruction or perforations in the cusps could occur. It can also aggravate and worsen the degree of pre-existing aortic regurgitation. The cusps may become thickened and develop sclerotic changes with aging. In the presence of associated hypertension, aortic regurgitation may occur. Rarely, blunt chest trauma can result in a tear of the aortic valve cusps and lead to aortic regurgitation.

AORTIC ROOT DISEASE

Aorta and the aortic root may be involved in the disease process, which may lead to significant dilatation of the aortic root *(42,43)*. The latter will stretch the aortic valve ring and make the cusps incompetent. The list of entities that can result in such a process include congenital aneurysm of the sinus of Valsalva, syphilitic aortitis, which is now quite uncommon, cystic medial necrosis with and without overt Marfan's syndrome, spondylitis, rheumatoid arthritis, Paget's disease, osteogenesis imperfecta, and hypertensive atherosclerotic aneurysm of the ascending aorta. The pathology will vary according to the disease entity involved. In many of these entities, the elastic tissue in the media of the aorta is destroyed, leading to expansion of the aorta. For instance, in the atherosclerotic aneurysm it has been shown that the media becomes infiltrated with macrophages, which elaborate metalloproteinases, leading to the destruction of the elastic tissue. Occasionally the aortic medial disease may make the aorta vulnerable to dissection, particularly in the presence of hypertension. In this instance the intima may tear on account of the hemodynamic stress, and the tear can extend and dissect through the media of the aorta. The dissection will result in two lumens in the aorta—one being the true lumen the other being a false lumen. When the dissection occurs in the ascending aorta and extends into the aortic root, the aortic valve cusps will lose support, and this will cause aortic regurgitation.

Pathophysiology of Chronic Aortic Regurgitation

The aortic valve closes at the end of systole when the left ventricular pressure begins to decline because of relaxation and falls below that of the aorta. The falling left ventricular pressure provides a low-pressure area, and the column of blood at the aortic root close to the aortic valve will tend to reverse the forward direction of flow and move toward the aortic valve. In the process it will be decelerated against the closed aortic valve, and the dissipation of the energy of the moving column of blood will cause the A2. If the aortic valve is not competent for any reason, then there will be backward flow of blood from the aorta to the left ventricle in diastole, which will start at the time of A2. This backward flow will occur under a relatively high-pressure gradient because the aortic diastolic pressure is significantly high soon after the closure of the aortic valve, whereas the left ventricular pressure would have fallen to close to zero at the onset of diastole. The high-pressure gradient will cause turbulence that will result in a predominantly high-fre-

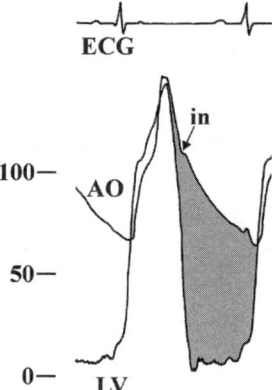

Fig. 5. Simultaneous recordings of electrocardiogram (ECG), the left ventricular (LV) and the aortic (AO) pressure curves from a patient with chronic aortic regurgitation. There is a high-pressure gradient between the AO and the LV during diastole (shaded area). The gradient is highest initially at the incisura (in), falling off gradually during the remainder of the diastole.

quency blowing-type murmur (Fig. 5). Following the rapid filling phase of diastole, the left ventricular diastolic pressure will begin to rise, and there will be a further rise in diastolic pressure of the left ventricle at the end of diastole due to atrial contraction augmenting filling. At the same time, the aortic diastolic pressure will gradually fall because of the peripheral runoff. Thus, the diastolic pressure gradient between the aorta and the left ventricle will be maximal at the beginning of diastole and will tend to fall gradually during diastole, reaching the minimal level toward the end of diastole. Thus, the decreasing diastolic gradient will have an effect on the diastolic murmur, which often will exhibit a decrescendo character starting at A2. During the rapid filling phase of diastole, the left ventricular pressure falls to zero and then rises. Thus, the pressure gradient between the aorta and the left ventricle may have an initial increase followed by a decrease. This transitory change in the pressure gradients may have an initial crescendo effect on the murmur followed by the typical decrescendo murmur.

The filling of the left ventricle during diastole will be augmented as a result of both the regurgitant volume of blood from the aorta and the normal pulmonary venous return through the mitral inflow. The left ventricle will enlarge because of the volume overload effect. The extent of rise in the filling pressure of the left ventricle will depend both on the severity of the regurgitation as well as on the compliance or distensibility of the left ventricle. In chronic aortic regurgitation, the left ventricle initially undergoes dilatation, and its compliance is generally preserved. This will help to keep the rise in the diastolic left ventricular pressure to a minimum *(42,45,46)*. On the other hand, the increased dimension of the left ventricle due to dilatation will increase the ventricular wall tension because the wall tension is directly proportional to the radius by the Laplace formula. The increased wall tension will increase the myocardial oxygen demand. This is one of the reasons that patients with aortic regurgitation may experience symptoms of exertional angina. The increase in the left ventricular wall tension is also a stimulus for secondary myocardial hypertrophy. In longstanding aortic regurgitation of more than moderate degree, therefore, the left ventricle will undergo secondary hypertrophy *(47)*.

Thus, in chronic severe aortic regurgitation the left ventricle is not only dilated and enlarged, but also significantly hypertrophied. The markedly hypertrophied and enlarged heart in aortic regurgitation is sometimes massive and referred to by the term "*cor bovinum.*" The increased wall thickness will help to reduce the wall tension slightly. The hypertrophic process is *eccentric* and is associated with replication of sarcomeres in series together with elongation of myofibers. The ratio of wall thickness to the radius of the cavity is maintained *(48)*. This is unlike the concentric hypertrophy that occurs in pressure overload states such as aortic stenosis, where the sarcomeres increase in parallel and the ratio of wall thickness to the radius of the cavity is increased *(49)*. The hypertrophy will, however, tend to make the left ventricle more stiff, and its compliance will become eventually diminished. This will result in further elevation of the left ventricular diastolic pressure. The increased left ventricular diastolic pressure will tend to interfere with subendocardial coronary perfusion. Since normal coronary flow occurs mostly in diastole, and because the arterial diastolic pressures are often low in significant aortic regurgitation secondary to compensatory peripheral vasodilatation, this will further compromise the coronary flow by reducing the coronary perfusion pressure. Although the reduced coronary reserve may not affect baseline left ventricular function, periods of increased metabolic demands induced by stress, exercise, and other activities may not be met by increased coronary flow. The increased myocardial oxygen demand together with decreased subendocardial perfusion will often result in some myocyte necrosis and replacement fibrosis. This will further depress the compliance of the left ventricle and cause an additional rise in the left ventricular diastolic pressure. This will further adversely affect the systolic left ventricular function as well *(42, 50–55)*.

Because the mitral valve is open in diastole, any elevation of the diastolic pressure before the *a wave* will lead to increased left atrial pressure. The elevated left atrial pressure will be transmitted to the pulmonary capillary bed and will cause symptoms of dyspnea. When the elevation of the left ventricular diastolic pressure is severe and associated with decreased left ventricular systolic function, the resulting high left atrial pressure will lead to aggravation of symptoms of dyspnea as well as cause orthopnea and paroxysmal nocturnal dyspnea.

Pathophysiology of Acute Severe Aortic Regurgitation

Unlike chronic aortic regurgitation, when the aortic regurgitation is severe and acute in onset, as may happen with rapidly progressive aortic valve endocarditis with a virulent and destructive pathogen, such as *Staphylococcus aureus*, or caused by a sudden rupture of a cusp or sudden disruption of a previously normal aortic valve prosthesis, the left ventricle will not have enough time to undergo compensatory dilatation. The severe regurgitation into the left ventricle is accommodated only with a significant elevation of the left ventricular diastolic pressure. The latter can not only rise to levels higher than the prevailing left atrial pressure in diastole, but also typically reach levels close to the aortic diastolic pressure. In fact, often by the end of diastole the left ventricular diastolic pressure becomes equal to the aortic diastolic pressure. The large regurgitant volume of blood from the incompetent aortic valve, together with the mitral inflow during the rapid-filling phase of diastole, often leads to an abrupt and large rise in the left ventricular diastolic pressure. The latter will have a significant deceleration effect on both the regurgitant column as well as the mitral inflow column of blood. This may result in the

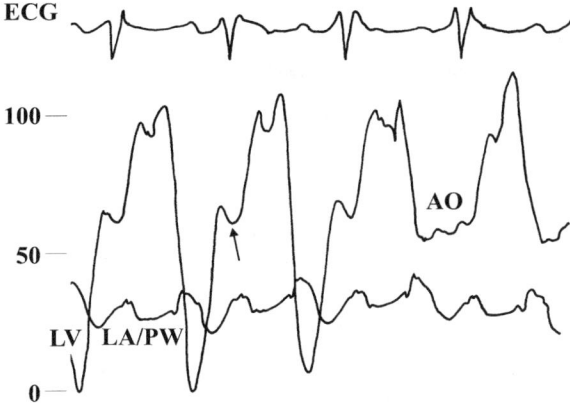

Fig. 6. Simultaneous recordings of the left ventricular (LV) and the indirect left atrial/pulmonary capillary wedge (LA/PW) pressures obtained at cardiac catheterization from a patient with acute severe aortic regurgitation. The aortic (AO) pressure is recorded while pulling back the catheter from the LV. The severity of the AO regurgitation and its acuteness do not allow enough time for the LV to undergo compensatory dilatation, thereby making the LV noncompliant. The LV diastolic pressure rises quickly with early diastolic inflow exceeding the LA pressure and continues to rise and becomes equal at end-diastole to the diastolic AO pressure (arrow).

production of an S3. In addition, the rapidly rising left ventricular diastolic pressure, when it exceeds the left atrial pressure in mid-diastole, will tend to close the mitral valve prematurely (Fig. 6). The premature closure of the mitral valve can be seen quite easily in M-mode recordings of the echocardiograms. The premature mitral closure will make the S1 soft. This has been discussed previously under S1 *(56,57)*.

The large volume of regurgitant aortic diastolic flow will give rise to predominantly low- and medium-frequency aortic regurgitation murmur, making it harsher in quality. In addition, the rapidly rising left ventricular diastolic pressure will limit the regurgitant flow by diminishing the pressure difference between the aorta and the left ventricle. This will make the murmur somewhat shorter. In the presence of a sinus tachycardia with the associated shortening of the diastole, one could misinterpret the harsh diastolic murmur to be a systolic ejection murmur.

Auscultatory Features in Aortic Regurgitation

1. The high-pressure gradient between the aorta and the left ventricle during diastole generally tends to give the aortic regurgitation murmur the classic high-frequency blowing quality. The beginner may mistake the murmur for the breath sound. Thus, aortic regurgitation murmur is best auscultated for, with the breath held at the end of expiration, preferably with the patient sitting up and leaning forward.
2. The aortic regurgitation murmur usually starts with the A2 and is often decrescendo in character. This follows the decreasing pressure gradient, which is maximal at the beginning of diastole and gradually diminishes toward the end of diastole. It usually can be mimicked by the following:

Lubbb.........Phoooooooooo

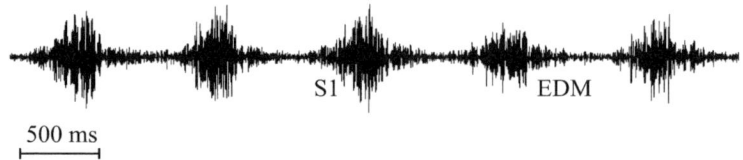

Fig. 7. Digital display of a magnetic audio recording from a patient with acute severe aortic regurgitation taken at the apex area. The first heart sound is very low in amplitude (soft). There is a systolic ejection murmur followed by a decrescendo high-frequency diastolic murmur (EDM) of the aortic regurgitation.

3. Occasionally the initial crescendo effect of the increasing pressure gradient (during the rapid filling phase) may not be heard leaving a slight pause after A2. It may then sound like:

    1...............2-haaaaa

4. The murmur may have low and medium frequencies if the degree of regurgitation is moderate to severe. This is especially the case in acute and severe aortic regurgitation where the murmur could sound somewhat harsh in quality (Fig. 7).
5. The aortic regurgitation murmur is generally heard over the "*sash area*," which extends from the second right interspace along the left sternal border to the apex.
6. The location of the maximal loudness can vary. It is along the left sternal border in most instances where valvular disease is the cause of the regurgitation. When the aortic root is dilated and the dilatation is the principal cause of the regurgitation, the murmur may tend to be equally loud or louder in the second and third right interspace compared to the left sternal border area.
7. Rarely, the aortic regurgitation murmur may only be heard best in certain unusual locations. When it is heard best in the left axillary area it goes by the name of *Cole-Cecil murmur (58)*. This may also occur in short, stocky individuals in whom the left ventricular apex is somewhat high in the axilla.
8. The aortic regurgitation murmur can occasionally sound quite musical and *dove cooing* in quality. When this occurs it is probably because of some aortic valve structure resonating and vibrating at a fixed frequency. This can be demonstrated on a phonocardiogram, which will show the even frequency (Fig. 8).
9. The loudness of the aortic regurgitation murmur does not usually have much bearing on the severity of the regurgitation. Sometimes severe aortic regurgitation may have soft murmurs.
10. When the regurgitation is significant (moderately severe or severe) and its jet is directed toward the anterior mitral leaflet, then the mitral valve may be prevented from opening fully. This will then cause a functional mitral stenosis, resulting in the production of a diastolic rumble at the apex. This is called the *Austin Flint rumble*. It is usually mid-diastolic and has predominant low frequencies like the mitral stenosis rumble (Fig. 9). The presence of this murmur is indicative of significant aortic regurgitation and requires that the regurgitant jet be directed toward the mitral leaflets. When the jet is directed toward the interventricular septum, as may sometimes happen, then the Austin Flint rumble will not be present despite a severe degree of aortic regurgitation. The Austin Flint murmur characteristically starts during the rapid filling phase of mitral inflow. Therefore, there is usually a pause between the S2 and the onset of the Austin Flint rumble. The latter is maximally loud at the left ventricular apex area *(22–26,59)*.

Chapter 8 / Heart Murmurs: *Part II*

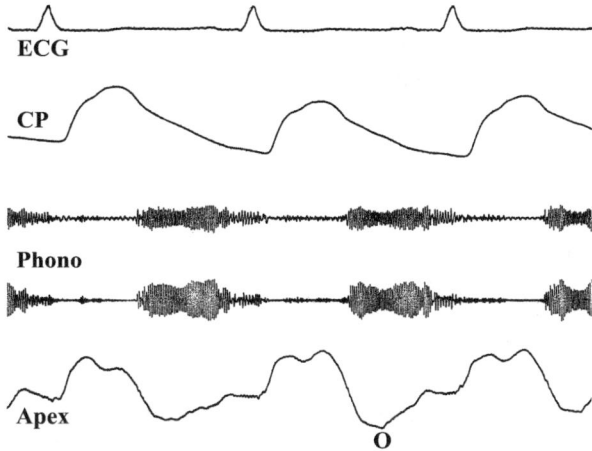

Fig. 8. Simultaneous recordings of electrocardiogram (ECG), carotid pulse (CP), apexcardiogram (Apex), and phonocardiogram (Phono) taken at the lower left sternal border area from a patient with significant aortic regurgitation and a dove-cooing musical murmur. The Phono shows the even frequencies of the diastolic murmur characteristic of the musical quality. The aortic regurgitation murmur as expected precedes the O point of the Apex, which corresponds to the mitral valve opening.

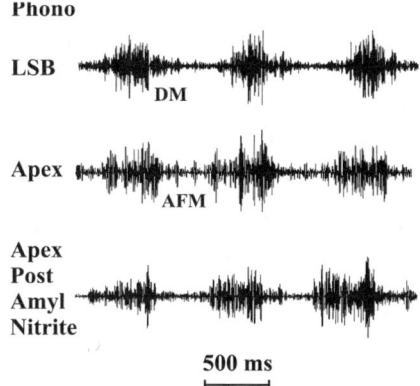

Fig. 9. Digital display of magnetic audio recordings taken from the left sternal border (LSB) area, the apex area (Apex) at rest, and following amyl nitrite inhalation (Apex Post Amyl Nitrite) from a patient with severe aortic regurgitation. The early diastolic decrescendo murmur of aortic regurgitation (DM) is seen to follow the systolic ejection murmur at the LSB. The diastolic murmur of Austin Flint (AFM) at the Apex noted at rest is not seen in the Post Amyl Nitrite recording.

11. The Austin Flint rumble needs to be distinguished from the low-frequency components of the aortic regurgitation murmur. The latter may sometimes be transmitted to the apex area. However, these low-frequency components of the aortic regurgitation murmur usually start with the A2 without any appreciable pause.
12. Often when the aortic regurgitation is mild or faint, the intensity of the murmur can be increased by increasing the peripheral resistance. This can be done at the bedside by asking the patients to squeeze their hands to clench their fingers and at the same time squat as well. This will tend to raise the blood pressure as well as the venous return and bring out the faint aortic regurgitation murmurs *(60)*.

13. When aortic regurgitation is moderate to severe, there is an increased diastolic volume, which will have a Starling effect on the left ventricle. This will lead to rapid ejection of an increased stroke volume. This may result in an ejection murmur during systole. Sometimes the ejection murmur can be quite loud.

PULMONARY REGURGITATION

Pulmonary valve regurgitation may occur either with pulmonary hypertension or with normal pulmonary artery pressures.

Pulmonary Hypertensive Pulmonary Regurgitation

When there is pulmonary hypertension of whatever cause, the pulmonary valves become easily incompetent. The reason for this is twofold. One is the elevated pulmonary diastolic pressure itself. The second reason is the pulmonary artery dilatation that eventually results from the high pulmonary pressures. The pulmonary valve ring is stretched, and the valve becomes easily regurgitant as a result.

Normotensive Pulmonary Regurgitation

The pulmonary valve can become incompetent in the presence of normal pulmonary artery pressures because of either valvular pathology or disease of the pulmonary artery. Congenitally the pulmonary valve may be absent, malformed, or have fenestrations. The pulmonary valve may become the seat of infective endocarditis. This is most likely associated with intravenous drug abuse. The pulmonary valve may also be made iatrogenically incompetent following pulmonary valvotomy. This is often seen in patients operated for Fallot's tetralogy. Occasionally the valve cusps may be quite normal, and there may be idiopathic dilatation of the pulmonary artery. The latter can stretch the valve ring and result in pulmonary valve regurgitation.

Pathophysiology of Pulmonary Regurgitation

Pulmonary regurgitation causes hemodynamic burden on the right ventricle similar to what happens on the left side with aortic regurgitation. The backward flow of blood into the right ventricle during diastole increases the right ventricular volume in diastole, causing a right ventricular volume overload. As a result, the right ventricle often enlarges and undergoes dilatation. The enlarged right ventricle can take over a large area anteriorly and sometimes form the apex beat.

The pressure difference under which the turbulent flow occurs as well as the degree of regurgitation will determine the predominant frequency of the resulting murmur. The pressure difference is between the pulmonary diastolic pressure and the right ventricular diastolic pressure. This is maximal at S2 at the onset of diastole and diminishes gradually toward the end of diastole, giving a decrescendo feature.

When the pulmonary artery pressure is high as in pulmonary hypertension, then the actual pressure difference is significantly high, and the resulting murmur will have predominantly high frequencies very similar to aortic regurgitation.

When the pulmonary artery pressure is normal, however, the murmur will be low in frequency because of turbulent flow occurring at low levels of pressure difference. Initially the right ventricular pressure falls more rapidly during the rapid filling phase than the pulmonary artery pressure. Then it quickly rises, giving a short crescendo–decrescendo shape to the gradient. The murmur will start after the P2 but will sound more like a rumble, somewhat short in duration.

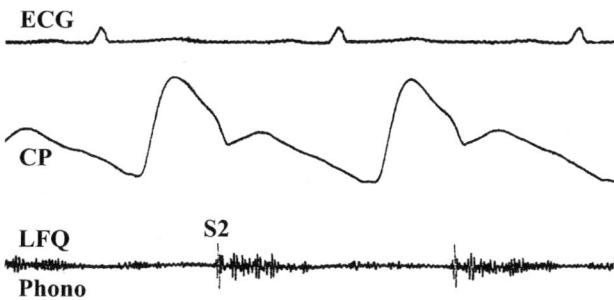

Fig. 10. Simultaneous recordings of electrocardiogram (ECG), carotid pulse (CP), and phonocardiogram (Phono) taken in the low-frequency (LFQ) range (50–100 Hz) over the third left interspace at the left sternal border from a patient with posttraumatic pulmonary regurgitation with normal pulmonary artery pressures. The murmur begins right after S2 and lasts through early diastole and is predominantly a low-frequency murmur.

When the regurgitation is severe and longstanding, then secondary hypertrophy of the right ventricle can occur, leading to somewhat decreased right ventricular compliance. This may lead to elevation of the right ventricular diastolic pressures. When the *pre-a wave* pressure is elevated, it will result in elevation of the right atrial and jugular venous pressures. In addition, the decreased compliance can result in sudden deceleration of both the regurgitant column of blood as well as the tricuspid inflow at the end of the rapid-filling phase. This can therefore result in the production of a right-sided S3. This is more likely to occur when there has been pre-existing right ventricular hypertrophy, as in patients with tetralogy of Fallot who have undergone pulmonary valvotomy as part of the tetralogy correction.

Auscultatory Features of Pulmonary Regurgitation

In the presence of pulmonary hypertension, the pulmonary regurgitation murmur assumes a high-frequency decrescendo character. It will start with P2 and blowing and decrescendo in quality very similar to the aortic regurgitation murmur. The S2 split may be narrow or wide. The P2 may be even loud and palpable at the second left interspace. The murmur is best heard over the second, third, and fourth left interspace and occasionally over the left sternal border area. The maximum loudness is often over the third left interspace. This murmur, when heard in a patient with severe mitral stenosis and secondary pulmonary hypertension, is referred to as the *Graham Steell murmur (1,61–65)*. But features are relatively the same however the pulmonary hypertension is caused. It is often indistinguishable from aortic regurgitation by the auscultatory features alone.

When the pulmonary artery pressures are normal, the turbulence occurring under low-pressure gradients produces predominantly a low-frequency murmur *(66)*. It sounds like a rumble starting after a brief pause after A2. The S2 split may be variable and occasionally wide, but generally physiological. The maximal loudness is over the third and fourth left interspace at the left sternal border. The murmur often is short and somewhat decrescendo to the ear (Fig. 10). There may be an associated ejection systolic murmur when the right ventricular stroke volume is increased because of the volume overload effect. Both the systolic and diastolic murmurs may be shown to increase in intensity on inspiration. There may be associated pulmonary ejection clicks *(67)*.

CLINICAL ASSESSMENT OF DIASTOLIC MURMURS

Evaluation of Symptoms

Because diastolic murmurs are often not very loud and sometimes very highly localized, as in mitral stenosis, they can be easily missed. Therefore, it is not common for patients with diastolic murmurs to present merely as problem of diagnosis of the cause of the murmur. More than likely they will be referred for other symptoms. A carefully obtained clinical history and its proper interpretation often will give clues as to what possibilities need to be considered. Symptoms of orthopnea and/or paroxysmal nocturnal dyspnea would imply high left atrial pressures *(62)*. Orthopnea occurs because of the gravitational shift of intravascular volume from the lower extremities raising the central blood volume and, therefore, the filling pressures in the left atrium. The nocturnal dyspnea occurs because of the elevation of the left atrial pressure occurring after a few hours of sleep at night, which is caused by the redistribution of fluid volume in the body compartments. The extravascular fluid enters the vascular compartment during sleep and increases the blood volume, leading to the rise in left atrial pressure. The classic paroxysmal nocturnal dyspnea, which occurs with left ventricular failure, is usually relieved with erect posture and does not occur more than once a night *(62)*. Patients with significant aortic regurgitation who develop symptoms of left ventricular decompensation may give this history. In significant mitral stenosis, the left atrial pressure will remain high and can cause orthopnea. However, nocturnal dyspnea will tend to be somewhat atypical in that it will not clear up quickly on assuming an erect posture. Patients may also complain that they may be waking up dyspneic more than once during the night. Symptoms suggestive of acute pulmonary edema needing emergency attention can occur if atrial fibrillation should develop suddenly in a patient with significant mitral obstruction from any cause *(1)*. It can also occur in severe aortic regurgitation. Low-output symptoms such as fatigue and lassitude may be present in significant mitral stenosis. Syncopal episodes and presyncopal episodes may occur in mitral obstruction because of tumors such as atrial myxoma. Characteristically these may be positionally aggravated, particularly in the left lateral decubitus position *(8)*. Systemic embolic episodes are characteristic for mitral stenosis with atrial fibrillation. This may occur to a lesser extent in atrial myxoma. Severe pulmonary hypertension of whatever cause will often produce symptoms of low output as well as episodes of syncope or presyncope, which may be exertional because of the inability of these patients to increase their cardiac output with exercise as a result of the high pulmonary vascular resistance *(62)*.

Clues from the Arterial Pulse, Precordial Pulsations, and the Venous Pulse

The clues that can be derived from the careful examination of the arterial pulse, venous pulse, and precordial pulsations are many, and these in turn can be used in conjunction with the auscultatory findings to confirm suspected lesions. Tight mitral obstruction and severe pulmonary hypertension are conditions characterized by low-amplitude pulse because of low stroke volume. Aortic regurgitation, which usually is associated with large stroke volume, will be characterized by large-amplitude pulsations both peripherally and in the carotids. The carotid artery pulsation may be visible from a distance (*Corrigan's pulse*). Jugular venous pressure and the pulse contour may indicate the presence or absence of abnormal right heart hemodynamics. How various stages of pulmonary hypertension and the presence of significant tricuspid regurgitation affect the venous pulse contours was discussed in detail in Chapter 4. The assessment of what dominates the precordial pulsation will also point to the appropriate lesions to be suspected. Left ventricular impulse is often normal in pure mitral stenosis. Hyperdynamic left ventricular impulse, forming a wide area with rapid and large-amplitude displacement together with marked precordial or sternal retraction, is often characteristic of significant aortic regurgitation. Right ventricular volume and/or pressure overload states may often be reflected by right ventricular impulse, which may be detected by subxiphoid palpation. Rarely, a large right ventricle because of significant volume overload, as may be seen in atrial septal defect or pulmonary regurgitation, may form the apex beat with characteristic lateral retraction.

The Auscultatory Assessment of Diastolic Murmurs

The auscultatory assessment of diastolic murmurs presupposes that the heart sounds have been assessed, including the S1 and S2, and that extra sounds, such as opening snap, S4, S3, and ejection clicks, have identified and characterized.

Next, the murmur itself is assessed with reference to the following:

1. Its predominant frequencies—whether rumbling and low pitched or high pitched and blowing in character.
2. Its timing in diastole—whether it is early diastolic, mid-diastolic, or presystolic.
3. Its length in diastole is also assessed to determine whether it occupies most of diastole or only part of diastole.
4. If it occupied only part of diastole, whether it occupies early to mid-diastole or mid- and late diastole.
5. Its audible shape—whether it is decrescendo or crescendo.
6. Its location of maximal loudness.
7. Finally, whether or not inspiratory increase in intensity or loudness is present.

The presence of a loud S1 and an opening snap will be a clue to the presence of mitral stenosis, and its characteristic murmur can then be looked for. Identification of a well-localized long diastolic low-pitched rumble over the apex beat will be confirmatory. The presence of a typical aortic ejection click may be a clue to the presence of an abnormal bicuspid aortic valve, and the characteristic decrescendo blowing early diastolic murmur with the maximal intensity over the sash area will be confirmatory. The presence of a pulmonary ejection click that becomes soft on inspiration and louder on expiration may be a clue and point to the cause of a low-pitched diastolic murmur over the second and third left interspace as being pulmonary regurgitation with normal pulmonary pressures. A fixed split S2 associated with signs of a large right ventricle may identify an atrial septal defect as the cause of a low-pitched diastolic rumble with maximal loudness over the lower left sternum and over the xiphoid area secondary to tricuspid inflow. Palpable loud P2 over the second left interspace and the associated early blowing diastolic murmur maximal over the second and third left interspace will point to the presence of pulmonary regurgitation associated with pulmonary hypertension. When the precordial pulsations and the arterial pulse are diagnostic of significant aortic regurgitation, the presence of a mid-diastolic low-pitched rumble over the left ventricular apex area will be suggestive of an *Austin Flint rumble*. The latter will also indicate the presence of severe degree of aortic regurgitation.

When aortic regurgitation is detected and the murmur is equally loud over the right of the sternum, the presence of aortic root disease as the cause of the aortic regurgitation should be suspected. When mitral stenosis is diagnosed and confirmed by auscultation, one should still look for the presence of aortic regurgitation because rheumatic heart disease often involves the aortic valve. Its presence must be determined by auscultation.

(For additional examples review Phono Files 1–18 and Mitral Stenosis: Echo Phono File 8 under Heart Murmurs Part 2 on the Companion CD.)

CONTINUOUS MURMURS

A murmur is considered to be continuous when it bridges systole and diastole, extending past the S2. In other words, a continuous murmur lasts through all of systole and goes beyond S2 into a significant portion of diastole, although it may fade away and become inaudible in the later part of diastole. It is very rare that a continuous murmur will last throughout systole and extend into all of diastole *(68)*.

Continuous murmurs represent a continuous turbulent blood flow where the cause of the turbulence extends beyond systole into diastole. Thus, continuous murmurs may be expected to occur in the following circumstances:

1. When there is communication between a high-pressure vessel and a low-pressure vessel or a chamber so that a persistent pressure gradient is present throughout systole and diastole, allowing continuous shunting of blood with turbulent flow
2. When there is marked increase in velocity of blood flow, resulting in turbulence over a local area or region either for physiological or pathological reasons
3. When there is a localized constriction in an artery with poor collateral flow to the distal segment, resulting in a pressure gradient that extends beyond systole into diastole *(68,69)*

Communication Between a High-Pressure Vessel and a Low-Pressure Vessel or Chamber

Arteriovenous shunt surgically produced in a patient requiring hemodialysis for renal failure therapy is a good example of a high-pressure vessel (artery) directly communicating with a low-pressure vessel (vein). Such a shunt bypasses the intervening capillary bed. Occasionally arteriovenous fistulous communications may be present congenitally or may form following some local trauma. In all these instances the communication or the shunt allows a pressure gradient between the two vessels to persist throughout systole and diastole, resulting in a turbulent flow. It is invariable that when such a shunt is open and functional, one will be able to hear a continuous murmur over the vein and its immediate tributaries receiving the flow. The murmur may be accompanied by a continuous thrill over the same area. The frequency of the murmur will depend not only on the level of the pressure gradient but also on the amount of actual flow. If the communication is large and between large vessels such as the aorta and the pulmonary artery, for instance, through a persistent ductus arteriosus, then the turbulence will be influenced by both the pressure gradient and the actual flow. The resulting murmur will have mixed frequencies, including both the high and the low frequencies. In addition, the murmur may exhibit an accentuation in systole because of the higher pressure gradient *(68,70)*.

The high-pressure vessel is generally an artery where the pressure is relatively high during both systole and diastole. Around the heart, the high-pressure vessel could be the aorta or the coronary artery with a normal origin, whereas the low-pressure area could be the pulmonary artery, abnormal coronary artery arising from the pulmonary artery, the right atrium, or the right ventricle.

Rarely, in the presence of mitral obstruction associated with an atrial septal defect (*Lutembacher syndrome*), the left atrial pressures may be significantly elevated compared to the right atrium, and the continuous flow through the atrial septal defect may produce a continuous murmur *(71)*. This is, however, very rare. In certain pulmonary diseases some bronchial artery collaterals to pulmonary artery branches may develop. The disorders where these may develop include bronchiectasis and sequestration of lung. Broncho-pulmonary collaterals do develop more commonly in cyanotic congenital heart diseases with reduced pulmonary flow such as tetralogy of Fallot *(6)*.

The maximum loudness of the murmur is usually over the receiving vessel or chamber. In the case of the persistent ductus, it is over the pulmonary artery; on the surface of the chest this usually corresponds to the second left interspace. If the receiving chamber is the right ventricular outflow tract, then the maximum loudness of the murmur may be over the third and fourth left interspace; when it is the mid-right ventricle, the maximum loudness will be lower sternal and the xiphoid area. If the receiving chamber is the right atrium, then the maximal loudness will be the right sternal edge or to the right of the lower sternum *(69)*.

In the case of aorto-pulmonary communications, the pulmonary vascular resistance may become significantly elevated, resulting in elevated pulmonary artery pressures. If this should occur, then the shunt will diminish because of diminishing pressure gradient, and the murmur will become short and may eventually disappear when the pulmonary pressures become systemic. In addition, the shunt flow may actually reverse in direction, leading to the development of cyanosis. In persistent ductus arteriosus, because the ductus joins the aorta beyond the origin of the left subclavian artery, the lower limbs will tend to become cyanotic, whereas the head and face and the upper extremities will be spared (*differential cyanosis*) *(38)*.

The following is a partial list of communications, arranged according to the feeding vessel.

1. From the aorta
   a. Persistent ductus arteriosus
   b. Aorto-pulmonary window
   c. Congenital sinus of Valsalva aneurysm with fistulae
2. From the coronary artery:
   a. Coronary arteriovenous fistulae draining into the right atrium, right ventricle, or pulmonary artery
   b. Anomalous origin of the left coronary artery from the pulmonary artery
3. Other arteriovenous communications
   a. Broncho-pulmonary collaterals
   b. Chest wall arteries–pulmonary vessels

Increased Velocity of Blood Flow

Physiological causes of rapid blood flow leading to continuous murmurs include cervical venous hum because of rapid venous inflow through the internal jugular vein *(72, 73)* and mammary souffle heard in pregnant women close to term or immediately postpartum during the lactating period *(74)*. Increased blood flow locally leading to continuous murmurs can occur under a variety of pathological causes, which include hemangiomas, neoplasms with hypervascularity, such as a hepatic carcinoma, and renal cell carcinoma. In general, these murmurs have more low-frequency components because of large blood flow volume. The location of maximal loudness will be related to the sites of the vessels involved *(68)*.

Arterial Obstruction

Most local obstruction in arteries generates only a systolic murmur because of the fact that the distal segment usually receives enough collateral flow, which helps to maintain relatively the same diastolic pressure as in the segment proximal to the stenosed area. Thus, arterial obstructions associated with continuous murmurs mean that the collateral flow to the distal segment is poor, resulting in a persistent gradient, which extends from systole through to diastole. Continuous murmurs secondary to localized obstructions of this nature are known to occur in aortic arch vessel occlusions, in *Takayasu's disease*, in atherosclerotic disease of the carotid vessels, occasionally in coarctation of aorta, as well as in main pulmonary artery stenosis and peripheral pulmonary artery stenosis.

Certain specific lesions producing continuous murmurs will be discussed further.

PERSISTENT DUCTUS ARTERIOSUS

Ductus arteriosus is a vascular channel that is normally present in the fetus connecting the aorta just distal to the left subclavian artery to the pulmonary trunk near the origin of the left pulmonary artery. In the unaerated lungs of the fetus, the pulmonary capillaries are shut down. The pulmonary vascular resistance is equal to the systemic resistance. The mixed venous and placental blood from the right ventricle passes through the ductus into the descending aorta. At the same time, part of the mixed venous and the placental blood goes through the foramen ovale to the left side and is pumped by the left ventricle into the ascending aorta supplying the head and the upper extremities. At birth, the expansion of the lungs and alveolar oxygenation lead to rapid lowering of the pulmonary vascular resistance. The ductus normally closes functionally during the first 24 h after birth. It becomes anatomically closed within a few weeks after birth. Closure may be delayed in premature as well as hypoxemic full-term infants. The left-to-right shunt through the ductus is dependent on the pulmonary vascular resistance. The pulmonary vascular resistance tends to be low in the premature infant, and the excessive flow through the ductus can cause congestive heart failure in the premature infant. In the hypoxemic infant, the pulmonary vascular resistance is usually high, raising the pulmonary artery pressure. The ductus in this instance will therefore not cause a continuous murmur *(75)*.

Occasionally the ductus remains open in the infant and persists into adulthood. Maternal rubella in the first trimester has a close association with a persistent ductus. Persistent ductus can occur either alone or associated with other anomalies, such as a ventricular septal defect or coarctation of the aorta. The degree of left-to-right shunt will depend on both the pulmonary vascular resistance as well as the size of the ductus.

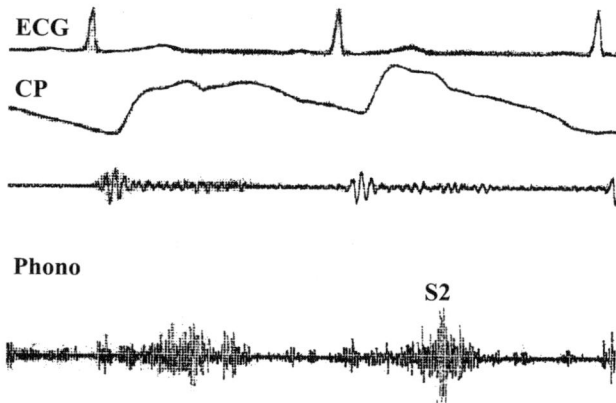

Fig. 11. Simultaneous recordings of electrocardiogram (ECG), carotid pulse, and phonocardiogram (Phono) taken over the second left interspace at the left sternal border from a patient with persistent ductus arteriosus. The Phono recording shows the murmur peaking around the second heart sound (S2).

The left-to-right shunt through the persistent ductus will cause volume overload of the left atrium and the left ventricle, leading to their enlargement. This will cause the apical impulse to be hyperdynamic and formed by the left ventricle. The arterial pulse will have a large amplitude with a rapid rise and a wide pulse pressure. The aortic diastolic pressure will fall to lower levels because of the large communication to the pulmonary artery with significantly lower vascular resistance *(38,70)*.

Persistent ductus generally causes no symptoms after the first year of life until perhaps the third decade. In the majority of patients the persistent ductus is associated with pulmonary pressures at levels considerably lower than the systemic pressures. In about 5% of patients the pulmonary vascular resistance may become significantly elevated, leading to pulmonary hypertension with *Eisenmenger's syndrome (63)*. This tends to occur in early adult life. The shunt will become right-to-left when the pulmonary vascular resistance is high. Because the ductus joins the aorta distal to the left subclavian, the cyanosis associated with reverse shunt will affect the lower extremities, and the *differential cyanosis and clubbing* may point to the diagnosis on mere inspection.

Auscultatory features in persistent ductus arteriosus include the following:

1. The flow to the pulmonary artery during early systole is usually from the right ventricle. But in late systole and in diastole, the flow through the ductus increases. The turbulent flow under significant pressure difference is produced in late systole and during diastole. Therefore, the typical ductus murmur is a continuous murmur, which increases in intensity around the second heart sound and fades away toward the end of diastole (Fig. 11) *(38,70)*.
2. When there is a large volume of flow, the ductus murmur is harsh and *"machinery"*-like or "train in a tunnel"-like and is associated with significant accentuation in later systole. They may also be associated with discrete "eddy" sounds, which may sometimes be like clicks or crackles *(76)*.
3. When the ductus is small, the flow may occur under a high-pressure gradient with a high velocity. This may give rise to a high-frequency continuous murmur.

4. The maximal loudness of the ductus murmur is usually over the second left interspace. The second best location for loudness is the first left interspace. This is an important differential point, which will help to distinguish persistent ductus from other causes of continuous murmurs *(59,70)*.
5. When the flow through the ductus is large enough to produce significant left ventricular enlargement, one may hear low-frequency short mid-diastolic rumble at the apex suggestive of increased mitral inflow.
6. The S2 may be paradoxically split on inspiration when the left-to-right shunt is large because of the reversed sequence caused by delayed A2. The A2 delay is best explained by the low systemic impedance consequent to a large communication (ductus), which exposes the entire pulmonary vascular bed to the aorta.
7. When pulmonary vascular resistance becomes elevated, initially the pulmonary diastolic pressures rise. This will abolish the diastolic pressure gradient between the aorta and the pulmonary artery, abolishing the diastolic portion of the murmur. This will leave the ductus murmur pansystolic. Eventually when the pulmonary systolic pressures also become elevated, the murmur will become shorter and shorter in systole. Finally, other auscultatory signs of pulmonary hypertension may become evident. These will include pulmonary ejection sounds, loud P2, single or closely split S2, and occasionally pulmonary regurgitation murmurs *(Graham Steell murmur)*
8. Since the pulmonary vascular resistance tends to be high in the neonatal period, a persistent ductus may only cause a systolic murmur initially, and typical continuous murmur may occur only when the pulmonary vascular resistance falls to normal levels *(38,75)*.

AORTO-PULMONARY WINDOW

The defect is often rather large round or oval and is usually between the adjacent parts of the aortic root and the main pulmonary artery, probably because of a gap in the development of the partition of the embryonic truncus arteriosus. The pathophysiology is very similar to the patent ductus. It is less common and tends to be associated with a higher incidence of pulmonary hypertension (Eisenmenger's syndrome). The murmur may therefore not be continuous, and both the upper and the lower extremities will show cyanosis. When the size of the defect is not large, the signs can be very similar to those of persistent ductus. However, the location of maximal loudness of the continuous murmur is lower and often over the second and third left interspace *(38,77)*.

SINUS OF VALSALVA ANEURYSM

Congenital aneurysms of the sinus of Valsalva are a result of focal defect in the media of the aortic sinus. They start as blind diverticulum, which may elongate and enlarge. They can grow like a windsock. Eventually they can rupture into the adjoining cardiac chamber. These aneurysms most often arise in the right coronary or the noncoronary sinus. They need to be distinguished from diffuse dilatation of the sinus as may occur in Marfan's syndrome. Aneurysm involving the right coronary sinus communicates with the right ventricle and occasionally the right atrium. Aneurysms of the noncoronary sinus communicate with the right atrium.

The pathophysiological effects of these aneurysms depend on how rapidly the rupture (leading to fistula formation) occurs resulting in the left-to-right shunt, the amount of flow through the fistula, and the chamber or chambers receiving the shunt *(38,78)*. If the communication develops gradually, the onset of symptoms will be insidious. If rupture occurs acutely, patient may present with sudden-onset chest discomfort and dyspnea. Congestive heart failure may subsequently develop after a variable period of several hours to several days *(78)*. Right atrium and the right ventricle will become volume overloaded and enlarged if the rupture occurs into the right atrium. The right ventricle will show volume overload if rupture occurs into that chamber. Because of the left-to-right shunt at the right heart level, the pulmonary venous return will always be higher than normal, leading to volume overload of the left atrium and the left ventricle. The arterial pulse will show rapid aortic runoff with wide pulse pressure, large amplitude, and rapid upstroke. The jugular venous pressure will reflect the raised right ventricular *pre-a wave* pressure, and the contour will show equal x' and y *descents*. If right ventricular failure occurs, tricuspid regurgitation may develop, which may be reflected in the jugulars. Rarely, a large aneurysm bulging into the right ventricular outflow may cause signs of obstruction.

These congenital aneurysms may be well visualized in two-dimensional echocardiographic images with color flow Doppler mapping, and their communication sites may be precisely defined.

Auscultatory Features

Once the communication is established, the congenital aneurysms of the sinus of Valsalva will lead to continuous murmurs. The location of maximal loudness will depend on the chamber into which the left-to-right shunt drains. If the communication is into the right atrium, the maximal loudness of the murmur is at the lower sternum and close to the right sternal edge and occasionally to the right of the sternal edge. Rupture into the right ventricle causes the murmur to be loudest at the lower left sternal border area, and when it communicates into the right ventricular outflow tract, the murmur may be loudest at the left sternal edge but at a higher level (third left interspace). The murmur may be louder either in systole or diastole. Rarely, right ventricular contraction may decrease the shunt in systole, resulting in accentuation of the murmur in diastole. If the shunt is large, then the murmur will have both high and low (mixed) frequencies. The low frequencies will arise from the large volume flow.

CORONARY ARTERIOVENOUS FISTULAE

Coronary arteriovenous malformations are isolated congenital anomalies. They may arise from either the right or the left coronary artery, and the majority of them drain into the right heart. The sites of drainage may be the right atrium, the coronary sinus, or the right ventricle. Rarely, they may drain into the main pulmonary artery. The coronary artery that forms the fistula is often dilated and sometimes tortuous. Rarely, the fistulous coronary artery branch may steal flow from the normal coronary artery because of the lower pressure. Myocardial ischemia is, however, rare. The left-to-right shunt generally is not very large, and the diagnosis may be considered when the continuous murmur is fairly localized and the maximal loudness of the continuous murmur is at an atypical site. The location of maximal loudness will depend on the site of drainage of the fistula. If the receiving chamber is the right atrium, the maximal loudness is at the lower sternal area and often at the upper or lower right sternal border. When the fistula drains into the right ventricle, the site of maximal loudness is over the xiphoid area or the lower sternum or the lower left sternal border area. When the fistula drains into the right ventricular outflow tract, the murmur is loudest at the third and the fourth left interspace. When it drains into the main pulmonary artery, the murmur is loudest at the second and third left interspace. The murmur often tends to be soft. The murmur may have diastolic accentuation because coronary flow occurs more during diastole than during systole. Occasionally systolic compression of the fistulous coronary by the contracting myocardium may significantly decrease the systolic portion of the continuous murmur *(79)*.

VENOUS HUM

The venous hum is generally caused by rapid flow through the internal jugular and the subclavian veins as they join the superior vena cava. It generally gives rise to a continuous roar and occasionally may have a whining quality. It is usually heard over the supraclavicular area between the clavicular and the sternal heads of the sternomastoid muscle. It tends to be louder on the right side. The bell of the stethoscope is most suited to listening for the venous hum because it will provide the best air seal in this region. The murmur is often heard in young children and occasionally in pregnant women. The venous hum can be brought out even in the normal adult by causing slight angulation of the internal jugulars by turning the head to the opposite side and tilting it slightly upward. Anemia and hyperthyroidism often lead to very rapid circulation and cause venous hums in adults. In these instances the venous hum may be audible without any need to turn the patient's head. The characteristic feature of the venous hum is that it can be temporarily abolished by digital pressure applied over the middle of the sternomastoid muscle so as to compress the internal jugular vein that runs underneath it. The site of digital pressure must obviously be above the site of auscultation. Releasing the jugular compression will temporarily increase the intensity of the venous hum. The venous hum also tends to be louder in the sitting position and tends to disappear in the supine position. The diastolic component of the murmur is often louder. When the venous hum is very loud, it may be transmitted to the infraclavicular area and may be mistaken for a persistent ductus arteriosus. Occasionally the high-frequency components of the murmur may be selectively transmitted to the infraclavicular area, and then it may be mistaken for aortic regurgitation murmur *(72,73)*.

MAMMARY SOUFFLE

This is a result of rapid and increased flow through the arteries in the breasts of pregnant women close to term or during lactation postpartum. The mammary arteries may be dilated. The murmur usually has a systolic accentuation and can be abolished by local pressure or pressure applied just lateral to the breast *(74)*.

CLINICAL ASSESSMENT OF CONTINUOUS MURMURS

A murmur must be considered continuous if it goes through S2 and extends into diastole. Most continuous murmurs do not extend throughout diastole. They generally fade away during the later part of diastole. When a continuous murmur is heard, assessment of the following will be important in arriving at the probable cause of the murmur:

1. The location of maximal loudness of the murmur
2. The location of the second best area of loudness of the murmur

3. The effect of internal jugular compression on the loudness of the murmur, especially when the murmur is audible over the second and third interspace
4. Whether the murmur is harsh and has a lot of low frequencies
5. Signs pertaining to the arterial pulse, which may suggest early runoff as in aortic regurgitation with large-amplitude bounding pulses
6. Signs of left ventricular volume overload, as suggested by a wide-area left ventricular apex beat, which is also hyperdynamic
7. Presence of mitral inflow rumble (low-pitched mid-diastolic murmur audible over a left ventricular apex area)
8. Abnormal jugular venous pressures and or contours
9. If S2 is split, whether it is normal or wide and physiological, fixed or reversed
10. Systemic signs such as cyanosis and its distribution

The three general causes of continuous murmurs need to be kept in mind in the differential diagnosis, namely:

1. Communication between high-pressure vessel and a low-pressure vessel or chamber
2. Marked increase in localized flow
3. Localized arterial obstruction with poor collateralization to the distal segment

The radiation of the murmur as usual is not as important as the location of maximal loudness. In children and young adults with thin chest, loud venous hum could be heard over a large area of the chest because of the wide area of transmission. The location of maximal loudness helps in identifying the receiving chamber (or vessel) in arteriovenous-type communications. The most important lesion among these is a persistent ductus arteriosus.

The features about persistent ductus arteriosus worth noting are:

1. The maximal loudness of the ductus murmur is over the second left interspace, and the second best area of loudness for the ductus murmur is the first left interspace, where it can be equally loud. If the murmur is equally loud over the third left interspace and not over the first left interspace, then communications of other types draining into the pulmonary artery or pulmonary outflow tracts should be considered and not a persistent ductus.
2. The ductus murmur increases in intensity around S2 and fades away in diastole.
3. When flow is large, the murmur is harsh.
4. One may often hear discrete crackling "eddy" sounds.
5. S2 may be paradoxically split.

Other Points to Consider

If internal jugular compression abolishes the murmur temporarily, then a venous hum is suggested. When the maximal loudness is over the lower sternal and xiphoid area, then communications draining into the mid-right ventricle must be considered. When the maximal loudness is over the right sternal edge or right of the sternum, the right atrium is likely to be the receiving chamber. When the murmur is harsh in the presence of an abnormal arteriovenous communication, it usually indicates a significant shunt with a lot of flow. Presence of signs of an enlarged left ventricle with hyperdynamic impulse and a mitral inflow rumble would indicate excessive flow through the mitral valve. This would indicate that the left-to-right shunt through the communication is significant.

Peripheral signs simulating aortic regurgitation, such as those of large-amplitude pulses with wide pulse pressure (bounding arterial pulses with early runoff) together with hyperdynamic and enlarged left ventricle, could be produced in situations with severe anemia or arteriovenous communications, which are large with significant shunt. These signs are also exaggerated if the aorta itself is involved in the communications such as through a persistent ductus arteriosus, aorto-pulmonary window, and congenital sinus of Valsalva aneurysm with fistulae.

Abnormal jugular contours and elevated jugular venous pressure with acute onset of symptoms and signs of rapidly progressive congestive failure in the presence of a loud continuous murmur would point to a lesion such as ruptured sinus of Valsalva aneurysm communicating with the right atrium or the right ventricle.

Coronary arteriovenous fistulae may be considered when signs of a large left-to-right shunt are absent and the continuous murmur is localized to an atypical site.

Localized arterial occlusions may be considered if arterial pulses are poorly felt or absent. This may affect the carotid vessels and vessels of the upper extremities in the case of *Takayasu's disease*.

PERICARDIAL FRICTION RUB

Acute pericarditis may occur as a result of infection of viral origin, secondary to underlying collagen vascular disease, such as rheumatoid arthritis and lupus erythematosus, secondary to trauma, typically post-cardiac-surgery, following acute myocardial infarction, in uremia, and sometimes secondary to invasive tumors. In all these states the cardiac motion against the inflamed pericardium with its two surfaces—the visceral and the parietal—will give rise to generation of friction noise, which is termed the pericardial friction rub. Often the diagnosis of acute pericarditis can be confirmed if a typical pericardial friction rub is heard. The rub could be transient and may be missed and sometimes absent because of accumulation of fluid between the two surfaces of the pericardium, preventing friction. The pericardial effusion, as a result of the inflammation, may, however, be detected by echocardiography. The friction rub is also sometimes quite localized either over the lower sternal border area or the apex. Occasionally it may be heard over a wide area of the precordium. Sometimes it may be audible only in certain patient positions.

The pericardial friction rub typically has three phases: systolic (because of ventricular contraction), diastolic (due to ventricular relaxation and expansion during diastole), and atrial systolic (secondary to atrial contraction at the end of diastole). The noise is usually scratchy or squishy and will show the three phases. Occasionally it may be harsh and have mixed frequencies, may simulate a murmur, and may be difficult to distinguish, particularly if the atrial systolic phase is absent. The systolic component is generally always present and may sometimes be the only component, especially when the rhythm is atrial fibrillation. Pericardial friction rubs always tend to accentuate on inspiration because the pericardium is distorted and pulled by the inspiratory expansion of the lungs and the descent of the diaphragm. This sign therefore needs to be looked for by careful auscultation during inspiration whenever friction rub is suspected. The usual left-sided murmurs, on the other hand, will not increase on inspiration *(80–82)*.

INNOCENT MURMURS

The term innocent murmur is used when the conditions that lead to the production of the murmur are entirely benign to the exclusion of significant organic abnormalities. The turbulence that accounts for these murmurs is often a result of normal or rapid flow, and the murmur may be entirely systolic and occasionally continuous and very rarely mid-diastolic.

Systolic Murmurs

The systolic murmurs that may qualify under this category are ejection in type and often short in duration. They may be heard variably over the precordium either at the second and third left interspace or over the lower left sternal border and at the apex area. They may occur in young children and young adolescents or in adults above the age of 50 yr. In the former it may arise from either the aortic or the pulmonary outflow tracts. In some young subjects with narrow antero-posterior diameter of the chest, the normal flow through the pulmonary outflow, which may be associated with some turbulence, may cause short ejection murmurs, which may be heard over the chest because of close proximity. In some children they may be quite vibratory and humming, as described by Still as *"twanging string"* murmur. It is usually best heard between the left sternal border and the apex. While they are accentuated by increased cardiac output, the frequency spectrum of these murmurs appears to be more related to the age of the patient and the left ventricular dimensions rather than the flow velocities *(83)*. The vibratory nature of the murmur may actually be related to vibration of structures like some congenital intracardiac bands, which may stretch across the ventricular cavity unattached to the valves *(38,83–86)*.

In adults over the age of 50 yr, benign ejection murmurs are again relatively common and may be a result of some roughening or sclerosis of the aortic valve cusps, aortic root dilatation, or distortion caused by atherosclerosis and hypertension; in some patients they may also be a result of an angulated septum (sigmoid septum), which may be seen on the two-dimensional echocardiographic images to be slightly hypertrophied at proximal level because of co-existing hypertension and lead to the production of outflow turbulence *(86,87)*.

The markers of the benign nature of these systolic murmurs are:
1. They are ejection in type and generally short in duration with early peak.
2. The murmur may be musical and humming or vibratory, which is hardly ever the case with organic semi-lunar valvular stenosis or obstructive outflow tracts.
3. The murmur will diminish in intensity on standing because of decrease in venous return and may actually disappear.
4. The murmur will also diminish in intensity during the strain phase of Valsalva maneuver.
5. The murmur will not be associated with ejection clicks.

Continuous Murmurs

Continuous murmurs, which may be considered benign, are usually caused by excessive and rapid blood flow. Venous hum heard in children and adults with anemia and/or thyrotoxicosis and mammary souffle heard in postpartum lactating women belong to this category. Venous hum can sometimes be loud and heard over a large area in the upper chest, especially in children. It often is a low-pitched roar. Occasionally it may sound high in frequency, particularly in the presence of anemia. It usually can be eliminated temporarily by occluding digital pressure over the internal jugular vein. Mammary souffle can be eliminated by local pressure applied just lateral to the breast *(72–74)*.

MID-DIASTOLIC MURMURS

In some young adults and children, the physiological S3 may have some vibrations, which may have some duration to it and may sound like a short rumble but has the same significance as the physiological S3 *(86)*.

(For additional examples review Phono files 19–31 under Heart Murmurs Part 2 on the Companion CD.)

REFERENCES

1. Wood P. An appreciation of mitral stenosis: I Clinical features. Br Med J 1954;1:1051.
2. Wood P. An appreciation of mitral stenosis: II Investigations and results. Br Med J 1954;1:1113.
3. Craige E. Phonocardiographic studies in mitral stenosis. N Engl J Med 1957;257:650.
4. Criley JM, Chambers RD, Blaufuss AH, Friedman NJ. Mitral stenosis: mechanico-acoustical events. American Heart Association Monograph 1975;46:149–159.
5. Lutembacher R. De la stenose mitrale avec communication interauriculaire. Arch Mal Coeur 1916; 9:237.
6. Perloff JK. The Clinical Recognition of Congenital Heart Disease. Philadelphia, PA: W.B. Saunders, 2003.
7. Angelino PF, Garbagni R, Tartara D. [The Lutembacher syndrome: clinical and hemodynamic observations before and after surgery.]. Arch Mal Coeur Vaiss 1961;54:511–524.
8. Nasser WK, Davis RH, Dillon JC, et al. Atrial myxoma. I. Clinical and pathologic features in nine cases. Am Heart J 1972;83:694–704.
9. Nasser WK, Davis RH, Dillon JC, et al. Atrial myxoma. II. Phonocardiographic, echocardiographic, hemodynamic, and angiographic features in nine cases. Am Heart J 1972;83:810–823.
10. Fortuin NJ, Craige E. Echocardiographic studies of genesis of mitral diastolic murmurs. Br Heart J 1973;35:75–81.
11. Otto CM. Mitral stenosis. In: Otto CM, ed. Valvular Heart Disease. Philadelphia, PA: W.B. Saunders, 2004.
12. Rahimtoola SH, Durairaj A, Mehra A, Nuno I. Current evaluation and management of patients with mitral stenosis. Circulation 2002;106:1183–1188.
13. Wooley CF, Klassen KP, Leighton RF, Goodwin RS, Ryan JM. Left atrial and left ventricular sound and pressure in mitral stenosis. Circulation 1968;38:295.
14. Criley JM, Feldman IM, Meredith T. Mitral valve closure and the crescendo presystolic murmur. Am J Med 1971;51:456–465.
15. Criley JM, Hermer AJ. The crescendo presystolic murmur with atrial fibrillation. N Engl J Med 1971; 285:1284.
16. Hada Y, Amano K, Yamaguchi T, et al. Noninvasive study of the presystolic component of the first heart sound in mitral stenosis. J Am Coll Cardiol 1986;7:43–50.
17. Perloff JK. The physiological mechanisms of cardiac and vascular physical signs. J Am Coll Cardiol 1983;1:184–198.
18. Perloff JK, Harvey WP. Auscultatory and phonocardiographic manifestations of pure mitral regurgitation. Prog Cardiovasc Dis 1962;5:172–194.
19. Ayers CR, Boineau JP, Spach MS. Congenital complete heart block in children. Am Heart J 1966;72: 381–390.
20. Rytand DA. Auricular diastolic murmur with heart block in elderly patients. Am Heart J 1946;32:579.
21. Coombs CF. Rheumatic myocarditis. Q J Med 1908;2:26.
22. Flint A. On cardiac murmurs. Am J Med Sci 1862;44:29.
23. Landzberg JS, Pflugfelder PW, Cassidy MM, Schiller NB, Higgins CB, Cheitlin MD. Etiology of the Austin Flint murmur. J Am Coll Cardiol 1992;20:408–413.
24. Reddy PS, Curtiss EI, Salerni R, et al. Sound pressure correlates of the Austin Flint murmur. An intracardiac sound study. Circulation 1976;53:210–217.

25. O'Brien KP, Cohen LS. Hemodynamic and phonocardiographic correlates of the Austin flint murmur. Am Heart J 1969;77:603–609.
26. Fortuin NJ, Craige E. On the mechanism of the Austin Flint murmur. Circulation 1972;45:558–570.
27. De Leon AC, Harvey PW. Pharmacological agents and auscultation. Mod Concepts Cardiov Dis 1975; 44:23–28.
28. Bousvaros GA, Stubington D. Some Auscultatory and phonocardiographic features of tricuspid stenosis. Circulation 1964;29:26-33.
29. Leake.H. Rheumatic tricuspid stenosis. Acta Med Scand 1958;161:109.
30. Wooley CF, Fontana ME, Kilman JW, Ryan JM. Tricuspid stenosis. Atrial systolic murmur, tricuspid opening snap, and right atrial pressure pulse. Am J Med 1985;78:375–384.
31. Carabello BA, Crawford FA, Jr. Valvular heart disease. N Engl J Med 1997;337:32–41.
32. el-Sherif N. Rheumatic tricuspid stenosis. A haemodynamic correlation. Br Heart J 1971;33:16–31.
33. Ewy GA. Tricuspid valve disease. In: Alpert JS, Dalen JE, Rahimtoola SH, eds. Valvular Heart Disease. Philadelphia, PA: Lippincott Williams and Wilkins, 2000:377–392.
34. Ashman H, Zaroff LI, Baronofsky I. Right atrial myxoma. Diagnosis during life: successful surgical removal. Am J Med 1960;28:487–496.
35. Waxler EB, Kawai N, Kasparian H. Right atrial myxoma: echocardiographic, phonocardiographic, and hemodynamic signs. Am Heart J 1972;83:251–257.
36. Gotzsche H, Falholt W. Ebstein's anomaly of the tricuspid valve; a review of the literature and report of 6 new cases. Am Heart J 1954;47:587–603.
37. Roberts WC. A unique heart disesae associated with a unique cancer: carcinoid heart disease. Am J Cardiol 1997;80:251–256.
38. Perloff JK. The Clinical Recognition of Congenital Heart Disease. Philadelphia, PA: W.B. Saunders, 1979–1981;279,312.
39. Wooley CF. The spectrum of tricuspid regurgitation. American Heart Association Monograph 1975;46:139–148.
40. Leatham A, Gray IR. Auscultatory and phonocardiographic signs of atrial septal defect. Br Heart J 1956;18:193.
41. Olson LJ, Subramanian R, Edwards WD. Surgical pathology of pure aortic insufficiency: a study of 225 cases. Mayo Clin Proc 1984;59:835–841.
42. Carabello BA. Progress in mitral and aortic regurgitation. Prog Cardiovasc Dis 2001;43:457–475.
43. Rahimtoola SH. Aortic regurgitation. Valvular heart disease. In: Braunwald.E, ed. Atlas of Heart Diseases, Vol. 11. Philadelphia, PA: Current Medicine, 1997;7, 9.
44. Fedak PW, Verma S, David TE, Leask RL, Weisel RD, Butany J. Clinical and pathophysiologicalal implications of a bicuspid aortic valve. Circulation 2002;106:900–904.
45. Bonow RO, Carabello B, de Leon AC, Jr., et al. Guidelines for the management of patients with valvular heart disease: executive summary. A report of the American College of Cardiology/American Heart Association Task Force on Practice Guidelines (Committee on Management of Patients with Valvular Heart Disease). Circulation 1998;98:1949–1984.
46. Bonow RO. Chronic aortic regurgitation. In: Alpert JS, Dalen JE, Rahimtoola SH, eds. Valvular Heart Disease. Philadelphia, PA: Lippincott Williams & Wilkins, 2000:245–268.
47. Fielitz J, Hein S, Mitrovic V, et al. Activation of the cardiac renin-angiotensin system and increased myocardial collagen expression in human aortic valve disease. J Am Coll Cardiol 2001;37:1443–1449.
48. Gaasch WH, Carroll JD, Levine HJ, Criscitiello MG. Chronic aortic regurgitation: prognostic value of left ventricular end-systolic dimension and end-diastolic radius/thickness ratio. J Am Coll Cardiol 1983;1:775–782.
49. Carabello BA. Concentric versus eccentric remodeling. J Card Fail 2002;8:S258–263.
50. Borer JS, Truter S, Herrold EM, et al. Myocardial fibrosis in chronic aortic regurgitation: molecular and cellular responses to volume overload. Circulation 2002;105:1837–1842.
51. Bonow RO. Chronic aortic regurgitation. Role of medical therapy and optimal timing for surgery. Cardiol Clin 1998;16:449–461.
52. Otto CM. Aortic regurgitation. In: Otto CM, ed. Valvular Heart Disease. Philadelphia, PA: W.B. Saunders, 2004.
53. Vatner SF, Shannon R, Hittinger L. Reduced subendocardial coronary reserve. A potential mechanism for impaired diastolic function in the hypertrophied and failing heart. Circulation 1990;81: III8–114.

54. Vatner SF, Hittinger L. Coronary vascular mechanisms involved in decompensation from hypertrophy to heart failure. J Am Coll Cardiol 1993;22:34A–40A.
55. Hittinger L, Mirsky I, Shen YT, Patrick TA, Bishop SP, Vatner SF. Hemodynamic mechanisms responsible for reduced subendocardial coronary reserve in dogs with severe left ventricular hypertrophy. Circulation 1995;92:978–986.
56. Reddy PS, Leon DF, Krishnaswami.V, O'Toole JD, Salerni R, Shaver JA. Syndrome of acute aortic regurgitation. American Heart Association Monograph 1975;46:166–174.
57. Wigle ED, Labrosse CJ. Sudden, severe aortic insufficiency. Circulation 1965;32:708–720.
58. Cole.R, Cecil AB. The axillary diastolic murmur in aortic insufficiency. Bull Johns Hopkins Hosp 1908;19:353.
59. Constant J. Bedside Cardiology. Boston, MA: Little, Brown and Company, 1976.
60. McCraw DB, Siegel W, Stonecipher HK, Nutter DO, Schlant RC, Hurst JW. Response of heart murmur intensity to isometric (handgrip) exercise. Br Heart J 1972;34:605–610.
61. Steell G. The murmur of high pressure in the pulmonary artery. Med Chronicle 1888;9:182.
62. Wood P. Diseases of the Heart and Circulation. Philadelphia, PA: J.B.Lippincott Co, 1956.
63. Wood.P. The Eisenmenger syndrome or pulmonary hypertension with reversed central shunt. Br Heart J 1963;2:701.
64. Perloff JK. Auscultatory and phonocardiographic manifestations of pulmonary hypertension. Prog Cardiovasc Dis 1967;9:303.
65. Grossman.W, Braunwald E. Pulmonary hypertension. In: Heart Disease: A Textbook of Cardiovascular Medicine. Philadelphia, PA: W.B. Saunders Co, 1988:793–818.
66. Bousvaros GA, Deuchar DC. The mumur of pulmonary regurgitation which is not associated with pulmonary hypertension. Lancet 1961;2:962–964.
67. Hultgren HN, Reeve R, Cohn K, McLeod R. The ejection click of valvular pulmonic stenosis. Circulation 1969;40:631–640.
68. Myers JD. The mechanisms and significances of continuous murmurs. Am Heart Association Monograph 1975;46:201–208.
69. Huffman T, Leighton RF, Goodwin RS, Ryan JM, Wooley CF. Continuous murmurs associated with shunts in the acyanotic adult. An anatomic classification. Am J Med 1970;49:160–169.
70. Gibson GA. Persistence of the arterial duct and its diagnosis. Edinburgh Med J 1900;8:1.
71. Ross J, Jr, Braunwald E, Mason DT, Braunwald N, Morrow AG. Inter-atrial communication and left atrial hypertension. A cause of continuous murmur. Circulation 1963;28:853.
72. Cutforth R, Wiseman J, Sutherland RD. The genesis of the cervical venous hum. Am Heart J 1970;80: 488–492.
73. Jones FL, Jr. Frequency, characteristics and importance of the cervical venous hum in adults. N Engl J Med 1962;267:658–660.
74. Tabatznik B, Randall TW, Hersch C. The mammary souffle of pregnancy and lactation. Circulation 1960; 22:1069–1073.
75. Zuberbuhler JR, Lenox CC, Park SC, Neches WH. Continuous murmurs in the newborn. Physiologic principles of heart sounds and murmurs: American Heart Association Monograph 1975;46:209–214.
76. Hubbard TF, Neis DD. The sounds at the base of the heart in cases of patent ductus arteriosus. Am Heart J 1960;59:807–815.
77. Morrow AG, Greenfield LJ, Braunwald E. Congenital aortopulmonary septal defect. Clinical and hemodynamic findings, surgical technic, and results of operative correction. Circulation 1962;25: 463–476.
78. Morgan JR, Rogers AK, Fosburg RG. Ruptured aneurysms of the sinus of Valsalva. Chest 1972;61: 640–643.
79. Morgan JR, Forker AD, O'Sullivan MJ, Jr, Fosburg RG. Coronary arterial fistulas: seven cases with unusual features. Am J Cardiol 1972;30:432–436.
80. Harvey WP. Auscultatory findings in diseases of the pericardium. Am J Cardiol 1961;7:15–20.
81. Spodick DH. Pericardial friction. Characteristics of pericardial rubs in fifty consecutive, prospectively studied patients. N Engl J Med 1968;278:1204–1207.
82. Spodick DH. Pericardial rub. Prospective, multiple observer investigation of pericardial friction in 100 patients. Am J Cardiol 1975;35:357–362.
83. Donnerstein RL, Thomsen VS. Hemodynamic and anatomic factors affecting the frequency content of Still's innocent murmur. Am J Cardiol 1994;74:508–510.

84. Still GF. Common Disorders and Diseases of Childhood. London, UK: Frowde, Hodder and Stoughton, 1909.
85. Joffe HS. Genesis of Still's innocent systolic murmur. Br Heart J 1992;67:206.
86. Tavel ME. Innocent murmurs. American Heart Association Monograph 1975; 46:102-106.
87. Dalldorf FG, Willis PW, 4th. Angled aorta ("sigmoid septum") as a cause of hypertrophic subaortic stenosis. Hum Pathol 1985;16:457–462.

9 Elements of Auscultation

Contents
- THE STETHOSCOPE
- AUSCULTATION METHOD
- REFERENCES

In order to get the most and useful information, auscultation of the heart should be focused and done in a methodical way and not just carried out in a haphazard manner. Generally by the time one is ready to auscultate, the diagnostic possibilities must have been narrowed down considerably. This is achieved by the continuous synthesis of the analysis of what has been detected by examination of the venous pulse, the arterial pulse, and the precordial pulsations in relation to the patient's presenting symptoms and the possibilities suggested by them. Thus, an experienced clinician must know what to expect on auscultation or what to listen for before auscultation is even begun. Auscultation is used to confirm or rule out diagnoses that are already being considered. Only a few conditions are diagnosed by auscultation alone. For instance, auscultation may be the only way to diagnose the presence of mild mitral regurgitation because of prolapsed mitral valve leaflets or mild pulmonary valvular stenosis with the typical pulmonary ejection click. In certain conditions, auscultation may not add much to the diagnosis that is already suspected, for instance, chronic stable angina with no prior infarction.

THE STETHOSCOPE

Use of an optimum and well-designed stethoscope is important for proper auscultation, as is the auscultator's head that fits in between the two earpieces. Generally the frequency range of heart sounds does not extend beyond 1000 Hz. It must be noted that the bell of the stethoscope picks up low frequencies while the diaphragm picks up the high frequencies. Understanding the frequency characters of the various heart sounds and murmurs heard in both the normal and the abnormal cardiac states will allow one to use the stethoscope appropriately for their detection. The ideal bell chest piece should be shallow with a large internal diameter to pick up low frequencies. The diaphragm should be thin and stiff. An x-ray film is not stiff enough to be a good diaphragm. Pressing the bell over the chest wall will make the skin taut and make it behave like a diaphragm and may result in bringing out higher frequencies. The optimum tubing of the stethoscope should be made of smooth vinyl or rubber about 10–12 in. or 25 cm in length, and the internal diameter should be about 3/16 in. Most commercially available stethoscopes (Littman, Harvey, Leatham, Rappaport-Sprague) will satisfy these requirements. The metal headpieces should be rotated so that the eartips face anteriorly toward the external auditory meatus because the external ear canals are normally oriented slightly backwards. Finally, the earpieces should be comfortably large.

AUSCULTATION METHOD

Auscultation needs to incorporate the following elements:
1. Listening for one thing at a time and one thing at a time only
2. Listening for specific things with predetermined mental filter with the use of cadence (or vocal simulation)
3. Application of principles based on sound transmission as related to the site of origin (not related to the traditional areas of auscultation)
4. Recognition of location of maximal loudness of sound and/or murmur and not merely the radiation
5. Effect of gradient versus effect of flow on frequency and character of the murmurs
6. Logical application of behavior of timing of sounds based on proper understanding of physiological alterations
7. Application of the concepts of mechanisms
8. Appropriate use of bedside maneuvers and vasoactive agents

Listening for One Thing at a Time and One Thing at a Time Only

This is extremely important and allows one to focus on all normal and abnormal heart sounds as well as on any murmur that may be heard. One needs to start auscultation by first assessing the S1 and S2. In fact, S2 may be assessed first because it demarcates systole from diastole. When one listens for the S2, one should literally ignore everything else until the S2 has been properly assessed. This means listening for S2 and its components all over the precordium, moving from the base to the apex, sequentially over all the areas including the second left interspace, the third left interspace, the second right interspace, the lower left sternal border area, the apex, the area between the apex, and the left sternal border and, if considered necessary, over the xiphoid area as well. Similarly one can focus on S1 and then other sounds, such as ejection click, opening snap (OS), S3, and S4, as well as murmurs, sequentially.

Listening for Specific Things With Predetermined Mental Filter

A specific cadence or rhythm is sometimes produced by the various heart sounds and murmurs, which often helps in their recognition. This has been mentioned in relation to the various sounds and murmurs (Fig. 1). This method often helps in the recognition of the OS and how widely it is separated from the S2, the S4, the S3, the presence of A2-P2 and OS, the identification of the ejection murmur, and the presence of mitral diastolic murmur. Obviously these are often specifically looked for, depending on the clinical possibilities being considered. For instance, one may specifically listen for an S3 when suspecting a dilated cardiomyopathy or mitral regurgitation. In this instance, one actually applies the specific mental filter, as it were, with the cadence of S3 in mind, to try to detect its presence or absence. Similarly, one may specifically listen for a mitral diastolic murmur in a patient already found to have a loud M1 and OS to detect the presence of mitral stenosis. In this instance, the cadence of the mitral diastolic murmur will apply.

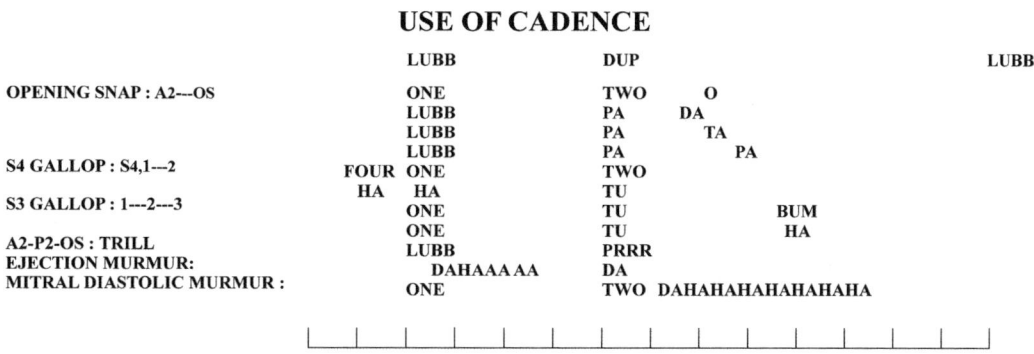

Fig. 1. Use of cadence. The cadence or rhythm produced by the various abnormal heart sounds and murmurs that can be imitated by vocal simulation of syllables are shown. Normal S1 and S2 are represented by syllables LUBB and DUP (shown at the top). The time lines are indicated at the bottom to approximate the length of systole and diastole of an average cardiac cycle. Each of the various abnormal sounds and murmurs is listed in the column on your left. The appropriate syllables are indicated against each of them individually according to their time of occurrence during the cardiac cycle. The cadence for each of the individual abnormal sound or murmur can be simulated vocally by using the syllables in the background rhythm of a cardiac cycle. In the case of the OS, the variations in the S2–OS intervals (short, medium, and late) correspond to three different syllables (PA..DA, PA....TA and PA......PA).

Application of Principles Based on Sound Transmission Related to the Site of Origin

By now it must be clear to everyone who has reviewed the previous sections on auscultation that the reference to the so-called traditional areas—mitral area referring to the apex, aortic area with reference to the second right interspace, and pulmonary area with reference to the second left interspace—involves incorrect terminology and is therefore best avoided. It is better to describe the sounds or murmurs with reference to their location in terms of the actual interspace (e.g., the second left interspace) on the chest or using chest wall reference terms such as the left lower sternal border, lower sternum, apex area, and xiphoid area. It should be recognized that the true aortic area is actually the sash area extending from the second right interspace across the left sternal border to the apex, and the true pulmonary area normally is over the second and third left interspace, which may extend into the lower sternum and sometimes to the apex, particularly in situations when the right ventricle becomes enlarged and actually forms the apex beat, as determined by the presence of a lateral retraction. The sound transmission of A2 and P2 to the chest will be such that they will be heard over the true aortic and pulmonary areas, respectively, depending on the individual patient. This concept allows us to formulate the "*rule of the split S2 at apex.*"

S2 split at the apex would indicate one of the following:

1. It may be from a loud P2 and therefore indicative of the presence of pulmonary hypertension.
2. If the P2 is not loud and there is no evidence of pulmonary hypertension, then the right ventricle may be enlarged as in volume overload (e.g., atrial septal defect) forming the apex.
3. P2 is normal and audible at apex because of a thin chest (e.g., in children).

4. The split S2 effect is being mimicked by a normal single A2 followed by another sound such as an OS or S3.

The rule then can be applied in the specific patient to derive the appropriate conclusions regarding the split S2 at the apex and its significance.

In situations of a split S2, to detect the sequence, whether it is A2 followed by the P2 or whether it is P2 followed by the A2, similar conceptual thinking can be applied. The A2 is the component that will remain audible at the normal apex area, which is usually formed by the left ventricle, whereas the P2 will either be absent or become softer and almost inaudible as when one moves over to the apex area. By noting whether it is the first or second component that becomes softer when one moves inching from the base to the apex while auscultating, one can develop the skills to decide what the sequence of the two components is in any given patient. This may be useful in situations where the patient is not able to follow instructions about breathing phases.

Recognition of Location of Maximal Loudness of Sound and/or Murmur

The location where a murmur or a sound radiates and therefore is heard does not have any diagnostic value. On the other hand, the location of maximal loudness is often very helpful and gives us clues as to what the sound or murmur is likely to be. Several examples can be given in this regard. The maximal loudness of an OS is usually between the left sternal border and the apex, whereas the maximal loudness of S3 is usually at the apex.

The regurgitation murmur caused by a ventricular septal defect (VSD) is maximally loud at the lower left sternal border, whereas the mitral regurgitation murmur is usually maximally loud over the apex. In acute septal rupture because of myocardial infarction, the murmur may be loudest at the apex. However, it is also equally loud medial to the apex. This is in contrast to acute mitral regurgitation, where the murmur may be loudest at the apex but is equally loud lateral to the apex and not medial to the apex. These points relative to the location of maximal loudness obviously have diagnostic significance. When aortic regurgitation murmur is as loud over the right sternal border as it is over the left sternal border, then aortic root dilatation may be suspected as the cause of the aortic regurgitation. With regard to continuous murmur, the location of maximal loudness correlates best with the chamber that receives the left-to-right shunt. For instance, if the continuous murmur is maximally loud over the second left interspace, then the receiving chamber is most likely the pulmonary artery. If the murmur is loudest at the third left interspace, the right ventricular outflow tract is most likely the receiving chamber.

Effect of Gradient vs Effect of Flow on Frequency and Character of Murmurs

It has been mentioned previously that the frequency of the murmur has a relationship to both flow as well as the pressure gradient involved in the turbulence. This relationship is such that the higher the pressure gradient, the higher the frequency, and the greater the flow, the greater the low frequency. The features of various murmurs stem from this relationship, and this helps in understanding their character. They are as follows:

1. The harshness of the ejection murmurs.
2. Low pitch of the mitral stenosis rumble.
3. The blowing character of the early diastolic murmur of aortic regurgitation.
4. The high frequency of the pulmonary hypertensive pulmonary regurgitation and the low pitch of the congenital pulmonary regurgitation

5. The harshness and the decrescendo character of acute severe mitral regurgitation secondary to ruptured chordae.
6. If a high-frequency murmur (e.g., mitral regurgitation) is harsh and has a lot of medium and low frequencies, it will suggest a lot of flow as well as indicate the regurgitation to be most likely hemodynamically significant or severe.

Logical Application of Behavior of Timing of Sounds Based on Proper Understanding of Physiological Alterations

Physiological alterations that occur with simple maneuvers such as standing can often be applied during auscultation to help distinguish certain sounds. Thus, one needs to understand the logical reason behind these. Often standing can be used to tell splitting of A2 and P2 from A2 and OS. A2-OS split separates more on standing, whereas A2-P2 tends to narrow. The reason for this is the decreased venous return, which lowers the left atrial pressure, thereby causing OS to occur later. The same maneuver can also be used to tell M1-A1 from S4-S1. The lower preload on standing leads to prolongation of the isovolumic phase of contraction, making the A1 come later, thereby separating it more from M1. The S4, on the other hand, with decreased left atrial pressure may become softer and may tend to come closer to M1.

Application of the Concepts of Mechanisms

Various maneuvers ranging from simple standing and squatting to the administration of amyl nitrite inhalation are sometimes carried out at the bedside while auscultating for their effects to help distinguish sounds and murmurs in various conditions. It is important to understand the concepts involved in each instance so that the auscultation can be carried out appropriately to achieve the proper conclusion. Some of these are listed below.

1. S2 components A2 and P2 and how they are affected by the following, namely, QRS delay, mechanical ventricular function, and impedance, e.g., post-Valsalva effect on S2 split to distinguish atrial septal defect vs pulmonary hypertension with right ventricular failure
2. Effect of long diastole (postextrasystolic pause) on ejection vs Regurgitation murmurs
3. Changing S1 intensity in complete atrioventricular (A-V) block (A-V dissociation)
4. Pulmonary ejection click getting softer on inspiration
5. Change of murmur intensity with standing and squatting in hypertrophic obstructive cardiomyopathy and mitral valve prolapse with mitral regurgitation
6. Effect of the Valsalva maneuver on the murmur of hypertrophic obstructive cardiomyopathy
7. Amyl nitrite inhalation to distinguish Austin Flint rumble in aortic regurgitation from organic mitral stenosis

The Use of Bedside Maneuvers and Vasoactive Agents

BEDSIDE MANEUVERS

Simple bedside maneuvers applied in appropriate situations can be quite useful in sorting out lesions in which the distinction is not clearly apparent. Again, understanding the physiological changes induced by the maneuvers is a preliminary step in understanding their likely effects on a given clinical lesion. Under this heading we will discuss the effect of respiration, the application of the Valsalva maneuver, the effect of changes in postures such as standing and squatting, and finally the effect of sustained handgrip or isometric exercise *(1–4)*.

Effect of Respiration

The effect of inspiration is to increase the venous return by increased negative intrathoracic pressure. It also expands the pulmonary vasculature, thereby decreasing the pulmonary impedance *(5)*. All right-sided events related to flow through the right heart and right ventricular volume will be expected to increase or intensify on inspiration. In addition to the effect on the timing of the P2, which is delayed, and the slight opposite effect on the timing of the A2, all pulmonary and tricuspid murmurs as well as right-sided S3, tricuspid inflow rumble, and S4 will intensify on inspiration. The inspiratory accentuation of the tricuspid regurgitation murmur goes by the name of *Carvallo's sign (6)*.

One exception is the pulmonary ejection click secondary to congenital pulmonary valvular stenosis *(7)*. In these patients the pulmonary artery pressure is usually very low. During inspiration the increased venous return into a hypertrophied and somewhat noncompliant right ventricle raises the right ventricular end-diastolic pressure during right atrial contraction. This may exceed the pulmonary artery diastolic pressure. This in effect would cause doming of the pulmonary valve even before ventricular contraction starts. Thus, with ventricular systole as the column of blood is set into motion, the valve being maximally domed, there is no sudden deceleration against the valve itself, and therefore no sound. It must be noted, however, that the pulmonary ejection sound associated with pulmonary hypertension will not be influenced by respiration because the pulmonary arterial diastolic pressure is often quite high and higher than the right ventricular diastolic pressures.

It must also be noted that the respiratory changes in venous return are exaggerated in the sitting and standing positions when the venous return is normally low. Thus, in order to fully appreciate the effect of respiration, it would be important to compare the effects in both the supine and the erect positions *(8)*. For instance, the respiratory variations of wide physiological splitting in young children or adults may be difficult to distinguish accurately in the supine position. On the other hand, the movements of the two components will be better appreciated in the sitting or standing position. This will help in avoiding misinterpretation of a wide physiological split of the S2 as a fixed splitting of the S2, a distinction that is of utmost importance.

Valsalva Maneuver

The Valsalva maneuver involves attempted forceful exhalation against a closed glottis. The effects occur in two phases: one during the strain phase and the other during the post-strain-release phase *(8–12)*. It is usually performed by asking the patient to take a medium breath and hold the breath and forcefully strain or bear down as if sitting on the toilet. One needs to ensure that the patient is in fact straining by placing one's hand on the patient's abdomen to see whether the abdominal muscles become tense. One can also instruct the patient to push the abdominal muscles against the hand. A controlled way of performing the Valsalva maneuver is to have the patient blow through a rubber tube attached to an aneroid manometer to keep the pressure around 40 mmHg during the period of straining. When performed appropriately, the intrathoracic pressure will become elevated together with elevations of the end-diastolic ventricular pressures. The pulmonary vessels empty into the left atrium, initially raising the arterial pressure slightly. Soon the increased intrathoracic pressure will significantly decrease the venous return.

The cardiac output and the systemic arterial pressure will fall with sympathetic stimulation, resulting in increased heart rate. Patient is normally asked to strain for about 10 s. When in the supine position, most patients will tolerate the maneuver. However, one should not perform this maneuver in the setting of active ischemic symptoms or acute coronary syndrome.

The effect of the strain phase is to considerably diminish the venous return and filling. Thus, all events and murmurs dependent on flow and filling will diminish. However, in two clinical states, the decrease in ventricular dimension may become critical enough to aggravate the lesion. One is mitral valve prolapse, where the decreased ventricular size will allow earlier onset of prolapse and mitral regurgitation, resulting in the murmur starting earlier and becoming longer. The murmur intensity may not necessarily increase. If there is a whoop, however, it may get louder. The other condition is hypertrophic cardiomyopathy with obstruction. In this condition the murmur will be expected to increase in intensity because the obstruction tends to become worse because of earlier and easier contact of the anterior mitral leaflet with the hypertrophied septum *(12)*.

The second part of the effect of the Valsalva maneuver occurs during the post-strain-release phase. During this phase, there is an immediate increase in venous return and flow, which will increase the right-sided volume for the first three to four beats and subsequently also the left ventricular volume. Thus, an immediate return to baseline will be seen on the right-sided events and murmurs, whereas the left-sided events and murmurs will gradually return to the baseline. The post-Valsalva effect on the P2 in distinguishing pulmonary hypertension with right ventricular dysfunction from atrial septal defect was referred to earlier.

Valsalva Maneuver in the Assessment of Left Ventricular Function

During the strain phase, with the drop in output and blood pressure there will often be a marked sympathetic stimulation resulting in a tachycardia. When the strain is released, the increased venous inflow—initially into the right side, later into the left heart—will result in increased cardiac output. The ejection of increased volume into a constricted vascular system will result in a significant rise in the arterial pressure, causing an overshoot. The overshoot will be accompanied by reflex bradycardia.

Patients with left ventricular failure and pulmonary congestion do not drop their filling much during the straining, and the blood pressure remains flat with very little change in the heart rate. This response is termed the *square-wave response*. Patients with left ventricular dysfunction who are not in overt failure also often have an abnormal response. They tend to have resting increase in sympathetic tone and fail to exhibit the overshoot in blood pressure as well as the reflex bradycardia. This can be detected at the bedside by taking the resting systolic blood pressure and keeping the cuff inflated about 25 mmHg above the resting systolic pressure during the strain and for 20–30 s after the release. If one detects Korotkoff sounds coming through, one can infer that there has been an overshoot in blood pressure. Failure to achieve an overshoot of 25 mmHg has been correlated with resting left ventricular dysfunction with decreased ejection fraction of 40 ± 10% *(11,13)*.

Postural Changes

Standing. Assumption of the standing posture from the supine position will have the effect of decreasing the venous return and causing the ventricular volume and output to fall together with a drop in the arterial pressure *(14)*. Events and murmurs dependent on filling and flow will be expected to diminish. Lesions that are critically affected by decrease in dimensions such as mitral regurgitation secondary to the prolapsed mitral leaflets and hypertrophic cardiomyopathy with obstruction will be expected to show the obvious changes. The prolapse will tend to occur earlier. This will be reflected in clicks moving closer to the S1 and the murmur of mitral regurgitation starting earlier and perhaps lasting longer. They may also variably change in intensity. The obstruction in hypertrophic cardiomyopathy will be expected to be either brought on or made worse by this erect posture. This will affect the murmur intensity directly in relation to either the development of the outflow gradient or the accentuation of a resting gradient.

The effect of standing in distinguishing the S2-OS from a split A2-P2 was referred to earlier. This is achieved by the decreased venous return resulting in lowering of the left atrial pressure, which causes the OS to occur later.

Squatting. The hemodynamic changes of squatting include an immediate increase in venous return and an increase in aortic pressure. The latter probably results from the compression of the lower limb arteries, thereby causing some reflex bradycardia. The sum effects of these changes will be to increase the filling volume on both sides together with an increase in the blood pressure.

If a patient is unable to squat, one can mimic the hemodynamic changes by passively bending the knees of the patient toward the abdomen while the patient remains supine. This maneuver also is quite useful in hypertrophic cardiomyopathy with obstruction, where the gradient will diminish along with the murmur intensity because of the increased left ventricular size and the elevated aortic pressure *(1,15)*. In mitral valve prolapse, the prolapse will start later. This will result in the click occurring later in systole. The mitral regurgitation murmur will either disappear or become significantly softer.

Exercise

Light walking exercise can be quite useful in bringing out very soft mitral diastolic murmurs in patients with severe mitral stenosis and low cardiac output with secondary pulmonary hypertension. Patients can be instructed to walk back and forth a few times and then asked to lie quickly in the left lateral decubitus position. They must be immediately auscultated before the effect of the exercise wears off. It is also useful in distinguishing wide-split S2 in severe pulmonary hypertension and right ventricular dysfunction and/or failure from atrial septal defect. Exercise will further widen the split in right ventricular failure.

Isometric exercise can also be applied. This exercise must be done for at least 60–90 s to achieve changes in sympathetic tone with increase in heart rate, cardiac output, and blood pressure *(16)*. These effects are best seen in the supine position. As opposed to aerobic exercise, such as walking on a treadmill, isometric exercise will result in marked increase in the systemic arterial resistance. The filling pressure will rise in the left ventricle, augmenting events related to ventricular filling such as left-sided filling sounds (S3 and the S4) *(17)*. The elevated left atrial pressure will cause the OS, if present, to occur earlier. The mitral diastolic murmur of mitral stenosis will become augmented. The effect in hypertrophic obstructive cardiomyopathy will be variable because of the opposing effects of the increased heart rate and the increased blood pressure on the gradient.

The most useful effect will be in bringing out an aortic regurgitation murmur that is not obvious clinically. The effect on mitral regurgitation will be to increase the regurgitation and the intensity of the murmur. Instructing the patient to squat and squeeze at the same time both of their hands thereby performing isometric contraction can also be a very useful maneuver in making faint aortic regurgitation murmurs become easily audible.

Transient Arterial Occlusion

This technique involves simultaneously inflating two sphygmomanometer cuffs placed around each arm of the patient to keep the systolic pressure 20–40 mm above that of the resting systolic pressure of the patient for a duration of about 20 s. This maneuver does not increase the aortic pressure, but increases the aortic impedance *(8,18)*. The effect will be to augment left-sided regurgitations such as mitral regurgitation, ventricular septal defect, and aortic regurgitation. This test does not require the patient's cooperation and is reported to be better than squatting.

VASOACTIVE AGENTS

Vasoactive agents, which have been used in the past to clarify difficult murmurs in cardiac auscultation, include vasopressor agents and amyl nitrite *(19–24)*. Vasopressors such as phenylephrine must be administered intravenously by infusion with careful monitoring of blood pressure. Because of this they are somewhat cumbersome to use, and we have not found the need for their application. Isometric handgrip exercise and/ or squeeze and squat maneuver will give a reasonable increase in peripheral arterial resistance and blood pressure to provide equivalent information in its place. Therefore, their application will not be discussed further.

Amyl nitrite, however, is still used in cardiological practice in selected instances to clarify certain clinical states. It is reasonably easy to use and quite safe when administered appropriately with the patient in the supine position, keeping the patient supine until its effects wear off. For this reason we will discuss its application here.

Amyl nitrite is a volatile ester of nitrous acid. When administered to the patient it causes a significant decrease in peripheral arterial resistance within a few seconds after inhalation because of arterial and arteriolar dilatation. It is usually dispensed in a cloth-covered ampule, which can be broken holding it inside gauze with a gloved hand. The patient must be supine and warned to expect to smell some vapors with a sweet almond-like fragrance (some compare it to that of dirty socks). The patient should be asked to take two or three whiffs of this by breathing in while the broken ampule is held close to the patient's nostrils. The administration must be done after baseline auscultation. It is preferable to have someone other than the examiner administer and monitor the systolic blood pressure by the use of a sphygmomanometer cuff and call the level of the blood pressure as the drug takes effect. When properly administered, it will result in a fall in the systemic blood pressure with a reflex tachycardia secondary to the sympathetic stimulation. The hypotensive effect usually wears off in 1–2 min. The hemodynamic effects include increase in cardiac output because of increased venous return caused by venoconstriction. This effect is different from that of nitroglycerin, which causes venodilatation. The venoconstriction is secondary to the reflex sympathetic stimulation caused by the hypotension. Other effects include increased ventricular contractility and increase in ejection velocity. A small rise in the pulmonary artery pressure may also occur because of increased venous return *(20,25,26)*. These significant circulatory effects result in modifications of the intensity of the murmur and its duration, depending on the nature of the lesion.

The effect of amyl nitrite inhalation on the behavior of the various murmurs encountered in both congenital and acquired lesions can be summarized briefly as follows:

1. Amyl nitrite, by increasing forward flow and the velocity of ejection, will increase the intensity of ejection murmurs caused by fixed outflow obstruction (the right-sided outflow obstruction at the valvular or infundibular level with intact ventricular septum and the left ventricular outflow obstruction). This effect can be used to differentiate the tetralogy of Fallot from pulmonary stenosis with right-to-left shunt at the atrial level *(23,24)*. In the presence of the tetralogy, the decrease in the systemic pressure will allow more right-to-left shunting through the ventricular septal defect. This will decrease the forward flow through the pulmonary outflow tract, decreasing the murmur intensity. The murmur of pulmonary stenosis with intact ventricular septum, on the other hand, will increase in intensity *(21)*.
2. Amyl nitrite is classically used to bring out or intensify the long ejection murmur of the hypertrophic cardiomyoathy. Both the drop in the peripheral resistance and the tachycardia with decreased ventricular size will accentuate the outflow obstruction and the murmur.
3. Amyl nitrite will decrease mitral regurgitation by virtue of the increased net forward flow and decreased peripheral resistance *(19)*.
4. In patients with ventricular septal defect (VSD) and normal pulmonary artery pressures, the effect will be similar to that in mitral regurgitation. It will diminish the shunt and the murmur. In VSD with large flow and pulmonary hypertension, there could be a different effect of increasing the flow through the defect because of a disproportionately greater fall in the pulmonary vascular resistance compared to that of the systemic resistance.
5. The response in mitral valve prolapse can be variable. The effect of more complete emptying and increased forward flow may result in critical left ventricular dimension for prolapse to occur earlier in systole because of smaller ventricular size. The late systolic murmur secondary to mitral regurgitation may disappear and be replaced with an early systolic murmur. Rarely, a patient may develop pansystolic mitral regurgitation. If only a mid-systolic click is audible, the click will move earlier in systole.
6. Innocent systolic pulmonary outflow murmur will be expected to increase because of increased flow.
7. Amyl nitrite classically will diminish aortic regurgitation and its murmur because of decreased peripheral resistance. When the aortic regurgitation is severe, the associated apical low-frequency diastolic murmur (*Austin Flint murmur*) will either be abolished or become softer as a result of the reduction of the severity of aortic regurgitation following amyl nitrite. The effect on the murmur of organic mitral stenosis is to increase its intensity because of the increased cardiac output and mitral flows.
8. The venous hum and the continuous murmur from pulmonary artetiovenous fistulae intensify after amyl nitrite because of excess flow. On the other hand, the murmurs of persistent ductus arteriosus and systemic arteriovenous fistulae shorten and become less loud. When the persistent ductus is associated with pulmonary hypertension, the diastolic component of the continuous murmur will be absent. In these patients, the systolic murmur will also be expected to shorten and become softer.

REFERENCES

1. Cochran PT. Bedside aids to auscultation of the heart. JAMA 1978;239:54–55.
2. Crawford MH, O'Rourke RA. A systematic approach to the bedside differentiation of cardiac murmurs and abnormal sounds. Curr Probl Cardiol 1977; 1:1–42.
3. Dohan MC, Criscitiello MG. Physiologicalal and pharmacological manipulations of heart sounds and murmurs. Mod Concepts Cardiovasc Dis 1970;39:121–127.

4. Lembo NJ, Dell'Italia LJ, Crawford MH, O'Rourke RA. Bedside diagnosis of systolic murmurs. N Engl J Med 1988;318:1572–1578.
5. Harrison DC, Goldblatt A, Braunwald E, Glick G, Mason DT. Studies on cardiac dimensions in intact, unanesthetized man. I. Description of techniques and their validation. II. Effects of respiration. III. Effects of muscular exercise. Circ Res 1963;13:448–467.
6. Perloff JK. The physiological mechanisms of cardiac and vascular physical signs. J Am Coll Cardiol 1983;1:184–198.
7. Hultgren HN, Reeve R, Cohn K, McLeod R. The ejection click of valvular pulmonic stenosis. Circulation 1969;40:631–640.
8. Grewe K, Crawford MH, O'Rourke RA. Differentiation of cardiac murmurs by dynamic auscultation. Curr Probl Cardiol 1988;13:669–721.
9. Gorlin R, Knowles JH, Storey CF. The Valsalva maneuver as a test of cardiac function. Pathologic physiology and clinical significance. Am J Med 1957;22:197.
10. Elisberg EI. Heart rate response to the Valsalva maneuver as a test of circulatory integrity. JAMA 1963;186:200–205.
11. Little WC, Barr WK, Crawford MH. Altered effect of the Valsalva maneuver on left ventricular volume in patients with cardiomyopathy. Circulation 1985;71:227–233.
12. Stefadouros MA, Mucha E, Frank MJ. Paradoxic response of the murmur of idiopathic hypertrophic subaortic stenosis to the Valsalva maneuver. Am J Cardiol 1976;37:89–92.
13. Zema MJ, Caccavano M, Kligfield P. Detection of left ventricular dysfunction in ambulatory subjects with the bedside Valsalva maneuver. Am J Med 1983;75:241–248.
14. Rapaport E, Wong M, Escobar EE, Martinez G. The effect of upright posture on right ventricular volumes in patients with and without heart failure. Am Heart J 1966;71:146–152.
15. Nellen M, Gotsman MS, Vogelpoel L, Beck W, Schrire V. Effects of prompt squatting on the systolic murmur in idiopathic hypertrophic obstructive cardiomyopathy. Br Med J 1967;3:140–143.
16. McCraw DB, Siegel W, Stonecipher HK, Nutter DO, Schlant RC, Hurst JW. Response of heart murmur intensity to isometric (handgrip) exercise. Br Heart J 1972; 34:605–610.
17. Cohn PF, Thompson P, Strauss W, Todd J, Gorlin R. Diastolic heart sounds during static (handgrip) exercise in patients with chest pain. Circulation 1973;47:1217–1221.
18. Lembo NJ, Dell'Italia LJ, Crawford MH, O'Rourke RA. Diagnosis of left-sided regurgitant murmurs by transient arterial occlusion: a new maneuver using blood pressure cuffs. Ann Intern Med 1986; 105:368–370.
19. Barlow J, Shillingford J. The use of amyl nitrite in differentiating mitral and aortic systolic murmurs. Br Heart J 1958;20:162–166.
20. Beck W, Schrire V, Vogelpoel L, Nellen M, Swanepoel A. Hemodynamic effects of amyl nitrite and phenylephrine on the normal human circulation and their relation to changes in cardiac murmurs. Am J Cardiol 1961;8:341–349.
21. de Leon AC, Jr, Harvey WP. Pharmacologic agents and auscultation. Mod Concepts Cardiovasc Dis 1975;44:23–28.
22. Ronan JA, Jr. Effect of vasoactive drugs and maneuvers on heart murmurs. American Heart Association Monograph 1975;46:183–186.
23. Schrire V, Vogelpoel L, Beck W, Nellen M, Swanepoel A. The effects of amyl nitrite and phenylephrine on the intracardiac murmurs of small ventricular septal defects. Am Heart J 1961;62:225–236.
24. Vogelpoel L, Schrire V, Nellen M, Swanepoel A. The use of amyl nitrite in the differentiation of Fallot's tetralogy and pulmonary stenosis with intact ventricular septum. Am Heart J 1959;57:803–819.
25. de Leon AC, Jr, Perloff JK. The pulmonary hemodynamic effects of amyl nitrite in normal man. Am Heart J 1966;72:337–344.
26. Perloff JK, Calvin J, Deleon AC, Bowen P. Systemic hemodynamic effects of amyl nitrite in normal man. Am Heart J 1963;66:460–469.

10 Pathophysiological Basis of Symptoms and Signs in Cardiac Disease

CONTENTS

PATHOPHYSIOLOGY OF MITRAL REGURGITATION
PATHOPHYSIOLOGY OF AORTIC REGURGITATION
PATHOPHYSIOLOGY OF MITRAL STENOSIS
PATHOPHYSIOLOGY OF AORTIC STENOSIS
PATHOPHYSIOLOGY OF MYOCARDIAL ISCHEMIA/INFARCTION
PATHOPHYSIOLOGY OF HYPERTENSIVE HEART DISEASE
PATHOPHYSIOLOGY OF DILATED CARDIOMYOPATHY
PATHOPHYSIOLOGY OF HYPERTROPHIC OBSTRUCTIVE
   CARDIOMYOPATHY
PATHOPHYSIOLOGY OF ATRIAL SEPTAL DEFECT
PATHOPHYSIOLOGY OF DIASTOLIC DYSFUNCTION
PATHOPHYSIOLOGY OF CONSTRICTIVE PERICARDITIS
PATHOPHYSIOLOGY OF CARDIAC TAMPONADE
APPENDIX
REFERENCES

In this chapter, the pathophysiological basis of symptoms and signs will be reviewed in the major categories of cardiac lesions seen mainly in adult patients, including both regurgitant and stenotic valvular lesions; cardiomyopathies, both dilated and hypertrophic; hypertensive heart disease; ischemic heart disease; and pericardial lesions with diastolic restriction. The only congenital lesion addressed is atrial septal defect, because more often than not it causes problems only in adults.

PATHOPHYSIOLOGY OF MITRAL REGURGITATION

Chronic Mitral Regurgitation

Mitral regurgitation is a volume overload state for the left ventricle because during diastole the ventricle receives not only the normal pulmonary venous return, but also the extra volume of blood, which goes into the left atrium during systole. The left ventricle thus has two outlets for systolic emptying in mitral regurgitation, namely, the aorta and the left atrium. The volume overload would result in left ventricular dilatation and enlargement. The left ventricular dilatation is accompanied initially by better compliance of the left ventricle, which helps to maintain relatively normal left ventricular diastolic pressure despite the large volume of blood entering the left ventricle during diastole. The left atrium also becomes enlarged when the regurgitation is significant. The left atrial enlargement is accompanied by increased compliance of the left atrium, which helps to maintain a normal left atrial pressure.

The two-outlet system allows supernormal emptying and therefore supernormal ejection fraction when the ventricular function is normal and preserved. The ejection fraction can still be maintained at near-normal levels, even when some left ventricular dysfunction develops because of the systolic advantage that the left ventricle has. The systolic tension is therefore maintained at normal levels *(1–4)*.

The increased diastolic tension caused by increased dimension (radius) will act as a stimulus to hypertrophy. The hypertrophy is often eccentric rather than concentric *(5)*. This will decrease the diastolic compliance of the left ventricle, leading to a rise in the diastolic left ventricular filling pressure. The raised diastolic pressure in the left ventricle may impede good subendocardial perfusion because the majority of coronary flow occurs in diastole. The decreased subendocardial perfusion may eventually lead to subendocardial fibrosis in late stages, which may further depress the compliance and begin to raise the *pre-a wave* pressure. Because the latter forms the baseline filling pressure over which the *a* and *v wave* buildup occurs in the atrium, the raised *pre-a wave* pressure will further raise the *v wave* pressure height in the left atrium. The upper normal left ventricular diastolic pressure for the end of diastole (*post- a wave*) is usually 12–15 mmHg, whereas the upper normal left ventricular *pre-a wave* pressure is 5–8 mmHg. The normal *v wave* in the left atrium may be between 12 and 18 mmHg. In chronic mitral regurgitation, even when the regurgitation is severe, the left atrial *v wave* height may only be mild to moderately elevated (20–35 mmHg). This would mean a persistent pressure difference between the left ventricle and the left atrium throughout systole, causing the regurgitant flow to last until the very end of systole and well into the isovolumic relaxation phase. The murmur, therefore, usually lasts for the whole of systole (thus termed pansystolic) and all the way to the S2 and slightly even beyond the S2. In addition, the gradient remains relatively large and constant from the beginning of systole to its end, giving rise to a plateau high-frequency systolic murmur.

Elevated left atrial pressure will cause some secondary pulmonary hypertension. This, together with the decreased left ventricular compliance and diastolic dysfunction, will eventually lead to systolic dysfunction, causing reduced stroke volume and ejection fraction (Fig. 1) *(1–4)*.

Acute Mitral Regurgitation

If the mitral regurgitation is severe and acute in onset as with ruptured chordae, then there may not be enough time to develop compensatory dilatation of either the left atrium or the left ventricle. The large volume of regurgitant blood entering a relatively stiff and nondilated left atrium will result in a steep rise in the *v wave* pressure in the left atrium (sometimes as high as 50–70 mmHg). The entry of a large volume of blood during diastole into a nondilated left ventricle will tend to raise the diastolic filling pressure in the left ventricle. The raised *pre-a wave* pressure may further add to the *v wave* height. The high *v wave* buildup in the left atrium during systole would mean a decreased and rapidly falling pressure difference between the left ventricle and the left atrium toward the later part of systole. This will in turn limit the regurgitant flow during the later part of systole, making the regurgitant flow and the murmur decrescendo. In addition, the excess flow would cause more low and medium frequencies, making the murmur sound harsher (Fig. 2) *(6–8)*.

Chapter 10 / Pathophysiological Basis of Symptoms and Signs

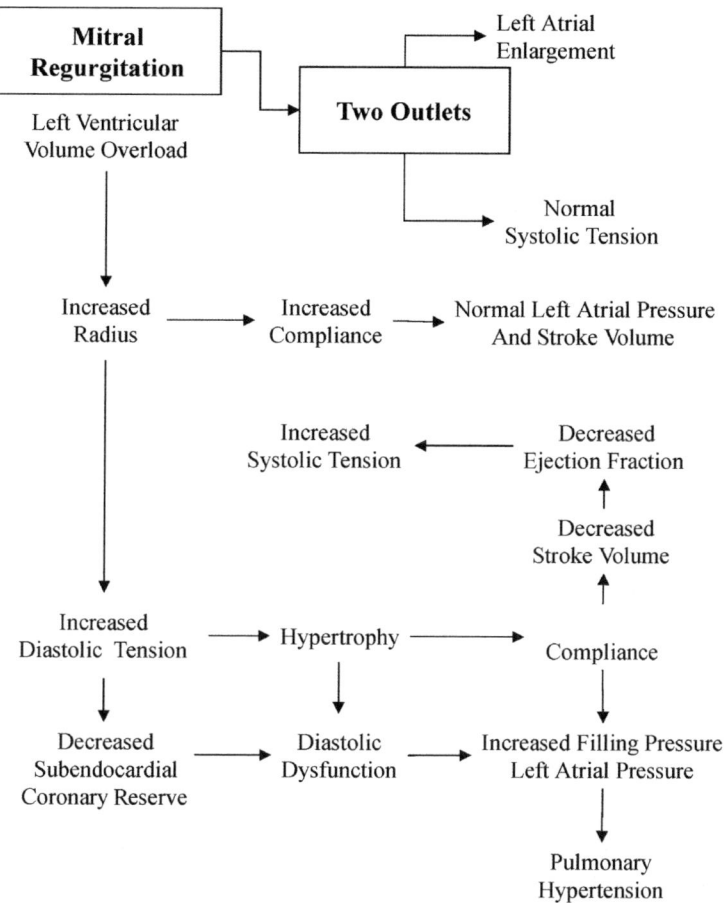

Fig. 1.

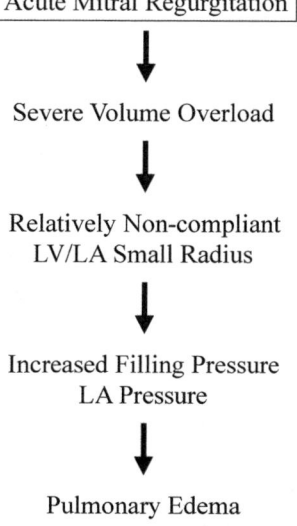

Fig. 2.

Table 1
Chronic Mitral Regurgitation

Pathophysiological changes	Clinical symptoms/signs
• Two outlets • Systolic advantage • Increased LV and LA compliance	• Long asymptomatic period
• Increased LA size	• Atrial fibrillation • Palpitation
• Increased LA pressure	• Dyspnea • Pulmonary congestion
• Reduced ejection fraction (late sign) • Pulmonary hypertension	• Low-output symptoms
• LV volume overload • Increased radius	• Hyperdynamic apex • Displaced/large area apex
• Retrograde flow from high-pressure LV into low-pressure LA	• Systolic murmur predominantly high frequency
• Increased flow across mitral valve in diastole due to (normal return + regurgitant flow)	• S3 • Mid-diastolic rumble

Signs of Severity

- Low normal pulse volume
- LV enlargement
- Wide split S2 due to an early A2
- Harsh low/medium frequencies in the regurgitation murmur iindicating a lot of flow
- S3 rumble (inflow rumble)
- Signs of pulmonary hypertension

LV, left ventricular; LA, left atrial.

Clinical Symptoms and Signs in Mitral Regurgitation

The pathophysiological changes as related to the clinical symptoms and signs in mitral regurgitation, together with clinical indicators of the severity of mitral regurgitation, are given in Table 1.

Even significant degrees of mitral regurgitation, when chronic, can be tolerated for many years because the left atrial pressure is kept at near- normal levels and the stroke volume and cardiac output maintained. Thus, there is often a long latent period when the patient remains asymptomatic. The left atrial enlargement may eventually lead to the development of atrial arrhythmias, especially atrial fibrillation. This may cause symptoms of palpitation. When the left atrial pressure begins to rise, patients may develop symptoms of dyspnea on exertion. When the left atrial pressure is significantly elevated, symptoms of pulmonary congestion, such as orthopnea and/or nocturnal dyspnea, may develop. When the mitral regurgitation is severe and acute or abrupt in onset, significant elevations in the left atrial pressure could occur, leading to dramatic symptoms of pulmonary congestion including pulmonary edema.

The enlarged left ventricle with supernormal ejection fraction in the early stages will lead to a hyperdynamic displaced large-area left ventricular apical impulse. The systolic advantage that the left ventricle has on account of the two outlets for systole often helps to maintain near-normal ejection fraction for a long time, and thus the apex beat is unlikely to be sustained. The increased flow across the mitral valve in diastole secondary to the normal pulmonary venous return, together with the regurgitant flow, would give rise to an S3 or a mid-diastolic rumble at the apex, especially when the mitral regurgitation is severe.

Reduced ejection fraction and significant pulmonary hypertension are often late signs if present, and then may be associated with low-output symptoms of fatigue and lassitude.

If mitral regurgitation is detected, the presence of some or all of the following signs (Table 1) would indicate that the mitral regurgitation is in fact severe: low normal pulse volume, large-area displaced hyperdynamic left ventricular apex beat, wide split S2 due to the early occurrence of the aortic component of S2, harshness of regurgitant murmur because of excessive flow adding some low and medium frequencies to the usual high frequencies of the regurgitant murmur, S3 and/or inflow mid-diastolic rumble at the apex, signs of pulmonary hypertension such as elevated jugular venous pressure with or without abnormal contour, sustained right ventricular impulse palpable in the subxiphoid area, and loud or palpable pulmonary component of the S2.

PATHOPHYSIOLOGY OF AORTIC REGURGITATION

Chronic Aortic Regurgitation

If the aortic valve is not competent for any reason, then there will be backward flow of blood from the aorta to the left ventricle in diastole, which will start at the time of A2. This backward flow will occur under a relatively high-pressure gradient because the aortic diastolic pressure is significantly high soon after the closure of the aortic valve, whereas the left ventricular pressure would have fallen close to zero at the onset of diastole. The high-pressure gradient will cause turbulence that will result in a predominantly high-frequency blowing-type murmur (*see* Chapter 8, Fig. 5). Because the diastolic pressure gradient is high at the onset of diastole and continues to fall gradually during diastole, reaching the minimal level at the end of diastole, the murmur also has a decrescendo character.

Aortic regurgitation also is a volume overload lesion for the left ventricle since the filling of the left ventricle during diastole will be augmented because of both the regurgitant volume of blood from the aorta and the normal pulmonary venous return through the mitral inflow (Fig. 3). The left ventricle will therefore enlarge because of the volume overload effect. The Starling effect of increased stretch caused by the dilatation and the volume overload will not only increase the contractility but also augment the stroke volume. Unlike mitral regurgitation, the left ventricle has only one outlet to eject blood, i.e., through the aorta. Thus, it does not have a systolic advantage. The ejection fraction thus does not become supernormal. The increased stroke volume increases the systolic pressure. Peripheral tissue perfusion is maintained by compensatory vasodilatation. This would contribute to the decrease in the arterial diastolic pressure.

The extent of rise in the filling pressure of the left ventricle will depend both on the severity of the regurgitation and on the compliance or distensibility of the left ventricle.

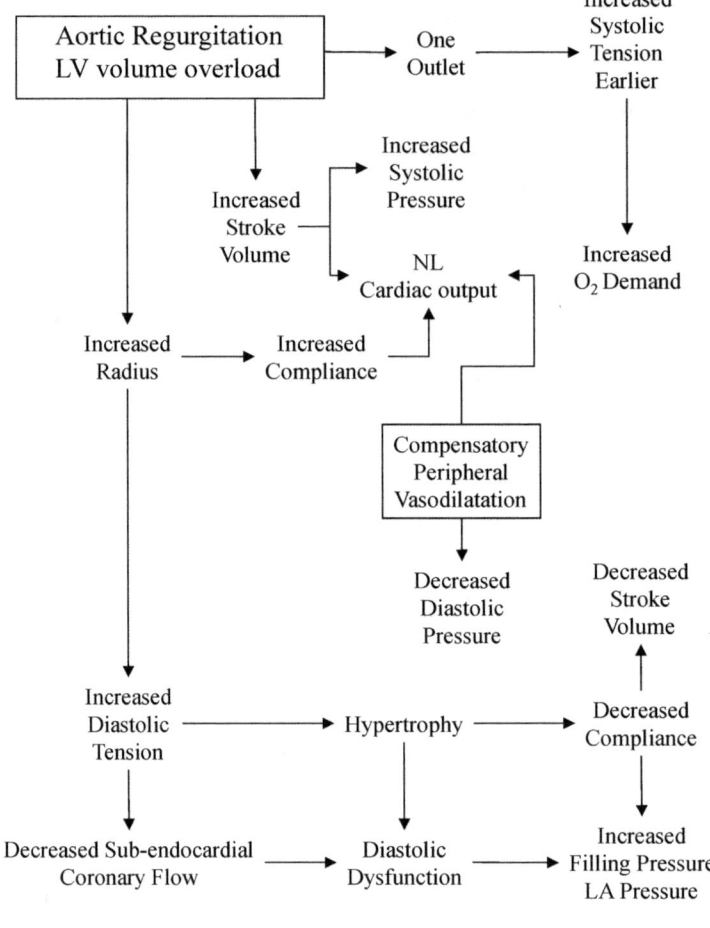

Fig. 3.

In chronic aortic regurgitation, the left ventricle initially undergoes dilatation, and its compliance is generally preserved. This will help to keep the rise in the diastolic left ventricular pressure to a minimum *(1,4,9)*. On the other hand, the increased dimension of the left ventricle because of dilatation will increase the ventricular wall tension. This is understandable since the wall tension is directly proportional to the radius according to the Laplace formula (*see* Appendix). The increased wall tension will increase the myocardial oxygen demand. This is one of the reasons that patients with aortic regurgitation may experience symptoms of exertional angina. The increase in the left ventricular wall tension is also a stimulus for secondary myocardial hypertrophy. In longstanding aortic regurgitation of more than moderate degree, therefore, the left ventricle will undergo secondary hypertrophy. Activation of the renin–angiotensin system has been shown to be involved in this process *(10)*. The hypertrophy is eccentric and is associated with replication of the sarcomeres in series together with the elongation of the myofibers. The ratio of wall thickness to the radius of the cavity is maintained *(11)*. This is unlike the concentric hypertrophy that occurs in pressure overload states where the sarcomeres increase in parallel and the ratio of wall thickness to the radius of the cavity is increased *(5)*. Thus, in chronic severe aortic regurgitation the left ventricle is not only dilated and enlarged,

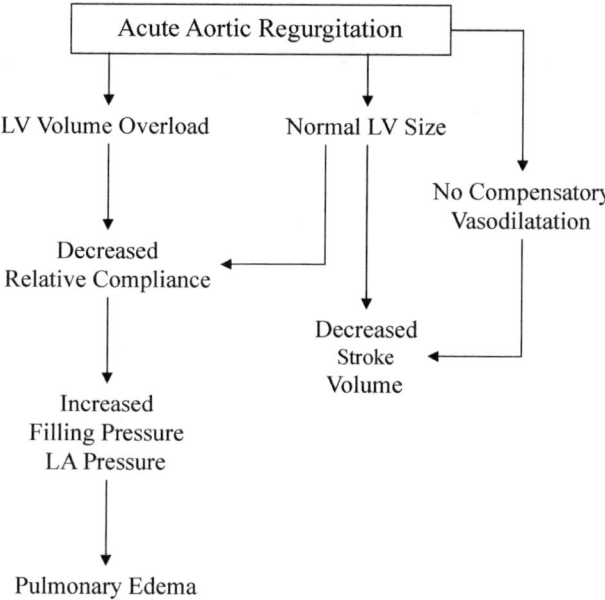

Fig. 4.

but also significantly hypertrophied. The markedly hypertrophied and enlarged heart in aortic regurgitation is sometimes massive (*cor bovinum*). The increased wall thickness will help to reduce the wall tension slightly. The hypertrophy will, however, tend to make the left ventricle more stiff, and its compliance will be diminished. This will result in further elevation of the left ventricular diastolic pressure. The increased left ventricular diastolic pressure will tend to interfere with subendocardial coronary perfusion. The increased myocardial oxygen demand together with decreased subendocardial perfusion will often result in some myocardial necrosis and replacement fibrosis. This will further depress the compliance of the left ventricle and cause an additional rise in the left ventricular diastolic pressure. This will further adversely affect the systolic function *(4,9,12–16)*.

Because the mitral valve is open in diastole, any elevation of the diastolic pressure before the *a wave* will lead to increased left atrial pressure. The elevated left atrial pressure will be transmitted to the pulmonary capillary bed and will cause symptoms of dyspnea. When the elevation of the left ventricular diastolic pressure is severe and associated with decreased left ventricular systolic function, the resulting high left atrial pressure will lead to aggravation of symptoms of dyspnea as well as cause orthopnea and paroxysmal nocturnal dyspnea (Fig. 3).

Acute Severe Aortic Regurgitation

When the aortic regurgitation is severe and acute in onset, the left ventricle will not have enough time to undergo compensatory dilatation (Fig. 4). The severe regurgitation into the left ventricle is accommodated only with a significant elevation of the left ventricular diastolic pressure. The latter can not only rise to levels higher than the prevailing left atrial pressure in diastole but also typically reach levels close to the aortic diastolic pressure. In fact, often by the end of diastole the left ventricular diastolic

Table 2
Chronic Aortic Regurgitation

Pathophysiological changes	Clinical symptoms/signs
• LV volume overload	• Hyperdynamic LV apex
• Increased radius	• Displaced large area apex
• Increased duration of systolic tension	• Sustained apex
• Increased systolic pressure	• Large-amplitude carotid pulse
• Lower diastolic pressure	• Normal upstroke
• Peripheral vasodilatation	• Wide pulse pressure
	• Peripheral signs of aortic regurgitation
• Retrograde flow through aortic valve with a high-pressure gradient	• Murmur predominantly high frequency
	• Decrescendo diastolic
• Regurgitant jet preventing mitral valve from opening freely	• Austin Flint rumble (relative mitral stenosis)
• Increased filling pressure	• Dyspnea
• Increased LA pressure	• Paroxysmal nocturnal dyspnea/orthopnea
• Increased O_2 demand	• Angina
• Decreased subendocardial perfusion	

LA, left atrial; LV, left ventricular.

pressure may become equal to the aortic diastolic pressure. The large regurgitant volume of blood from the incompetent aortic valve, together with the mitral inflow during the rapid filling phase of diastole, often lead to an abrupt and large increase in the left ventricular diastolic pressure. The latter will have a significant deceleration effect on both the regurgitant column as well as the mitral inflow column of blood. This may result in the production of an S3. In addition, the rapidly rising left ventricular diastolic pressure when it exceeds the left atrial pressure in mid-diastole may close the mitral valve prematurely (see Chapter 8, Fig. 6). The premature closure of the mitral valve can be seen quite easily in M-mode recordings of the echocardiograms. The premature mitral closure will contribute to the S1 becoming soft or even absent.

The large volume of regurgitant aortic diastolic flow will give rise to predominantly low- and medium-frequency aortic regurgitation murmur, making it harsher in quality. In addition, the rapidly rising left ventricular diastolic pressure will limit the regurgitant flow by diminishing the pressure difference between the aorta and the left ventricle. This will make the murmur somewhat shorter *(17–19)*.

Clinical Symptoms and Signs in Aortic Regurgitation

The left ventricular enlargement in significant aortic regurgitation will tend to cause a displaced wide area left ventricular apex beat, which will be hyperdynamic. It may also become sustained if the duration of high systolic wall tension is increased. This is likely to happen because the left ventricle has no special systolic advantage, unlike mitral regurgitation (Table 2). Many of the peripheral signs of aortic regurgitation stem from the large stroke volume, increased ejection velocity and momentum together with decreased peripheral resistance, and widened pulse pressure with low diastolic pressure secondary to retrograde flow into the left ventricle and peripheral vasodilatation (see Chapter 2) *(20)*.

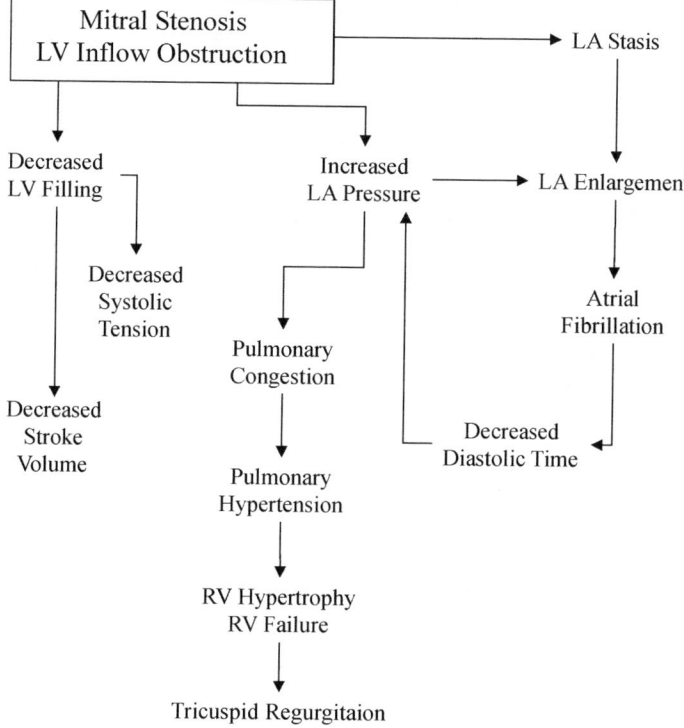

Fig. 5.

The high diastolic pressure gradient between the left ventricle and the aorta will make the murmur predominantly high frequency and blowing in character. It is also decrescendo because the gradient continues to fall as diastole proceeds. The regurgitant jet from the aorta may prevent full opening of the anterior mitral leaflet when it is severe, causing a state of functional mitral stenosis. This may cause turbulence in the mitral inflow, in turn giving rise to a mid-diastolic low-frequency murmur, the *Austin Flint rumble*. The presence of this murmur will also indicate that the degree of aortic regurgitation is severe or significant *(21,22)*. Increased left ventricular diastolic pressure, for various reasons mentioned previously, will cause elevation of the left atrial pressure and therefore the pulmonary capillary wedge pressures, thereby contributing to the symptoms of dyspnea, paroxysmal nocturnal dyspnea, and orthopnea. The increased myocardial O_2 demand because of increased left ventricular wall tension together with decreased coronary perfusion pressure secondary to decreased aortic diastolic pressure and increased left ventricular intracavitary diastolic pressure will contribute to the symptoms of angina.

PATHOPHYSIOLOGY OF MITRAL STENOSIS

Mitral stenosis is a left ventricular inflow obstructive lesion. The consequences of mitral inflow obstruction are twofold:

1. Underfilling of the left ventricle, which will cause low stroke volume if the obstruction is severe and low left ventricular systolic tension
2. Increased left atrial pressure and left atrial stasis and hence left atrial enlargement (Fig. 5)

When there is any significant obstruction to flow at the mitral valve, the left atrial pressure will be elevated because of the obstruction and the flow through the valve in diastole will occur under a higher *v wave* pressure gradient. The more severe the obstruction or the stenosis, the more persistent will be the elevation in the left atrial pressure. The pressure gradient between the left atrium and the left ventricle will tend to persist throughout diastole. The diastolic flow occurring under a higher and a persistent pressure gradient will contribute to a turbulent flow, which may last throughout diastole. The normal left atrial *v wave* pressure is usually about 12–15 mmHg. When there is significant mitral stenosis, the *v wave* pressure may be elevated up to 25–30 mmHg (*see* Chapter 8, Fig. 1). However, the pressure gradient noted even with severe mitral stenosis is still fairly low in terms of the absolute mmHg elevation. On the other hand, the volume of flow through the mitral valve is always significant because the entire stroke volume of the heart will have to go through the mitral valve in diastole. Thus, a large volume going through the mitral valve under relatively low levels of pressure will be expected to give rise to turbulence, which will produce predominantly low-frequency murmur, the characteristic diastolic rumble.

The elevated left atrial pressure and left atrial stasis will lead to left atrial enlargement, which over a period of time would contribute to the development of atrial fibrillation. The rapid ventricular response during atrial fibrillation and resulting tachycardia will shorten the diastolic filling period. By impeding the left atrial emptying, this will further tend to increase the left atrial pressure.

The elevated left atrial pressure will get transmitted to the pulmonary capillary bed, causing symptoms of pulmonary congestion. Elevation of pulmonary venous pressure eventually will lead to secondary rise in the pulmonary arterial pressure. Persistent and significant elevation of the pulmonary arterial pressure would lead to right ventricular hypertrophy. When the pulmonary hypertension is significant and longstanding, the right ventricle, which remains compensated initially, will eventually fail with right ventricular dilatation. This will eventually lead to the development of significant tricuspid regurgitation *(2,23–26)*.

Clinical Symptoms and Signs in Mitral Stenosis

The elevated left atrial pressure transmitted to the pulmonary capillary bed will cause symptoms of dyspnea, paroxysmal nocturnal dyspnea, and even orthopnea (Table 3). The latter may be atypical, for these patients will have a raised left atrial pressure most of the time when the mitral obstruction is significant. Therefore, they may never feel comfortable enough to go to sleep once they are woken up from sleep because of dyspnea, and furthermore they may wake up with dyspneic sensation more than once in a night. These features are not seen in classical paroxysmal nocturnal dyspnea because of left ventricular failure where patients usually are able to fall asleep again after they have been up on their feet or up for a while in a recumbent position with their feet dangling. Furthermore, the classical paroxysmal nocturnal dyspnea does not occur more than once in a night.

When atrial fibrillation supervenes because of the various factors mentioned, risk of systemic embolism becomes high. Symptoms will pertain then to the embolic sites or organs. In addition, patients may complain of palpitation as well as record an increase in their level of symptoms and decrease in exertional tolerance because of further rise in the left atrial pressure caused by shortened diastolic filling time related to the rapid

Table 3
Mitral Stenosis

Pathophysiological changes	Clinical symptoms/signs
• Raised LA pressure	• Dyspnea
	• Othropnea
	• Paroxysmal nocturnal dyspnea
• LA stasis	• Atrial fibrillation
• LA enlargement	• Palpitation
	• Systemic embolism
• Pulmonary hypertension	• Low-output symptoms
• RV failure	• Peripheral congestion/edema
• Rapid heart rate	• Poorly tolerated
• Shortening of diastole (e.g., *atrial fibrillation*)	• Pulmonary congestion
• Further rise in LA pressure (e.g., pregnancy)	
• Underfilled LV	• Normal apex
	• Carotid pulse Low normal volume
• Mitral closure at higher point of LV pressure because of higher LA pressure	• Loud S1 "closing snap"
• Entire LV stroke volume flowing through stenotic valve in diastole at low pressures	• Diastolic murmur
	• Low frequency rumble
• The higher the LA pressure (i.e., the more severe the stenosis), the earlier the mitral valve opening	• S2 – OS interval severity

LA, left atrial; LV, left ventricular; OS, opening snap; RV, right ventricular.

heart rate. Sometimes a patient may develop acute pulmonary edema with sudden onset of rapid atrial fibrillation.

The apex beat is usually normal because the left ventricle is in fact normal except for underfilling. The first heart sound may be loud and may become palpable. The loud M1 in mitral stenosis is due to the fact that the mitral closure point occurs at a higher left ventricular pressure because of the raised left atrial pressure. The loud S1 may become palpable. The opening snap of the mitral valve tends to occur earlier in diastole when the mitral stenosis is severe because of higher left atrial pressure. The diastolic murmur of mitral stenosis is predominantly low in frequency as a result of the fact that the entire left ventricular output goes through the mitral valve in diastole and at relatively low levels of pressure gradients.

PATHOPHYSIOLOGY OF AORTIC STENOSIS

Aortic stenosis is a lesion that causes left ventricular outflow tract obstruction. This causes the pressure in the left ventricle to rise to overcome the obstruction. The aortic pressure even in the most severe degree of obstruction (>75 mmHg pressure gradient across the aortic valve) may be maintained close to normal (systolic pressure of about

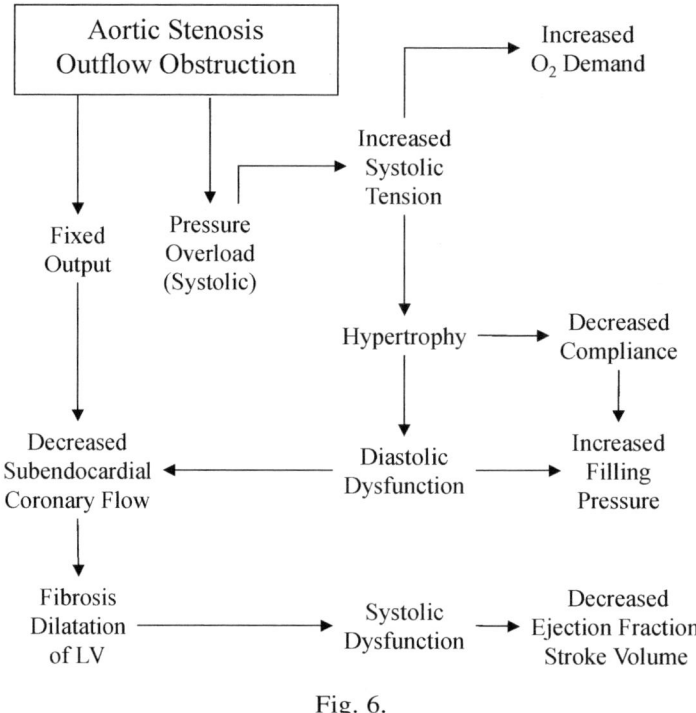

Fig. 6.

100–120 mmHg). Depending on the severity, the left ventricular systolic pressure can therefore be as high as 200–250 mmHg. This of course will place a systolic pressure load on the left ventricle. It will raise the systolic tension, thereby increasing the oxygen demand of the myocardium. In addition, the left ventricular pressure takes a longer time to fall to the level of the aortic diastolic pressure. Therefore, the stroke volume is ejected over a longer period of time (prolonged ejection time). The momentum with which the pressure pulse is delivered to the arterial system is slow because of the obstruction. The prolonged slow ejection is felt in the carotid pulse, which has a slow and sustained rise. The left ventricle will be unable to increase the cardiac output because of the fixed nature of the obstruction. With exertion the cardiac output will not sufficiently rise and the peripheral vasodilatation caused by the muscular exertion may actually cause the aortic and the arterial pressure to fall. The increased systolic tension will tend to be a good stimulus to left ventricular hypertrophy. The increased wall thickness is an attempt at normalizing the left ventricular wall tension because the latter is inversely related to the wall thickness (by Lamé's modification of the Laplace relationship). But the hypertrophy is often not enough to reduce or normalize the wall tension completely. The hypertrophied left ventricle is stiffer and therefore will offer more resistance to ventricular filling. The decreased left ventricular compliance leads to increased left ventricular diastolic or filling pressures. The increased intraventricular diastolic pressures will offer more resistance to the subendocardial capillary flow. Over a period of time unrelieved severe obstruction can lead to chronic subendocardial ischemia, which can in turn lead to myocardial necrosis and replacement fibrosis. Eventually the left ventricle may also begin to dilate and when decompensation sets in, left ventricular systolic function will also deteriorate with reduced ejection fraction (Fig. 6) *(1,2,5,10,16,27)*.

Table 4
Aortic Stenosis

Pathophysiological changes	Clinical symptoms/signs
• Obstruction at the valve	• Slow, rising carotid pulse
• Increased systolic tension + slow fall in tension because of prolonged ejection	• Sustained LV apex
• Decreased LV compliance	• S4 and atrial kick
• Increased O_2 demand • Decreased subendocardial flow	• Angina
• Fixed output	• Syncope/presyncope on exertion
• Increased LV filling pressure	• Dyspnea • Paroxysmal nocturnal dyspnea/orthopnea
• Dilatation	• Displaced, large-area LV apex
• Decreased stroke volume	• Low-volume pulse • Low-output symptoms

LV, left ventricular.

Clinical Symptoms and Signs in Aortic Stenosis

In normals, most of the stroke volume is ejected during the first third of systole, causing a rapid rise in the aortic pressure giving rise to a rapid upstroke. In aortic stenosis, this rapid ejection cannot occur. In fact, it takes all of systole to eject the same volume. The decreased mass or volume ejected per unit time leads to considerable decrease in ejection momentum despite increased velocity of ejection. In addition, the increased velocity of flow caused by the significant pressure gradient between the left ventricle and the aorta caused by the stenosis produces a Venturi effect on the lateral walls of the aorta. This has the effect of significantly reducing the net pressure rise in the aorta. Thus, the rate of rise of the arterial pressure pulse is slow in aortic stenosis. The net effects on the arterial pulse in valvular aortic stenosis are diminished amplitude (small), slow ascending limb (*parvus*), and a late and poorly defined peak (*tardus*). When the stenosis is very severe and accompanied by failing ventricle, the upstroke and the pulse may be poorly felt, if felt at all (*pulsus tardus et parvus*, meaning late, slow, and small).

Increased left ventricular systolic wall tension may cause the left ventricular apex beat to become sustained. Decreased left ventricular compliance may lead to the production of an *atrial kick* and /or a fourth heart sound. (S4).

Increased myocardial oxygen demand caused by the increased left ventricular systolic wall tension and the decreased subendocardial capillary flow aggravated by the raised left ventricular diastolic pressures would contribute to the symptoms of angina. Because of the fixed cardiac output, exertional hypotension, and syncope and presyncope may also occur. The increased left ventricular filling pressures, transmitted to the pulmonary capillary bed, will give rise to symptoms of dyspnea, paroxysmal nocturnal dyspnea, and orthopnea as well as pulmonary congestion.

Eventually when the left ventricle becomes dilated and begins to fail, the dilated enlarged left ventricle can give rise to a large area apex beat. The associated low cardiac output symptoms may be reflected in a very low amplitude arterial pulse (Table 4).

PATHOPHYSIOLOGY OF MYOCARDIAL ISCHEMIA/INFARCTION

Although myocardial ischemia or infarction could occur in the absence of coronary artery disease and may be caused by other factors such as vasospasm (e.g., patients with *vasospastic* or *Prinzmetal's angina*) and coronary emboli (e.g., systemic embolism in patients with atrial fibrillation and mitral stenosis), still its most common cause is atherosclerotic disease of the coronaries. When an atheromatous plaque in a coronary artery develops a crack or a rupture, it results in the formation of an occlusive thrombus, leading in turn to acute ischemic injury of the myocardium supplied by that artery. When the ischemia is of sufficiently long duration (usually more than 20 min), then a myocardial infarction could result.

Both contractility and relaxation will be impaired in the ischemic or infarcted myocardial segments. In addition, the affected myocardium will become less compliant and relatively stiffer, offering resistance to filling in diastole. When the compliance of the left ventricle is significantly reduced, then the normal left ventricular filling in diastole will be accompanied by a significant rise in the diastolic filling pressures. The increased filling pressures will have a beneficial effect on the nonischemic or noninfarcted segments, inducing them to be stretched more, thereby increasing their contractility. This will have a beneficial effect in maintaining a normal stroke volume. However, the increased filling pressures will also have a detrimental effect on the subendocardial capillary flow. It may aggravate or cause subendocardial ischemia. This, in turn, can further decrease the ventricular compliance and further raise the diastolic filling pressures.

If the ischemia or infarction involves a large area of the left ventricular myocardium, then the decreased contractility of the ischemic segments will be expected to be associated with a decreased ejection fraction, increased end systolic volume, and decreased stroke volume. The greater the increase in the end-systolic volume, the poorer becomes the clinical outcome. Clinical symptoms of heart failure may develop when more than 25% of the myocardium is involved, and cardiogenic shock may result if more than 40% of the myocardium is infarcted. The latter of course carries with it a high mortality rate.

The infarcted area, particularly when large, can undergo excessive thinning before formation of a firm scar. This process, when it occurs without additional myocardial necrosis, is termed infarct expansion. Pathologically this involves myocyte and tissue loss with disruption of normal myocardial cells in the infarct zone.

The ischemic or infarcted segments could be *dyskinetic* and therefore bulge out during systole. This will tend to increase the left ventricular dimension. The resultant increase in the radius will raise the left ventricular wall tension by the Laplace relationship. The increased wall tension could become a stimulus for hypertrophy of the healthy segments of the myocardium. Hypertrophy will eventually lead to further decrease in the left ventricular compliance.

The noninfarcted myocardium could also undergo dilatation. This is a consequence of the degree of elevation of the filling pressures and the underlying systolic and diastolic left ventricular wall tension. In addition to the loading conditions, it is also dependent on the size of the infarct and the patency of the infarct related artery.

These changes in both the infarcted and the noninfarcted myocardium, which involve varying degrees of hypertrophy and dilatation resulting in changes in the shape and size

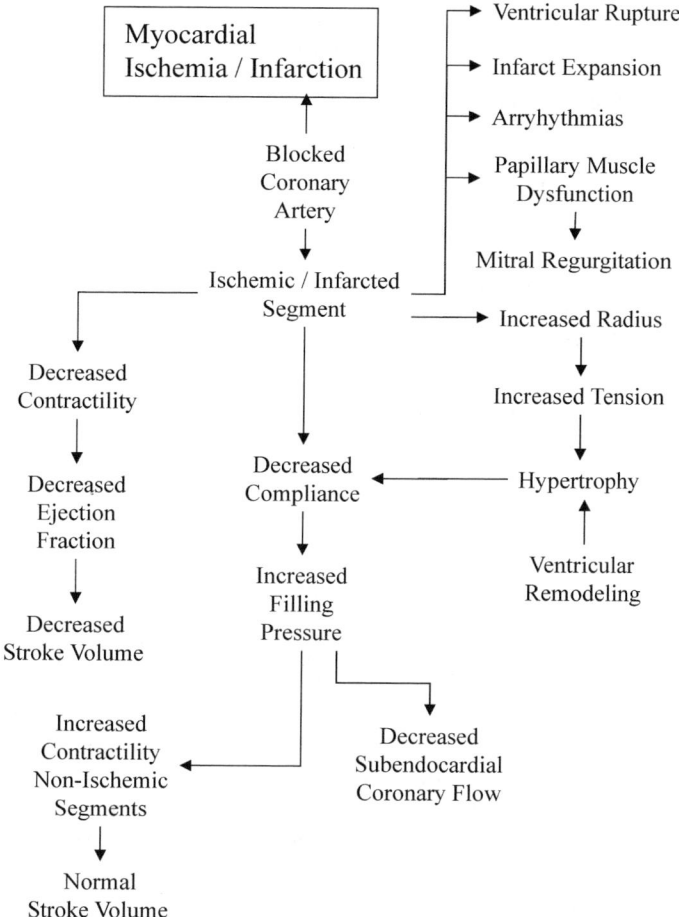

Fig. 7.

of the ventricle, is termed *ventricular remodeling*. The early and sustained activation of the various neurohormones, including the renin–angiotensin and the aldesterone pathway, has been shown to be intimately involved in the remodeling that the myocardium undergoes following a myocardial infarction. The blockade of this pathway with angiotensin-converting enzyme inhibitors has been shown to prevent the adverse myocardial remodeling, thereby improving the clinical outcome.

The complications that can follow significant myocardial ischemia/infarction include ventricular arrhythmias, ventricular rupture, papillary muscle dysfunction, and mitral regurgitation. The inhomogeneous repolarization that occurs in the ischemic myocardium and the presence of high sympathetic stimulation accompanying acute ischemia or infarction set the conditions favoring the production of the ventricular arrhythmias. When the myocardium underlying a group of papillary muscle is ischemic or infarcted, then the mitral leaflets would tend to become incompetent. The resulting papillary muscle dysfunction will cause varying degrees of mitral regurgitation (Fig. 7) *(28–44)*.

Table 5
Myocardial Ischemia/Infarction

Pathophysiological changes	Clinical symptoms/signs
• Decreased LV compliance	• S4
• Increased LV filling pressure	• Dyspnea
	• Pulmonary congestion
• Decreased supply	• Angina
• Decreased subendocardial flow	
• Increased tension	
• Increased O_2 demand	
• Reduced ejection fraction	• Sustained LV apex
• Increased duration of systolic tension	
• Papillary muscle dysfunction	• Mitral regurgitation murmur

LV, left ventricular.

Clinical Symptoms and Signs in Myocardial Ischemia/Infarction

The decreased left ventricular compliance caused by various factors discussed earlier would favor the production of a fourth heart sound (S4) as long as the left atrium is healthy and the sinus rhythm is preserved. The increased filling pressures in the left ventricle by transmission will raise the pulmonary capillary pressures, thereby causing pulmonary congestion and symptoms of dyspnea. Anginal symptoms will be expected on account of the various factors that increase the myocardial oxygen demand in the face of decreased supply caused by coronary occlusion. When the ejection fraction is decreased and significant left ventricular dysfunction is present, then the increased duration of the raised left ventricular systolic wall tension will cause the left ventricular apical impulse to become sustained. When the papillary muscle dysfunction supervenes, one can also hear a mitral regurgitation murmur (Table 5). When significant left ventricular dysfunction and failure develop together with elevated left atrial pressure, an S3 may also be heard.

PATHOPHYSIOLOGY OF HYPERTENSIVE HEART DISEASE

Significant and longstanding hypertension, whether secondary or primary, can lead to cardiac pathological changes and give rise to signs and symptoms. The sequence of these changes pertaining to the heart will be reviewed without attempting to review all of the vascular changes that lead to eventual target-organ damage in other parts of the body, including the brain and the kidney.

Hypertension, the essential or the primary type, is a fairly common disorder. The disorder is characterized by a reduction in the caliber as well as in the number of small arterioles, resulting in increased peripheral vascular resistance. While hypertension by itself can produce significant cardiac changes leading to symptoms and signs, it is also a significant risk factor for the development of atherosclerosis. Therefore, it can aggravate symptoms and signs of ischemic heart disease. The endothelial relaxation factor, nitric oxide, is not produced adequately because of the endothelial dysfunction that accompanies hypertension. This will cause poor coronary vasodilatation reserve. In addition, the increased systolic pressure will raise the systolic left ventricular wall tension, thereby increasing the myocardial oxygen demand. The increased wall tension is also a stimulus for left ventricular hypertrophy. The hypertrophied left ventricle is less compliant, thereby raising the left ventricular filling pressures. The latter will compromise the subendocardial capillary flow. This will over a period of time contribute to the development of fibrosis, particularly in the subendocardium. As a result of this, the filling pressures will further rise. The elevated filling pressures could cause the symptoms of pulmonary congestion because of the transmission of pressures to the left atrium and the pulmonary capillary bed. At this stage, the systolic function may still be well preserved with good ejection fraction. In fact, hypertension is an important condition, which is often associated with symptoms of congestive failure in the presence of preserved systolic left ventricular function. Eventually in longstanding cases with significant untreated hypertension, the left ventricle will begin to dilate and enlarge and result in systolic dysfunction.

The interaction of the arterial system with the left ventricular function also needs some clarification. This interaction is a direct result of the properties of the peripheral arteries pertaining to their effects on the arterial wave reflection and pulse wave transmission (*see* Chapter 2). The properties of the proximal arterial system in healthy young individuals are such that the pulse pressure generated by ventricular ejection is not very high. Also, the component of wave reflection returns to the central aorta in diastole, raising the diastolic coronary perfusion pressure without causing any increase in the systolic load on the ventricle. With aging, however, both the aorta and the arterial system in general become stiffened. The stiffening of the aorta itself contributes to the increased pulse pressure generated by the ventricular ejection. In addition, the stiffened arteries lead to increased pulse wave velocity. This will result in early return of the reflected pressure wave from the periphery to the heart. As long as the left ventricle is compensated, this will add to the late systolic pressure rise and increase the pressure load on the left ventricle without compromising the aortic forward flow. In fact, early wave reflection is an important contributor to the development of systolic hypertension in the elderly.

When the left ventricle is dilated and its function compromised, it will be unable to accommodate for the early pressure wave reflection. This will negatively impact on the forward aortic flow out of the left ventricle, with early deceleration of the flow eventually resulting in decreased ejection time and diminished stroke output. While these peripheral arterial effects could play a role in any patient with compromised left ventricular function, it is particularly relevant in the elderly hypertensive patient developing failure. Recognition of this factor is important in view of its therapeutic implications. Reduction of wave reflection with the use of appropriate vasodilataory agents becomes an important therapeutic goal in the treatment of hypertension.

Often the raised left atrial pressures will lead to left atrial enlargement and can cause the development of atrial arrhythmias, particularly atrial fibrillation, which can aggravate or precipitate heart failure symptoms (Fig. 8). When ischemic heart disease is coexistent, papillary muscle dysfunction and mitral regurgitation can also supervene.

Clinical Symptoms and Signs in Hypertensive Heart Disease

Hypertension may remain silent for a long time and may go undetected because of a lack of specific symptoms associated with it. Therefore, it is called the silent killer. It may be detected, however, in patients being evaluated for symptoms of atypical chest pain,

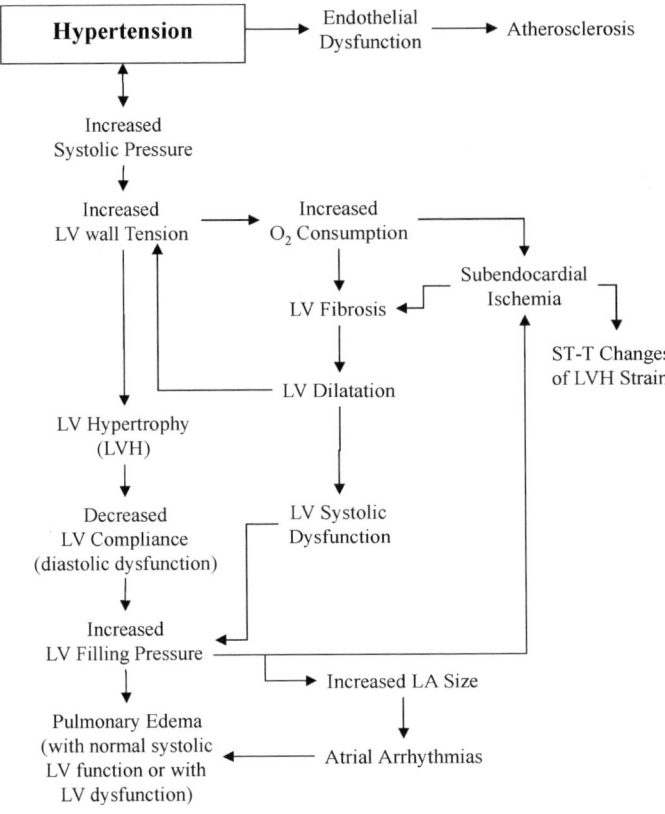

Fig. 8.

angina, dyspnea, or palpitation. The increased myocardial oxygen demand, the increased left ventricular diastolic filling pressure, as well as the elevated left atrial pressure could be contributing to these symptoms. The strong left atrial contraction evoked by the hypertrophied and less compliant left ventricle in those patients with healthy left atria may give rise to a fourth heart sound and/or a palpable atrial kick in the apex beat. The apical impulse may be sustained only when the systolic pressure is very high or when the left ventricular ejection fraction is decreased. The second heart sound is usually narrowly split and may occasionally show reverse splitting with delayed A2. The latter may occur when severe hypertension is accompanied by ischemia as well. The hypertrophy of the left ventricle may be associated with the voltage criteria of left ventricular hypertrophy on the electrocardiogram (ECG). The subendocardial ischemia and the development of fibrosis in the late stages would explain the repolarization (ST-T waves) changes on the ECG (left ventricular hypertrophy strain pattern) (Table 6) *(14,16,45–50)*.

PATHOPHYSIOLOGY OF DILATED CARDIOMYOPATHY

Dilated cardiomyopathy refers to intrinsic myocardial disease. The etiology is often idiopathic, while in others it may be related to definable etiological factors such as ethanol-related myocardial damage or a definite viral myocarditis. Whatever may be the etiology, the hallmark of the disorder is a dilated poorly contracting left ventricle, and

Table 6
Hypertension

Pathophysiological changes	Clinical symptoms/signs
	• Asymptomatic for long time
• Increased systolic LV wall tension	• Atypical chest pain
• Increased O_2 demand	• Angina
• Increased LV filling pressure	• Dyspnea
• Decreased subendocardial flow	• Palpitation
• Increased left atrial pressure	
• Decreased LV compliance	• S4/atrial kick
• Severe hypertension or decreased LV systolic function	• Sustained LV apex
• Subendocardial ischemia ± fibrosis	• ECG—repolarization abnormalities
	• LVH strain pattern

LV, left ventricular; ECG, electrocardiogram; LVH, left ventricular hypertrophy.

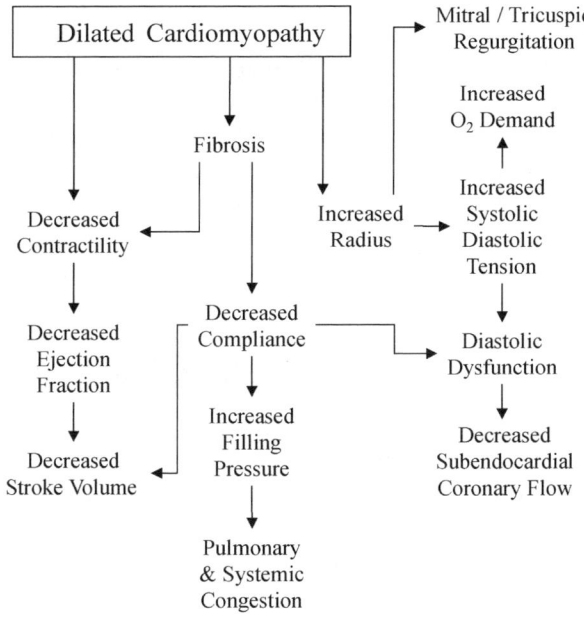

Fig. 9.

the process might involve equally the right ventricle. The increased radius caused by the dilatation would increase the oxygen demand by raising the left ventricular wall tension both during systole and diastole. The diastolic dysfunction would contribute to decreased left ventricular compliance. Other factors that may be involved in the decrease of the ventricular compliance include myocardial fibrosis in longstanding cases. The decreased compliance will lead to increased filling pressures in the ventricle. This would account for both systemic and pulmonary congestion. In addition, it will contribute to decreased subendocardial capillary flow. That will further cause abnormal rise in the filling pressures (Fig. 9).

Table 7
Dilated Cardiomyopathy

Pathophysiological changes	Clinical symptoms/signs
• Increased radius	• Displaced large-area LV apex
• Increased duration of systolic tension • Reduced ejection fraction	• Sustained LV apex
• Increased LV/RV filling pressures	• Dyspnea/edema
• Decreased stroke volume	• Low-volume (amplitude) pulse • Low-output symptoms
• Severe reduction in ejection fraction	• Poorly felt apex beat

LV, left ventricular; RV, right ventricular.

Clinical Symptoms and Signs in Dilated Cardiomyopathy

The increased radius will cause a large-area displaced left ventricular apical impulse. If the contractility is significantly reduced, then the accompanying decreased ejection fraction will give rise to a sustained apical impulse. The increased left and right ventricular filling pressures will lead to pulmonary and systemic congestion, causing symptoms of dyspnea and peripheral edema. When the ejection fraction is significantly reduced, the stroke volume may be low and give rise to low-amplitude low-volume pulse. Severe decrease in ejection fraction and stroke volume may actually lead to a very poorly felt apical impulse (Table 7) *(51,52)*.

PATHOPHYSIOLOGY OF HYPERTROPHIC OBSTRUCTIVE CARDIOMYOPATHY

Hypertrophic cardiomyopathy is characterized by idiopathic hypertrophy of the ventricular myocardium, especially of the left ventricle, often with an asymmetrical involvement of the septum. The myocardium exhibits considerable disarray of the myocardial fibers. The intraventricular cavity is usually small. The left ventricle is often hypercontractile. The rapid ejection with increased ejection fraction will allow normal systolic tension to be maintained when there is no obstruction. The rapid and forceful ejection may, however, create a Venturi effect on the anterior mitral leaflet. The anterior mitral leaflet then may be pulled forward from its closed position during systole. The systolic anterior motion of the anterior leaflet may bring the leaflet into contact with the interventricular septum, thereby causing obstruction to the left ventricular outflow during the middle of systole. This anterior motion of the anterior mitral leaflet will make the mitral valve incompetent and allow mitral regurgitation to develop when obstruction to the left ventricular outflow tract is produced. In this condition, the obstruction to the left ventricular outflow is often dynamic. It may be exaggerated or increased under conditions of increased inotropic stimulation as may occur with sympathetic stimulation. It also can be increased by maneuvers that decrease the ventricular dimension, which will make mitral leaflet and septal contact to occur earlier in systole. If the septal hypertrophy is excessive and the intraventricular cavity is small, then obstruction could occur even

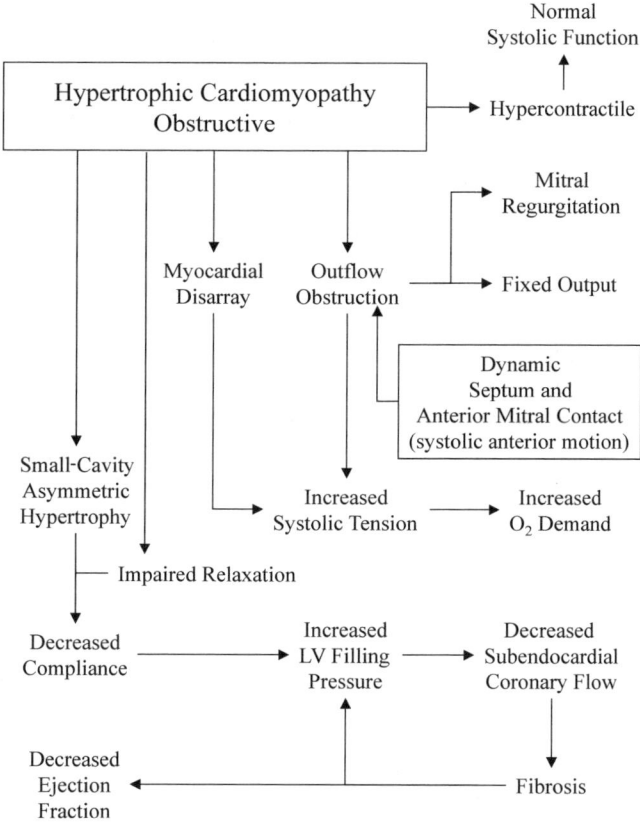

Fig. 10.

at rest. When there is significant obstruction during systole, then the left ventricular systolic wall tension will be increased. Increased left ventricular wall tension will increase myocardial oxygen demand.

The hypertrophy of the myocardium as well as the small left ventricular size will decrease the left ventricular compliance. This will increase the filling pressures in the left ventricle. The increased filling pressures will also impede subendocardial coronary capillary flow. The latter will contribute to the development of some myocardial fibrosis in the subendocardium. In longstanding cases, the left ventricular function could deteriorate with development of myocardial fibrosis, and the ejection fraction could actually fall. The decreased left ventricular systolic function, a late phenomenon, could further raise the diastolic filling pressures in the ventricle (Fig. 10) *(53–57)*.

Clinical Symptoms and Signs in Hypertrophic Obstructive Cardiomyopathy

The hypercontractile left ventricle with rapid ejection will give rise to a sharp and rapid rate of rise of the arterial pulse. In the presence of significant outflow obstruction, the pulse will either have normal or low amplitude. The increased left ventricular wall tension during systole accompanying significant obstruction will be associated with a sustained duration of the apical impulse. Decreased left ventricular compliance will evoke a strong atrial contraction and may result in the production of a fourth heart sound (S4). It may also cause an atrial kick to be felt at the apex. The dynamic nature of the obstruction between the anterior mitral leaflet and the interventricular septum will explain the varying loudness of the ejection murmur, depending on the degree of the obstruction. This can be brought out by change in the venous return and the resultant change in the left ventricular dimension caused by change in posture from a supine to the erect position. The murmur will be louder and longer on standing than when supine because the left ventricular size will be smaller in the standing position than when supine, causing the septal and mitral leaflet contact to occur earlier. In addition, the increase in the sympathetic tone caused by the assumption of the upright posture will help increase the contractility of the left ventricle. This will further increase the force of ejection. This will generate a greater Venturi effect on the mitral leaflet, pulling the anterior leaflet forward more forcefully. The aortic pressure is the distending pressure that will oppose the systolic anterior motion of the anterior mitral leaflet. Standing may actually cause a slight fall in the systemic arterial pressure, thereby decreasing this opposing force. For all these reasons, the ejection murmur tends to be longer and louder on standing than when supine.

The increased left ventricular diastolic filling pressures being transmitted to the pulmonary capillary bed will produce symptoms of pulmonary congestion. Depending on the severity of the elevation of the left atrial and the pulmonary venous pressures, these symptoms can consist of dyspnea, paroxysmal nocturnal dyspnea, and/or orthopnea. When the left atrial pressure is significantly increased and the left ventricular compliance markedly diminished, then abrupt deceleration of the early rapid diastolic inflow into the left ventricle could occur, causing the production of an S3.

The increased myocardial oxygen demand and the decreased subendocardial capillary flow could contribute to symptoms of angina.

When the obstruction to outflow is severe, the cardiac output becomes fixed and will not significantly increase on exertion. In fact, exercise-induced peripheral vasodilatation may actually drop the systemic arterial pressure further and may cause the obstruction to become worse because of the decreased (distending) aortic root pressure (i.e., the opposing force of the systolic anterior motion of the anterior mitral leaflet). This may manifest as symptoms of exertional presyncope or syncope. The mitral regurgitation that accompanies the systolic anterior motion of the anterior mitral leaflet during systole may vary in severity, depending on the degree of obstruction. The longstanding effects of mitral regurgitation and the elevated left atrial pressure could result in the development of atrial arrhythmias especially atrial fibrillation. These may manifest as symptoms of palpitation. The underlying myocardial disease and the pathological changes of myocardial disarray and fibrosis could also set conditions suitable for the development of ventricular arrhythmias (Table 8).

PATHOPHYSIOLOGY OF ATRIAL SEPTAL DEFECT

Atrial septal defect represents the lesion that allows left-to-right shunt at the atrial level. The right ventricular wall is normally thinner compared to the left ventricle. The pulmonary arterial resistance is significantly lower than the systemic vascular resistance. Therefore, the right ventricle is more compliant than the left ventricle. Because of these reasons, the right side offers less resistance to flow than the left side. So the left-to-right shunt is a natural consequence in the presence of a defect in the atrial septum.

Table 8
Hypertrophic Obstructive Cardiomyopathy

Pathophysiological changes	Clinical symptoms/signs
• Hypercontractile left ventricle	• Sharp carotid upstroke
• Outflow obstruction	• Normal or low-amplitude pulse
• Increased systolic tension with slow fall in tension	• Substained LV apex
• Decreased LV compliance	• Atrial kick • S4
• Dynamic nature of obstruction anterior leaflet MV and septum	• Ejection murmur varying in loudness
• LV size; systemic resistance—aortic pressure; contractility	• Murmur loader on standing • Murmur softer on squatting
• Increased LV filling pressure • LA pressure	• Dyspnea • Paroxysmal nocturnal dyspnea/orthopnea
• Increased O_2 demand • Decreased subendocardial flow	• Angina
• Increased LA pressure • Decreased compliance	• S3
• Fixed output	• Exertional syncope/presyncope
• Mitral regurgitation	• Atrial fibrillation • Palpitation
• Myocardial disease	• Ventricular arrhythmias

LV, left ventricular; LA, left atrial, MV, mitral valve.

The right atrium and the right ventricle will therefore receive the usual normal systemic venous return as well as this extra volume of blood received through the atrial septal defect. This leads to a volume overload state of the right ventricle. The large right ventricular stroke volume and the increased pulmonary flow is maintained for a long period of time (i.e., for many years) with normal or even low pulmonary arterial pressures. In some patients the large flow could be associated with slight or moderate increase in the pulmonary arterial pressures mainly related to the flow. The increased size of the dilated right ventricle will cause increased right ventricular wall tension by *Laplace relationship*. The increased wall tension being a stimulus for hypertrophy will result in right ventricular hypertrophy. The dilatation of the right ventricle may cause increased tension in the moderator band through which the right bundle normally reaches the free wall of the right ventricle. This may contribute to the right bundle branch block pattern that is commonly seen in patients with atrial septal defect. The longstanding shunt and the secondary right ventricular hypertrophy could lead to decreased right ventricular compliance, thereby raising the right ventricular filling pressures and therefore the right atrial pressures. The large pulmonary flow also means increased pulmonary venous inflow into the left atrium, contributing also to some left atrial enlargement.

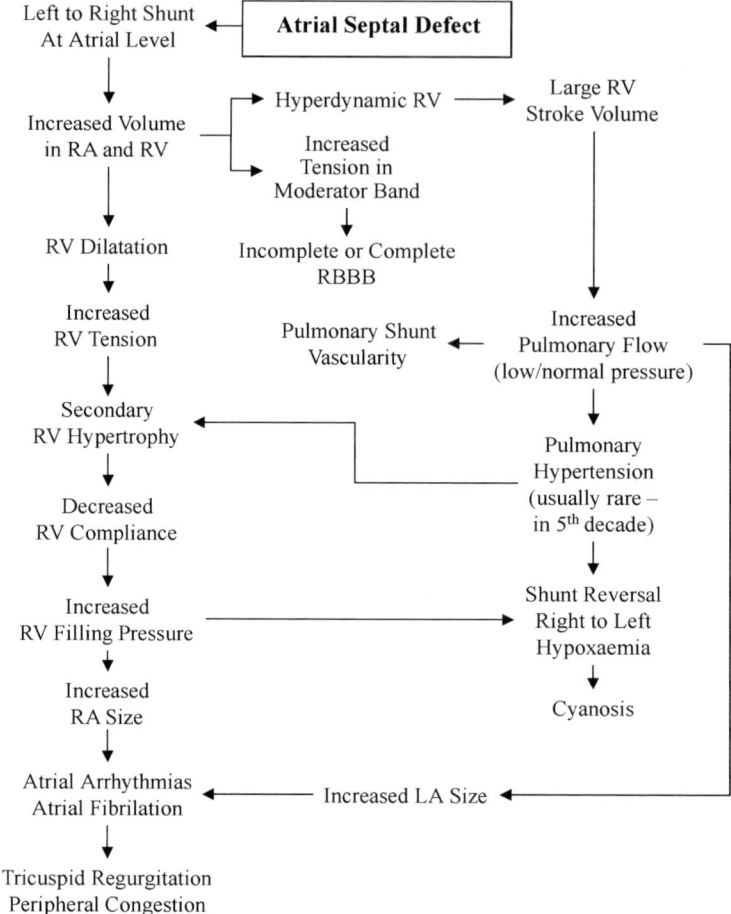

Fig. 11.

With increasing age the left ventricular compliance is decreased further. This will allow more preferential flow to the right side increasing the magnitude of the left-to-right shunt. The dilated atria would lead to the development of atrial arrhythmias and in particular atrial fibrillation. Because right ventricular dilatation automatically stretches the tricuspid valve ring, tricuspid regurgitation usually ensues. This is aggravated by the onset of atrial fibrillation, which usually heralds the symptoms and signs of peripheral congestion. The tendency for the development of atrial fibrillation and symptoms of heart failure is particularly increased after the fourth decade of life.

The rise in pulmonary vascular resistance caused by pulmonary vascular disease secondary to longstanding increase in the pulmonary flow is usually a very late phenomenon and is seen only in adults and in a small percentage of patients. If the pulmonary hypertension is significant then, it can further cause right ventricular hypertrophy and secondarily increase its filling pressures. The increased resistance in the pulmonary vascular bed together with increased right ventricular and right atrial filling pressures could then reverse the shunt and begin to produce cyanosis secondary to hypoxemia. This type of *Eisenmenger's syndrome* with atrial septal defect secundum is usually rare (Fig.11) *(58–62)*.

Table 9
Atrial Septal Defect

Pathophysiological changes	Clinical symptoms/signs
	• Maybe asymptomatic
• Not clearly explainable	• Vague symptoms, fatigue, palpitation, dyspnea
• Onset of atrial fibrillation	• Peripheral congestion
• RV volume overload	• Apex formed by right ventricle with lateral retraction
• Increased venous return on inspiration with decrease in left-to-right shunt and opposite changes on expiration	• Fixed split S2
• Increased pulmonary flow secondary to left-to-right shunt	• Ejection murmur II and III LICS • Tricuspid inflow rumble

LICS, left intercostal space.

Clinical Symptoms and Signs in Atrial Septal Defect

Atrial septal defect may not cause any significant symptoms and may be picked up by the presence of an ejection systolic murmur heard over the second left interspace caused by the increased pulmonary flow and/or a fixed splitting of the second heart sound (S2). The increased venous return on inspiration is accompanied by decreased left-to-right shunt flow. The opposite occurs with expiration, thereby keeping the pulmonary flow varying very little with respiration. This allows the A2 and P2 separation to remain constant and unchanging with respiration. While this explanation may be simple, there could be other factors involved. The murmur may sometimes be scratchy and harsh and sometimes may be absent.

Patients with atrial septal defect may also have vague symptoms of fatigue, palpitation, and shortness of breath, all of which may not be clearly explainable. The symptoms of peripheral congestion with the onset of atrial fibrillation are usually noteworthy. The left ventricle is usually underfilled and displaced posteriorly by the enlarged right ventricle. The enlarged right ventricle may in fact form the apical impulse and may be characterized by the presence of *lateral retraction*. A short mid diastolic inflow murmur may accompany the increased flow into the right side across the tricuspid valve, which may be audible over the lower sternal or xiphoid area. The murmur may increase in intensity on inspiration, indicating its tricuspid origin. The presence of such a flow murmur is usually indicative of a significant left-to-right shunt (Table 9) *(63–65)*.

PATHOPHYSIOLOGY OF DIASTOLIC DYSFUNCTION

Several factors can affect the compliance of the left ventricle, thereby affecting the filling characteristics as well as its diastolic filling pressures. These include the completeness of ventricular relaxation, the chamber size, the thickness of the wall, the composition of the wall (inflammation, infiltrate, ischemia or infarction, scars, etc.), the pericardium, and the right ventricular volume and pressure.

The diastolic filling consists of three consecutive phases, namely:

1. The early rapid filling phase, which is an active phase beginning with ventricular relaxation

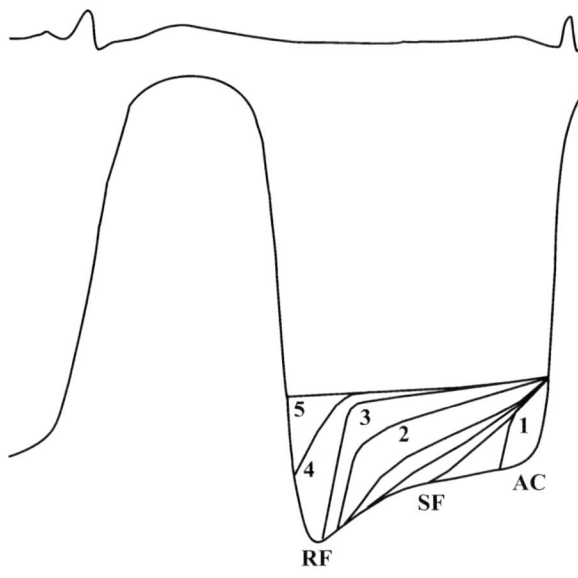

Fig. 12.

2. The slow filling phase
3. The atrial contraction phase during end-diastole

The degree of decrease in diastolic compliance may vary. In the early stages it may restrict only end-diastolic filling. It may evoke a strong atrial contraction to help achieve better filling and stretch of the ventricular myocardium. At this stage only the end-diastolic ventricular pressure will be increased and only the *a wave* pressure will be increased in the atrium. This will not significantly affect the mean atrial pressure because of the short duration of the *a wave*. When the degree of diastolic dysfunction is more advanced, it may begin to encroach on the slow filling phase of diastole as well. At this stage, the *pre-a wave* pressure will also be increased, thereby increasing the mean atrial filling pressure. The etiology of this type of diastolic restriction may be intraluminal as in systolic heart failure where the ventricle empties poorly because of decreased ejection fraction and therefore becomes overfilled quite early in diastole. It may be because of endocardial pathology as in idiopathic endomyocardial fibrosis or fibroelastosis, secondary to myocardial pathology of various etiologies, or because of pericardial causes including significant pericardial effusion and/or constrictive pericarditis. In all these situations the filling in the rapid filling phase is not impaired, but restriction affects the slow filling phase to end of diastole. The third type of restriction is when it involves all of diastole, beginning with the early rapid filling phase. This type of total diastolic restriction is characteristic of *cardiac tamponade*. The latter is usually the result of collection of fluid or blood in the pericardial space, which is under high pressure, thereby compressing the ventricles from the very onset of diastole. This type of restriction is rare in systolic heart failure except in some very rare instances of severe degree of heart failure (Fig.12 and Table 10).

Table 10
Diastolic Dysfunction

1. Decreased ventricular compliance in end-diastole only

2. Progressive stages of decreased compliance affecting the slow-filling phase of diastole, leading to eventual increase in mean atrial pressure

	Etiology
• Intraluminal	• Systolic failure
• Endocardial	
• Myocardial	
• Pericardial	• Pericardial effusion
	• Constriction

3. Filling restriction also involving the rapid filling phase of diastole (cardiac tamponade). Rarely, severe heart failure

PATHOPHYSIOLOGY OF CONSTRICTIVE PERICARDITIS

As a result of recurrent episodes of pericarditis or chronic pericarditis and especially those associated with certain specific pathogens, such as tuberculous pericarditis, the pericardium may mount excessive reaction and may eventually thicken, become fibrosed, and even become calcified. In the initial stages there may be pericardial effusion, but this eventually disappears and the thickened pericardium will become adherent to the underlying epicardium. A similar reaction can also follow traumatic, postsurgical, or radiation-induced pericarditis. Often, however, the etiology may be difficult to pinpoint and may be truly idiopathic. Occasionally patients may present during the transitional phase with both effusion and signs of constriction. The signs of constriction may actually become evident when the patient's hemodynamics fail to show improvement even after the effusion is drained. These patients may be termed to have *effusive–constrictive pericarditis*.

In constrictive pericarditis, the pericardium is very stiff and fibrotic and may even be calcified. The visceral pericardium is thickened (sometimes up to 1 cm thick) and adherent to the underlying myocardium. The thickened and fibrotic pericardium acts as a steel armor around the ventricles, preventing their full expansion. The ventricles could expand in early diastole, but as soon as their sizes reach the limits set by the thickened pericardium, the expansion is suddenly restricted and the filling comes to an abrupt end. No further expansion being possible, there is hardly any further filling during the later phases of diastole. The ventricular pressure that dips to zero at the onset of diastole suddenly rises to a peak and flattens out and stays elevated during the remainder of diastole, giving rise to the characteristic "*dip-plateau*" *square-root sign* of the filling pressures in the ventricles. Because the pericardium restricts both the right ventricle and the left ventricle alike, the filling pressures rise on both sides to similar levels. The increased diastolic ventricular pressures raise the mean pressures in both the atria. The raised right atrial pressure leads to the formation of systemic congestion, and the raised left atrial pressure would cause pulmonary congestion. The severe diastolic filling restriction would cause decreased stroke output. This will be felt as low-amplitude arterial pulse. The cardiac output may be maintained by a reflex increase in the heart rate (Fig. 13).

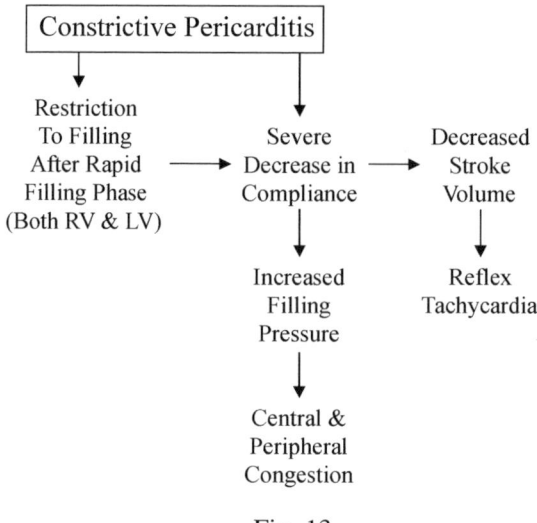

Fig. 13.

Clinical Symptoms and Signs in Constrictive Pericarditis

The jugular venous pressure is not only elevated because of the raised right atrial pressures, it shows the altered contour with a dominant *y descent*. This is because the *v wave* pressure head is raised with sudden restriction to filling at the end of the early rapid-filling phase. This abrupt deceleration to the rapid inflow into the ventricles also sets the stage for the production of an early S3, *the pericardial knock*. The elevation of the atrial pressures will result in central congestion and dyspnea as well as peripheral congestion leading to edema and ascites.

The venous pressure will rise on inspiration with the increased venous return as the right ventricular compliance is significantly decreased because of the pericardial restriction. This is the basis of *Kussmaul's sign*. In some patients with constrictive pericarditis, one may also have a pulsus parodoxus. This may happen for the reason that the inspiratory increase in the right ventricular filling pressure may produce some septal shift, causing decreased left ventricular filling and pressure, and therefore the stroke output on inspiration may fall and the opposite changes will occur on expiration and improve the left ventricular filling, thereby increasing the stroke output. These changes may be reflected in the arterial pressure with the pressure falling on inspiration and rising on expiration significantly. When the filling is considerably impaired, the decreased output will cause the arterial pulse to have low amplitude, and this may be associated with low-output symptoms of lassitude, fatigue, and weakness as well (Table 11).

PATHOPHYSIOLOGY OF CARDIAC TAMPONADE

When pericarditis occurs, the inflamed surfaces of both the pericardium and the epicardium moving against each other as a result of heart movement with each cardiac beat cause friction because of the roughened surfaces. This results in an audible pericardial friction rub. The friction rub may disappear as a result of the inflammation settling down and the surfaces becoming smooth again. This is a good sign. But the friction rub may also disappear as a result of fluid accumulation between the two surfaces, which acts as a buffer and eliminates the friction and the friction rub.

Chapter 10 / Pathophysiological Basis of Symptoms and Signs

Table 11
Constrictive Pericarditis

Pathophysiological changes	Clinical symptoms/signs
• Increased RV diastolic pressure	• Elevated JVP
• Restriction after rapid filling	• Dominant *y descent*
• Sudden deceleration of early diastolic inflow	• S_3 (early)
	• "Pericardial knock"
• Central and peripheral congestion	• Dyspnea
	• Acsites
	• Edema
• Severe decrease in compliance	• Kussmaul's sign
• Inspiratory increase in RV filling pressure	
• Inspiratory increase in RV filling pressure	• Pulsus paradoxus
• Septal shift	
• Decreased LV filling pressure	
• Decreased stroke volume	• Low-output symptoms

LV, left ventricular; JVP, jugular venous pulse;

If the fluid accumulation of whatever cause (viral pericarditis, malignancy, systemic lupus, uremia, etc.) is slow, the pericardium may adapt and dilate slowly, allowing the intrapericardial pressure to stay low. Therefore, a large effusion may be well tolerated by the patient if accumulated over a period of time. Although the intrapericardial pressure may remain low with large effusion, the volume pressure relationship of the pericardium is such that when it has reached its limits of compliance, further accumulation of even a small amount of fluid could suddenly raise the intrapericardial pressure quite dramatically, leading to cardiac tamponade. This change could occur within a short period of time.

When there is acute accumulation of pericardial fluid as seen in bleeding into the pericardial space secondary to trauma, ruptured myocardium post-myocardial-infarction or following aortic root dissection (type I), the pericardium will be unable to adapt to the sudden accumulation of volume and the intrapericardial pressure will rise acutely and cause cardiac tamponade.

In *cardiac tamponade*, the restriction involves all of diastole. The filling pressures are increased and equal in both the right and the left ventricles. The ventricles receive blood flow with great difficulty. All four chambers are boxed in a tight space with high fluid pressure in the pericardial space. The blood can enter the heart only when it leaves the heart, namely during systole. The blood that enters the atria during systole is with great difficulty transferred to the ventricles during diastole. The filling becomes inadequate invariably with low stroke output, which will result in reflex tachycardia (Fig. 14).

Clinical Symptoms and Signs in Cardiac Tamponade

The increased filling pressures contribute to symptoms of dyspnea and cause the venous pressure to be elevated. The jugular contour will show no *y descent* despite high venous pressure because the restriction involves all of diastole. The contour may show only an *x' descent*. That too may be difficult to discern but can be best recorded by Doppler flow over the jugular. The marked decrease in stroke volume will cause hypotension and low systolic and low pulse pressure in addition to causing low-output symptoms. The reflex sympathetic stimulation will be reflected in the presence of tachycardia (Table 12) *(66–72)*.

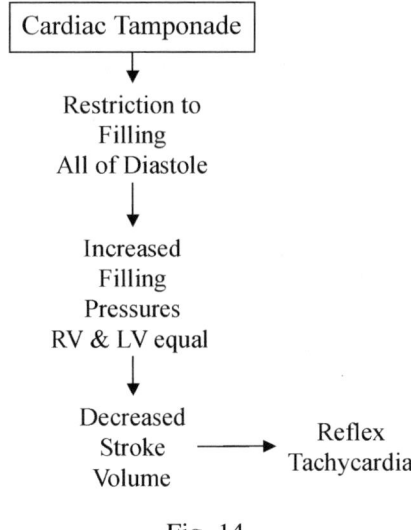

Fig. 14.

Table 12
Cardiac Tamponade

Pathophysiological changes	Clinical symptoms/signs
• Increased filling pressures	• elevated JVP
	• Dyspnea
• Restriction of all diastole including early rapid filling phase	• Absent *y descent*
	• *x' descent*
• Severe decrease in stroke volume	• Hypotension
	• Low pulse pressure
	• Low-output symptoms
• Sympathetic stimulation	• Tachycardia

JVP, jugular venous pulse.

In addition, in the majority of patients there will be a significant *pulsus paradoxus* (with an inspiratory drop in blood pressure of more than 15 mmHg). The increased inspiratory venous return to the right ventricle and the associated right ventricular expansion may shift the interventricular septum as in the case of the constrictive pericarditis. In this situation the pericardial fluid is squeezed and shifted to the left side, restricting expansion of the left ventricle during diastole. The effects of fluid shift may be seen as collapse or compression of relatively thin and low-pressure chambers like the right atrium or the right ventricle during diastole on a two-dimensional echocardiogram *(73,74)*.

In some patients with large pericardial effusions, the marked increase in cardiac size may at times cause some compression and atelectasis of the adjacent lung, resulting in a small well-defined area of bronchial breathing just below the tip of the left scapula. The same area may also be dull to percussion and show egophony (*Ewart's sign*). This sign, sometimes seen in patients with large pericardial effusions, may also be noted in patients with marked cardiomegaly of other causes. Because bronchial breathing and dullness may be present as a result of other pulmonary causes, this sign is not very specific.

Laplace's law
for a thin walled cylindrical shell.
Tension = P (pressure) × r (radius)

Lamé's equation
If the wall has a thickness, then circumferential wall stress is given by

$$\text{Tension} \propto \frac{P \text{ (pressure)} \times r \text{ (radius)}}{2h \text{ (wall thickness)}}$$

Fig. 15.

Table 13
Factors Determining Myocardial O_2 Consumption

- Heart rate
- Wall tension (Laplace's law)
- Systolic pressure, LV volume
- Contractility (inotropic state)

LV, left ventricular.

APPENDIX

Laplace's Law

Laplace's Law defines the relationship between the wall tension (T) and the pressure (P) and the radius (r) for a thin-walled cylindrical shell (Fig. 15).

The tension is directly related to the pressure and the radius.

If the wall has a thickness, then the circumferential wall stress is given by *Lamé's equation* (Fig. 15), where the wall tension (T) is related to the pressure (P) and the radius (r) and inversely related to the wall thickness (h).

In other words, hypertrophy of the wall is a compensatory mechanism, which tends to bring back the wall tension to near-normal levels. Dilatation or enlargement, on the other hand, significantly increases the wall tension. This relationship needs to be kept in mind for it operates in many disorders, both physiological and pathological. One of the important determinants of myocardial oxygen consumption is the wall tension developed in the left ventricle. The other factors include heart rate and contractility or inotropic state (Table 13).

Symptoms of High Left Atrial Pressure

High left atrial pressure, however produced, will lead to elevated pulmonary venous and capillary bed pressure. This in turn will cause symptoms of dyspnea. When the pressure is significantly elevated it can produce symptoms of orthopnea, which is dyspnea on assuming supine position relieved by raising the head or sitting up, as well as paroxysmal nocturnal dyspnea. The latter requires the sleep mechanism, and it usually occurs at night. The patient will give a history of waking up short of breath from sleep after having gone to sleep a few hours prior to the episode. Sitting up and dangling the feet or getting up and standing for a while relieves the dyspnea. The extravascular fluid shifts gradually into the vascular compartment during sleep. This expands the blood volume and raises the left atrial pressure. In normal subjects, the left ventricle accom-

Table 14
Clinical Features of Left Atrial and Pulmonary Hypertension

Symptoms of high left atrial pressure
- Dyspnea
- Orthopnea
- Paroxysmal nocturnal dyspnea
- Palpitation if in atrial fibrillation

Symptoms of pulmonary hypertension
- Low-output symptoms
- Exertional presyncope/syncope (from fixed output)
- Chest pain

Signs of pulmonary hypertension
- Loud P2 (may be palpable in II LICS)
- Narrow split S2
- Wide split S2 if RV failure
- Sustained subxiphoid impulse
- Elevated JVP
- JVP contours
    - $x' > y$ (RV compensated)
    - $x' = y$ (RV diastolic dysfunction with raised RV filling pressure)
    - $x' < y$ (early RV systolic failure)
    - y *descent* with large v *wave* (tricuspid regurgitation with RV dilatation)

JVP, jugular venous pulse; LICS, left intercostal space; RV, right ventricular.

modates the extra volume by increasing the output, and the consequent increase in renal blood flow increases the urine output. However, when the left atrial pressure is somewhat elevated already, this shift from the extravascular to the intravascular compartment is not tolerated and results in symptoms of pulmonary congestion. The classical paroxysmal nocturnal dyspnea occurs in patients with decompensated left ventricles. In mitral stenosis, where the left ventricle is underfilled and normal, one may get the history of paroxysmal nocturnal dyspnea. However, it is often atypical. The patient never gets comfortable completely after being up or tends to wake up more than once in the night because the left atrial pressure is significantly elevated because of the mitral obstruction (Table 14). Occasionally the patient with elevated left atrial pressure may complain of a nocturnal cough instead of dyspnea.

Clinical Signs of High Left Atrial Pressure

In the absence of mitral stenosis, high left atrial pressure secondary to heart failure will often be associated with the presence of a pathological S3.

The pulmonary congestion may result in basal rales or crepitations (crackles) when the lungs are auscultated. These crepitations result from the congestion of the smaller airways with swelling, resulting in the closure of the airways during expiration as the lungs collapse. With expansion of the lungs on inspiration, the closed airways snap open, causing these snapping sounds. These crackles, heard when the patient is supine, may sometimes clear up on patients assuming an erect posture because of a decrease in the venous return resulting in lowered left atrial pressure. When the pulmonary congestion is significant, it would require active therapy for improvement. When untreated or ineffectively treated, it may end in a vicious cycle of hypoxemia, worsening left ventricular function, further rise in left atrial pressure, and worse pulmonary congestion. Acute pulmonary edema may follow with marked shortness of breath associated with labored breathing with the use of the accessory muscles. Cyanosis may occur and the patient may start coughing up pink froth. Because of pulmonary venous congestion, the fluid is blood tinged, making it pink. The surfactant in the lung causes the fluid to bubble, hence the froth. Hypoxemia and low cardiac output will be associated with sinus tachycardia. Untreated, this may deteriorate. There could be gradual slowing of the heart rate, with the patient losing consciousness resulting in hypoxemic cardiorespiratory arrest.

The pulmonary signs of crackles, however, are not specific for high left atrial pressure and more often present in other causes of pulmonary disease, including pneumonia, chronic obstructive pulmonary disease, and pulmonary fibrosis. Furthermore, pulmonary edema can also occur in the absence of elevated left trial pressure.

Symptoms of Pulmonary Hypertension

When pulmonary hypertension is severe, the vascular changes that develop in the pulmonary arterial bed not only raise the pulmonary vascular resistance but also act as severe obstructive lesion peripherally reducing flow and output. This is further aggravated when the right ventricle becomes decompensated. The main symptoms of pulmonary hypertension are therefore one of low output. The output may become relatively fixed and fail to increase with exertion and may actually paradoxically fall, causing symptoms of presyncope and/or syncope with exertion. The oxygen saturation may also fall with exertion. The hypoxemia may also predispose to the development of arrhythmias. Often patients may also complain of vague atypical chest pain. The cause of this is not easily explainable (Table 14).

Signs of Pulmonary Hypertension

Pulmonary hypertension would cause the pulmonary component of the second heart sound (P2) to become more sharp and loud. The P2 may become palpable in the second left interspace, where it is often best heard. A palpable S2 (when confirmed to be a result of the loud P2 by auscultation) in the second left interspace usually is a good sign of pulmonary hypertension, and the pulmonary systolic pressure may be 75 mmHg or higher when this sign is present. The S2 split is usually narrow when the right ventricle is still compensated because the effect of the higher pulmonary impedance will be to bring the P2 earlier, making the split narrower. When the right ventricle is decompensated, however, the S2 split may become wide because of a delayed P2 component as a result of poor and delayed right ventricular relaxation. The split may not vary well with respiration when this happens; it may be confused with a fixed splitting of S2. However, following exercise or in the post-Valsalva strain phase, the S2 split can be shown to vary making this a useful maneuver during auscultation.

The increased right ventricular pressure and the consequent increase in its wall tension may give rise to a sustained right ventricular impulse on subxiphoid palpation. One may also feel along with it an atral kick because of a strong right atrial contraction. This is usually present only in the early compensated state of significant pulmonary hypertension.

Table 15
Signs of Wide Pulse Pressure with Decreased Peripheral Resistance

- Corrigan pulse (visible carotid pulse)
- Quincke's sign (increased capillary pulsation)
- Pistol shot sounds
- Duroziez's bruit (systolic and diasystolic bruit over femorals, brought out by compression)
- Collapsing pulse
- de Musset's sign (rocking head movement)
- Positive Hill's sign (blood pressure in the leg higher than in the arm >15 mm)

The decreased right ventricular compliance because of diastolic dysfunction and right ventricular hypertrophy will lead to increased right ventricular diastolic pressure. This is reflected in the right atrial and the jugular venous pressures. Thus, pulmonary hypertension will often lead to elevated jugular venous pressure and abnormal jugular venous pulse contour. This has been discussed in detail in Chapter 4. Here it suffices to summarize the sequence of jugular contour changes in pulmonary hypertension. In the presence of pulmonary hypertension, the jugular venous pulse contour of $x' > y$ indicates compensated right ventricular function, $x' = y$ indicates right ventricular diastolic dysfunction with raised filling pressures, $x' < y$ indicates early right ventricular systolic failure, and *y descent* with large *v wave* denotes tricuspid regurgitation and right ventricular dilatation (Table 14).

Signs of Wide Pulse Pressure With Decreased Peripheral Resistance

These are listed in Table 15.

Splitting of the Second Heart Sound

The respiratory variations in the timing of both the A2 and the P2 components of the S2 and their effects on the splitting of the S2 are shown in Fig. 16.

IN NORMALS

In the normals, the sequence of the components is A2 followed by P2 because the left ventricle is a more powerful chamber. Its contraction and relaxation are much faster than that of the right ventricle. On inspiration, there is decreased intrathoracic pressure with increased venous return to the right side. The lungs expand and the pulmonary impedance falls. Thus, the increased right ventricular volume and the decreased pulmonary impedance make the P2 come later on inspiration. The expansion of the lungs on inspiration diminishes the pulmonary venous return to the left heart. This may make the A2 come slightly earlier on inspiration. The effect of these changes on inspiration is to make the A2 and the P2 move away from each other, resulting in a split. The reverse changes occur on expiration. The A2 comes later, and the P2 comes earlier. The components come together with the splitting narrowing.

RIGHT BUNDLE BRANCH BLOCK (RBBB)

In RBBB the right ventricular electrical depolarization is delayed; therefore, the right ventricular mechanical events are also delayed by the same amount. Otherwise the variations are the same as in the normal. The right ventricular delay causes a wider

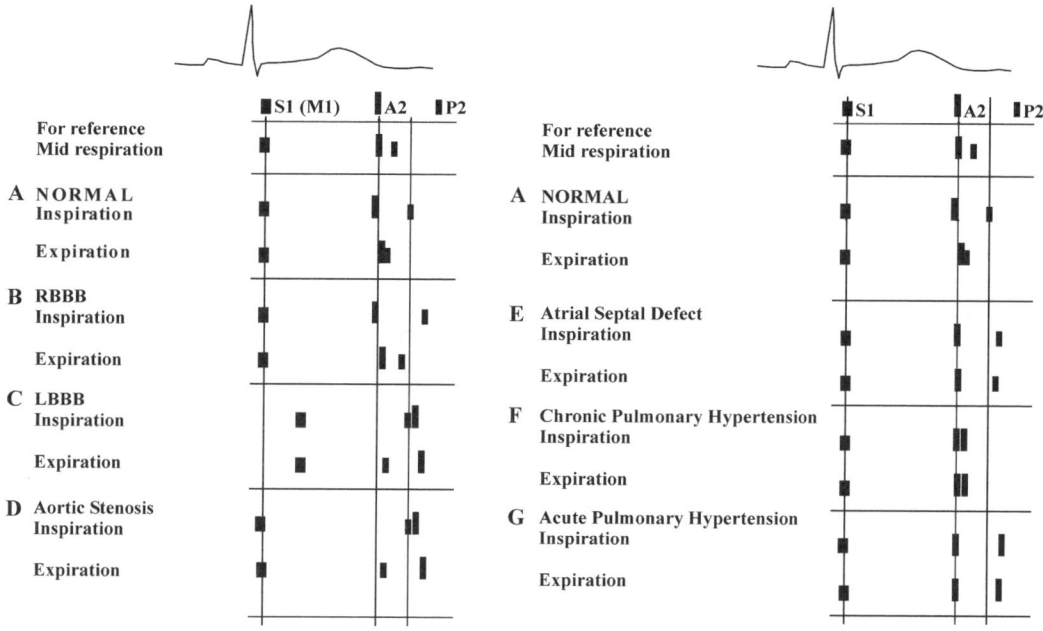

Fig. 16.

splitting of S2 because of delayed P2 on inspiration. The P2 does not come close to A2 during expiration. Thus, the split remains on expiration (*audible expiratory splitting*), although there is significant movement in A2- P2 intervals with respiration.

LEFT BUNDLE BRANCH BLOCK (LBBB)

In LBBB, the left ventricular depolarization and mechanical events are delayed. Therefore, both the mitral component of the S1 (M1) and the A2 are delayed. This delay causes the A2 to occur after P2, resulting in an abnormal sequence. This leads to a reversal of the splitting on inspiration called "*paradoxical splitting*." The P2 moves as in the normal, but because of the delay in A2, the two components come together during inspiration and move away from each other during expiration.

AORTIC STENOSIS

In aortic stenosis, a paradoxical splitting of the S2 can occur as a result of delayed A2 (closure of aortic valve). This is not because of an electromechanical delay as in LBBB, but rather because of increased ejection time as a result of the stenotic valve causing outflow obstruction. Unlike the case in LBBB, the M1 in this case is not delayed. Ischemia can also cause similar change.

ATRIAL SEPTAL DEFECT

In atrial septal defect, there is a left-to-right shunt across the atrial septum. The respiratory variations in the venous return and the consequent right-sided filling are compensated by the variations in the shunt with the result that the right ventricle receives more or less the same amount of blood on both inspiration and expiration. In addition, the overfilled pulmonary arterial bed from the left-to-right shunt does not allow any significant changes in the pulmonary impedance on inspiration. The left-sided filling also remains relatively the same for similar reasons. This results in a relatively fixed splitting of A2 and P2.

CHRONIC PULMONARY HYPERTENSION

In chronic pulmonary hypertension, the P2 becomes louder because of significant increase in the pulmonary arterial pressure and the high pulmonary arterial resistance. The high pulmonary impedance does not drop much with inspiration. This will result in a P2 that occurs somewhat early and does not change much with respiration. This will result in a narrow split of the S2 or a single S2.

ACUTE PULMONARY HYPERTENSION

In acute pulmonary hypertension as seen in large acute pulmonary embolism, the P2 is not only loud but in fact may be delayed, resulting in a wide-split S2. It may remain wide until full compensatory mechanisms come into play. The wide split may become normal eventually unless recurrent embolism leads to the development of chronic pulmonary hypertension.

REFERENCES

1. Bonow RO, Carabello B, de Leon AC, et al. ACC/AHA guidelines for the management of patients with valvular heart disease. A report of the American College of Cardiology/American Heart Association. Task Force on Practice Guidelines (Committee on Management of Patients with Valvular Heart Disease). J Am Coll Cardiol 1998;32:1486–588.
2. Carabello BA, Crawford FA, Jr. Valvular heart disease. N Engl J Med 1997;337:32–41.
3. Carabello BA. The pathophysiology of mitral regurgitation. J Heart Valve Dis 2000;9:600–608.
4. Carabello BA. Progress in mitral and aortic regurgitation. Prog Cardiovasc Dis 2001;43:457–475.
5. Carabello BA. Concentric versus eccentric remodeling. J Card Fail 2002;8:S258–263.
6. DePace NL, Nestico PF, Morganroth J. Acute severe mitral regurgitation. Pathophysiology, clinical recognition, and management. Am J Med 1985;78:293–306.
7. Roberts WC, Braunwald E, Morrow AG. Acute severe mitral regurgitation secondary to ruptured chordae tendineae: clinical, hemodynamic, and pathologic considerations. Circulation 1966;33:58–70.
8. Ronan JA, Jr., Steelman RB, DeLeon AC, Jr., Waters TJ, Perloff JK, Harvey WP. The clinical diagnosis of acute severe mitral insufficiency. Am J Cardiol 1971;27:284–290.
9. Bonow RO. Chronic aortic regurgitation. In: Alpert JS, Dalen JE, Rahimtoola SH, eds. Valvular Heart Disease. Philadelphia, PA: Lippincott Williams & Wilkins, 2000:245–268.
10. Fielitz J, Hein S, Mitrovic V, et al. Activation of the cardiac renin-angiotensin system and increased myocardial collagen expression in human aortic valve disease. J Am Coll Cardiol 2001;37:1443–1449.
11. Gaasch WH, Carroll JD, Levine HJ, Criscitiello MG. Chronic aortic regurgitation: prognostic value of left ventricular end-systolic dimension and end-diastolic radius/thickness ratio. J Am Coll Cardiol 1983;1:775–782.
12. Borer JS, Truter S, Herrold EM, et al. Myocardial fibrosis in chronic aortic regurgitation: molecular and cellular responses to volume overload. Circulation 2002;105:1837–1842.
13. Otto CM. Aortic regurgitation. In: Otto C, ed. Valvular Heart Disease. Philadelphia, PA: W.B. Saunders, 2004.
14. Vatner SF, Shannon R, Hittinger L. Reduced subendocardial coronary reserve. A potential mechanism for impaired diastolic function in the hypertrophied and failing heart. Circulation 1990;81:III8–14.
15. Hittinger L, Mirsky I, Shen YT, Patrick TA, Bishop SP, Vatner SF. Hemodynamic mechanisms responsible for reduced subendocardial coronary reserve in dogs with severe left ventricular hypertrophy. Circulation 1995;92:978–986.
16. Vatner SF, Hittinger L. Coronary vascular mechanisms involved in decompensation from hypertrophy to heart failure. J Am Coll Cardiol 1993;22:34A–40A.

17. Reddy.P.S, Leon DF, Krishnaswami.V, O'Toole JD, Salerni.R, Shaver JA. Syndrome of acute aortic regurgitation. American Heart Association Monograph 1975;46:166–174.
18. Wigle ED, Labrosse CJ. Sudden, severe aortic insufficiency. Circulation 1965;32:708–720.
19. Meadows WR, Vanpraagh S, Indreika M, Sharp JT. Premature mitral valve closure: a hemodynamic explanation for absence of the first sound in aortic insufficiency. Circulation 1963;28:251–258.
20. Sapira JD. Quincke, de Musset, Duroziez, and Hill: some aortic regurgitations. South Med J 1981;74: 459–467.
21. Reddy PS, Curtiss EI, Salerni R, et al. Sound pressure correlates of the Austin Flint murmur. An intracardiac sound study. Circulation 1976;53:210–217.
22. Constant J. Bedside Cardiology. Boston, MA: Little, Brown and Company, 1976.
23. Wood P. An appreciation of mitral stenosis I. Clinical features. BMJ 1954;1:1051–1113.
24. Wood P. An appreciation of mitral stenosis II Investigations and results. BMJ 1954;1:1113–1124.
25. Rahimtoola SH, Durairaj A, Mehra A, Nuno I. Current evaluation and management of patients with mitral stenosis. Circulation 2002;106:1183–1188.
26. Otto CM. Mitral stenosis. In: Otto CM, ed. Valvular Heart Disease. Philadelphia, PA: W.B. Saunders, 2004.
27. Gould KL, Carabello BA. Why angina in aortic stenosis with normal coronary arteriograms? Circulation 2003;107:3121–3123.
28. Braunwald E, Antman EM, Beasley JW, et al. ACC/AHA guidelines for the management of patients with unstable angina and non-ST-segment elevation myocardial infarction. A report of the American College of Cardiology/American Heart Association Task Force on Practice Guidelines (Committee on the Management of Patients With Unstable Angina). J Am Coll Cardiol 2000;36:970–1062.
29. Braunwald E, Antman EM, Beasley JW, et al. ACC/AHA guideline update for the management of patients with unstable angina and non-ST-segment elevation myocardial infarction—2002: summary article: a report of the American College of Cardiology/American Heart Association Task Force on Practice Guidelines (Committee on the Management of Patients With Unstable Angina). Circulation 2002;106:1893–1900.
30. Corti R, Fuster V, Badimon JJ. Pathogenetic concepts of acute coronary syndromes. J Am Coll Cardiol 2003;41:7S–14S.
31. Forrester JS, Wyatt HL, Da Luz PL, Tyberg JV, Diamond GA, Swan HJ. Functional significance of regional ischemic contraction abnormalities. Circulation 1976;54:64–70.
32. Fuster V, Corti R, Fayad ZA, Schwitter J, Badimon JJ. Integration of vascular biology and magnetic resonance imaging in the understanding of atherothrombosis and acute coronary syndromes. J Thromb Haemost 2003;1:1410–21.
33. Pfeffer MA, Braunwald E. Ventricular remodeling after myocardial infarction. Experimental observations and clinical implications. Circulation 1990;81:1161–1172.
34. St John Sutton M, Lee D, Rouleau JL, et al. Left ventricular remodeling and ventricular arrhythmias after myocardial infarction. Circulation 2003;107:2577–2582.
35. Swan HJ, Forrester JS, Diamond G, Chatterjee K, Parmley WW. Hemodynamic spectrum of myocardial infarction and cardiogenic shock. A conceptual model. Circulation 1972;45:1097–110.
36. Antman EM, Anbe DT, Armstrong PW, et al. ACC/AHA guidelines for the management of patients with ST-elevation myocardial infarction—executive summary. A report of the American College of Cardiology/American Heart Association Task Force on Practice Guidelines (writing committee to revise the 1999 guidelines for the management of patients with acute myocardial infarction). J Am Coll Cardiol 2004;44:671–719.
37. Boersma E, Mercado N, Poldermans D, Gardien M, Vos J, Simoons ML. Acute myocardial infarction. Lancet 2003;361:847–858.
38. Libby P. Current concepts of the pathogenesis of the acute coronary syndromes. Circulation 2001;104: 365–381.
39. Goodman SG, Langer A, Ross AM, et al. Non-Q-wave versus Q-wave myocardial infarction after thrombolytic therapy: angiographic and prognostic insights from the global utilization of streptokinase and tissue plasminogen activator for occluded coronary arteries-I angiographic substudy. GUSTO-I Angiographic Investigators. Circulation 1998;97:444–450.
40. White HD, Norris RM,. Brown MA,Brandt PW, Whitlock RM, and Wild CJ. Left ventricular end-systolic volume as a major determinant of survival after recovery from myocardial infarction. Circulation 1987;76:44–51.

41. Sadanandan S, Buller C, Menon V, et al. The late open artery hypothesis—a decade later. Am Heart J 2001;142:411–421.
42. Pfeffer MA, Lamas GA, Vaughan DE, Parisi AF, Braunwald E. Effect of captopril on progressive ventricular dilatation after anterior myocardial infarction. N Engl J Med 1988;319:80–86.
43. Weisman HF, Bush DE, Mannisi JA, Weisfeldt ML, Healy B. Cellular mechanisms of myocardial infarct expansion. Circulation 1988;78:186–201.
44. Pfeffer.MA. Left ventricular remodeling after acute myocardial infarction. Ann Rev Med 1995;46: 455–466.
45. Laskey WK, Kussmaul WG. Arterial wave reflection in heart failure. Circulation 1987;75:711–722.
46. London GM, Guerin A. Influence of arterial pulse and reflective waves on systolic blood pressure and cardiac function. J Hypertens Suppl 1999;17:S3–6.
47. Nichols WW, O'Rourke MF. McDonald's Blood Flow in Arteries. London, UK: Edward Arnold, 1998.
48. O'Rourke MF, Kelly R, Avolio A. The Arterial Pulse. Philadelphia, PA: Lea & Febiger, 1992.
49. Westerhof N, O'Rourke MF. Haemodynamic basis for the development of left ventricular failure in systolic hypertension and for its logical therapy. J Hypertens 1995;13:943–952.
50. Hein S, Arnon E, Kostin S, et al. Progression from compensated hypertrophy to failure in the pressure-overloaded human heart: structural deterioration and compensatory mechanisms. Circulation 2003; 107:984–991.
51. Deedwania PC. The key to unraveling the mystery of mortality in heart failure: an integrated approach. Circulation 2003;107:1719–1721.
52. Braunwald E, Bristow MR. Congestive heart failure: fifty years of progress. Circulation 2000;102: IV14–23.
53. Braunwald E, Morrow AG, Cornell WP, Aygem MM, Hilbish TF. Idiopathic hypertrophic subaortic stenosis. Clinical, hemodynamic and angiographic manifestations. Am J Med 1960;29:924.
54. Glancy DL, Shepherd RL, Beiser D, Epstein SE. The dynamic nature of left ventricular outflow obstruction in idiopathic hypertrophic subaortic stenosis. Ann Intern Med 1971;75:589–593.
55. Murgo JP, Alter BR, Dorethy JF, Altobelli SA, McGranahan GM, Jr. Dynamics of left ventricular ejection in obstructive and nonobstructive hypertrophic cardiomyopathy. J Clin Invest 1980;66:1369–1382.
56. Ross J, Jr, Braunwald E, Gault JH, Mason DT, Morrow AC. The mechanism of intra-ventricular pressure gradient in idiopathic hypertrophic subaortic stenosis. Circulation 1966;34:558.
57. Sherrid MV, Gunsburg DZ, Moldenhauer S, Pearle G. Systolic anterior motion begins at low left ventricular outflow tract velocity in obstructive hypertrophic cardiomyopathy. J Am Coll Cardiol 2000;36:1344–1354.
58. Perloff JK. The Clinical Recognition of Congenital Heart Disease. Philadelphia, PA: W.B. Saunders, 2001.
59. Campbell M. Natural history of atrial septal defect. Br Heart J 1970;32:820–826.
60. Craig RJ, Selzer A. Natural history and prognosis of atrial septal defect. Circulation 1968;37:805–815.
61. Therrien J, Dore A, Gersony W, et al. CCS Consensus Conference 2001 update: recommendations for the management of adults with congenital heart disease. Part I. Can J Cardiol 2001;17:940–959.
62. Wood P. The Eisenmenger syndrome or pulmonary hypertension with reversed central shunt. Br Heart J 1963;2:701.
63. Aygen MM, Braunwald E. The splitting of the second heart sound in normal subjects and in patients with congenital heart disease. Circulation 1962;25:328–345.
64. Perloff JK, Harvey WP. Mechanisms of fixed splitting of the second heart sound. Circulation 1958; 18:998–1009.
65. O'Toole JD, Reddy PS, Curtiss EI, Shaver JA. The mechanism of splitting of the second heart sound in atrial septal defect. Circulation 1977;56:1047–1053.
66. Dornhorst A, Howard P, Leathart GL. Pulsus paradoxus. Lancet 1952;1:746–748.
67. Gibson R. Atypical constrictive pericarditis. Br Heart J;21:583.
68. Ranganathan N, Sivaciyan V. Jugular venous flow velocity pattern, application to bedside recognition of jugular venous pulse contour and right heart hemodynamics. Am J Noninvas Cardiol 1993;7: 75–88.
69. Reddy PS, Curtiss EI, O'Toole JD, Shaver JA. Cardiac tamponade: hemodynamic observations in man. Circulation 1978;58:265–272.
70. Shabetai R, Fowler NO, Guntheroth WG. The hemodynamics of cardiac tamponade and constrictive pericarditis. Am J Cardiol 1970;26:480–489.

71. Wood P. Chronic constrictive pericarditis. Am J Cardiol 1961;7:48–61.
72. Bilchick KC, Wise.RA. Paradoxical physical findings described by Kussmaul: pulsus paradoxus and Kussmaul's sign. Lancet. 2002;359:1940–1942.
73. Fowler NO, Gabel M, Buncher CR. Cardiac tamponade: a comparison of right versus left heart compression. J Am Coll Cardiol 1988;12:187–193.
74. Spodick.DW. Pericardial diseases. In: Braunwald.E, Zipes.D, Libby.P, eds. Heart Disease. Philadelphia, PA: W.B. Saunders, 2001:1823–1876.

11 Local and Systemic Manifestations of Cardiovascular Disease

Franklin Saksena, MD

CONTENTS

> GENERAL OBSERVATIONS
> CONGENITAL SYNDROMES/DISEASES
> VASCULAR DISEASES
> VALVULAR HEART DISEASE
> ENDOCRINE AND METABOLIC DISEASES
> INFLAMMATORY DISEASES
> DISEASES OF CONNECTIVE TISSUE AND JOINTS
> PHARMACOLOGICAL AGENTS
> MUSCULOSKELETAL DISEASES
> TUMORS
> SYNOPSIS
> REFERENCES

A good deal of information about cardiovascular diseases can be obtained by the thorough inspection of a patient using only the unaided senses. Inspection is a frequently overlooked aspect of cardiovascular physical diagnosis. This chapter discusses the recognition of the local and systemic manifestations of cardiovascular disease under the following headings: general observations, congenital syndromes, vascular diseases, valvular heart disease, endocrine and metabolic diseases, inflammatory diseases, diseases of connective tissue and joints, pharmacological agents, musculoskeletal diseases, and tumors. Associated cardiovascular findings are placed in brackets.

GENERAL OBSERVATIONS

The patient's height, weight, degree of alertness, skin, nails, and clothing are initially evaluated *(1)*.

Height

A tall thin patient with an arm span exceeding the height, ectopia lentis, long thin fingers, hyperextensible joints, and high arched palate suggests *Marfan syndrome*. Such patients often have aortic regurgitation, dissecting aneurysm of the aorta, and mitral valve prolapse *(2)* (Fig. 1A,B).

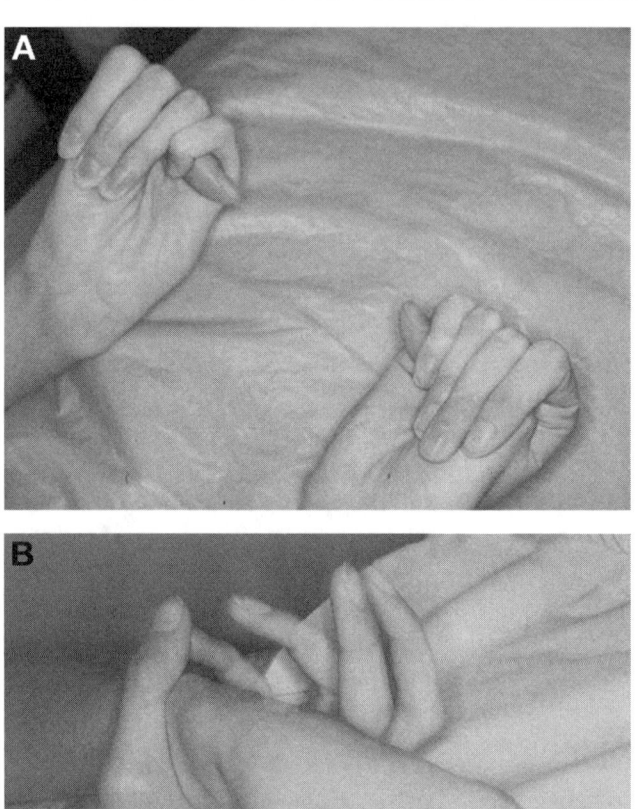

Fig. 1. (**A,B**) Twenty-seven-yr-old female with Marfan syndrome showing arachnodactyly (positive thumb and wrist signs). Her arm span = height = 73 in. She had aortic insufficiency and a dilated aortic root measuring 6 cm in diameter.

The characteristic features of *Turner syndrome* (coarctation of the aorta) are: female patients, <5 ft height with webbing of the neck, widely spaced nipples, and long fourth finger *(3)*.

Weight

Obese patients have a body mass index exceeding 26 kg/m^2. Obesity localized to the abdomen (android or central type) has a higher incidence of hypertension and diabetes *(4)*.

A large protuberant abdomen may result from central obesity or ascites. Patients with ascites may have liver disease or less commonly right heart failure *(5)*.

Weight gain or loss can be visually assessed by noting the changing position of the belt buckle markings, how well the clothing fits or whether a wedding ring is too loose or too tight *(1)*.

Degree of Alertness

Patients who fall asleep frequently during an interview may have *sleep apnea syndrome*. Such patients may or may not be obese and may have coexisting polycythemia, cor pulmonale, or systemic hypertension *(6)*.

Skin

Skin color alterations and edema provide useful clues in the detection of underlying cardiovascular disease. Alterations in skin color may be a result of cyanosis, polycythemia, anemia, periodic facial flushing, jaundice, or bronzed pigmentation.

Cyanosis is a bluish discoloration of the skin that occurs when there is at least 5 g% of reduced hemoglobin circulating in the capillaries and venules. Cyanosis may be of central, peripheral, or mixed origin.

Central cyanosis is often associated with clubbing and polycythemia. It is visually detected when the arterial saturation is less than 80% and is best seen under the tongue *(7)*. Central cyanosis is seen in patients with intracardiac right-to-left shunts (e.g., tetralogy of Fallot, Eisenmenger's syndrome), Pulmonary arteriovenous (A-V) fistula, or intrapulmonary shunts (e.g., chronic obstructive lung disease, pulmonary infarction).

Differential cyanosis may occur in persistent ductus arteriosus with right-to left-shunting of blood. The cyanosis may be more pronounced in the legs and left arm than in the right arm and head. Coexisting coarctation of the aorta will aggravate this differential cyanosis *(8,9)*. If transposition of the great vessels coexists with a persistent ductus arteriosus with right-to-left shunting, then cyanosis is more prominent in the upper extremities and head than in the lower extremities *(9a)*.

Peripheral cyanosis is seen in low-output states or localized venous obstruction. Thus, it is common in congestive heart failure, Raynaud's disease, or vena caval obstruction. It may be detected in the ears, nailbeds, or the lips. Clubbing and polycythemia are absent *(9)*.

Patients with polycythemia have a ruddy complexion and brick red conjunctiva. Polycythemia is of primary or secondary origin. Secondary polycythemia is seen in patients with arterial hypoxemia because of right-to-left intracardiac shunting or secondary to intrapulmonary shunting (e.g., COPD). There is an increased incidence of myocardial infarction and thrombo-embolism in patients with primary polycythemia *(10)*. Secondary polycythemia is rarely a cause of myocardial infarction *(10a)*.

Anemia is best detected by looking for conjunctival pallor *(11)*. Nailbed and palmar crease pallor are unreliable signs of anemia *(11)*. Anemia may account for a pulmonary flow murmur, *bruit de diable*, venous hum, and high-output failure. Although the cardiac output is almost always raised when the hemoglobin is <6 g% *(12)*, high-output failure may occur at higher levels of hemoglobin concentration in the presence of underlying ventricular dysfunction.

Periodic flushing of the skin of the face, neck, and chest is seen in patients with *carcinoid syndrome*. Patients with carcinoid syndrome have a high incidence of tricuspid regurgitation and pulmonic stenosis *(13)*.

Jaundice may be detected as a yellowish tint of the skin, the subglossal mucosa, or sclera and is usually mild in cardiac disease. Jaundice is seen in patients with (1) hepatic congestion because of right heart failure, tricuspid regurgitation, or constrictive pericarditis or (2) hemolysis associated with prosthetic valve dysfunction.

Patients with *hemochromatosis* have iron and melanin deposits in the skin producing a diffuse slate grey or bronzed appearance especially prominent in the face, neck, and distal parts of the extremities. Diabetes and hepatic dysfunction frequently co-exist along with a restrictive or a dilated cardiomyopathy *(14).*

Multiple *café au lait macules* larger than 1.5 cm in diameter occur in neurofibromatosis. Other skin lesions consist of neurofibromas, axillary, or inguinal freckling. These skin lesions are randomly distributed but appear most commonly over the back and chest. Neurofibromatosis (von Recklinghausen's disease) is associated with hypertension because of renal artery stenosis or pheochromocytoma *(15).* Cardiac neurofibromas may produce outflow tract obstruction *(16).*

Bilateral edema of the legs is seen in heart failure, venous insufficiency, venous thrombosis, lymphoedema, hypoalbuminemia, or severe anemia *(17).* Of the causes of bilateral leg edema, only heart failure is associated with an elevated jugular venous pressure *(17).* Unilateral leg edema is usually a result of local venous obstruction. Edema of the upper extremity is seen in superior vena cava syndrome, subclavian vein thrombosis, thoracic outlet syndrome, or lymphatic obstruction because of breast cancer *(17,18).* Edema of the hand may be caused by all the causes mentioned for upper extremity edema as well as local causes such as infection or trauma *(19).* The shoulder–hand syndrome as a cause of hand edema is rarely seen now.

Nails

The nails are examined for clubbing, subungual hemorrhages, subungual fibromas, and any distinctive color.

Subungual hemorrhages (*splinter hemorrhages*) are seen in endocarditis and usually involve the middle portion of the nail. Subungual hemorrhages may also be seen in trauma, vasculitis, or systemic embolism *(20,21).*

Subungual fibromas (hands, feet) are a feature of tuberous sclerosis *(22).*

White nails (*Terry nails*) are in my opinion commonly seen in chronic hepatic congestion resulting from heart failure but may also be seen in liver cirrhosis *(23). Blue–gray nails* are seen in hemochromatosis (cardiomyopathy), Wilson's disease (cardiomyopathy), and ochronosis (aortic or mitral valvular disease) *(24). Black nails* are seen in Cushing's syndrome (hypertension) *(24).*

Onycholysis (*Plummer's nails*) is seen in hyperthyroidism, but may also occur in trauma, psoriasis, or syphilis *(25).* A red lunula is associated with heart failure, but is also seen in psoriasis and collagen diseases *(26).*

Gait

A high steppage gait is seen in muscular dystrophy (cardiomyopathy), whereas sensory ataxia and pes cavus are seen in Friedreich's ataxia (cardiomyopathy).

Tabes dorsalis, a manifestation of tertiary syphilis, is characterized by sensory ataxia, Argyll Robertson pupil, and optic atrophy (aortic regurgitation).

A festinating gait with orthostatic hypotension is seen not only in Parkinson's disease, but also in the Shy–Drager syndrome *(27).*

CONGENITAL SYNDROMES/DISEASES

Inspection of the head and/or hands *(8)* is often useful in detecting congenital disorders associated with underlying heart disease. In this section I will mention the Down,

Leopard, Noonan, Williams', Osler–Weber–Rendu, and Holt–Oram syndromes, as well as tuberous sclerosis and cyanotic congenital heart disease. The importance of clubbing will be discussed under the latter heading.

Down Syndrome

Down syndrome occurs in 1 of 1000 newborns and is characterized by a vacant expression on the face, mental retardation, slanting of the palpebral fissures, Brushfield spots, small ears, macroglossia, a simian crease, and a small fifth digit *(28)* (The associated congenital heart defects are A-V canal, ventricular septal defect, and tetralogy of Fallot) *(29)*.

LEOPARD Syndrome

Patients with this syndrome have *Lentigenes* (1- to 5-mm brown macules on back, thorax, and neck), *Electrocardiographic* conduction defects, *Ocular* hypertelorism, *Pulmonic* stenosis (and other cardiovascular system abnormalities such as hypertrophic cardiomyopathy), *Abnormalities of genitalia* (hyopgonadism), *Retardation* of growth, and *Deafness* of sensorineural origin *(30)* (Fig. 2). Patients with LEOPARD syndrome are predisposed to sudden death if there is coexistent hypertrophic cardiomyopathy *(31)*.

Noonan Syndrome

This syndrome consists of hypertelorism, mental retardation, high arched palate, webbing of neck, a simian crease, and cryptorchidism (the associated congenital heart defect is pulmonic stenosis) *(32,33)*.

Tuberous Sclerosis

This entity is inherited as an autosomal dominant trait (1:10,000) and diagnosed by detecting angiofibromata of the lower half of the face (adenoma sebaceum). There is often a history of mental retardation, seizure disorder, and multiple subungual fibromas. These patients often have a rhabdomyoma, which may occasionally obstruct the right ventricular or left ventricular outflow tract *(22)*.

Williams' Syndrome

Patients with this syndrome have a large forehead, upturned nose, a long philtrum, an enlarged overhanging upper lip, deformed teeth, puffy cheeks, and a friendly disposition (an elfin-like appearance). The voice is hoarse and has a metallic tone *(34)*. The associated lesion is supravalvular aortic stenosis and patients may occasionally have pulmonary artery branch stenosis *(35)*.

Osler–Weber–Rendu Syndrome

This autosomal dominant entity is characterized by capillary angiomata of the tongue and lips *(36)* (Fig. 3). Epistaxis and gastrointestinal bleeding may also occur (The associated lesion is pulmonary A-V fistula) *(37)*.

Holt–Oram Syndrome

This is an autosomal dominant condition in which patients with a secundum atrial septal defect have various hand abnormalities such as a long first proximal phalanx (fingerized thumb) or a missing thumb or an extra digit *(38)*.

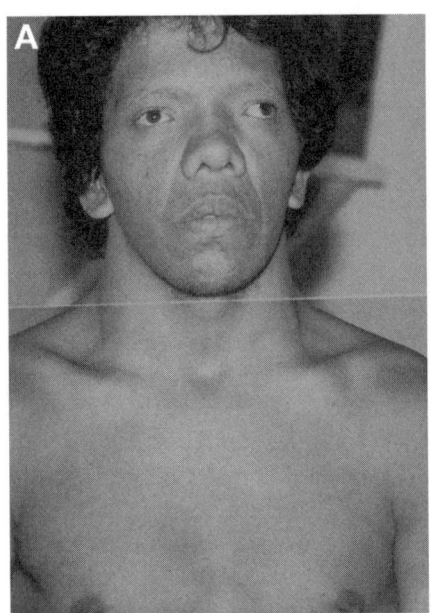
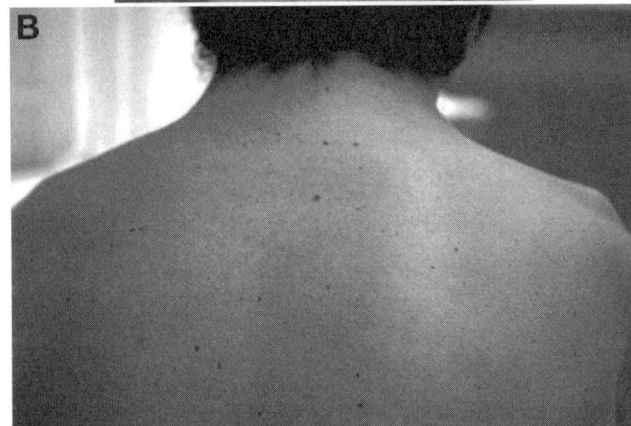
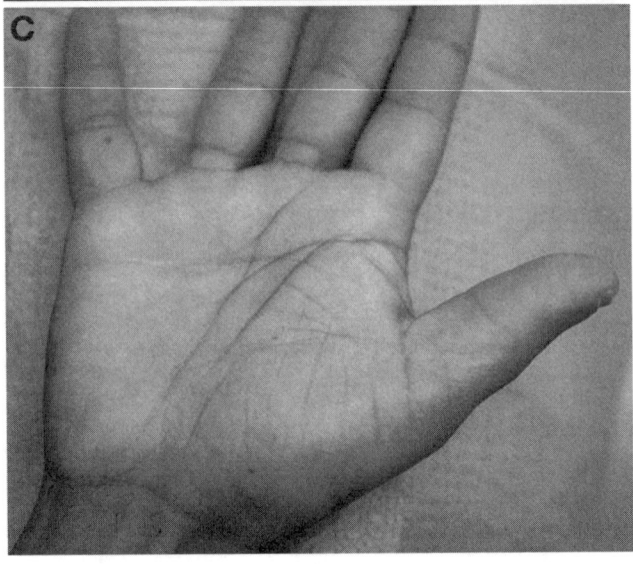

Chapter 11 / Manifestation of Cardiovascular Disease

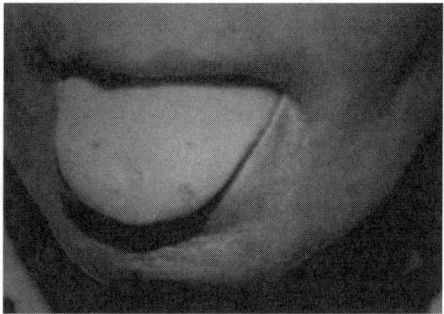

Fig. 3. (Color Plate 5, following p. 270) Osler–Weber–Rendu syndrome. This 44-yr-old female had capillary angiomata on the tongue and telangiectasia of the cheeks. There was no history of epistaxis or gastrointestinal bleeding.

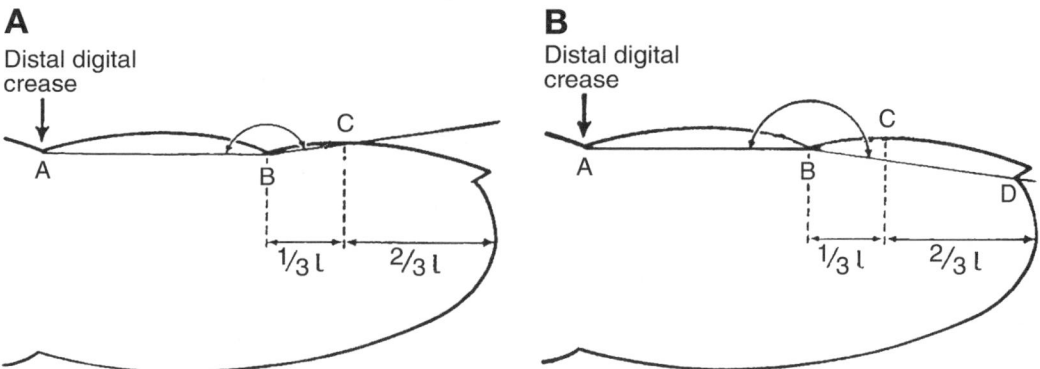

Fig. 4. **(A)** The profile nailbed angle ABC is depicted (normal = 150–170°). **(B)** The hyponychial nailbed angle ABD is seen (normal = 178–192°). (Modified from ref. *40*.)

Cyanotic Congenital Heart Disease

Patients with clubbing, cyanosis, and polycythemia often have cyanotic congenital heart disease (tetralogy of Fallot, tricuspid atresia with right-to-left shunt at atrial level, or Eisenmenger's syndrome).

Clubbing is a very important physical finding in the detection of cardiopulmonary disease and needs some discussion as to its detection and usefulness.

The normal angle that the nail plate makes with the adjacent skin fold is 150–170° *(39)* (Fig. 4A) and the hyponychial angle (nail plate to distal nail angle) is 178–192° *(40)* (Fig. 4B). In clubbing, the nail bed angle or profile angle exceeds 180° and the hyponychial angle is increased. Normally there is a window formed between the thumbnails when they are held together and seen in profile. In clubbing, the hyponychial angle is increased and the window between the two pressed-together thumbnails is lost (*Shamroth's clubbing sign*) *(41)*.

Fig. 2. *(Opposite page)* Thirty-five-yr-old Mexican male with features of leopard and Noonan syndromes showing chest wall lentigines, webbing of the neck, hypertelorism **(A,B)**, and a variant of a simian crease **(C)**. He had mental retardation and pulmonary stenosis.

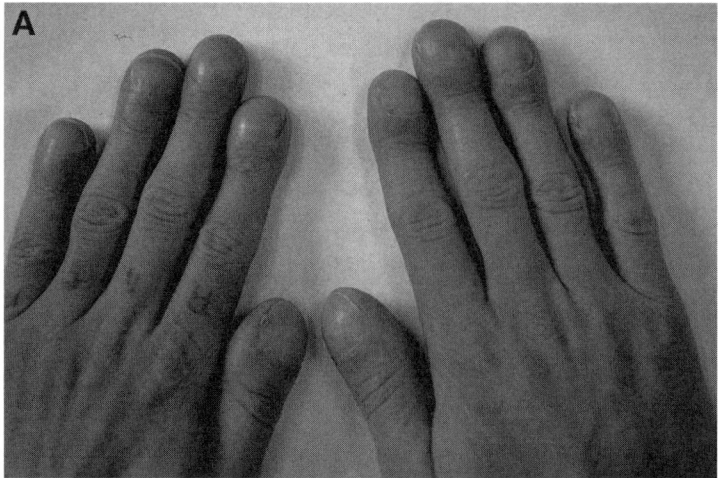
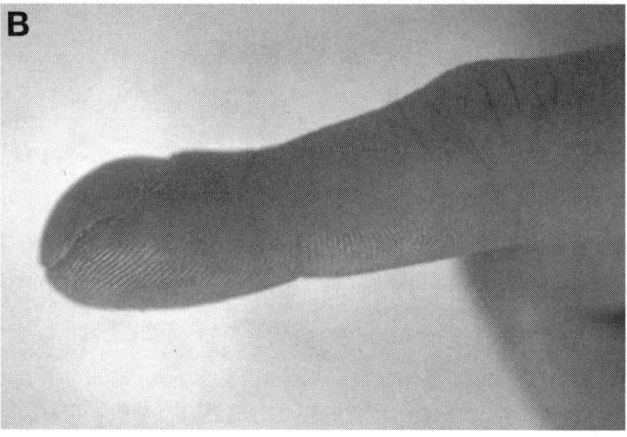

Fig. 5. Tetralogy of Fallot: A 23-yr-old man with polycythemia (hemoglobin 21 g%) and advanced clubbing (hyponychial angle 210°) and cyanosis. The hands show (**A**) subcuticular edema and (**B**) bulbous fingertips. Right ventricular pressure was 135/1; pulmonary artery pressure 13/5. There was a ventricular septal defect with a. pulmonary:systemic blood flow ratio of 0.8.

A useful measure of early clubbing is to determine if the ratio of the distal phalangeal depth to the interphalangeal joint depth in the index finger exceeds 1.0 (normal ratio using a micrometer is 0.9) *(42)*. This distal/interphalangeal ratio may also be visually assessed at the bedside with a "shadowgram" of the finger in profile *(43)*.

Subcuticular edema and ballotability of the nail itself are often present, but may be a late sign of clubbing *(44)*. Clubbing needs to be distinguished from nail beaking. In nail beaking the nail is curved, the hyponychial angle is preserved, and there is loss of pulp tissue *(45)*. Nail beaking is not associated with cardiac disease *(46)*.

Clubbing of the fingers is usually associated with pulmonary disease (80% of cases), with cardiac disease accounting for 10–15% of cases *(47)*. Cardiovascular associations include right-to-left shunts (e.g., tetralogy of Fallot, transposition of the great vessels), infective endocarditis (IE) *(47)* (Fig. 5), myxoma of left atrium *(48)*, and rarely an infected abdominal aortic graft *(49)*.

Unilateral finger clubbing is seen in aortic or subclavian aneurysm or, rarely persistent ductus arteriosus with right-to-left shunting and an absent aortic arch *(50)*.

Differential clubbing, in which clubbing is more prominent in the feet than in the hands, occurs in persistent ductus arteriosus when there is a right-to-left shunt or an infected abdominal aortic graft *(49)*.

VASCULAR DISEASES

Coronary Artery Disease

Coronary artery disease may be suspected if any of the cardiac risk factors are present (hypertension, hyperlipidemia, smoking, diabetes, obesity) or in the presence of a diagonal ear crease sign, prior mediastinal radiation, progeria, polycythemia, Tangier disease, or in a cocaine user.

HYPERTENSION

Hypertension may be detected by a funduscopic examination. Hypertensive retinopathy is graded by the *Keith–Wagner–Barker criteria (51)*:

Grade 1: There is generalized narrowing of the arterioles, with the A-V ratio falling to one-third from the normal value of two-thirds.

Grade 2: There is further narrowing of the arterioles with focal areas of spasm.

Grade 3: The arteriolar walls thicken and take on a copper wire appearance. Hemorrhages and exudates appear.

Grade 4: The arterioles thicken further and appear like silver threads. There are pronounced A-V nicking, hemorrhages, and exudates, and papilledema is now seen.

HYPERLIPIDEMIA

Hyperlipidemia may be suspected if there is arcus corneae or xanthomas are seen. Arcus corneae is a gray-yellow band up to 1.5 mm wide that may surround the rim of the cornea. It occurs with aging, but if seen before the age of 40 in a Caucasian may be a marker of coronary artery disease *(52)*.

Xanthomas are seen in hyperlipidemia as follows.

Hypercholesterolemia

Eyelid xanthomas (*xanthelasma*) are multiple soft elevated yellow plaques that usually occur near the inner canthi bilaterally. About 50% of patients will have normal lipid levels, and the rest have elevated serum cholesterol (Fredrickson type II) *(53)*.

Tendon xanthomas are yellow papular–nodular lesions found on the dorsum of the feet, the achilles' tendon, or on the extensor tendons over the metacarpals (type II) *(54)*.

Hypertriglyceridemia

Eruptive xanthomas are discrete yellow papular lesions surrounded by a red base and are most commonly found on the buttocks, back, elbows, and knees (Fig. 6). These lesions may be mistaken for acne. The lesions appear in crops and may coalesce to form plaques. Eruptive xanthomas usually appear when the plasma triglyceride exceeds 1000 mg/dL *(55)*. *Lipemia retinalis* may be detected when the plasma triglycerides are greater than 3000 mg/dL *(56)*. A milky white serum occurs when the plasma triglycerides are greater than 600 mg/dL *(57)*. Eruptive xanthoma may thus be seen in Fredrickson Types I, III, and V.

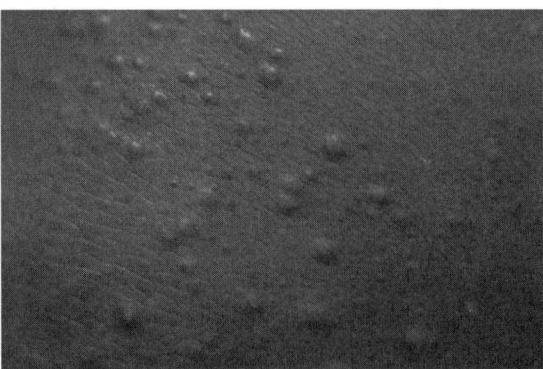

Fig. 6. (Color Plate 6, following p. 270) Eruptive xanthoma: The skin lesions were seen over the back and chest and resemble acne. Serum triglyceride level was >2000 mg%.

Dysbetalipoproteinemia (Type III)

Patients with this disorder have elevated serum cholesterol and triglyceride levels and exhibit characteristic *palmar xanthoma*. Palmar xanthomas consist of yellow infiltrations of the palmar and digital creases of the hand *(58)*.

Tuberous xanthomas and eruptive xanthomas may also be seen in dysbetalipoproteinemia *(58)*. Tuberous xanthomas are flat or elevated yellow nodules surrounded by a red margin seen mainly on the knees or elbows.

SMOKING, OBESITY AND DIABETES

Patients who are smokers may exhibit tobacco-stained fingers, a tobacco odor to the clothing, or cigarette burns on their clothing. Excessive and premature wrinkling (especially "crow's feet" around the eyes) is seen in heavy smokers, but can also be seen in nonsmokers chronically exposed to sunlight *(59)*.

Central obesity with a waist measurement exceeding 35 in. in a woman and 40 in. in a man represents another easily recognizable coronary risk factor *(60)*.

Diabetes may be suspected by detecting vascular changes on funduscopic examination and the presence of small vessel disease in the feet.

OTHER CONDITIONS WITH INCREASED RISK FOR CORONARY ARTERY DISEASE (MYOCARDIAL INFARCTION)

The diagonal *ear crease sign* is said to be a marker for coronary artery disease, but its utility is controversial *(61)*. If seen in patients younger than 40 yr, I believe other coronary artery risk factors should be looked for.

Patients who have received extensive *radiation therapy to the mediastinum* may show atrophy of the paravertebral muscles of the back as well as chronic radiation dermatitis. Such patients have a higher incidence of coronary artery stenosis *(62)*.

Progeria is characterized by premature aging, best seen by examining the face. The skin is thin and translucent and lacks wrinkles. There is also alopecia and dwarfism. These patients usually die before the age of 15 of a myocardial infarction *(63)*.

Patients with primary polycythemia have a higher incidence of coronary artery disease *(9)*.

Tangier disease (hypoalphalipoproteinemia) is a very rare condition characterized by very low high-density lipoprotein cholesterol and low total cholesterol blood levels *(64)*. Cholesterol esters are deposited on the tonsils, producing a characteristic orange tiger-striped appearance. These patients have premature coronary artery disease *(65,66)* and peripheral neuropathy *(67)*.

Cocaine use may be suspected if there is perforation of the nasal septum *(68)*, speckled enamel loss on the buccal surfaces of the teeth *(69)*, skin popping, or venous track sites. Cocaine use is associated with myocardial ischemia or necrosis, hypertension, or endocarditis *(70)*.

Pseudoxanthoma elasticum (PXE) is characterized by a network of closely grouped yellow papules (plucked chicken skin appearance). The skin is lax and hangs in folds. PXE occurs in the neck, axilla, abdomen, and thighs *(71)*. There may be associated angioid streaks and retinal hemorrhages. PXE is associated with mitral valve prolapse, hypertension, peripheral vascular disease, and premature coronary artery disease *(72)*, the latter being a common cause of early death *(72)*.

Scars of a median sternotomy, radial artery, or saphenous vein-harvesting sites point to prior coronary artery bypass surgery.

Unilateral Internal Carotid Artery Disease

Internal carotid artery disease may be suspected if the external carotid or unilateral arcus signs are present along with a *Hollenhorst plaque* seen on fundoscopy. Patients with internal carotid artery stenosis have an increase in blood flow in the ipsilateral external carotid artery, so that its superficial temporal artery branch is more prominent than on the nonobstructed side (*Olivarius's external carotid sign*) *(73)*. This is a useful sign, especially if combined with greater prominence of the ipsilateral brow arterial pulse *(73)*.

Unilateral arcus is very rare and suggests internal carotid artery stenosis on the nonarcus side *(74)* provided that ocular hypotony has been excluded *(75)*.

A Hollenhorst plaque is a cholesterol-laden crystal that embolizes to a retinal arteriole usually from an ipsilateral atherosclerotic internal carotid artery or less often from the aorta or cardiac valves *(75)*. These emboli are pale yellow and refractile.

Temporal Arteritis

This occurs in patients over the age of 50 and is characterized by scalp tenderness in the temporal area followed occasionally by scalp necrosis. The superficial temporal artery is tender and pulseless and feels ropy. There may be lingual gangrene and jaw claudication. Polymyalgia rheumatica may coexist. Blindness may occur in ≤5 mo after the onset of symptoms *(75a)*.

Cholesterol Emboli to the Lower Extremities

These emboli originate from an atherosclerotic descending aorta in which plaques may break off from the aorta either spontaneously, following surgical manipulation of the aorta *(76)* or angiography or associated with the use of anticoagulants *(77)* or fibrinolytic agents *(78)*. Cholesterol emboli may present as *livedo reticularis*, gangrene, or *the purple toe syndrome*. Livedo reticularis is a red pruritic macular eruption resembling the imprint of fine wire mesh on the skin of the legs and especially the feet. The foot pulses are usually present, but often diminished *(79)*. The purple toe syndrome is characterized by multiple bluish-red toes and palpable arterial pulses *(76,79)*.

Buerger's Disease (Thromboangiitis Obliterans)

Buerger's disease is a nonatherosclerotic inflammatory obliterative disease characterized by thrombotic occlusion of the small and medium-sized vessels of the lower extremities and, less commonly, the upper extremities. Gangrene of one or more digits may occur. Buerger's disease has usually been regarded as occurring mostly in males less than 40 yr of age who are heavy smokers. Recent studies *(80)* show that Buerger's disease is now more common in the 40- to 60-yr age group and that the male:female ratio has dropped from 9:1 to 3:1. Thirty percent of patients have an associated superficial thrombophlebitis *(80)*.

Raynaud's Phenomenon

Patients with *Raynaud's phenomenon* have reversible digital artery spasm precipitated by cold or emotional stress. The digits become pallid, then blue, and on rewarming or relief of the emotional stress become hyperemic. It is most commonly associated with collagen vascular disease (scleroderma or disseminated lupus erythematosus), but may also be associated with Buerger's disease, primary pulmonary hypertension, or thoracic outlet syndromes *(81)*.

Patients with scleroderma and Raynaud's phenomenon may show digital ischemia, fingertip necrosis (rat-bite lesions), and even autoamputation *(82)*.

Superior Vena Cava Syndrome

Obstruction of the superior vena cava may be caused by encroachment of the superior vena cava by an intrathoracic tumor *(83)* or an aortic aneurysm *(84)* or thrombosis associated with a transvenous pacemaker *(85)*. Patients may have a ruddy complexion aggravated by recumbency, bluish-red discoloration of the upper chest and neck, edema of the head and neck and upper extremities, neck vein distention, venous stars, and collateral veins on the anterior chest wall. The extent and location of these collateral veins depend on how rapidly the obstruction occurs and whether the obstruction of the superior vena cava occurs above, at, or below the azygos vein *(83)*.

Subclavian Vein Thrombosis

Subclavian vein thrombosis gives rise to a swollen arm, distended veins in the arms, and cyanosis. Because the arm may be painful to move, eliciting *Pemberton's sign* (suffusion of face with arms held above the head) *(86)* is, I believe, impractical.

Inferior Vena Cava Syndrome

Obstruction of the inferior vena cava may occur because of a malignancy or an underlying thrombophlebitis or thrombosis *(87)*. Distended venous collaterals are seen on the lateral aspect of the abdominal wall. There may be bilateral leg edema. Coexistent ascites points to an inferior vena caval obstruction superior to the renal veins *(87)*.

VALVULAR HEART DISEASE

Only the more advanced forms of valvular heart disease may be visually detected:
1. Tricuspid regurgitation: Tricuspid regurgitation may be suspected on observation if there are ear lobe pulsations, a prominent *v wave* in the jugular venous pulse, as well as hepatic pulsations.

Chapter 11 / Manifestation of Cardiovascular Disease 373

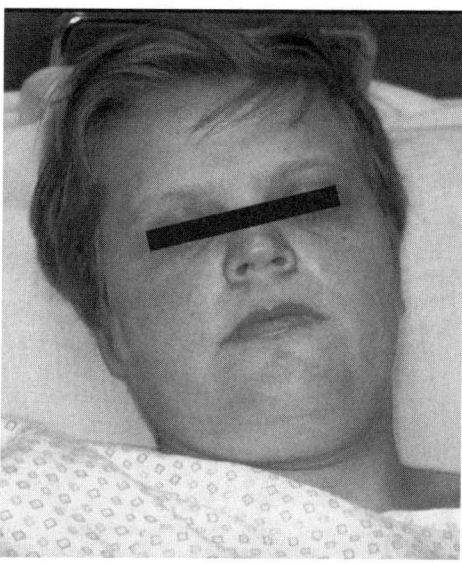

Fig. 7. (Color Plate 7, following p. 270) Mitral facies: 35-yr-old Polish female P1 G6 Ab4 showing a malar flush. She had mitral stenosis and mitral regurgitation.

2. Mitral stenosis: Caucasian patients with mitral stenosis may have venous telangiectasia of the cheeks (malar flush) because of a low-output state and an elevated pulmonary vascular resistance *(88)* (Fig. 7).
3. Aortic regurgitation: A patient may be suspected of having aortic regurgitation if he presents with dyspnea, a head that shakes with each arterial pulsation (*de Musset's sign*), and prominent arterial pulsations in the neck.

ENDOCRINE AND METABOLIC DISEASES

A careful examination of the face will detect patients with acromegaly, thyroid disease, Cushing's disease, amyloidosis, gout, and ochronosis.

Acromegaly

Acromegaly is detected by looking at the head and the hands. These patients have a lantern jaw, coarsening of the facial features (best determined by comparing old photographs), widely spaced teeth, macroglossia, and spade-shaped hands (Fig. 8) Acromegaly is associated with hypertension of the low-renin type *(89)*. There is an increased incidence of premature coronary atherosclerosis in acromegaly because of coexistent diabetes and hypertension.

Hyperthyroidism

Patients with hyperthyroidism are often detected by looking at the face. There may be lid lag, exophthalmos, ophthalmoplegia, and temporal muscle wasting. Other features include palmar erythema, warm moist palms, fine tremor of the outstretched hands, proximal myopathy, pretibial myxedema, and an enlarged thyroid (Fig. 9). The patient may appear restless and show evidence of weight loss by wearing loose-fitting clothes.

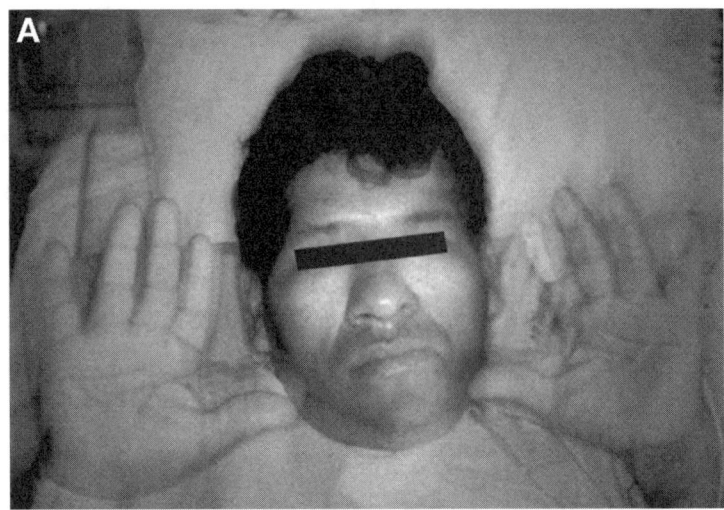
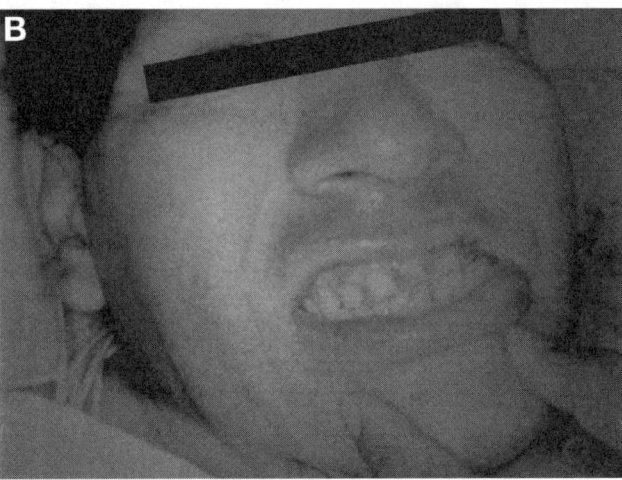

Fig. 8. Acromegaly: 40-yr-old man admitted to the hospital with an acute anterior wall myocardial infarction. He had a lantern jaw, coarse facial features, (**A**) spade-like hands, and (**B**) widely spaced teeth.

Hyperthyroidism may be associated with a high-output failure, atrial fibrillation, or a cardiomyopathy *(90)*. Some elderly patients with hyperthyroidism may not have the above eye or skin changes, but present with heart failure or atrial fibrillation (apathetic hyperthyroidism).

Myxedema

Peri-orbital puffiness, brittle hair, dry skin, slowing of cerebration, low husky voice, macroglossia, and delayed relaxation of heel reflexes are the main clinical features of myxedema (Fig. 10) Thyroid-replacement therapy may lead to a striking improvement of the facies. Myxedema is associated with pericardial effusion, which rarely leads to cardiac tamponade *(91)*.

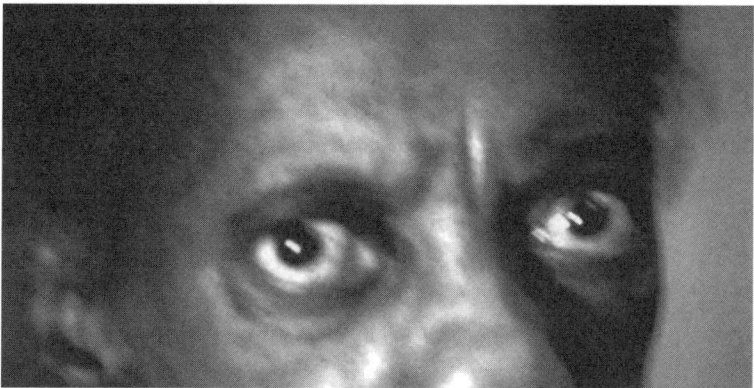

Fig. 9. Hyperthyroidism: 60-yr-old female with lid retraction, exophthalmos, and facial muscle wasting.

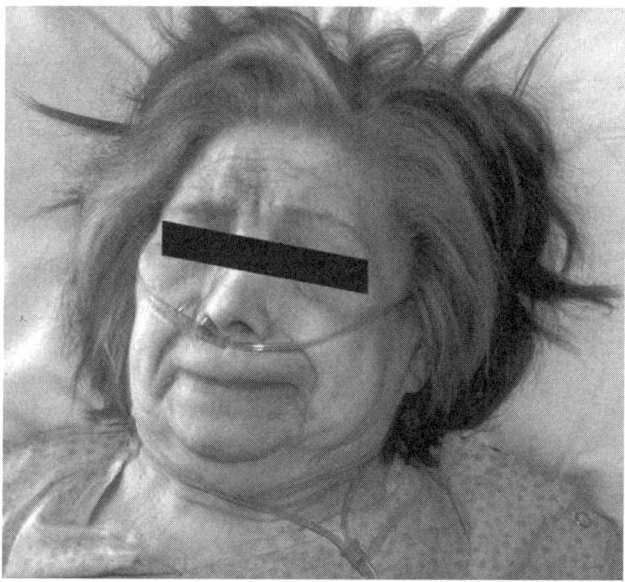

Fig. 10. Myxedema: 80-yr-old female admitted in heart failure. She had stopped taking her thyroid medicine a year before. She has a pasty face, some periorbital puffiness, dry skin, and coarse hair. Thyroid-stimulating hormone level was 100 µU/mL.

Cushing's Disease

Moon facies, buffalo hump, truncal obesity with thin limbs, and red abdominal striae are the usual features of Cushing's disease. It is associated with hypertension in 80% of cases *(92)*.

Amyloidosis

Primary or hereditofamilial amyloidosis may involve the deposition of an amyloid protein consisting of light-chain immunoglobulins in the heart, skin, or tongue *(93)*. Patients with amyloidosis may have waxy yellow translucent papules and plaques on the

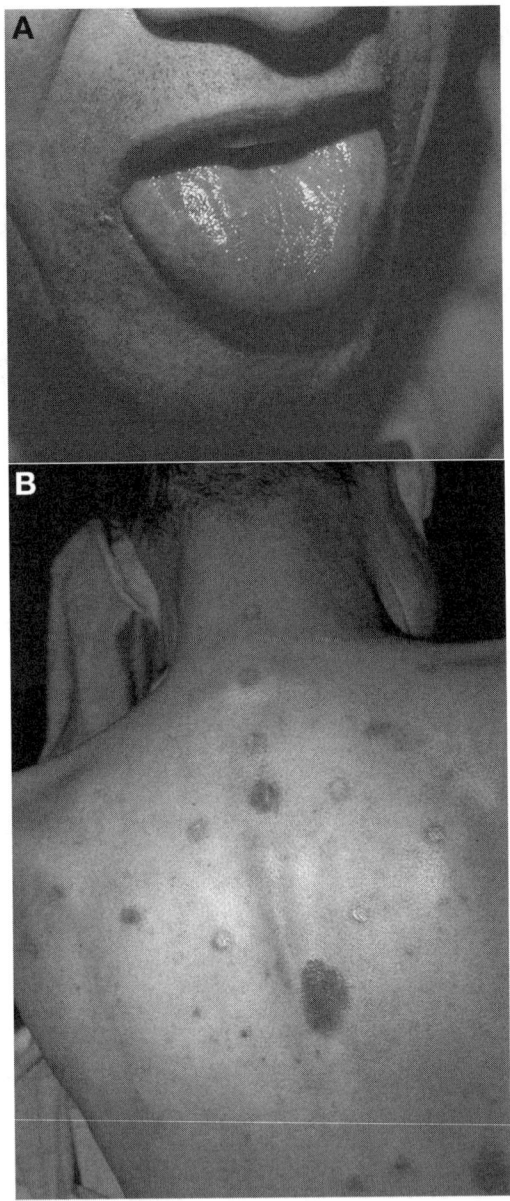

Fig. 11. Amyloidosis: 60-yr-old man with (**A**) large tongue and (**B**) brown maculopapular lesions on the back. He was admitted in heart failure because of a restrictive cardiomyopathy. Echocardiography showed biventricular hypertrophy and a sparkling appearance to the myocardium. He had biopsy-proven amyloidosis.

eyelids, naso-labial folds, and mouth *(94)*. Purpura frequently occurs in these areas after minor trauma *(94)*. The tongue may be diffusely or irregularly enlarged *(94)*. Restrictive cardiomyopathy is often seen in amyloidosis *(93,94)* (Fig. 11).

Hemochromatosis

(*See* General Observations, Skin Color on p. 364.)

Gout

The patient may have gouty tophi (urate deposits) on the ears or the small joints of the hand. Rarely, urate deposits may involve the heart valves or the conducting system, causing complete heart block *(95)*. Patients with gout, via its association with elevated serum uric acid levels, have a higher incidence of hypertension *(96)* and possibly coronary artery disease *(97)*.

Alkaptonuria (Ochronosis)

Alkaptonuria (*Ochronosis*) is a defect in tyrosine metabolism in which homogentisic acid is deposited in the skin, joints, ear, and the mitral and aortic valves. The skin on the ears gradually darkens, and the fingernails show a blue-gray discoloration. Aortic stenosis is the most significant lesion associated with it *(98)*.

INFLAMMATORY DISEASES

Inflammation may be caused by chemical or physical agents or infections. In this section infective endocarditis (IE), syphilis, and sarcoidosis will be discussed.

Infective Endocarditis

Patients with IE may or may not have evidence of recreational drug use (e.g., skin popping, venous tracks). Systemic manifestations of IE are said to be less frequent now, but are still quite common in poorer patients, who are often late in coming to get medical attention. The fundi may show flame-shaped hemorrhages and Roth spots (microinfarct of the retina). The hand may reveal *Osler nodes* (red subcutaneous nodules 2 mm in size on the tips of the fingers, thenar or hypothenar areas that disappear after a few days) *(99)*. Splinter nailbed hemorrhages may be seen, but can also occur with local trauma, vasculitis, or systemic embolism *(20)*. *Janeway lesions* are painless red macules or nodules seen on the palms or soles of the feet *(100)* (Fig. 12). Clubbing may occur in late cases of IE *(99)*. Petechial hemorrhages are seen in the conjunctiva, palate, buccal mucosa, and extremities *(17)*.

Syphilis

Patients with tertiary syphilis may have a saddle-shaped nose, optic atrophy, Argyll Robertson pupil, and evidence of aortic regurgitation.

Sarcoidosis

Patients with sarcoidosis may have skin and cardiac involvement. The skin lesions that involve the face may take two forms: red papules around the eyes, nose, and mouth, which are pruritic and do not ulcerate; purple plaques that produce a bulbous nose, thickened cheeks, and thickened ears (lupus pernio) *(101)*. There may also be erythema nodosum (red nodules on the legs) *(101)*. Twenty percent of patients with sarcoidosis have cardiovascular findings at autopsy *(102,103)*. Clinical manifestations include congestive heart failure, ventricular tachycardia, complete heart block, or cor pulmonale *(102,103)*.

DISEASES OF CONNECTIVE TISSUE AND JOINTS

In this section, inherited disorders of the connective tissue (Ehlers–Danlos syndrome, osteogenesis imperfecta, Marfan syndrome, pseudoxanthoma elasticum) and immune-

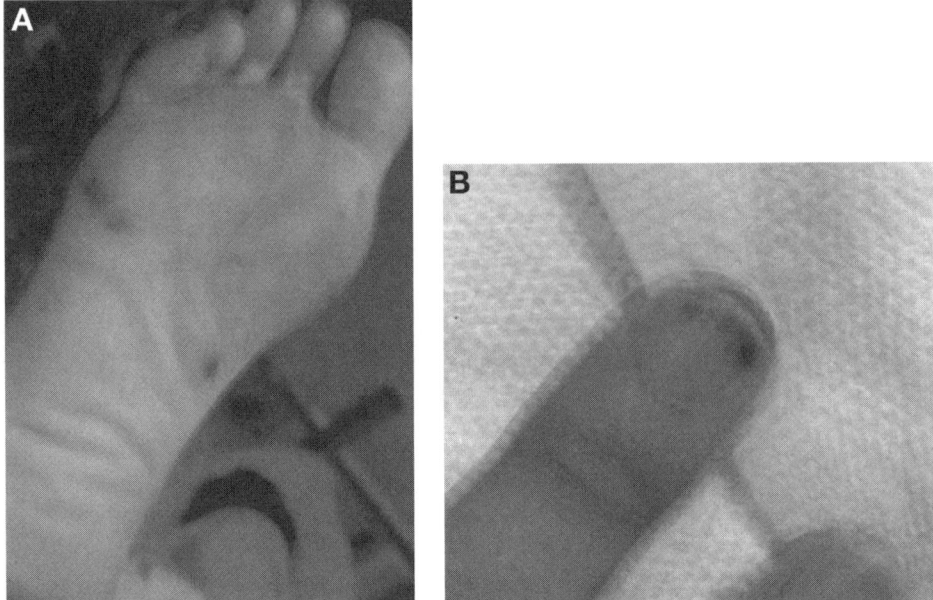

Fig. 12. Infective endocarditis: 50-yr-old drug addict admitted with fever and mitral regurgitation. She had (**A**) Janeway lesions on the soles of her feet (Color Plate 8, following p. 270) and (**B**) subungal hemorrhages. There was vegetation on the mitral valve.

mediated diseases of the connective tissue (systemic lupus erythematosus [SLE], scleroderma, polyarteritis nodosa, rheumatic fever, ankylosing spondylitis, and Reiter's syndrome) are discussed.

Ehlers–Danlos Syndrome

Usually Ehlers–Danlos syndrome is characterized by excessive mobility of joints and a thin stretchable skin. However, in type 4 Ehlers–Danlos syndrome these findings are attenuated and patients have bruises and pigmented scars over the bony prominences. Patients with type 4 Ehlers-Danlos syndrome may have an aortic aneurysm and rupture as well as mitral valve prolapse *(103a)*.

Osteogenesis Imperfecta

Patients with osteogenesis imperfecta have a decrease in bone mass and thus a tendency to have multiple bone fractures on minor trauma. Blue sclera and kyphoscoliosis are seen along with aortic and mitral regurgitations. (*See also* page 384 under section on "Musculoskeletal Diseases").

Marfan Syndrome

(*See* General Observations, Height on p. 361.)

Pseudoxanthoma Elasticum

(*See* Coronary Artery Disease, Pseudoxanthoma Elasticum on p. 371.)

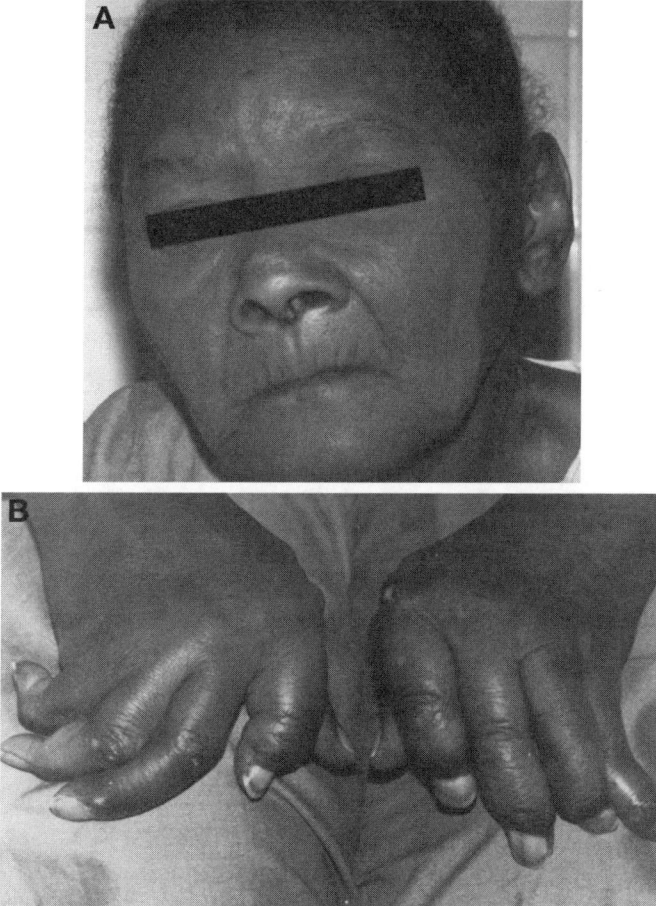

Fig. 13. (Color Plate 9, following p. 270) Mixed connective tissue diseases (lupus, rheumatoid arthritis, scleroderma). **(A)** The patient had a mask facies with puckering of skin around lips and malar depigmentation. **(B)** The patient's hand showed ulnar deviation of the metacarpophalangeal (MP) joints as well as a taut shiny skin.

Systemic Lupus Erythematosus SLE

The diagnosis of SLE may often be made by inspection of the face and the hands. In Caucasians, 10–61% (average 45%) of patients with SLE will have a characteristic malar butterfly skin lesion consisting of a red confluent maculopapular eruption with fine scaling involving the nose and cheeks *(104)*. However, in black patients with SLE there is depigmentation in the malar area. (Fig. 13) The dorsum of the hands may show red plaques or confluent red papules that spare the skin creases of the joints *(105)*. Because vasculitis is a feature of SLE, leg ulcers or livedo reticularis may be seen. Raynaud's phenomenon occurs in 27% of SLE cases *(104)*.

SLE is associated with clinically evident pericarditis in 25% of cases, hypertension in 16%, cardiomyopathy in 10%, symptomatic coronary arteriosclerosis in 10%, pulmonary hypertension in 5%, and ,rarely, aortic or mitral regurgitation or complete A-V block *(106–108)*.

Scleroderma

Patients with scleroderma may initially develop Raynaud's phenomenon and then skin changes involving the face and hands. Facial edema occurs followed by the development of smooth, shiny taut skin, resulting in a loss of facial wrinkling, puckering of the skin around the mouth, and difficulty in opening the mouth wide.

The dorsum of the hands may also show skin tightening and the development of flexion contractures of the inter-phalangeal (I-P) joints (claw hand). Focal areas of skin necrosis may be seen on the fingertips (rat-bite necrosis) *(82)*. Loss of one or more of the distal phalanges may ensue. *Telangiectasia* is frequently seen in the skin of the face and the limbs *(109)*. Patients with scleroderma commonly have pulmonary hypertension, symptomatic pericarditis in 15% of cases *(110)*, and depressed left ventricular function in less than 5% of cases *(111)*.

Dermatomyositis

Patients with dermatomyositis develop a dusky heliotrope eruption in the periorbital areas and may have facial fold erythema *(112)*. Violaceous papules are seen over the knuckles (*Gottron's papules*), which are virtually pathognomonic of dermatomyositis *(113)*. Raynaud's phenomenon and proximal muscle weakness also occur.

Patients with dermatomyositis may develop myocarditis leading to congestive heart failure. Pericarditis and heart block rarely occur *(114)*.

Polyarteritis Nodosa

Polyarteritis nodosa is a necrotizing arteritis involving the small and medium-sized arteries of the body. Visual findings are somewhat limited because skin lesions are seen in only 15% of cases *(115)*. There may be subcutaneous red nodules following the course of a leg artery, which may ulcerate and become necrotic. Livedo reticularis may be seen over the thighs. There is often hypertension and congestive heart failure, and although coronary arteritis occurs in 50% of cases, myocardial infarction is uncommon *(116)*.

Rheumatic Fever

Rheumatic fever remains quite common in developing countries. Boyd described rheumatic fever as a disease that licks the joints and bites the heart. The visible manifestations of rheumatic fever are *erythema marginatum*, subcutaneous nodules, and Jaccoud's syndrome. Erythema marginatum is a pink circular eruption with a pale center and raised red margins usually seen on the trunk, limbs, or axillae. It often precedes carditis and joint involvement. Erythema marginatum may occur in 10–25% of cases of rheumatic fever *(117)*. Subcutaneous nodules are uncommon. They occur around the elbow, knuckles, and spinous processes and usually signify cardiac involvement *(118)*. *Jaccoud's syndrome* is a rare rheumatoid-arthritis-like deformity of the hand following one or more attacks of rheumatic fever *(119)*. Patients with rheumatic fever may develop a pancarditis in the acute stage consisting of (1) valvulitis (mitral regurgitation or occasionally aortic regurgitation), (2) myocarditis and ,rarely, heart block, and (3) pericarditis. Subsequently, mitral stenosis occurs in the established case of rheumatic heart disease.

Ankylosing Spondylitis

Patients with ankylosing spondylitis have limited mobility of the spine (Schober test) *(120)*, which eventually becomes rigid (*bamboo spine*). The mobility of the sacroiliac joint is reduced and chest expansion limited. Aortic regurgitation is seen in 3–10% of cases of longstanding ankylosing spondylitis *(120)*. Complete heart block is very rarely seen *(120)*.

Reiter's Syndrome

The diagnosis of Reiter's syndrome (conjunctivitis, arthritis and urethritis) may also be considered in the presence of keratoderma blenorrhagica, the latter occurring in 60% of cases of Reiter's syndrome *(121)*. Keratoderma blenorrhagica occurs on the soles of the feet or the palms of the hand, mostly in Caucasian males. The skin lesions consist of red macules that become hyperkeratotic waxy papules with a central zone of yellow surrounded by a red halo. The papules coalesce to form plaques with subsequent crusting. Aortic regurgitation may occur in 60% of cases of Reiter's syndrome *(121)*. Complete heart block occurs rarely *(121)*.

PHARMACOLOGICAL AGENTS

Nifedipine

The side effects of nifedipine include postural hypotension, pedal edema, and gum hyperplasia. Pedal edema may occur with higher doses (>60 mg/d) in 5–10% of cases *(122)*. Gum hyperplasia may occur in 38% of patients who have been on nifedipine for 3 mo or more *(123)*. Patients with poor dental hygiene are more liable to have gum hyperplasia. Dilantin and cyclosporine are other drugs that may give rise to gum hyperplasia *(124)*.

Angiotensin-Converting Enzyme Inhibitors

These drugs produce rapid swelling of the face, tongue, and larynx (angioedema) in 0.2% of cases. It is more common in black patients and may be fatal *(125,126)*.

Anticoagulants
(Heparin, Coumadin)

Heparin-induced skin necrosis may be seen in the arms and is attributed to hypersensitivity angiitis *(127)*. Bleeding into the skin or mucous linings is readily detected if the heparin dose is excessive or in the rare instance of heparin-induced thrombocytopenia *(128)* (Fig. 14).

Coumadin may also rarely (0.01%) produce extensive purpuric areas of skin necrosis involving the breasts, thighs, and extremities *(129)*. It is common in middle-aged obese females *(129)*.

Anticoagulants may also give rise to retroperitoneal bleeding and can be detected by seeing bruising of the flanks (*Grey Turner's sign*) (Fig. 15) or around the umbilicus (*Cullen's sign*) *(130)* (Fig. 16). Swelling of the tongue as a result of bleeding may also be seen if a patient is overanticoagulated.

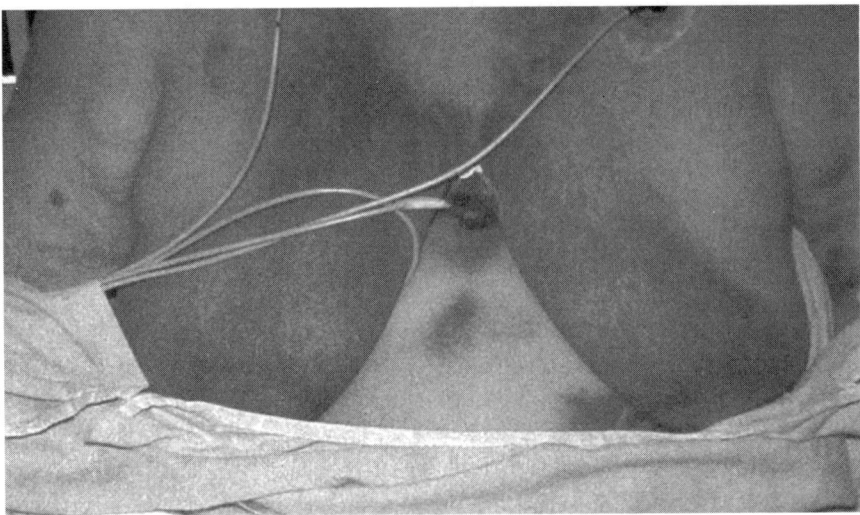

Fig. 14. Heparin-induced thrombocytopenia: 80-yr-old female who developed an extensive area of ecchymosis over the anterior chest wall and severe thrombocytopenia. Four days previously she had received (direct current) DC shock for ventricular tachycardia as well as heparin for an acute myocardial infarction. She had received heparin for a deep vein thrombosis in the past without any ill effects.

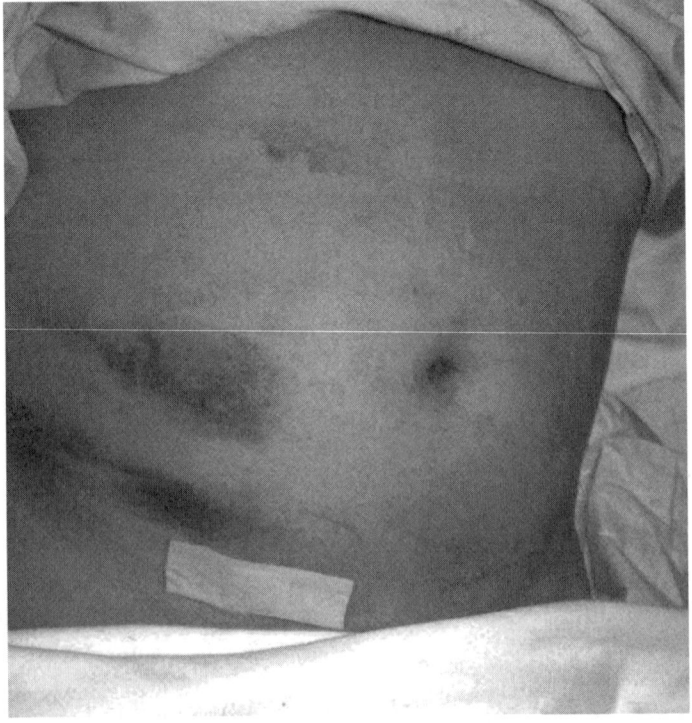

Fig. 15. Grey Turner's sign: 60-yr-old female with retroperitoneal bleeding following the use of heparin. Extensive ecchymoses seen in the right flank.

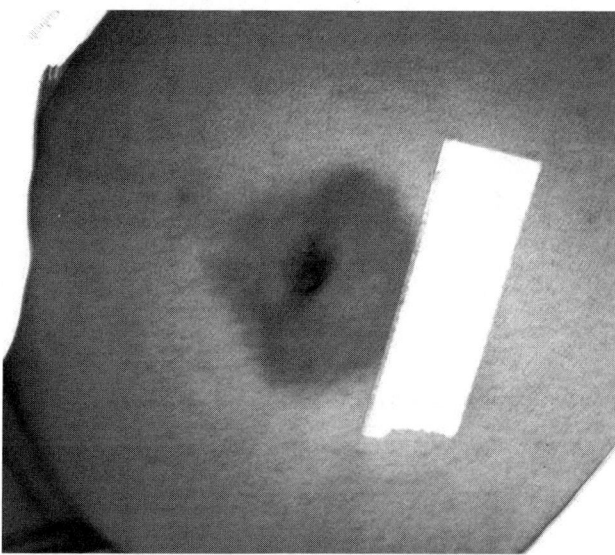

Fig. 16. Cullen's sign. This patient came into the hospital with retroperitoneal bleeding because of coumadin overdose. Ecchymosis is seen around the umbilicus. Prothrombin time was 110 s.

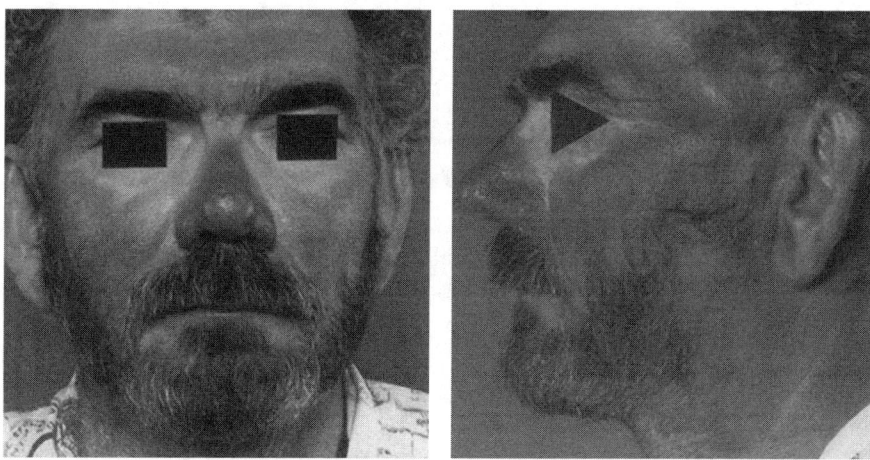

Fig. 17. (Color Plate 10, following p. 270) Amiodarone skin toxicity. There is a blue-gray dermal melanosis of the face, which partially improved 18 mo after amiodarone was stopped. (From ref. *132*.)

Amiodarone

Patients on long-term high-dose amiodarone (600 mg/d for 2 yr) may develop a blue-gray dermal melanosis of the face, especially of the areas exposed to the sun *(131)*. It may take several months for the skin discoloration to resolve after stopping the drug because of its long half-life *(132,133)* (Fig. 17). A lupus-like syndrome has also been reported with amiodarone *(134)*. Hyperthyroidism, hypothyroidism, liver dysfunction, and pulmonary fibrosis are other side effects of amiodarone *(131)*.

Procaine Amide

A lupus-like syndrome may occur with the use of procaine amide, but the butterfly rash is rarely seen *(135)*. Pericarditis may also occasionally be seen *(136)*.

Hydralazine

This drug may also produce a lupus-like syndrome and rarely a pericarditis *(136)*. A malar butterfly rash is more often seen than in procaine-amide-induced lupus *(136)*.

Alpha-Methyldopa

This drug may produce a lupus-like syndrome but without the malar butterfly rash *(135)*.

Digitalis, Spironolactone, Estrogens

Gynecomastia is seen occasionally with these drugs.

Recreational Drugs

Venous tracks or skin-popping sites (Fig. 18A,B) are some of the suggestive findings in a drug abuser. Additional findings in a cocaine abuser are described elsewhere *(68)*, including its association with coronary artery disease and hypertension *(70)*. Venous tracks may be seen in drug users who repeatedly inject heroin intravenously. They are usually found in the forearm or less commonly the neck. Heroin addicts are at risk for IE.

Skin-popping sites are rounded scars, 1–3 cm in diameter, seen on the legs and arms of drug abusers who inject heroin or cocaine subcutaneously. Extensive cellulitis and scarring on the thighs occur with deep and repeated subcutaneous drug injections (Fig. 18C).

MUSCULOSKELETAL DISEASES

Muscular Dystrophies

Myotonic dystrophy is the most common of the muscular dystrophies. This autosomal dominant disease shows characteristic facial features (a thin narrow face with drooping eyelids, frontal baldness) and muscle weakness of the neck, hands, and extremities. The patient has a high steppage gait and difficulty in grasp relaxation (*myotonia*). Fifty percent of such patients have a cardiomyopathy *(137)* and occasionally complete heart block *(138)*.

Duchenne dystrophy is a sex-linked recessive entity seen in boys characterized by proximal muscle weakness, waddling gait, and pseudohypertrophy of the calf muscles. Cardiomyopathy or atrial arrhythmias are often present *(138)*.

The Kearns–Sayre syndrome is characterized by ophthalmoplegia, short stature, and retinitis pigmentosa and is associated with complete heart block and cardiomyopathy *(34)*.

Friedreich's Ataxia

Patients with Friedreich's ataxia are characterized by pes cavus, nystagmus, and sensory ataxia. Cardiomyopathy is seen in more than 50% of cases *(138)*.

Osteogenesis Imperfecta

In this autosomal dominant entity, patients have multiple bone fractures, bowing of the long bones, kyphoscoliosis, pectus excavatum, and blue sclera (from loss of scleral collagen). Aortic or mitral regurgitation may be found in patients with osteogenesis imperfecta *(139,140)*.

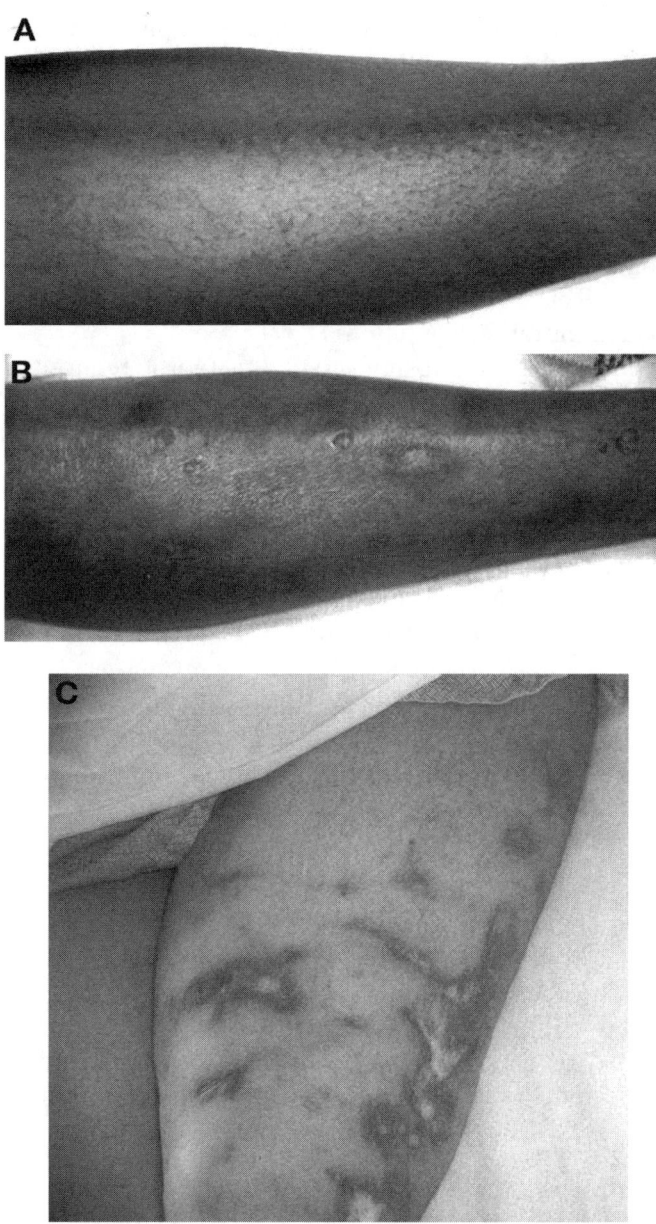

Fig. 18. Signs of drug addiction: (**A**) venous tracks in arm; (**B**) skin-popping sites in leg; (**C**) extensive cellulitis and scarring of thigh because of extensive subcutaneous injections of heroin.

Thoracic Cage Deformities

Thoracic cage deformities may provide a clue to the presence of underlying cardiovascular diseases. A patient with the *straight-back syndrome* (transverse diameter: anteroposterior ratio of >3 and loss of normal kyphosis) may have an innocent pulmonary flow murmur, which may be confused with pulmonic stenosis or an atrial septal defect *(141)*.

A shield chest is a broad chest with widely spaced nipples and an increased angle between manubrium and the body of the sternum. It is seen in *Turner syndrome* (coarctation of aorta) *(3)* and LEOPARD syndrome (pulmonic stenosis) *(30)*.

Pectus carinatum (pigeon chest) is associated with Marfan syndrome (aortic regurgitation, dissecting aneurysm) *(2)*.

Pectus excavatum is seen in Marfan syndrome *(2)*, Noonan syndrome (pulmonary stenosis) *(32)*, homocysteinuria (coronary artery disease), Ehlers–Danlos syndrome (aortic dissection, spontaneous aortic rupture, and mitral valve prolapse) *(34)*, gargoylism (mitral valve disease, ischemic heart disease, cardiomyopathy) *(34)*, and osteogenesis imperfecta (aortic and mitral regurgitation) *(139)*.

A bamboo spine is seen in ankylosing spondylitis (aortic regurgitation) *(120)*.

Kyphoscoliosis occurs in Friedreich's ataxia (cardiomyopathy) *(138)*, gargoylism *(34)*, neurofibromatosis (hypertension, outflow tract obstruction) *(15)*, and osteogenesis imperfecta *(139)*.

A barrel-shaped chest (transverse/antero-posterior (AP) diameter ratio of 1) is an unreliable sign of chronic obstructive lung disease, because it can also be found in the elderly patients without chronic obstructive lung disease *(142)*.

Paget's Disease of Bone

Patients with *Paget's disease* may have a progressive increase in hat size (because of a thickening skull), a decline in height (because of kyphoscoliosis) as well as saber shins *(143)*. Aortic stenosis *(144)* and left ventricular systolic dysfunction *(145)* occur in moderately severe Paget's disease of bone, whereas high-output failure occurs in patients with more extensive osseous involvement *(145)*.

TUMORS

Atrial myxomas may be considered in the differential diagnosis of clubbing *(48)*. The LAMB syndrome (Lentigines, Atrial myxoma, Mucocutaneous myxomas, Blue nevi) comprises 7% of all atrial myxomas and consists of lentiginous macules of the face or "freckling," atrial myxoma, mucocutaneous myxomas of the breast and skin, and blue nevi *(146,147)*. Rhabdomyomas are seen in tuberous sclerosis in 66% of cases *(22)*. Neurofibromas of the heart are seen in neurofibromatosis (von Recklinghausen's disease) *(16)*.

SYNOPSIS

Step 1: Detection of the Physical Signs

General Observations

Is the patient excessively tall or short? Body build should be noted. Is the patient alert or somnolent? Are there any abnormalities in the gait? Note the clothing for evidence of weight change or tobacco use.

Head

Are there any facial features to suggest a collagen or endocrine disorder such as butterfly eruption or exophthalmos, respectively? A mask-like face may suggest parkinsonism, scleroderma, or myotonia dystrophica, whereas a vacant expression suggests Down syndrome.

Are the eyes widely spaced apart (hypertelorism)? Do the conjunctiva appear pale or brick red? Are there any xanthelasma, waxy eyelid plaques, or drooping eyelids? Is the sclera discolored (e.g., blue or yellow)? Is there an Argyll Robertson pupil or subluxation of the lens? Is there an arcus corneae (unilateral or bilateral)? Fundi should be checked for hypertension, diabetes, dyslipidemias, or embolic changes because of carotid artery disease or IE.

Is there unilateral temporal artery prominence to suggest ipsilateral carotid disease or temporal arteritis? Skin findings such as malar flush, angiofibromata, slate gray pigmentation because of amiodarone, lupus pernio, facial edema, or premature aging should be noted.

The mouth should be inspected for dental hygiene or enamel erosions, gum hyperplasia, widely spaced teeth, macroglossia, tongue angiomata, or sublingual cyanosis. Are there any tonsillar lesions to suggest Tangier disease? Are there any petechiae on the hard palate? Is the nose saddle-shaped? Do the ears show evidence of gout, alkaptonuria, or a diagonal crease sign?

Neck

Is there any webbing of the neck? Is the thyroid enlarged? Are there any surgical scars to suggest carotid or thyroid operations? Is there unilateral or bilateral jugular venous distention? Plucked chicken skin appearance of the neck?

Chest

Are there any deformities of the thoracic cage such as kyphoscoliosis, straight-back syndrome, pectus excavatum, shield chest, or bamboo spine? Are there any surgical scars (thoracotomy, pacemaker, intravenous access site, or vascular surgery)? Are the ribs or sternum still intact? Are there any venous collaterals on the chest wall to suggest Superior Vena Cava (SVC) syndrome? Is there gynecomastia?

Upper Extremity

The hand should be examined for:
1. Size and shape: acromegaly (spade-like), Marfan syndrome (arachnodactyly), rheumatoid arthritis with an ulnar drift, Ehlers–Danlos syndrome with hyperextensible joints, Holt–Oram syndrome with *fingerized thumb*. Absent digits or deformed digits are also noted. Is there clubbing?
2. Edema: superior vena cava syndrome, thoracic outlet syndrome.
3. Neuromuscular disease: myotonia dystrophica, fine tremor of hyperthyroidism.
4. Color change: nicotine staining, cyanosis of nail beds, Raynaud's phenomenon, Osler's nodes, Janeway lesions, tissue necrosis associated with vasculitis.
5. Nail abnormalities: splinter hemorrhages, Terry nails, red lunula, onycholysis, subungual fibromas.
6. Palmar changes: palmar erythema, simian crease, and yellow palmar creases.
7. Temperature change: warm hands (e.g., hyperthyroidism) or cold hands (e.g., vasculitis, arterial occlusion).

Any xanthomas (elbows, hands). Any surgical scars (brachial artery cutdown, radial artery harvesting site for coronary artery bypass graft)? Any venous tracks from intravenous drug abuse?

Abdomen

Is there ascites or central obesity? Is the liver enlarged, tender, or pulsating? Are there prominent venous collaterals because of inferior vena cava (IVC) obstruction? Any signs of red abdominal striae of Cushing's disease; flank or periumbilical ecchymoses?

Back

Deformities such as kyphoscoliosis or bamboo spine are noted. The skin lesions of neurofibromatosis or eruptive xanthoma are often seen here. Is any radiation dermatitis associated with paravertebral muscle atrophy noted?

Lower Extremities

Skin lesions of erythema marginatum (thighs), erythema nodosum (legs), keratoderma blenorrhagica, or Janeway lesions (soles of feet) are noted. Are skin-popping sites (legs, thighs) seen?

Is there leg swelling (unilateral or bilateral)? Does the swelling pit, or is it firm? Note evidence of pseudohypertrophy of calf muscles and saber shins. Xanthomas of the nodular or tendinous type should be noted. Check for evidence of vascular insufficiency and gangrene of toes.

Step 2: Correlation of Physical Signs With a Cardiovascular Entity

Congenital Heart Disease

It is known that certain syndromes are associated with specific congenital cardiac conditions. Thus diagnosis of some of these syndromes from general physical signs would immediately suggest the appropriate specific associated congenital cardiac defect. Syndromes and associated defects are indicated in the following list.

- Holt–Oram syndrome (atrial septal defect)
- Down syndrome (A-V communis, ventricular septal defect, tetralogy of Fallot)
- Turner syndrome (coarctation of the aorta)
- Central cyanosis, polycythemia, and clubbing, pointing to a right-to-left shunt

Vascular Disease

Hypertension, hyperlipidemia, smoking, diabetes, and obesity are detectable as coronary artery disease risk factors. Ischemic heart disease may also be suspected in the presence of an ear crease sign, evidence of mediastinal radiation, progeria, polycythemia, PXE, Tangier disease, acromegaly, and in a cocaine addict. Sleep apnea, polyarteritis nodosa, von Recklinghausen's disease, Cushing's syndrome, acromegaly, and gout are associated with hypertension.

Arcus corneae, xanthoma, and lipemia retinalis suggest hyperlipidemia. Hyperlipidemia is seen in acromegaly and myxedema. Olivarius's sign, unilateral arcus corneae, and a Hollenhorst plaque occur in internal carotid artery disease.

Marfan and Ehlers–Danlos syndromes are associated with aortic aneurysms/rupture. Sleep apnea, sarcoidosis, scleroderma, and tricuspid regurgitation are associated with pulmonary hypertension. The Shy–Drager syndrome gives rise to postural hypotension.

Limb ischemia/necrosis may be because of atherosclerosis, cholesterol embolism, Buerger's disease, diabetes, Raynaud's phenomenon, or a collagen disease.

Facial edema, neck vein distention, prominent venous collateral circulation on the chest wall, and venous stars are seen in the superior vena cava syndrome, whereas prominent abdominal venous collateral circulation, leg edema, and possibly ascites point to the inferior vena cava syndrome.

Patients with the Osler–Weber–Rendu syndrome may have pulmonary A-V fistula.

Infective Endocarditis

The physical signs are *Roth spots*, retinal hemorrhages, subungual hemorrhages, petechiae involving the conjunctiva or palate, *Osler's nodes*, and *Janeway lesions*. Valvular heart disease may also be present.

Valvular Heart Disease

Some syndromes and conditions are specifically associated with certain valvular dysfunctions. Thus detection of these on general physical signs would immediately point the appropriate associated valvular lesion that needs to be considered. They are listed as follows.

- Carcinoid syndrome, pulmonary hypertension (tricuspid regurgitation)
- Carcinoid, LEOPARD, and Noonan syndromes (pulmonic stenosis)
- Osteogenesis imperfecta, PXE, and Marfan syndrome, infective endocarditis (mitral regurgitation)
- PXE, Ehlers–Danlos syndrome, and Marfan syndrome (mitral valve prolapse)
- Marfan, Reiter's, ankylosing spondylitis, tertiary syphilis, infective endocarditis, and osteogenesis imperfecta (aortic regurgitation).
- Ochronosis and Paget disease of bone (aortic stenosis)
- LEOPARD syndrome (hypertrophic cardiomyopathy)
- Williams' syndrome (supravalvular aortic stenosis)

Heart Failure

Patients with heart failure may have peripheral cyanosis, edema, neck vein distention, leukonychia, and mild jaundice (hypertension, coronary artery disease, valvular heart disease, myocarditis, cardiomyopathy, or pericardial disease may be the underlying cause). High-output failure is seen in Paget's disease of bone and hyperthyroidism.

Myocardial and Pericardial Disease

Myocardial and or pericardial disease will be the cardiac lesion to be considered when physical signs suggest some of the following disorders: hemochromatosis, muscular dystrophy, Friedreich's ataxia, hyperthyroidism, amyloidosis (cardiomyopathy), rheumatic fever, Reiter's syndrome (myocarditis), scleroderma, dermatomyositis, sarcoidosis (pericarditis), and myxedema (pericardial effusion and possibly tamponade).

Heart Block

Increased risk of development of delays and blocks in the electrical conduction of the heart may be suggested when general physical signs lead to the detection of the following disorders: sarcoidosis, gout, rheumatic fever, Reiter's syndrome, SLE, and ankylosing spondylitis.

Cardiac Tumors

The presence of cardiac tumors such as atrial myxoma or rhabdomyoma may have to be considered when systemic examination reveals signs of the following: neurofibromatosis (neurofibromas of the heart), tuberous sclerosis (rhabdomyoma), and the *LAMB syndrome* (atrial myxoma).

ACKNOWLEDGMENT

The author is indebted to the secretarial skills of Mrs. Ruby N. Stubbs-Stamps.

REFERENCES

1. Fitzgerald FT, Tierney LM Jr. The bedside Sherlock Holmes. West J Med 1982;137:169–175.
2. Pyeritz RE. The Marfan syndrome. Ann Rev Med 2000;51:481–510.
3. Rudolph AM, Hoffman JIE, Rudolph CD. In: Rudolph's Pediatrics, 20th Ed. Stamford, CT: Appleton & Lange, 1996:1782.
4. Clinical guidelines on the identification evaluation and treatment of overweight and obesity in adults—the evidence report—NIH. Obes Res Suppl 1998;2:51S–209S.
5. Ruyon BA. Cardiac ascites. J Clin Gastroenterol 1988;10:410–412.
6. Fraser RS, Colman N, Muller NL, ParÈ PD. Obesity hypoventilation syndrome. In: Fraser & Pare's Diagnosis of Diseases of the Chest, 4th Ed. Philadelphia, PA: W.B. Saunders, 1999:3053.
7. Lin YT, Yeh L, Oka Y. Pathophysiology of general cyanosis. NY State J Med 1977;77:1393–1396.
8. Silverman ME, Hurst JW. The hand and the heart. Am J Cardiol 1968;22:718–728.
9. Blount SG, Jr. Cyanosis: pathophysiology and differential diagnosis. In: Friedberg CK, ed. Pathophysiology and Differential Diagnosis in Cardiovascular Disease. New York, NY: Grune & Stratton, 1971;89–99.
9a. Aziz K, Sanyal SS, Goldblatt E. Reversed differential cyanosis. Br Heart J 1968;30:288–290.
10. Saif MW, Khan U, Greenberg BR. Cardiovascular manifestations of myeloproliferative disorders: a review of the literature. Hosp Phys 1999;(July):43–54.
10a. Grant P, Patel P, Singh S. Acute myocardial infarction secondary to polycythemia in a case of cyanotic congenital heart disease. Int J Cardiol 1985;9:108–110.
11. Nardone DA, Roth KM, Mazur DJ, et al. Usefulness of physical examination in detecting the presence or absence of anemia. Arch Intern Med 1990;150:201–204.
12. Wade OL, Bishop JM. Cardiac Output and Regional Blood Flow. Oxford: Blackwell, 1962:187.
13. Strickman NE, Rossi PA, Massumkhani GA, et al. Carcinoid heart disease: a clinical pathologic and therapeutic update. Curr Probl Cardiol 1982;6:4–42.
14. Porter J, Cary N, Schofield P. Hemochromatosis presenting as congestive cardiac failure. Br Heart J 1995;73:73–75.
15. Karnes PS. Neurofibromatosis: a common neurocutaneous disorder. Mayo Clin Proc 1998;73:1071–1076.
16. Alaeddini J, Frater RW, Shirani J. Cardiac involvement in neurofibromatosis. Tex Heart Inst J 2000; 27:218–219.
17. Friedberg CK. Edema and pulmonary edema. In: Friedberg CK, ed. Pathophysiology and Differential Diagnosis in Cardiovascular Disease. New York, NY: Grune and Stratton, 1971:40–71.
18. Berry TJ. The Hand as a Mirror of Systemic Disease. Philadelphia, PA: F.A. Davis, 1963:193–204.
19. Byrne JJ. The Hand: Its Anatomy and Diseases. Springfield, IL: Charles C Thomas,1959:194–195.
20. Daniel CR, Sams WM, Scher RK. Nails in systemic disease. In: Scher RK, Daniel CR, eds. Nails: Therapy, Surgery, and Diagnosis. Philadelphia, PA: W.B. Saunders Company, 1990:167–191.
21. Doughty RN, Haydock DA, Wattie J, et al. Systemic embolism from a large ascending aortic aneurysm. Circulation 1998;97:1421–1422.
22. Weiner DM, Ewalt DH, Roach ES, et al. Tuberous sclerosis complex: a comprehensive review. J Am Coll Surg 1998;187:548–561.

23. Holzberg M, Walker HK. Terry's nails: revised definition and new correlations. Lancet 1984;1: 896–899.
24. Fitzpatrick TB, Johnson RA, Wolff K. Blue-gray nails. In: Color Atlas and Synopsis of Clinical Dermatology, 3rd Ed. New York, NY: McGraw-Hill, 1997: 498–499.
25. Friedberg IM, Vogel LN. Thyrotoxicosis — onycholysis. In: Werner & Ingbar's The Thyroid, 6th Ed. Philadelphia, PA: J.B. Lippincott, 1986:732.
26. Terry RC. Red half moons in cardiac failure. Lancet 1954;11:842–844.
27. Cuetter AC, Pearl W, Ferrans VJ. Neurological conditions affecting the cardiovascular system. Curr Probl Cardiol 1990;15:475–568.
28. Rudolph AM, Hoffman JIE, Rudolph CD. Down syndrome. In: Rudolph's Pediatrics, 20th Ed. Stamford, CT: Appleton & Lange, 1996:298.
29. Tandon R, Edward JE. Cardiac malformation associated with Down syndrome. Circulation 1973;47:1349–1355.
30. Gorlin RJ, Anderson RC, Blaw M. Multiple lentigenes syndrome. Am J Dis Children 1969;117:652–662.
31. Woywodt A, Welzel J, Haase H, et al. Cardiomyopathic lentiginosis/LEOPARD syndrome presenting as sudden cardiac arrest. Chest 1998;113:1415–1417.
32. Grumbach MM, Conte FA. Noonan's syndrome. In: William's Textbook of Endocrinology, 9th Ed. Philadelphia, PA: W.B. Saunders, 1998:1355.
33. Burch M, Sharland M, Shinebourne E, at al. Cardiologic abnormalities in Noonan syndrome. Phenotypic diagnosis and echocardiographic assessment of 118 patients. J Am Coll Cardiol 1993;22: 1189–1192.
34. Sternberg MA, Neufeld HN. Physical diagnosis in syndromes with cardiovascular disease. In: Friedberg CK, ed. Physical Diagnosis in CVS Disease. New York, NY: Grune & Stratton, 1969:16–40.
35. Zalzstein E, Moes CAF, Musew NN, et al. Spectrum of cardiovascular anomalies in Williams-Beuren syndrome. Pediatr Cardiol 1991;12:219–223.
36. Peery WH. Clinical spectrum of hereditary hemorrhagic telangiectasia (Osler-Weber-Rendu disease). Am J Med 1987;82:989–997.
37. Swanson KL, Prakash UBS, Stanson AW. Pulmonary arteriovenous fistulas: Mayo Clinic experience. Mayo Clin Proc 1999;74:671–680.
38. Basson CT, Solomon SD, Weissman B, et al. The clinical and genetic spectrum of the Holt-Oram syndrome (heart-hand syndrome). N Engl J Med 1994;330:885–891.
39. Lovibond JL. The diagnosis of clubbed fingers. Lancet 1938;1:363–364.
40. Regan GM, Tagg B, Thomson ML. Subjective assessment and objective measurement of finger clubbing. Lancet 1967;1:530–532.
41. Shamroth L. Personal experience. S Afr Med J 1976;50:297–300.
42. Waring WW, Wilkinson RW, Wiebe RA, et al. Quantitation of digital clubbing in children. Measurements of casts of the index finger. Am Rev Respir Dis 1971;104:166–174.
43. Bentley D, Moore A, Schwachman H. Finger clubbing: a quantitative survey by analysis of the shadograph. Lancet 1976;2:164–167.
44. Lovell RRH. Observation on the structure of clubbed fingers. Clin Sci 1950;9:299–317.
45. Carroll DG, Jr. Curvature of the nails, clubbing of the fingers and hypertrophic pulmonary osteoarthropathy. Trans Am Clin Clim Assoc 1971;83:198–208.
46. Schneiderman H. Digital clubbing because of idiopathic pulmonary fibrosis. Consultant 1996;36: 1249–1256.
47. Coury C. Hippocratic fingers and hypertrophic osteoarthropathy. A study of 350 cases. Br J Dis Chest 1960;54:202–209.
48. Goodwin JR. Diagnosis of left atrial myxoma. Lancet 1963;1:464–467.
49. Hansen-Flaschen J, Nordberg J. Clubbing and hypertrophic osteoarthropathy. Clin Chest Med 1987; 8:287–298.
50. Dorney ER. Unilateral clubbing of the fingers because of absence of the aortic arch. Am J Med 1955; 18:150–154.
51. Kanski JJ. Clinical Ophthalmology, 4th Ed. Oxford: Butterworth, 1999:495–497.
52. Barchiesi BJ, Eckel RH, Ellis PP. The cornea and disorders of lipid metabolism. Survey Ophthalmol 1991;36:1–22.
53. Allander E, Bjornsson OJ, Kolbeinsson A, et al. Incidence of xanthelasma in the general population. Int J Epidermiol 1972;1:211.

54. Parker F. Xanthomas and hyperlipidemia. J Am Acad Dermatol 1985;13:1–30.
55. Borrie P, Slack J. A clinical syndrome characteristic of primary Type IV-V hyperlipoproteinemia. Br J Dermatol 1974;90:245–253.
56. Polano MK. Xanthomatoses. In: Fitzpatrick TB, Eisen OZ, Wolff K, eds. Dermatology in Medicine, 4th Ed., Vol 2. New York, NY: McGraw-Hill, 1993:1910.
57. Glueck CJ. Triglyceride analysis in hyperlipidemia. In: Rifkind BM, Levy RI, eds. Diagnosis and Therapy. New York, NY: Grune & Stratton, 1977:22.
58. Brewer MB, Zech LA, Gregg RE, et al. Type III hyperlipoproteinemia: diagnosis, molecular defects, pathology and treatment. Ann Int Med 1983;98:623–640.
59. Daniell MW. Smoker's wrinkles: a study in the epidemiology of crow's feet. Ann Intern Med 1971;75:873–880.
60. Pouliot MC, Després JP, Lemieux S, et al. Waist circumference and abdominal sagittal diameter: best simple anthropometric indexes of abdominal visceral adipose tissue accumulation and related cardiovascular risk in men and women. Am J Cardiol 1994;73:460–468.
61. Eber B, Delgado P. More on the diagonal earlobe crease as a marker of coronary artery disease; Am J Cardiol 1993;72:861.
62. Stewart JR, Fajardo LF, Gillette SM, et al. Radiation injury to the heart. Special feature — late effects. Consensus conference. Int J Radiation Oncology Biol Phys. 1995;31:1205–1211.
63. George WM. Cutaneous findings related to cardiovascular disorders. Int J Derm. 1998;37:161–172.
64. Fredrickson DS, Altrocchi PH. Tangier disease. In: Aronson SM, Volk BW, eds., Cerebral Sphingolipidoses. New York, NY: Academic Press, 1962:343–357.
65. Mahley RW, Weisgraber KH, Farese RV, Jr. Disorders of lipid metabolism. In: William's Textbook of Endocrinology, 9th Ed. Philadelphia, PA: W.B. Saunders, 1998:1134.
66. Komuro R, Yamashita S, Sumitsuji S, et al. Tangier disease with continuous massive and longitudinal diffuse calcification in the coronary arteries. Circulation 2000;101:2446–2448.
67. Pietrini V, Ruzzuto N, Vergani C. Neuropathy in Tangier disease: a clinicopathologic study and a review of the literature. Acta Neurol Scand 1985;72:495–505.
68. Warner EA. Cocaine abuse. Ann Intern Med 1993;119:226–235.
69. Krutchkoff DJ, Eisenberg E, O'Brien JE, et al. Cocaine-induced dental erosions (lett). N Engl J Med 1990;322:408.
70. Pitts WR, Lange RA, Cigarroa JE, et al. Cocaine-induced myocardial ischemia and infarction: pathophysiology, recognition and management. Prog Cardiovasc Dis 1997;40:65–76.
71. Franks AG, Jr. Cutaneous aspects of cardiopulmonary disease. In: Fitzpatrick TB, Eisen AZ, Wolff K, Austen KF, eds., Dermatology in General Medicine, 3rd Ed. New York, NY: McGraw-Hill Book Co, 1997:1981.
72. Lebwohl M, Halperin J, Phelps RG. Brief report: occult pseudoxanthoma elasticum in patients with premature cardiovascular diease. N Engl J Med 1993;329:1237–1239.
73. Fischer CM. Facial pulses in internal carotid artery occlusion. Neurology 1970;20:476–478.
74. Smith JL, Susac JO. Unilateral arcus senilis: sign of occlusive disease of the carotid artery. JAMA 1973;226:676.
75. Sapira JD. An internist looks at the fundus oculi. Disease A Month 1984;30:1–64.
75a. Hellmann DB. Temporal arteritis. A cough, toothache and tongue infarction. JAMA 2002;287:2996–3000.
76. Blackshear JL, Jahanger A, Owenburg WA, et al. Digital embolization from plaque-related thrombus in the thoracic aorta: identification with transesophageal echocardiography and resolution with warfarin therapy. Mayo Clin Proc 1993; 68:268–272.
77. Feder W, Auerbach RM. "Purple toes": an uncommon sequela of oral coumadin therapy. Ann Int Med 1961;55:911–917.
78. Pettelot G, Bracco J, Barrillon D, et al. Cholesterol embolization. Unrecognized complication of thrombolysis. Circulation 1998;97:1522.
79. Falanga V, Fine MJ, Kapor WN. The cutaneous manifestations of cholesterol crystal embolization. Arch Dermatol 1986;122:1194–1198.
80. Olin JW, Young JR, Graor RA, et al. The changing clinical spectrum of thromboangiitis obliterans (Buerger's disease). Circulation 1990; 82(Suppl IV):IV-3–IV-8.
81. Spittell JA, Jr. The vasospastic disorders. Curr Probl Cardiol 1984;8:5–27.
82. Fitzpatrick TB, Johnson RA, Wolff K. Vasculitis. Color Atlas and Synopsis of Clinical Dermatology, 4th Ed. New York, NY: McGraw-Hill, 2001:373–377.

83. Ricca J. Obstruction of the superior vena caval system: an extensive review. NY State J Med 1959; 59:4171–4177.
84. Parish JM, Marschlke RF, Dines DE, et al. Etiologic considerations in superior vena cava syndrome. Mayo Clin Proc 1981;56:407–413.
85. Blackburn T, Dunn M. Pacemaker-induced superior vena cava syndrome: consideration of management. Am Heart J 1988;116:893–896.
86. Wallace C, Siminoski K. The Pemberton sign. Ann Intern Med 1996;125:568–569.
87. Berlin L, Waldman I, Fong JK. Occlusion of the inferior vena cava. A major roentgenographic abnormality with minor clinical manifestations. JAMA 1965;194:136–138.
88. Wood P. An appreciation of mitral stenosis. Br Med J 1954; 1:1051, 1113.
89. Thorner MO, Vance ML. Acromegaly. In: William's Textbook of Endocrinology, 9th Ed. Philadelphia, PA: W.B. Saunders, 1998:298–299.
90. McKenzie JM, Zakarija M. Hyperthyroidism. In: LJ De Groot, Saunders WB, eds., Endocrinology, 3rd Ed. Philadelphia, PA: W.B. Saunders, 1995:676–712.
91. Manolis AS, Varriale P, Ostrowski RM. Hypothyroid cardiac tampanode. Arch Intern Med 1987; 147:1167–1169.
92. David DS, Grieco MH, Cushman P. Adrenal glucocorticoids after 20 years. A review of their clinically relevant consequences. J Chron Dis 1970;22:637–711.
93. Gertz MA, Lacy MQ, Dispensieri A. Amyloidosis: recognition, confirmation, prognosis and therapy. Mayo Clin Proc 1999;74:490–494.
94. Braverman IM. Amyloidosis. In: Skin Signs of Systemic Disease, 3rd Ed. Philadelphia, PA: W.B. Saunders, 1998:190–197.
95. Pund EE, Hawley RL, McGee HJ, et al. Gouty heart. N Engl J Med 1960;263:835–838.
96. Messerli FH, Frohlich ED, Dreslinski GL, et al. Serum uric acid in essential hypertension. Ann Intern Med 1980;93:817–821.
97. Maxwell AJ, Bruinsma KA. Uric acid is closely linked to vascular nitric oxide activity. Evidence for mechanism of association with cardiovascular disease. J Am Coll Cardiol 2001;38:1850–1858.
98. Kenny D, Ptacin M, Bamrah VS, et al. Cardiovascular ochronosis: a case report and review of the medical literature. Cardiology 1990;77:477–483.
99. Scheld WM, Sande MA. Endocarditis and intravascular infections. In: Mandell GL, Bennett JE, Dolin R, eds. Principles and Practice of Infectious Diseases, 4th Ed. New York, NY: Churchill Livingstone, 1995:748.
100. Proudfit WL. Skin signs of infective endocarditis. Am Heart J 1983;106:1451–1453.
101. James DG, Neville E, Siltzback LE, et al. A worldwide review of sarcoidosis. Ann NY Acad Sci 1976; 278:321–334.
102. Matsui Y, Iwai K, Tachibana T, et al. Clinical pathological study of fatal myocardial sarcoidosis. Ann NY Acad Sci 1976;278:455–469.
103. Roberts WC, McAllister HA, Ferrans VJ. Sarcoidosis of heart. Am J Med 1977;63:86–108.
103a. Pepin M, Schwarze U, Superti-Furga A, et al. Clinical and genetic features of Ehlers–Danlos syndrome type IV, the vascular type. N Engl J Med 2000;342:673-680.
104. Wallace DJ, Hahn BH, eds. Dubois' Lupus Erythematosus, 6th Ed. Philadelphia, PA: Lippincott, William & Wilkins, 2001:622.
105. Fitzpatrick TB, Johnson RA, Wolff K, et al. DLE. In: Color Atlas and Synopsis of Clinical Dermatology, 4th Ed. New York, NY: McGraw-Hill, 2001:361–367.
106. Moder KE, Miller TD, Tazelaar HD. Cardiac involvement in systemic lupus erythematosus. Mayo Clin Proc 1999;74:275–284.
107. Doherty NE, Siegel RJ. Cardiovascular manifestations of systemic lupus erythematosus. Am Heart J 1985;110:1257–1265.
108. Roberts WC, High ST. The heart in systemic lupus erythematosus. Curr Probl Cardiol 1999;24:1–56.
109. Braverman IM. Scleroderma. In: Skin Signs of Systemic Disease, 3rd Ed. Philadelphia, PA: W.B. Saunders, 1998:235–241.
110. Follansbee WP. The cardiovascular manifestation of systemic sclerosis (scleroderma). Curr Probl Cardiol 1986;11:245–298.
111. Anuari A, Graninger W, Schneider B, et al. Cardiac involvement in systemic sclerosis. Arthritis Rheum 1992;35:1356–1361.
112. Katayama I, Sawada Y, Nishioka K. Facial fold erythema—dermatomyositis: seborrheic pattern of dermatomyositis. Br J Derm 1999;140:978–979.

113. Plotz PH, Moderator. Current concepts in the idiopathic inflammatory myopathies: polymyositis, dermatomyositis and related disorders. Ann Intern Med 1989;111:143–157.
114. Braunwald E. Dermatomyositis in Heart Disease, 5th Ed. Philadelphia, PA: W.B. Saunders, 1997: 1779–1780.
115. Fitzpatrick TB, Johnson RA, Wolff K, et al. Polyarteritis nodosa. In: Color Atlas and Synopsis of Clinical Dermatology, 3rd Ed. New York, NY: McGraw-Hill, 1997:372–375.
116. Schrader ML, Hockman JS, Bulkley BH. The heart in polyarteritis nodosa: a clinico-pathologic study. Am Heart J 1985;109:1353–1359.
117. Sahn EE, Maize JC, Silver RM. Erythema marginatum: an unusual histopathological manifestation. J Am Acad Dermatol 1989;21:145–147.
118. Scott JT. Rheumatic fever. In: Copeman's Textbook of the Rheumatic Diseases, 5th Ed. Edinburgh: Churchill Livingstone, 1978;781–782.
119. Bywaters EGL. Relationship between heart and joint disease including 'rheumatoid heart disease' and chronic post-rheumatic arthritis (type Jaccoud). Br Heart J 1950;12:101–131.
120. Scott JT. Ankylosing spondylitis. In: Copeman's Textbook of the Rheumatic Diseases, 5th Ed. Edinburgh: Churchill Livingstone, 1978:513–516.
121. Weinberger HS, Ropes MW, Kulka JP, et al. Reiters syndrome; clinical and pathological considerations. A long term study of 16 cases. Medicine (Baltimore) 1962;41:35–91.
122. Freher M, Challapalli S, Pinto JV, et al. Current status of calcium channel blockers in patients with cardiovascular disease. Curr Probl Cardiol 1999;25:229–340.
123. Steele RM, Schuna AA, Schreiler RT. Calcium antagonist-induced gingival hyperplasia. Ann Intern Med 1994;120:663–664.
124. Mcraw SJ, Sheridan PJ. Medically induced gingival hyperplasia. Mayo Clinic Proc 1998;73:1196–1199.
125. Opie LH, Gersh BJ. Drugs for the Heart, 5th Ed. Philadelphia, PA: W.B. Saunders, 2001:118.
126. Lapostolle F, Borron SW, Bekka R, et al. Lingual angioedema after perindopril use. Am J Cardiol 1998;81:523.
127. Hirsh J, Dalen JE, Deykin D, et al. Heparin: mechanism of action, pharmacokinetics, dosing considerations monitoring, efficacy and safety. Chest 1992;102(suppl):337S–351S.
128. Warkentin TE. Heparin induced thrombocytopenia, part 1. The diagnostic clues. J Crit Illness 2002; 17:172–178.
129. Pineo GF, Hull RD. Adverse effects of coumadin anticoagulants. Drug Safety 1993;9:263–271.
130. Silen W. Cope's Early Diagnosis of the Acute Abdomen, 16th Ed. Oxford: Oxford University Press, 1983:119.
131. Harris L, McKenna WJ, Rowland E, et al. Side effects of long-term amiodarone therapy. Circulation 1983;67:45–51.
132. Blackshear JL, Randle HW. Reversibility of blue-gray cutaneous discoloration from amiodarone. Mayo Clin Proc 1991;66:721–726.
133. Sra J, Bremner S. Amiodarone skin toxicity. Images in cardiovascular medicine. Circulation 1998;97: 1105.
134. Sheikhzadeh A, Schafer V, Schnabel A. Drug induced lupus erythematosus by amiodarone. Arch Intern Med 2002;162:834–836.
135. Solinger AM. Drug related lupus. Clinical and etiological considerations. Rheum Dis Clin North Am 1988;14:187–202.
136. Wallace DJ, Hahn BH. Drug induced lupus. In: Dubuois' Lupus Erythematosus, 6th Ed. Philadelphia, PA: Lippincott, Williams & Wilkins, 2001:891–896.
137. Victor M, Ropper AH. Adams & Victor's Principles of Neurology, 7th Ed. New York, NY: McGraw-Hill, 2001:1145.
138. Perloff JK. The heart in neuromuscular disease. Curr Probl Cardiol 1986;11:511–557.
139. White NJ, Winearls CG, Smith R. Cardiovascular abnormalities in osteogenesis imperfecta. Am Heart J 1983;106:1416–1420.
140. Wong RS, Follis FM. Shively BK, et al. Osteogenesis imperfecta and cardiovascular diseases. Ann Thorac Surg 1995;60:1439–1443.
141. Datey KK, Deshmukh MM, Engineer SD, et al. Straight back syndrome. Br Heart J 1964; 26:614–619.
142. Pierce JA, Ebert RV. The barrel deformity of the chest, the senile lung and obstructive pulmonary emphysema. Am J Med 1958;25:13–22.

143. Bailey H. Demonstration of Physical Signs in Clinical Surgery,13th Ed. Bristol: John Wright & Sons Ltd, 1960;802.
144. Hultgren HN. Osteitis deformans (Paget's disease) and calcific disease of the heart valves. Am J Cardiol 1998;81:1461–1464.
145. Arnalich F, Plaza JA, Sabrino J, et al. Cardiac size and function in Paget's disease of bone. Int J Cardiol 1984;5:491–505.
146. Rhodes AR, Silverman RA, Harrist TJ, et al. Mucocutaneous lentigines, cardiomucocutaneous myxomas, and multiple blue nevi: the Lamb syndrome. J Am Acad Dermatol 1984;10:72–82.
147. Vidaillet Jr HJ, Seward JB, Fyke FE, et al. "Syndrome myxoma": a subset of patients with cardiac myxoma associated with pigmented skin lesions and peripheral and endocrine neoplasms. Br Heart J 1987;57:247–255.

Index

A
A1
  in aortic root aneurysm, 153
  in aortic valve stenosis, 153
  in bicuspid aortic valve, 153
  intensity, 153
  Abdominal aorta
  aneurysm, 35
  graft, 368, 369
  pulsations, transmitted, 135
A2
  in aortic regurgitation, 163
  decreased systemic impedance, 170
  delayed
    in aortic valvular stenosis, 169
    in HOCM, 169
    in ischemia, 170
    LBBB, 168–169
    mechanical, 169–170
    in severe hypertension, 170
  early
    MR, 172
  in heart failure, 162
  intensity, 162
  sequence identification, 176–177
  timing of abnormal, 164
  see also A2–P2 splitting
A2–P2 splitting
  in abnormal respiratory variations, 173–174
  in ASD, 100f, 172, 173f, 174, 174f
  audible expiratory split, 177–178
  in Eisenmenger's syndrome, 167
  in hypertension, pulmonary, 170, 171–172
  in ischemia, 170
  early A2/P2, 172–173
  electrical delay, 164, 165f
  fixed splitting, 173–174
  impedance
    delay secondary to effects of, 165–167, 166f, 167f
    pulmonary, 172
  mechanical delay, 159f, 164, 165f, 166–167, 166f, 167f
  normal respiratory variation, 161
  paradoxical splitting, 173, 355
  rule of split S2 at apex, 177, 311
  sequence identification, 176–177
  wide splitting (physiological), 167–168, 168f
ACE inhibitors, 381
Acquired cardiac disease, 5t
Acromegaly, 373, 374f
Acute infection, 9
Alkaptonuria, 377
Allen's test, 35
Alpha methyldopa, 384
Amiodarone, 383, 383f
Amyl nitrite
  aortic insufficiency, 362f
  aortic regurgitation, 318
  arterial dilatation, 31, 32f
  auscultation, 313
  Austin Flint murmur, 281–282, 313, 318
  mitral stenosis, 282
  mitral valve prolapse, 318
  MR, 318
  outflow obstruction (HOCM), 228
  persistent ductus arteriosus, 381
  pulmonary arteriovenous fistulae, 318
  pulmonary flow murmur, 318
  systemic arteriovenous fistulae, 318
  tetralogy of Fallot, 318
  venous hum, 318
  VSD, 262, 318
Amyloidosis, 375–376, 376f
Anacrotic shoulder, 23, 24f, 37
Android obesity, 362
Anemia, 263, 300
Angina
  atypical, 3
  chronic stable, 309
  exertional, 3, 54, 55, 285, 326
  Prinzmetal's (or variant), 3, 334
  typical, 3

Angioedema, 381
Angiotensin-converting enzyme inhibitors, 381
Ankylosing spondylitis, 381
Anomalous left coronary origin, 5, 249, 295
Anticoagulants (coumadin, heparin), 381, 382f, 383f

Aortic aneurysm, 35, 134, 372, 378, 388
    dissecting, 61–62
    root, A1, 153
Aortic area, true, 160f, 161, 311
Aortic coarctation
    blood pressure, 62–63
    in bruits, 39
    variations in, and bedside diagnosis, 35
Aortic compliance, 21
Aortic dissection
    blood pressure, 53
    pectus excavatum, 386
Aortic ejection click, 153, 154f, 155f, 224
Aortic insufficiency, 362f
    see also Aortic regurgitation
Aortic regurgitation
    acute, 286–287
    aortic dissection, 284
    aortic root causes, 284
    aortic valve prolapse, 284
    atherosclerotic aneurysm, 284
    A2 intensity, 163
    auscultatory features, 287–290, 288f, 289f
    bicuspid aortic valve, 283
    chronic, 284–285
    cystic medial necrosis of root, 284
    ineffective endocarditis, 284
    LV function in, 63
    mimickers, 36, 38, 41
    M1, 150–151
    osteogenesis imperfecta, 284
    Paget's disease, 284
    pathophysiology of
        acute severe, 286–287, 287f, 327–328
        chronic, 284–286, 285f, 325–327, 326f, 327f
    peripheral signs, 41–44, 43f
    popliteal pulse, 35
    precordial pulsations, 136
    severity, assessment of, 63
    signs and symptoms, 328–329, 328t
    sinus of Valsalva aneurysm, 7, 284
    spondylitis, 284
    syphilitic aortitis, 284
    trauma, 284
    valvular causes, 283–284, 373
Aortic root
    aneurysm, A1, 153
    aortic regurgitation, 284
    in severe aortic stenosis, 162
Aortic sinus rupture, 36, 38, 41
Aortic stenosis,
    A1, 153
    apical impulse, 126, 126f, 129f, 130f, 135f, 138
    A2, 162, 169
        pathophysiology of, 331–332, 332f
    Paget's disease, 386
    rheumatic heart disease, 224
    S4, 201–202
    signs and symptoms, clinical, 333, 333t
    S2 split, 355
    subvalvular, 224–229, 226f, 227f, 229f
    supravalvular, 38, 230, 389
Aortic valve disease, 30, 184, 265, 282
Aortic valve prolapse, 284
Aortic valvular stenosis, 169
Aorto-pulmonary window, 36
Apex cardiogram, 113, 114
Apical impulse
    in aortic stenosis, 126, 126f, 129f, 130f, 135f, 138
    area, 121, 137
    assessment, 120
    atrial kick, 128–129, 128f, 129f, 130f, 133f, 138
    character, 124–126, 125f, 126f, 127f, 128, 128f
    determinants, 118–119, 118f, 119f
    diffuse, 124
    double impulse, 131, 132f
    duration, 124–126, 127f, 137–138, 127126f
    dynamicity, 124, 125f, 138
    exaggerated A *wave,* 128
    formation of, governing principles, 115, 116f, 117, 117f
    heave, 125
    in high cardiac output, 124
    HOCM, 131
    hyperdynamic, 124, 125f
    in hypertension, severe, 128
    lateral retraction, 123

location, 120, 120f, 137
LV, 125f, 136
mechanics and physiology of, 113–115
medial retraction, 121
median retraction, 123
mid-systolic retraction, 131—132, 132f, 133f
palpable sounds and murmurs, 132
precordial pulsations, 136–138
rapid-filling wave, 125f, 130, 131f
RV, 122–123, 124, 135, 135f, 136, 138
sustained, 125–126, 126f, 128, 129f, 130f, 138
tapping apex, 132
triple impulse, 132
ventricular, 121–123, 123f
Arachnodactyly, 362f, 387
Arcus cornealis, 388
Argyll Robertson pupil, 364, 377, 387
Arterial pressure, mean, 346, 347t
Arterial pulse
amplitude, 19, 19t, 20f, 36
assessment, clinical, 34, 44–46
bruits, 38–39
contour, 19, 19t, 20f, 32, 33f, 38
determinants, 19t
LV pump, 21–22
peripheral signs, 41–44
physiology, 15–17
pressure in vessel, 18
proximal, 20–21
pulse deficit, 34
pulsus alternans, 39, 40f, 41
rate, 34
reflection, 18–19, 26–28, 29, 30–31
rhythm, 34
stroke volume, 22
symmetry, 34–36
upstroke, 23, 24f, 37–38
velocity, 25–26
vessel wall characteristics, 36
volume effect, 17
see also Ejection; Pulse wave
Arterial system, proximal, 20
Arteriosclerosis, 25
Arteriovenous communications, 24
Ascites, 162, 388, 389
Atrial contraction phase, 186f, 188
Atrial fibrillation
a wave, 84
JVP contour, 73f

M1, 146, 149
pulse deficit, 34
regurgitant systolic murmurs, 240, 242f, 244
S1, 282
Starling effect, loss of, 87, 88f
S2–OS interval, 183
x descent, 84
x′ descent, 69, 71, 86–87, 101, 282
y descent, 104
Atrial gallop, 200
Atrial kick, 128–129, 128f, 129f, 130f, 133f, 138
Atrial myxoma
left, 238, 279
mitral stenosis in, 6, 12, 147, 276
M1, 147
MR in, 238
right, 255, 258, 282–283
S3 (tumor plop), 195–196, 196f, 279
tricuspid obstruction in, 152, 255, 258, 282–283
tumors, 386, 390
Atrial septal defect (ASD)
jugular venous pressure, 100, 100f
pathophysiology of, 342–344, 344f
signs and symptoms, clinical, 345, 345t
S2 split, fixed, 178, 355–356
venous pulse contour, 100, 100f
Atrioventricular (A–V) block, 149, 197
Atrioventricular (A–V) dissociation
S1, 200
summation gallop, 197

Augmented gallop, 197
Auscultation
amyl nitrite, 318
bedside maneuvers, 313–314
concepts of mechanisms, application of, 313
exercise, 316–317
frequency and character of murmur, 312–313
inching, 312
isometric exercise, 316
maximum loudness, recognizing location of, 312
mental filter, predetermined, 310–311
methodology, 310
one thing at a time, listening for, 310
phenylephrine, 317

with physiologic alterations, 313
principles of sound transmission, 311–312
respiration effect, 314
squatting, 316
standing, 315–316
stethoscope, 309–310
transient arterial occlusion, 317
Valsalva maneuver, 314–315
vasoactive agents, 317
vasopressors, 317
Auscultatory gap, 52
Austin Flint murmur, 281–282, 288, 289, 289f, 294, 313, 318, 329
a wave, 80f, 81f, 84–85
in atrial fibrillation, 84

B

Ballistocardiography, 43
Bamboo spine, 386
Barrel-shaped chest, 386
Basal diastolic tension, 24, 25
Beaking, nail, 368
Berger's disease, 372, 389
Bernheim effect, 87f, 88, 90t, 92
Bicuspid aortic valve, 283
Bifid pulse, 30, 38, 46
Bisferiens pulse, 30, 31f
Black nails, 364
Blood pressure
in aortic dissection, 53
in aortic regurgitation, 44, 63
arterial occlusion, assessment of, 61–63
in atherosclerotic disease, 53, 62
blood flow, physiology of, 49–50
in cardiac tamponade, 56–57
in coarctation of aorta, 62–63
expiratory gain, 58
heart sound intensity, 64
inspiratory fall, 56–57
in LV function assessment, 63
manual assessment, 63–64
measurement
in clinical situations, 56–64
factors affecting, 53–54
interpretation of, 54–56
Korotkoff sounds, origin of, 39, 50–52
points worth noting, 52–53
overshoot, 28
pulsus alternans, determination of, 61
respiratory variation, 56
Valsalva maneuver, 58–61, 59f, 60f

Blue gray nails, 364
Brachial pulse, 35
Brachio-radial delay, 37
Broadbent sign, 134
Bronchial asthma, 58
Bruit de diable, 363
Bruits, 38
Buerger's disease, 372, 389

C

Café au lait macules, 364
Canadian Cardiovascular Society (CCS) classification, 4
Cannon wave, 104
Carcinoid syndrome, 254, 283, 363, 389
Cardiac disease
acquired, 4, 5t
assessment
diagnosis, 4–6, 5t
reasons for, 2
symptoms, appraisal of, 2–4
congenital, 388
symptoms, 2–4
Cardiac output, 31, 32f
Cardiac tamponade
blood pressure, 56–57
exaggerated dicrotic wave, 38
pathophysiology of, 348–349, 350f
pulsus paradoxus, 56–57
signs and symptoms, clinical, 349–350, 350t
Cardiac tumors, 8, 390
Cardiogenic shock, 254, 260, 334
Cardiomyopathies, 8, 12
Cardiomyopathy, dilated
pathophysiology of, 338–339, 339f
signs and symptoms, clinical, 340, 340t
Cardiovascular disease, general observations
degree of alertness, 363
gait, 364
height, 361–362, 362f
nails, 364
skin, 363–364
weight, 362
Carey Coombs murmur, 281
Carotid artery disease, unilateral internal, 371
Carotid pulse
amplitude, 36, 37
artifacts, 70
tracing, 16, 16f, 18f
upstroke, 37, 114
Carvallo's sign, 257

Index 401

Central cyanosis, 363, 388
Central obesity, 370
Chest pain, 3
Cholesterol emboli, of lower extremities, 371
Cleft chordae, 234, 234f, 238, 250, 254
Clubbing, 367–369, 377
Coanda effect, 38, 230
Cocaine use, 371
Cole–Cecil murmur, 288
Commissural chordae, 234, 234f
Conduction system disorders, 8
Congenital heart disease, 5t
   cyanotic, 367–369, 367f, 368f
Congenital syndromes/diseases, 364–365, 366f, 367–369, 368f
   see also individual listings
Connective tissue and joints, diseases of, 377–381
   see also individual listings
Constrictive pericarditis
   JVP, 73f, 91f, 100–101, 101f
   pathophysiology of, 347, 348f
   precordial pulsations, 134
   pulsus paradoxus, 57–58
   signs and symptoms, clinical, 348, 349t
   S3, pericardial knock, 194–195, 195f
Continuous murmurs
   aorto-pulmonary window, 298
   arteriovenous fistulae, 299–300
   arteriovenous shunt, 294–295
   causes, 294
   clinical assessment of, 300–302
   innocent, 303–304
   mammary souffle, 300
   pericardial friction rub, 302
   persistent ductus arteriosus, 296–298, 297f
   sinus of Valsalva aneurysm, 298–299
   venous hum, 300
Cor bovinum, 286, 327
Coronary arteriovenous fistulae, 299–300, 302
Coronary artery disease, 369–372
   risk factors, 369, 388
   see also individual listings
Cor pulmonale, 255, 363, 377
Corrigan's pulse, 36, 41
Coumadin, 381
Crista supraventricularis muscle, 220, 232, 264
Crow's feet, 370
Cullen's sign, 381, 383f
Cushing's disease, 375

cv wave, 86, 98
Cyanosis
   central cyanosis, 363, 388
   differential cyanosis, 363
   peripheral cyanosis, 363

D

DeMusset's sign, 42–43
Dermatomyositis, 380
Diabetes, 364, 370
Diastasis, 185
Diastolic dysfunction. *See* Left ventricular diastolic dysfunction
Diastolic flow, jugular venous, 70f, 71f, 82, 89, 92
Diastolic murmurs
   auscultatory assessment, 293–294
   clinical assessment, 292
Diastolic pressure, 50, 51, 52, 53, 54, 55
Diastolic ventricular filling
   atrial contraction phase, 188–189
   diastasis, 185
   rapid filling phase, 188–189, 190f
   restrictions, 73f, 81f, 94–96, 95f, 96f
   slow filling phase, 188, 190
Dicrotic notch, 18f, 19, 27, 28f, 29f, 39
Dicrotic wave, 27, 28, 30, 38
Differential cyanosis, 363
Digitalis, 384
Dissecting aortic aneurysm, 61–62
Dorsalis pedis artery, 34, 36
Double descents, 96–97, 98t, 104
Double diastolic descents, 84f, 104
Double gallop, 206
Down syndrome, 365, 388
DP/dt, 21, 23, 146
Duchenne dystrophy, 384
Duroziez's sign, 42
Dysbetalipoproteinemia (type III), 370

E

Ear crease (diagonal) sign, 370
Ebstein's anomaly
   JVP contour, 103
   precordial pulsations, 134
   T1, 152, 152f
   venous pulse contours in, 103
Eccentric jet, 153, 222
Ectopia lentis, 361
Edema
   bilateral leg, 364, 372
   unilateral legs, 364

upper extremity, 364
see also Pulmonary edema
Effusive-constructive pericarditis, 347
Ehlers–Danlos syndrome, 378, 388
Eisenmenger's syndrome
   A2–P2 splitting, 167
   cyanosis in, 363
   in pulmonary hypertension, 255
   in VSD, 262–263
Ejection
   contractility, 22–23, 24f
   duration of (ejection time), 19t, 27–28, 28f, 29f
   impedance, 23–24
   LV ejection time, 39, 40f
   momentum of (mv), 21, 31
   peripheral resistance, 24–25
   pre-ejection period, 39, 40f
Ejection click, 153, 154f, 155f, 156, 156f, 158
Ejection murmurs
   in aortic valve stenosis, 223–224, 224f, 225f
   of ASD, 231f
   in atrial fibrillation, 220
   in bicuspid aortic valve, 222, 223f
   cadence, 219
   characteristics of, 218–220, 219f, 220f
   in complete heart block, 222
   formation of, 218
   frequencies, 218–219
   HCM, 225–229, 226f, 227f, 229f
   impulse gradient, 217–218
   intensity, 219–220, 220f
   in large stroke volume, 222
   outflow tract, 220, 221f
   in post-extrasystolic beat, 220, 227f
   in proximal septal hypertrophy with angulated septum, 229–230
   pulmonary valvular stenosis, 230–232, 231f, 232f
   in rapid circulatory state, 221–222
   rhythm, 219, 219f
   in sigmoid septum, 222, 223f, 229
   in straight back syndrome, 222
   in subvalvular aortic obstruction, 224–229, 226f, 227f, 229f
   in subvalvular membranous stenosis, 225
   in subvalvular pulmonary stenosis, 232
   supravalvular aortic stenosis, 230
   supravalvular pulmonary stenosis, 232

ventricular ejection, normal physiology of, 217–218, 218f
Ejection sound, 153
Ejection velocity, 23, 25, 34
Endocrine and metabolic diseases, 373–377
   see also individual listings
Endothelial function, 24
Eruptive xanthoma, 369, 370f
Erythema marginatum, 380, 388
Erythema nodosum, 377, 388
Estrogens, 384
Ewart's sign, 350
Exaggerated ascents of waves, 104
Exophthalmos, 373, 375f, 386
Expansile pulsation, 35
External jugular vein, 67, 82
Extrapapillary subendocardial network, 236f, 237

F

Femoral artery, 42, 43, 43f
Festinating gait, 364
Flushing-periodic facial, 363
Flutter waves, 104
Fredrickson Types, 369
Friedreich's ataxia, 364, 384, 386, 389
Friedreich's diastolic collapse, 100

G

Gallavardin phenomenon, 224, 268
Gallop rhythms, 197, 205–206
Gargoylism, 386
Giant *a wave*, 104
Gottron's papules, 380
Gout, 377
Graham Steell murmur, 263
Grey Turner's sign, 381, 382f
Gum hyperplasia, 381

H

Hang-out interval, 166
Heart block, 389–390
   complete, 377, 381, 384
   second degree, 149
Heart failure, 389
   A2, 162
   JVP, 101, 104
   M1, 149
   severe, venous pulse contour in, 74, 101
   Valsalva maneuver, 60
Heart murmurs. *See* Murmurs
Heart size assessment, 267, 268

Heart sounds
    first, 64, 142 (*see also* S1)
    formation of, 141–142
    fourth, 128, 142, 200–202, 204 (*see also* S4)
    second, 64 (*see also* S2)
    third, 130, 141, 185 (*see also* S3)
    see also Auscultation
Height, 361–362, 362f
Hemochromatosis. *See* Skin color
Heparin, 381, 382f
Hepatic pulsation, 372
Hepato-jugular reflux, 106
Hill's sign, 43–44, 43f
Hollenhorst plaque, 371, 388
Holt–Oram syndrome, 365, 388
Hydralazine, 384
Hypercholesterolemia, 369
Hyperlipidemia, 369
Hypertelorism, 365, 367
Hypertension
    apical impulse in severe hypertension, 128
    A2–P2 splitting, 170, 171–172
    grades of, 369
    severe, 25, 128, 170, 338
    S4, 201
Hypertensive heart disease, 7–8
    acute pulmonary edema, 7, 338f
    pathophysiology of, 336–337, 338f
    signs and symptoms, clinical, 337–338, 339t
Hypertensive retinopathy, 369
Hyperthyroidism, 373–374
    apathetic, 374
Hypertriglyceridemia, 369, 370f
Hypertrophic cardiomyopathy (HCM)/hypertrophic obstructive cardiomyopathy (HOCM)
    amyl nitrite, effect of, 318
    apical impulse, 131
    arterial pulse contour, 32, 33f
    in A2, delayed, 169
        digoxin, effect of, 227
    diastolic function, 187
    ejection murmurs, 225–229, 226f, 227f, 229f
    exercise, effect of, 314, 316
    isoproterenol, effect of, 227
    midsystolic retraction, 131, 132, 133f
    Müller maneuver, effect of, 228
    non-obstructive, 12, 32
    pathophysiology of, 340–341, 341f, 343t
    pulse, 32, 33f
    SAM, 32, 225
    S4, 204
    signs and symptoms, clinical, 341–342, 343t
    squatting, effect of, 313, 314, 316
    standing, effect of, 313, 314, 315–316
    systemic resistance, effect of, 343t
    Valsalva maneuver, effect of, 313
Hypovolemic shock, 58

I

Idiopathic dilatation, mitral annular, 238
Idiopathic prolapsed mitral leaflet syndrome, 248
Impedance to ejection, 23
    pulmonary, 172
    systemic 165, 166, 170
Impulse, 21
Impulse cardiogram, 113, 114
Impulse gradient, 21, 217–218
Incident wave, 26, 27
Incisura, 166, 167
Ineffective endocarditis, 377, 378f, 389
Infarct expansion, 334, 335f
Infarction, myocardial, S3 in, 194
Inferior vena cava syndrome, 372
Inflammatory diseases, 377
    see also individual listings
Infundibulum, RV, 220, 232, 253, 261, 264
Innocent murmurs
    continuous, 303–304
    mid-diastolic, 304
    systolic, 303
Interstitial pulmonary fibrosis, 255–256
Ischemia, myocardial
    A2–P2 splitting, 170
    S3, 194
Ischemic heart disease, 7, 238
Ischemic limb, 389
Isovolumic contraction, 115, 117f, 118, 143, 146, 169, 171

J

Jaccoud's syndrome, 380
Janeway lesions, 377, 378f, 387, 388, 389
Jaundice, 363, 389
Joints. *See* Connective tissue and joints, diseases of

Jugular venous flow, 68, 72f, 73f, 74, 92
    diastolic, 82, 89, 92
    systolic, 82, 86, 89, 96, 98
Jugular venous pulse (JVP), 67–68
    assessment of, clinical, 107–111
    double descents, 96–97, 98t, 104
    flutter waves, 104
    giant *a wave*, 104
    normal, bedside recognition of, 72f, 81–82, 83f
    pressure, assessment of, 105–106, 105f
        hepato-jugular reflux, 106
            superior vena cava, obstruction of, 107
    single *y descent*, 104
    triple descent, 104
    velocity patterns, abnormal, 92
        in post-cardiac-surgery patients, 92, 93f, 94f
        in pulmonary hypertension, 92, 93f
        in ventricular filling, diastolic restriction, 73f, 81f, 94–96, 95f, 96f
    and venous flow events, 74–81, 75f–81f
    see also Right atrial pressure pulse
Jugular venous pulse (JVP) contour
    in ASD, 100, 100f
    in atrial fibrillation, 71, 73f
    in cardiomyopathy, 86, 89
    in constrictive pericarditis, 73f, 91f, 100–101, 101f
    differentiation from arterial pulse, 82
    double descents, 96–97, 98t, 104
    double diastolic descents, 84f, 104
    in Ebstein's anomaly, 103
    exaggerated ascents of waves, 104
    flutter waves, 104
    post-cardiac surgery, 92, 93f, 94f
    pulmonary hypertension, 86f, 87f, 98–99, 98t, 99f
    in RV infarction, 101–103
    in severe heart failure, 101, 104
    single *y descent*, 104
    triple descents, 104

K

Kearns–Sayre syndrome, 384
Keith–Wagner–Barker criteria, 369
Keratoderma blenorrhagica, 381, 388
Kinetic energy, 21
Kinetocardiogram, 114
Korotkoff sounds
    determination, 50
    factors affecting, 51–52
    interpretation, 53, 56
    mechanisms of origin, 50–52
    phases, 50, 51
    pulsus alternans, 39, 61
Kussmaul's sign, 89, 348, 349t
Kyphoscoliosis, 89, 378, 384, 386, 387, 388

L

LAMB syndrome, 386, 390
Lamé's equation, 17, 118, 351f
Laminar flow, 212, 213, 215
Laplace's equation or law, 17, 118, 351, 351f, 351t
Lateral retraction, 123
Left atrial pressure, elevated
    signs of, clinical, 352–353
    symptoms of, 351–352, 352t
Left atrium
    in acute mitral regurgitation, 150, 204, 213, 215, 240, 243, 245, 252, 280, 322
    in aortic stenosis, 202
    in diastolic murmurs, 292
    echocardiogram showing, 144, 246
        in mitral stenosis, 181
        at end of diastole, 190, 201
        left atrial myxoma, 296
        hypertrophic obstructive cardiomyopathy, 226
    enlarged, 239, 321, 322
    expansion of, 133, 134, 136
    fibrosis of, 129
    and gallop rhythm, 206
    large, 133, 183
    in mitral stenosis, 6
    in regurgitant murmurs, 233, 239f, 240f
    provoking Starling effect, 204
    in ventricular dysfunction, 199
    volume overload, 297, 299, 321
    v wave in, 240, 276, 280, 322
Left bundle branch block (LBBB), 164, 168–169, 355
Left ventricular compliance, 189, 332, 333, 334, 341, 342, 344
Left ventricular diastolic dysfunction
    pathophysiology of, 345–346, 346f, 347t
Left ventricular function
    afterload, 9, 21, 23, 41, 233
    apical impulse, 125f, 136

ejection time, 39
preload, 21, 23, 217
pump, 21–22
remodeling, 256, 335
Valsalva maneuver, 60–61, 315
Left ventricular hypertrophy
concentric, 240, 286, 322
eccentric, 240, 283, 286, 322, 326
LEOPARD syndrome, 365, 366f
Lid lag, 373
Limb ischemia, 389
Lipemia reticularis, 369
Livedo retinalis, 371, 379, 380
Lupus pernio, 377, 387
Lutembacher syndrome, 276

M
M1
in aortic regurgitation, 150–151, 151f
in atrial fibrillation, 146, 149
in atrial myxoma, 147
in A–V dissociation, 149
in heart failure, 149
intensity, 146
isovolumic phase, 150
in mitral stenosis, 147, 147f, 148f
in MR, 149–150
normal, 145–146, 145f
in PR interval, 147, 148f, 149, 149f
Starling mechanism, 150
Malar flush, 373, 373f, 387
Mammary souffle, 296, 300, 303, 304
Marfan's syndrome, 284, 388
see also Height
Mass. *See also* Stroke volume
medial retraction, 121
median retraction, 123
Mean arterial pressure, 25, 26, 31, 37, 50
Metabolic diseases. *See* Endocrine and metabolic diseases
Mid-diastolic murmurs
innocent, 304
Mid-systolic retraction (MSR), 131–132, 132f, 133f
Mid-systolic sound, 250
Mitral diastolic murmurs
abnormal mitral valve, 281
acute rheumatic fever, 281
aortic regurgitation, 281–282
causes, 275
characteristics of, 277–279, 278f
functional mitral stenosis, 281–282
increased diastolic inflow, 279–280
left atrial myxoma, 279, 280f
mitral stenosis, 276–277, 276f
Mitral regurgitation (MR)
acute severe, 7, 87f, 240, 241f
annular abnormalities, 238
in atrial myxoma, 238
A2 in, 243, 252
causes of, 237–239
characteristics of, 240, 241f, 242–243, 242f, 243f
chronic, 7, 239, 239f
leaflet and chordal abnormalities, 238
M1, 149–150
normal mitral valve and function, 233–237, 234f, 235f, 236f, 237f
papillary muscle and LV abnormalities, 238
in papillary muscle dysfunction, 248–250
pathophysiology of, 239–240, 239f
acute MR, 322, 323f, 324t
chronic MR, 321–322, 323f
precordial pulsations, 133–134, 136
in prolapsed mitral valve, 245, 246f–248f, 249
in rheumatic heart disease, 244
in ruptured chordae tendinae, 250–253, 251t, 252f, 253f
severity of, 243–244, 244f
S4 in acute MR, 252
signs and symptoms, clinical, 324–325, 324t
S2 in, 240, 241f, 242, 243, 244
Mitral stenosis
M1, 147, 147f, 148f
opening snap, 181–182
pathophysiology, 329–330, 329f, 331t
signs and symptoms, clinical, 330–331, 331t
in valvular heart disease, 373, 373f
Mitral stenosis murmur, 6
characteristics, 277–279, 278f
duration, 279
intensity, 278f, 279
presystolic crescendo, 279
Mitral valve
normal function, 233–234
premature closure, 328
Mitral valve prolapse, 309, 313, 315, 316
Momentum of ejection (mv), 21, 31
Müller maneuver, 228

Murmurs
    aortic stenosis, 223
    frequencies, 214–215
    grading intensity, 216
    hemodynamic factors, 214
    mitral stenosis, 213, 214
    MR, 213, 215
    pitch, 215, 216
    principles of murmur formation, 211–214
    systolic, 216–217
Muscular dystrophies, 384
Muscular-skeletal diseases, 384–386
    see also individual listings
Myocardial infarction, acute
    pulmonary edema, acute, 7, 9
    S3 in, 194
Myocardial ischemia/infarction
    in A2–P2 splitting, 170
    pathophysiology of, 334–335, 335f
    signs and symptoms, clinical, 336, 336t
    in S3, 194
Myotonic dystrophy, 384
Myxedema, 374, 375f
Myxoma, left atrial, 279, 368
Myxomatous degeneration, 251, 251t, 254

N

Nails, 364
Neurofibroma, 364, 386
Neurofibromatosis, 364, 386, 388
New York Heart Association, classification, 4
Nifedipine, 381
Nitric oxide, 24
Nitroglycerin, hemodynamic effect of, 281
Non-ejection click, 245, 246f, 248, 250, 266
Noonan syndrome, 365

O

Obesity, central (android), 370
Ochronosis, 364, 373, 377, 389
Olivarius's external carotid sign, 371, 388
Onycholysis, 364, 387
Opening snap (OS), 179–180, 179f, 180f
    in absence of mitral stenosis, 181–182
    clinical assessment, 184–185
    intensity, 184
    mechanism, 180–181, 181f
    S3 differentiation, 199–200
    timing, 182–183, 182f, 183f
    trill, 185, 186f
Ophthalmoplegia, 373, 384
Orthopnea, 292, 351

Osler nodes, 377
Osler–Weber–Rendu syndrome, 365, 367f, 389
Osteogenesis imperfecta, 378, 384
Ostium primum ASD, 238

P

P2
    delayed, 170
        in pulmonary artery dilatation, 172
        in pulmonary embolism (acute), 172
        in pulmonary hypertension, 167f, 171–172
        in pulmonary impedance, decreased, 172
        in pulmonary stenosis, 171
        RBBB, 171
        RV outflow obstruction, 171
        sequence identification, 176–177
    early, 173
    intensity, 163
    timing of abnormal, 164
    see also A2–P2 splitting
Paget's disease, 386
Palmar xanthomas, 370
Palpable sounds, 137
Papillary muscle dysfunction
    clinical features, 249–250
    in MR, 238
Paradoxical splitting of S2, 167, 168f
Parkinson's disease, 364
Paroxysmal nocturnal dyspnea, 248, 286, 292, 326f, 327
Pectus carinatum, 386
Pectus excavatum, 386
Pemberton's sign, 372
Percussion wave, 30, 32, 33f
Pericardial disease, 8
Pericardial effusion, 95f, 96, 98, 99, 302, 346
Pericardial friction rub, 302
Pericardial knock, 194
Pericarditis, 347–348, 348f, 349t
Periodic flushing, facial, 363
Peripheral cyanosis, 363
Peripheral resistance, 24–25
Peripheral vasodilatation, 24
Persistent ductus arteriosus
    auscultatory features, 297–298
    pathophysiology, 296–297
Petechial hemorrhages, 377
Pharmacological agents, 381–384
    see also individual listings

Pheochromocytoma, 364
Physical signs, detection
  abdomen, 388
  back, 388
  chest, 387
  general, 386
  head, 286–287
  lower extremities, 388
  neck, 287
  upper extremities, 387
Pickwickian syndrome, 256
Pigeon chest, 386
Pistol-shot sounds, 42
Plummer's nails, 364
Pneumonia, 9
Poiseuille law, 211
Polyarteritis nodosa, 378, 380, 388
Polycythemia
  primary, 370
  secondary, 363
Popliteal artery, 35
Post-cardiac surgery, 92, 93f, 94f
Posterior tibial artery, 34, 36
Postextrasystolic potentiation, 39, 41
Postural hypotension, 381, 388
Pre-*a wave* pressure, 82, 84f
Precordial pulsations
  in aortic regurgitation, 133–134, 134f, 136
  clavicular head pulsations, 134
  clinical assessment, 136–138
  in constrictive pericarditis, 134
  in Ebstein's anomaly, 134
  left parasternal impulse, 133
  left parasternal retraction, 133–134, 134f
  left 2nd and 3rd intercostals spaces, 135
  in MR, 133–134, 136
  right parasternal impulse, 134
  sternal movement, 133,
  sternal retraction, 136, 138
  subxiphoid impulse, 135, 135f, 138
Pre-ejection period (PEP), 39
Pregnancy, in S3, 190
Premature closure, of mitral valve, 328
Prinzmetal's angina, 3, 334
Procaine amide, 384
Progeria, 370
Prolapsed mitral valve, 309, 313, 315, 316
Protodiastolic gallop, 205
Proximal arterial system, 20–21
Pseudoxanthoma elasticum (PXE), 371

Pulmonary arteriovenous fistula, 383
Pulmonary artery dilatation
  left 2nd and 3rd intercostal spaces, 135
  P2, 172
Pulmonary disease, chronic obstructive, 58
Pulmonary edema, acute
  myocardial infarction, 7
Pulmonary ejection click, 153, 156, 156f
Pulmonary embolism
  acute, 9–11, 58
  S3, 194
Pulmonary hypertension, 92, 93f
  A2–P2 splitting, 170, 171–172
  causes, 8
  in Eisenmenger syndrome, 255
  etiological factors, 255–256
  in hyperkinetic circulation, 255
  in hypoventilation, 256
  in intracardiac shunts, 255
  JVP, 86f, 87f, 98–99, 98t, 99f
  in left-sided pathology, 255
  pathophysiology, 255
  P2, 171–172
  in pulmonary disease, 255–256
  in pulmonary embolism, 254, 356
  signs and symptoms of, 352t, 353
  in smoking, 255–256
  S2 split, 178, 356
  and tricuspid regurgitation, 255–256
  vasculitis in, 256
Pulmonary regurgitation
  auscultatory features, 291, 291f
  normotensive, 290
  pathophysiology of, 290–291
  in pulmonary hypertension, 290
  in pulmonary valvotomy, post, 290
  without pulmonary hypertension, 290
Pulmonary valve stenosis, 230
Pulmonic stenosis, 363, 365, 385
Pulsations. *See* Precordial pulsations
Pulse deficit, 34
Pulse pressure, wide, 35, 43, 44, 297, 299, 354, 354t
Pulse wave
  contour, 19, 20f
  transmission, 25–26
  see also Reflection
Pulsus alternans, 39, 40f, 41, 61
Pulsus paradoxus, 56–58
  in asthma, 58
  in cardiac tamponade, 56–57

in constrictive pericarditis, 57–58
in hypovolumic shock, 58
in pulmonary embolism, 58
Pulsus parvus, 37
Pulsus tardus, 37
Purple toe syndrome, 371

Q

Quadruple rhythm gallop, 206
Quincke's sign, 41

R

Radial compression test, 35
Radial pulse, in jugular assessment, 108
Radio-femoral delay, 34–35
Rapid filling phase, 186f, 188–189
Rapid filling wave, 130, 131f, 132, 138
Rat bite lesions, 372, 380
Raynaud's phenomenon, 372
Recreational drugs, 384, 385f
Red lunula, 364, 387
Reflection, 18–19, 29f
    clinical implications, 30–31
    coefficient, 26
    conditions governing, 31
    effects of, 26–28, 28t
    harmonics, 26, 27
    intensity, 28–29
Regurgitant systolic murmurs, 232
    in atrial fibrillation, 240, 242f, 244
    characteristics of, 233
    conditions for, 233
    in post-extrasystolic beat, 233
    in tricuspid regurgitation, 233
    see also Mitral regurgitation (MR)
Reiter's syndrome, 381
Remodeling, LV, 256, 335
Resistance vessels, 24
Retraction
    lateral, 123
    medial, 121, 123, 137
    median, 123
    mid-systolic, 131–132, 132f, 133f
    parasternum/sternum, 136
    systolic, marked, in AR, 134, 174f
Retrograde flow into jugulars, 78–79
Reverse splitting, 338
Reynolds formula, 214
Rheumatic fever, 380
Right atrial pressure pulse
    components of, recognizing in jugulars
        a wave, 80f, 81f, 84–85

        pre-*a wave* pressure, 82, 84f
        v wave, 80f, 84f, 88–89
        x descent, 72f, 77f, 83f, 84f, 85
        x' descent, 73f, 85–87, 86f, 88f
        y descent, 81f, 84f, 89–90
        y descent, exaggerated, 84f, 86f, 90–92, 90t, 91f
    contours, 68–70, 70f
    jugular venous inflow velocity patterns, 70–74, 71f, 72f, 73f, 74f
Right atrial pressure pulse contours, 68–70, 70f
Right atrial relaxation, 68, 69, 71, 72f, 74, 102, 104
Right bundle branch block (RBBB), 164, 171, 354–355
Right ventricular apical impulse, 122–123, 124, 135, 135f, 136, 138
Right ventricular compliance, 104, 256, 291, 348
Right ventricular diastolic dysfunction, 13, 354
Right ventricular diastolic filling
    atrial contraction phase, 188–189
    pre *a wave* pressure, 98
    rapid filling phase, 188
    restriction, 73f, 81f, 94–96, 95f, 96f
    slow filling phase, 188
Right ventricular infarction, 95f, 99
    venous pulse contours in, 101–103
Right ventricular infundibulum, 220, 232, 253, 261, 264
Right ventricular outflow obstruction, 171
Roth spots, 377, 389
Ruptured chordae tendineae, clinical features, 172
Rytand murmur, 280

S

S1
    aortic component, 143, 144f–145f
    assessment
        clinical, 156
        intensity (loudness), 157
    atrial component, 142
    mitral component, 142–143, 143f, 144f, 145f
    normal. *See* M1
    tricuspid component, 143
    variability of intensity, 149
    see also A1; T1

Index

S2
- abnormal, 162
- aortic component, A2, 325
- clinical assessment 174–175
- components, 167–168. *See also* aortic component, A2; pulmonary component, P2
- intensity, 162
  - in aortic regurgitation, 163
- in jugular assessment, 108
- mechanism, 158–159, 159f
- normal, 159–161, 160f
- paradoxical splitting of, 167, 168f
- pulmonary component, P2, 159f, 232
- splitting, 175–176
  - in acute pulmonary hypertension, 356
  - in ASD, 355–356
  - audible expiratory, 177–178
  - in chronic pulmonary hypertension, 356
  - fixed, 173
  - LBBB, 355
  - in normals, 354
  - paradoxical, 167
  - RBBB, 354–355
  - respiratory variation, 167–168, 168f
  - rule of split S2 at apex, 177, 311
  - sequence identification, 176–177
  - timing, respiratory variations in, 355f
  - wide physiological, 168
- systemic impedance, decreased, 168f, 170
- tambour sound, 162

S3, 185
- in atrial myxoma, 195–196, 196f
- clinical assessment, 198–199
- clinical features, 197–198, 198f
- in constrictive pericarditis, 194–195, 195f
- diastolic function, 185–187, 186f
- differentiation
  - from S2–OS, 199–200
  - from S2 split, 199
  - from tumor plop, 200
- external origin, 190
- filling phases, 186f, 188—189
- gallop rhythm, 205–206
- in HOCM, 187
- intermittent, 200
- mechanism of formation, 189–190, 190f
- in myocardial infarct (acute), 194
- in myocardial ischemia, 194
- persisting on standing, 195f, 199
- physiological, 190, 191f
- postextrasystolic beat, 187
- in pregnancy, 190
- in pulmonary embolism, 194
- in ventricular
  - aneurysm, 194
  - dysfunction, 188, 193, 193f, 206
  - overload, 191, 192f, 193
- right sided S3, 193, 194, 198, 199, 258, 283, 314

S4
- in aortic stenosis, 201–202
- clinical assessment, 204
- gallop rhythm, 205–206
- in hypertension, 201
- in LV dysfunction, 206
- mechanism of formation, 200–204, 201f, 202f, 203f
- in MR (acute), 204
- pre-requisites, 201
- split S1 differentiation, 205

Saber shins, 386, 388
Sail sound, 152
Sarcoidosis, 377
Sarcoplasmic reticulum (SR), 41
Schober test, 381
Scleroderma, 380
Second-degree A–V block, S1 in, 157
Semilunar valve regurgitation, 283
Shamroth's clubbing sign, 367
Shield chest, 386, 387
Shy–Drager syndrome, 364
Single ventricle, 264
Single *y descent,* 104
Sinus of Valsalva aneurysm
- auscultatory features, 299
- pathophysiology, 298–299

Skin color, 363–364
Skin popping sites, 384
Sleep apnea, 256, 388
Sleep apnea syndrome, 363
Slow filling phase, 188, 190
Smoking, 370
Spironolactone, 384
Splinter hemorrhages, 364, 387
Square root sign, 194
Square wave response, 60, 60f, 315
Starling mechanism, 124, 150, 233
Stethoscope, 309–310
Still's murmur, 222

Straight back syndrome, 163
Strain gauge manometer system, 15, 16f
Stroke volume, 22, 22f
Strut chordae, 235, 235f
Subclavian vein thrombosis, 372
Subcutaneous nodules, 377, 380
Subungual fibromas, 364, 365, 387
Subungual hemorrhages, 364
Subxiphoid impulse, 135, 135f, 138
Summation gallop
    in A–V block, 197
    in A–V dissociation, 197
    in sinus tachycardia, 197
Superior vena cava, and jugulars, 78, 79, 81, 92, 106
Superior vena cava, obstruction of, 107
Superior vena cava syndrome, 372
Supravalvular aortic stenosis, 38, 230, 389
Symptoms
    cardiac, 2–4
    classifications, CCS, NYHA, 4
Syphilis, 377
Systemic lupus erythematosis (SLE), 379, 379f
Systolic anterior motion (SAM) of MV, 23, 32, 225, 226
Systolic flow, jugular venous, 82, 86, 89, 96, 98
Systolic murmurs
    auscultatory assessment of, 266–269
    character, 266–267
    clinical assessment, 265–266
    diamond shape, 216
    duration, 216, 232, 267
    ejection murmurs, 267
    holosystolic, 216
    innocent, 303
    kite shape, 216
    pansystolic, 268
    plateau murmurs, 261
    quality, 268, 269
    timing, 216
Systolic pressure, 49–50, 52, 53, 61, 62, 63
Systolic time intervals, 39, 61

T

T1
    in Ebstein's anomaly, 152, 152f
    intensity, 151–152, 152f
Tabes dorsalis, 364
Takayasu's disease, 296
Tambour sound (S2), 162
Tamponade, cardiac
    blood pressure, 56–57
    exaggerated dicrotic wave, 38
    pathophysiology of, 348–349, 350f
    pulsus paradoxus, 56–57
    signs and symptoms, clinical, 349–350, 350t
Tangier disease, 371
Temporal arteritis, 34, 371
Temporal muscle wasting, 373
Tendon xanthomas, 369
Terry nails, 364, 387
Tetralogy of Fallot, 263, 290, 291
Thoracic cage deformities, 385–386
Thready pulse, 36
Thromboangiitis obliterans, 372
Tidal wave, 27, 32, 33f
Tricuspid diastolic murmur
    causes, 282
    characteristics of, 282
    right atrial myxoma, 282–283
    tricuspid stenosis, 282
Tricuspid regurgitation
    acute, 257
    annular abnormalities, 254
    in atrial myxoma, 255
    causes, 253
    characteristics, 257–258
    leaflet and chordal abnormalities, 254
    in normal PA pressure, 256–257
    pacemaker electrode, 255
    papillary muscle & RV wall pathology, 254–255
    pathophysiology, 253
    in pulmonary hypertension, 255–256
    in rheumatic heart disease, 258
    in valvular heart disease, 372
Tricuspid stenosis murmur
    characteristics, 282
    increased diastolic flow, 283
    pathophysiology, 282
Tricuspid valve anatomy, 253
Tricuspid valve prolapse, 283–284
Triple descents, 104
Trill, 185, 186f
Tuberous sclerosis, 365
Tuberous xanthomas, 370
Tumor plop (S3), 195–196, 196f, 279
Tumors, 386
Turbulent flow, 218, 275, 282, 290, 294

Turner syndrome, 388
Twanging string murmur, 303

U

Ulnar pulse, 35
Upstroke, 37–38

V

Valsalva maneuver, 314–315
   blood pressure response to, 58–61, 59f, 60f
   in heart failure, 60
   in LV function assessment, 60–61, 315
   in normals, 58
   square wave response, 60, 60f
   in S2 split, 178
Valvular heart disease, 372–373, 373f, 389
Vascular compliance (aorta), 21
Vascular disease, 388–389
   atherosclerotic, 62
Vascular resistance, 49
Venous hum, 300
Venous tracks, 384
Ventricular ejection
   during exercise, 218
   physiology, 217–218, 218f
Ventricular filling
   restrictions, 73f, 81f, 94–96, 95f, 96f
Ventricular outflow tracts, comparison of right and left, 220
Ventricular rate, rapid, 9
Ventricular relaxation
   in HOCM, 187
   in LV dysfunction (mild), 188
   in post-extrasystolic beat, 187
Ventricular remodeling, 335
Ventricular septal defect (VSD), 258
   amyl nitrite, effect of, 262
   characteristics of, 260–261, 261f
   clinical spectrum, 260
   congenital, 259–260
   hemodynamic severity, grade classifications, 260
   membranous, 258
   in myocardial infarction, 259, 260, 264–265, 265f
   perimembranous, 258
   pulmonary valvular stenosis, 230
   spontaneous closure, 259
   squatting, effect of, 262
   in tetralogy of Fallot, 263
   variations
      Eisenmenger reaction, 262–263
      large, 259, 262
      muscle, small, 262
      pulmonary stenosis, with, 263–264
      septal rupture, 264–265, 265f
      single ventricle, 264
      subpulmonic, 261
      vasoactive agents, effect of, 262
Venturi effect, 23, 37, 38, 226, 227–228
Vessel characteristics, of walls, 36
Volume effect, 17
Von Recklinghausen's disease, 364, 386, 388
V wave, 80f, 84f, 88–89

W

Water-hammer pulse, 42
Waterhammer theory, 51
Weight change assessment, 386
White coat syndrome, 55
White nails, 364
Wide pulse pressure, 354t
Wide splitting of S2, 178
William's syndrome, 365

X

Xanthomas, 369
X descent, 72f, 77f, 83f, 84f, 85
X' descent, 73f, 85–87, 86f–88f
   in atrial fibrillation, 69, 71, 86–87, 101, 282
   mechanism, 103

Y

Y descent, 81f, 84f, 89–90
   exaggerated, 84f, 86f, 90–92, 90t, 91f

About the Authors

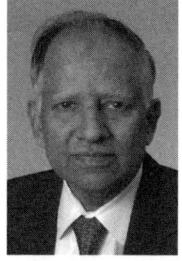

NARASIMHAN RANGANATHAN, MBBS, FRCP(C), FACP, FACC, FAHA, is an associate professor in medicine at the University of Toronto and a senior cardiologist at St. Joseph's Health Centre, Toronto, a university-affiliated community teaching hospital. A graduate in medicine from the University of Madras, India, Dr. Ranganathan trained in internal medicine in the Johns Hopkins Service at the Baltimore City Hospitals and in the State University of New York at Buffalo, in cardiology at Tulane University Medical School in New Orleans, and as research cardiology fellow at the Toronto General Hospital. He served as both an invasive and noninvasive cardiologist at St. Michael's Hospital, University of Toronto, from 1970 to 1989 and as chief of cardiology at St. Joseph's Health Centre, Toronto, from 1989 to 1998.

Dr. Ranganathan is a recipient of the W.T. Aikins Award for Excellence in teaching from the University of Toronto (1985) and has written many original papers published in peer-reviewed journals. He has organized several continuing medical education programs in Toronto during the last 28 years. His popular annual course on "The Art and Science of Cardiac Physical Examination" has always received enthusiastic and appreciative comments from attendees about its unique teaching methods.

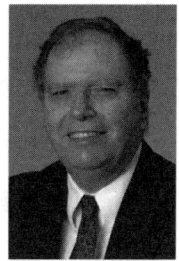

VAHE SIVACIYAN, BSc, MD, FRCP(C), received the degrees of bachelor of science in 1968 and doctor of medicine in 1972 from the University of Toronto. Dr. Sivaciyan did postgraduate work in internal medicine and cardiology at University of Toronto hospitals and at Albert Einstein School of Medicine in New York, where he was a cardiology fellow. He is certified in the specialties of internal medicine and cardiology by the Royal College of Physicians of Canada as well as by the American Boards of Internal Medicine and Cardiovascular Diseases.

Dr. Sivaciyan is an assistant professor at his alma mater, the University of Toronto, and has been actively involved in undergraduate as well as graduate teaching for over 20 years. He has done original research in areas pertinent to cardiac physical examination and has published in peer-reviewed journals.

Dr. Sivaciyan practices invasive cardiology at St. Michael's Hospital in Toronto and is a senior staff cardiologist and the director of the pacemaker program at St. Joseph's Health Centre, a university-affiliated community teaching hospital. He is a valued faculty member in the annual continuing medical education courses on "The Art and Science of Cardiac Physical Examination," "12-Lead ECG Interpretation," and "Cardiac Arrhythmias: Recognition and Management" offered at that institution. His particular interest in teaching has led him to lecture nationally and internationally.

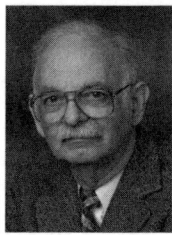

FRANKLIN B. SAKSENA, MD, CM, FACP, FRCP(C), FACC, FAHA, served as senior attending physician in the department of cardiology at Stroger Hospital of Cook County, Chicago, IL, for 32 years, where he was director of the cardiac catheterization lab for over 12 years, and for a period acting chief of cardiology. He remains active there as a voluntary attending physician. In addition, he is an assistant professor of medicine at both Northwestern University Medical School and Rush Medical School, and he continues a part-time private practice in cardiology and internal medicine at Swedish Covenant and St. Mary of Nazareth Hospitals.

Educated in England and Canada, he obtained his medical degree at Queen's University, Kingston, Ontario, Canada. He was a pulmonary fellow at The University of Chicago for two years and spent three years as a cardiology fellow (Northwestern Medical School and Toronto University hospitals).

He has won a number of awards for excellence in teaching cardiology and physical diagnosis to medical students and residents and continues to be much sought after by medical students and those in the MD–PhD program.

Dr. Saksena has written a monograph entitled *Hemodynamics in Cardiology: Calculations and Interpretations* (Praeger Scientific, New York, 1983). As a Sherlock Holmes enthusiast, he endeavors to apply Holmesian deductions to bedside diagnosis. He is also the author of *101 Sherlock Holmes Crossword Puzzles* (2000).

```
RC         Ranganathan,
683          Narasimhan.
.R25
2006       The art and science
             of cardiac physical
             examination.
                                    48708
$99.50
```

DATE			

SOUTH UNIVERSITY
709 MALL BLVD.
SAVANNAH, GA 31406

BAKER & TAYLOR

SOUTH UNIVERSITY LIBRARY